NURSING AND INFORMATICS
for the 21st Century
An International Look at Practice,
Trends and the Future

Edited by
Charlotte A. Weaver
Connie White Delaney
Patrick Weber
Robyn L. Carr

HIMSS Mission

To lead change in the healthcare information and management systems field through knowledge sharing, advocacy, collaboration, innovation, and community affiliations.

About the Editors

Charlotte A. Weaver, PhD, RN, is Chief Nurse Officer and Vice President of Patient Care Systems at Cerner Corporation, and serves as Adjunct Professor at the University of Kansas School of Nursing. She has over 35 years experience in the health care industry with 24 of those years specifically in health care information technology. Dr. Weaver joined the Product Management team at TDS in 1983 and then moved into IT management consulting in the late 1980s through to mid-1990s working in the U.S., Canada and Australia. Prior to joining Cerner in 1999, Dr. Weaver served as the Director of Information Services at the MetroHealth System in Cleveland implementing one of the first electronic medical record systems with physician order entry in the country. A frequent presenter at national and international conferences, Dr. Weaver is widely published in informatics, patient safety and quality, and evidence-based practice, and currently serves as IMIA NI-SIG chair on evidence-based practice.

Connie White Delaney, PhD, RN, FAAN, FACMI, is Dean of the School of Nursing at the University of Minnesota and also holds an appointment with the Medical School's Health Informatics Division of the Department of Laboratory Medicine and Pathology. She holds a dual appointment at the University of Iceland, Reykjavik, in the Faculty of Nursing and the Faculty of Medicine. Prior to August 2005, Dr. Delaney directed the Institute for Nursing Knowledge at The University of Iowa, Iowa City and held joint appointments in the College of Nursing and the School of Library and Information Science. Dr. Delaney is a fellow of the American Academy of Nursing. An internationally recognized health informatics scholar, Dr. Delaney is the only dean of nursing to be a fellow in the American College of Medical Informatics. She serves on the Board of Directors of the American Medical Informatics Association, is immediate past-chair of its Nursing Informatics Working Group, and has held numerous offices in professional organizations, including the American Nurses Association and the International Medical Informatics Association. Dr. Delaney has published over 80 books, chapters and articles, and holds a substantial record in funded grants and contracts.

Patrick Weber, MA, RN, is the Director and Principal of Nice Computing in Lausanne, Switzerland. He has over 30 years of health care experience, with more that 20 years in the field of health informatics. Mr. Weber has served as his country's national representative to IMIA—Nursing Informatics for over the past eight years, and is a recognized informatics leader across Europe. He has been a pivotal leader in the European Federation for Medical Informatics (EFMI) holding numerous offices in EFMI and in Switzerland's Nursing Association. Mr. Weber works actively with the European Union in the areas of informatics and world health. In addition, Mr. Weber works extensively across Europe and is a frequent collaborator on informatics projects across the European Union countries. He has numerous publications in both English and French, and is a frequent presenter at national and international conferences.

Robyn L. Carr, RGON, is Director of Informatics Project Contracting (IPC) & Associates, in Cambridge, New Zealand, and serves as Vice Chair of Health Informatics New Zealand (HINZ) and Vice Chair of International Medical Informatics Association—Nursing Informatics (IMIA-NI). She has over 40 years of experience in healthcare and in 1991 became one of the founding members of nursing informatics in New Zealand. Ms. Carr has been an active leader in nursing informatics in the Asia-Pacific region, as well as with the International Medical Informatics Association (IMIA), and New Zealand as the host country for the 2000 International Congress for Nursing Informatics meetings. In 2006, she will assume the chair of IMIA-Nursing Informatics-Special Interest Group. Robyn has co-authored *NINZ the First 10 Years,* published in 2000 and is co editor for "One Step Beyond: The Evolution of Technology and Nursing," 7th International Congress Nursing Informatics Proceedings, published by Springer-Verlag in 2000.

Contributors

Yvonne M. Abdoo, PhD, RN
Assistant Professor, Nursing Business and
  Health System
University of Michigan

Mari E. Akre, PhD, RN
Clinical Assistant Professor, College of
  Nursing
University of Wisconsin-Milwaukee

Rebecca Ambrosini, MSN, RN
Consultant
Corazon Consulting

Marion J. Ball, EdD
Vice President
Healthlink Incorporated
Adjunct Professor
Johns Hopkins School of Nursing

Liana Bera, Eng, PhD
Lecturer, Victor Papilian Faculty of Medicine
Lucian Blaga University of Sibiu

Karen Berg, RN, ANP, C
Director, Knowledge Integration,
  Knowledge and Discovery Department
Cerner Corporation

Helen J. Betts, EdD, RN
Dean, CHIRAD, School of Social Sciences
University College Winchester

Carol J. Bickford, PhD, RN, BC
Senior Policy Fellow, Nursing Practice
  and Policy
American Nurses Association

**Patricia Flatley Brennan, PhD, RN,
  FAAN, FACMI**
Moehlman Bascom Professor, School of
  Nursing and College of Engineering
University of Wisconsin-Madison

Kathleen M. Carley, PhD
Professor, Computation, Organization, and
  Society, Institute for Software Research
  International
Carnegie Mellon University

Robyn L. Carr, RGON
Vice Chair IMIA.NI, Vice Chair HINA,
  Company Director
Informatics Project Consulting & Associates

Barbara Carty, EdD, RN
Clinical Associate Professor, Nursing
  Department
New York University

Anne Casey, MSc, RN, FRCN
Royal College of Nursing of the
  United Kingdom

**James A. Cato, MSN, MHS, EdD
  (candidate), RN, CRNA**
Vice President, Chief Nursing Officer
Eclipsys Corporation

Mary Chambers, PhD
Professor
Kingston University/St. George's Hospital
  Medical School, South West London and
  St. George's Mental Health NHS Trust,
  Springfield University Hospital

**Stephen Chu, BAppSc (AdvNursing,
  Biomed), PhD, FACS**
Information Systems & Operations
  Management
University of Auckland

Thomas R. Clancy, PhD candidate, RN
Vice President, Professional Services,
  All Clinical Support Services and
  Long-term Care
Mercy Hospital

Amy Coenen, PhD, RN, FAAN
Associate Professor, College of Nursing
University of Wisconsin
Director, International Classification for
    Nursing Practice (ICNP®) Programme
USA & International Council of Nurses

Rita Collins, MEd, RGN, RM, RNT
Lecturer
School of Nursing & Midwifery

Helen R. Connors, PhD, RN, FAAN
Associate Dean, Academic Affairs,
    School of Nursing
University of Kansas
Executive Director
Kansas University Center for Healthcare
    Informatics

Moya Conrick, PhD, RN
Professor, Nursing, Nathan Campus
Griffith University

Robyn Cook, BBus, MBA, RN
Nurse Informatics Consultant, formerly,
    Manager, Clinical Informatics & Business
    Consulting, Information Services
    Department
South Western Sydney Area Health Service,
    Eastern Campus, Liverpool Hospital

Julie Creamer, MS, RN
Vice President, Operations and Quality,
    Quality Administration
Northwestern Memorial Hospital

Cheryl R. Croft, BSPA, RN, FCCJ
Chair, Information Services,
    Administration Department
Mayo Clinic

Grace T. M. Dal Sasso, DNs, RN
Associate Professor, Researcher, Nursing
    Informatics, Nursing Department
Federal University of Santa Catarina

**Connie White Delaney, PhD, RN, FAAN,
    FACMI**
Dean and Professor, School of Nursing
University of Minnesota
Professor, Faculty of Nursing and
    Faculty of Medicine
University of Iceland

Charles Docherty, PhD, RNT
Associate Professor, School of Nursing,
    Midwifery and Community Health
Glasgow Caledonian University

Melanie C. Dreher, PhD, RN, FAAN
Dean and Professor, College of Nursing
University of Iowa

Eva Edwin, MNSc, RN
Researcher, Senter for Sykepleietjenesten,
    Medisinsk Divisjon
Ullevål University Hospital

Margareta Ehnfors, PhD, RN
Professor, Department of Health Sciences
Örebro Univerity

Anna Ehrenberg, PhD, RN
Post-doc Fellow, Assistant Professor,
    Department of Caring Sciences
Örebro Univerity and Dalarna University

Sue Ela, MSN, RN
Senior Clinical Vice President
Aurora Health Care
President
Aurora Visiting Nurse Association of
    Wisconsin

Firdevs Erdemir, PhD, RN
Associate Professor, Department of Nursing
Baskent University

Wolfram Fischer, MSc, lic.oec.HSG
Zentrum für Informatik und wirtschaftliche
    Medizin

Annie Fogarty, MA, BHS
A+ Network Centre for Best Patient Outcomes
Auckland District Health Board

Mary-Jane Fry, BN, RN
Clinical Change Counselor, CHIME Project
Queensland Health

Carsten Giehoff, RN
Faculty of Business Management and Social
    Sciences
University of Applied Sciences Osnabrueck

Marc Glorieux, MSc, RN

Mary Gobbi, PhD, DipNEd
Senior Lecturer, School of Nursing and
    Midwifery
University of Southampton

William T.F. Goossen, PhD, RN
Researcher and Consultant
Acquest Research and Development

Brian Gugerty, DNS, RN
Director, Nursing Informatics
Siemens Medical Solutions Health Services
    Corporation

Mary E. Hagle, PhD, RN
Director
Aurora Health Care, Inc., Center for Nursing
    Research and Practice

Kaija Hämäläinen, PHN
Project Manager, Home and Elderly Care
Centre for Social and Health Services

Kara Hamilton, RGON
Charge Nurse, Vascular Services
Auckland District Health Board

**Doon Hassett, BBS, BN, GradDip
    Bus(Health Informatics)**
IS Service Representative, Information
    Services
Auckland District Health Board

Kristina Häyrinen, MSc
Researcher, Department of Health Policy
    and Management
University of Kuopio

Maria Heimisdóttir, PhD, MBA, MD
Chair, Electronic Patient Record Committee,
    Office of the Chief Medical Executive
Landspitali University Hospital

Barbara Hertzler, MS, RN
Executive Vice President and Chief
    Operating Officer
St. Joseph Mercy Oakland

Mark Hoffman, PhD
Director, Genomics Strategy
Cerner Corporation

**Michelle Honey, MPhil (Nursing), RGON,
    FCNA**
Senior Lecturer, School of Nursing
University of Auckland

Mary L. Hook, MS, APRN
Research Associate, Center for Nursing
    Research and Practice
Aurora Health Care, Inc.

**Evelyn J.S. Hovenga, PhD, RN, FACHI,
    FCHSE, FRCNA, MACS**
Professor, School of Information Systems
Central Queensland University

Diane L. Huber, PhD, RN, FAAN, CNAA, BC
Professor, College of Nursing
University of Iowa

Ursula Hübner, Dr. Rer. Nat.
Professor, Faculty of Business Management
    and Social Sciences
University of Applied Sciences Osnabrück

Dirk Hunstein, Dipl.-Pflegewirt
HSK Dr. Horst Schmidt Klinik, Department of
    Nursing Science and Development

Vilborg Ingolfsdottir, MPH, BScN
Chief Nursing Officer
Directorate of Health

Annikki Jauhiainen, PhD, RN
Principal Lecturer, Social and Health
    Professions
Iisalmi, Savonia Polytechnic

Josette F. Jones, PhD, RN
Assistant Professor, Environments for Health
Indiana University School of Nursing

Malina Jordanova, PhD
Institute of Psychology, Bulgarian Academy of
    Sciences, Acad. G. Bonchev

Myun-Sook Jung, PhD
Professor, Department of Nursing, College of
    Medicine
Gyeongsang National University

Alain Junger, MHS, RN
Director of Nursing Information System
    Leader
University Hospital of Lausanne (CHUV)

Martti Kansanen, PhD, MD
Administrative Medical Director,
    Administration Central Office
Kuopio University Hospital

Gail M. Keenan, PhD, RN
Associate Professor and Principal Investigator,
    Hands Research Project, Division of
    Nursing Business and Health Systems
University of Michigan-School of Nursing

**Esa Kemppainen, MSc (Eng)/Information
    Technology**
Hospital Engineer, Computer and Clinical
    Engineering
Kuopio University Hospital

**Karolyn Kerr, PhD candidate, MHSc,
    RGON**
Advisor, Health Information Strategy and
    Policy
Ministry of Health
PhD Student, Department of Information
    Systems and Operations Management
Auckland University

**Jeongeun Kim, PhD, RN, Informatics
    Nurse Specialist**
Assistant Professor, College of Nursing
Seoul National University

Tae Youn Kim, PhDc
Doctoral Candidate, School of Nursing
University of Pennsylvania

Angelina Kirkova, MSc Eng
College of Medicine at Higher Medical
    University Plovdiv

Penka Koltchakova, MSc Med.
Doctor, College of Medicine at Higher
    Medical University Plovdiv

Jorma Komulainen, MD
Department of Pediatrics
Kuopio University Hospital

Pirkko Kouri, MNSc, PHN
Senior Lecturer
Savonia Polytechnic Health Professions
    Kuopio

Karen Knecht, BSN, RN
Vice President, Clinical Solutions
Healthlink, an IBM Company

Nedialka Krasteva, DSc Med
Associate Professor, College of Medicine
Higher Medical University Plovidv

Angela M. Lambert, MBA, RN
Vice President, Adult Patient Care Services
MCG Health, Inc.

Norma M. Lang, PhD, RN, FAAN, FRCN
Aurora Professor of Healthcare Quality and
    Informatics, Wisconsin Distinguished
    Professor University of Wisconsin-
    Milwaukee College of Nursing
Lillian S. Brunner Professor of Nursing and
    Dean Emeritus
University of Pennsylvania School of Nursing

Gail E. Latimer, MSN, RN
Vice President, Chief Nursing Officer
Siemens Medical Solutions USA, Inc.

Derek Louey-Gung, B. App. Sc
Client Executive, Asia Pacific
Cerner Corporation

Sally P. Lundeen, PhD, RN
Dean and Professor
University of Wisconsin-Milwaukee
    College of Nursing

Heimar F. Marin, PhD, RN, FACMI
Professor, Nursing Informatics,
    Department of Nursing
Federal University of São Paulo

**Myriam Fernandez Martin, PhD Student in
    Nursing, RN**
Departmento de Enfermería
Universidad de Alicante
Cerner Corporation

Maria Cristina Mazzoleni, DR Ing
Fondazione Maugieri, IRCCS, Bioengineering
    Department

Nolwazi Mbananga, PhD
Executive Manager Informatics and
    Knowledge Management, Informatics and
    Knowledge Management Directorate
Medical Research of South Africa

Angela Barron McBride, PhD, RN, FAAN
Distinguished Professor and University
    Dean Emeritus
Indiana University School of Nursing

Margaret L. McClure, Ed.D, RN, FAAN
Professor, College of Nursing and School of
    Medicine
New York University

**Kathleen A. McCormick, PhD, RN, FAAN,
    FACMI**
Senior Scientist/Vice President, Health
    Department
SAIC

Anna M. McDaniel, DNS, RN, FAAN
Associate Professor, Director, Health
    Informatics Graduate Program
Indiana University School of Nursing and of
    Informatics

Barbara D. Meeks, MBA, RN
Vice President, Pediatric Patient Care Services
MCG Health Inc., Children's Medical Center
    Administration

Judith Fitzgerald Miller, PhD, RN, FAAN
Associate Dean for Graduate Programs &
    Research, Professor
Marquette University College of Nursing

Anne Moen, PhD, RN
Researcher, Special Advisor
Ullevål University Hospital, Senter for
    Sykepleietjenesten, Medisinsk Divisjon

Ioana Moisil, PhD
Senior Researcher and Professor, Computer
    Science and Automatic Control Department,
    Hermann Oberth Faculty of Engineering
Lucian Blaga University of Sibiu

Eloise Monger, BSc (Hons), RGN
School of Nursing and Midwifery
University of Southampton

Franca Mongiardi, MSc, RGN
Corporate Development
Tees and North East Yorkshire NHS Trust

Oyweda Moorer, MSN candidate, RN, BC
Program Director, Technology and Health
    Systems
Department of Veterans Affairs, Office of
    Nursing Service

Judy Murphy, BSN, RN, FACMI
Vice President, Information Services
Aurora Health Care

Lynn M. Nagle, PhD, RN
Senior Vice President, Technology &
    Knowledge Management
Mount Sinai Hospital

Ramona Nelson, PhD, RN, BC
Professor, Department of Nursing
Slippery Rock University

Karl Øyri, MNS, RN
Nurse Manager and Researcher,
    The Interventional Center
Rikshospitalet University Hospital

Anthony Michael Paget, MSc, RMN, RGN
Lecturer in Health Informatics, School of
    Health Science
University of Wales Swansea

Hyeoun-Ae Park, PhD, RN, FACMI
Professor, College of Nursing
Seoul National University

Neal Patterson, MBA
Co-founder, Chair, and Chief Executive
    Officer
Cerner Corporation

Daniel J. Pesut, PhD, RN, APRN, BC, FAAN
Professor and Associate Dean for Graduate
    Programs, Environments for Health
    Department
Indiana University School of Nursing

Jari Porrasmaa, MSc
Software Designer, IT Services Centre
University of Kuopio

Danny Rathgeber, MBA, Graduate Dipl Management, Graduate Dipl Critical Care, Certificate Coronary Care, Certificate Cardiothoracic
Nurse Executive Officer, Melbourne Health
Royal Melbourne Hospital

Donna L. Reck, MSN, RN, BC
Chief Nursing Officer
Penn State Milton S. Hershey Medical Center,
    Nursing Administration

Cathy Rick, MSN, RN, CNAA, FACHE
Program Director, Technology and Health
    Systems, Office of Nursing Service
Department of Veterans Affairs

Liliana Rogozea, PhD, MD
Associate Professor, Faculty of Medicine
University of Transilvania Brasov

Virginia K. Saba, EdD, RN, FAAN, FACMI
Distinguished Scholar, Department of Nursing
    and Health Sciences
Georgetown University

Julita Sansoni, PhD
Professor, Public Health, Nursing Department
University of Rome

Kaija Saranto, PhD
Professor, Department of Health Policy
    and Management
University of Kuopio

Harold H. Scott, BS Computer Science (Hons), MA Management and Supervision
Vice President Information Services,
    Chief Information Officer
MCG Health Inc.

Bjoern Sellemann, Dipl-Pflegewirt (FH)
Faculty of Business Management and
    Social Sciences
University of Applied Sciences, Osnabrueck

Joyce Sensmeier, MS, RN, BC, CPHIMS, FHIMSS
Vice President, Informatics
Healthcare Information and Management
    Systems Society (HIMSS)

Walter Sermeus, PhD, RN
Professor, School of Public Health
Catholic University Leuven

Arvydas Seskevicius, PhD
Dean, Faculty of Nursing
Kaunas University of Medicine

Fintan Sheerin, BNS, PGDipEd, RMHN
School of Nursing & Midwifery

Roy L. Simpson, RN, C, FNAP, FAAN
Vice President, Nursing Informatics
Cerner Corporation

Nicola T. Shaw, BSc(Hons), PhD, MBCS
Research Scientist
Centre for Healthcare Innovation &
    Improvement

José Siles González, PhD, RN
Professor, Departmento de Enfermería
Universidad de Alicante

Diane J. Skiba, PhD, FAAN, FACMI
Professor, School of Nursing
University of Colorado at Denver and
    Health Sciences Center

Patricia Sodomka, MS, FACHE
Senior Vice President, Patient and Family
    Centered Care
MCG Health Inc.
Director, Center for Patient and Family
    Centered Care
Medical College of Georgia

Anne Spencer, BA(Hons), RN
Nursing and Midwifery Informatician
Portsmouth Hospitals NHS Trust, Queen
    Alexandra Hospital Cosham

Hans Springer, BSc, RN
School of Health
Hogeschool INHOLLAND

Heather Strachan, MSc, Dip. N, RGN, MBCS
Interim Director of Nursing and Healthcare Governance
NHS Argyll and Clyde

Renée M. Stratton, MS
Project Manager
Walther Cancer Institute, Indiana University School of Nursing

Marianne Tallberg, PhD, RN, MA, PHN
Docent, Department of Nursing Science
Kuopio University,

Asta Thoroddsen, MSc, RN
Associate Professor, Faculty of Nursing
University of Iceland

Marita G. Titler, PhD, RN, FAAN
Director, Research, Quality and Outcomes Management, Department of Nursing Services and Patient Care
University of Iowa Hospitals and Clinics

Eric Vande Walle, MS, BN, BInformatics
Chair, National Professional Nursing Informatics Working Group and Nurse Director
A.Z.St-Lucas Bruges (Hospital) Nursing Department

Torun Vedal
Special Advisor, Psykiatrisk Divisjon
Ullevål University Hospital

Jorge Gonzalez Vivo, MD
Physician Executive
Cerner Corporation, Latin America and Caribbean

Amy Walker, MS, RN
Nursing Informatics Consultant, formerly, Chief Clinical Informatics Officer
Adventist Health Systems, AHS Information Services

Judith J. Warren, PhD, RN, BC, FAAN, FACMI
Associate Professor, Director of Nursing Informatics
Kansas University Center of Healthcare Informatics, University of Kansas School of Nursing

Graham Watkinson, EdD, RN, PGCE, MIHPE
Assistant Director of Public Health
Western Sussex NHS Primary Care Trust

Charlotte A. Weaver, PhD, RN
Chief Nurse Officer and Vice President Patient Care Systems
Cerner Corporation

Mike Weaver, PhD, PGDipR, PGCTLHE
Doctor, School of Nursing and Midwifery
University of Southhampton

Patrick Weber, MA, RN
Director
Nice Computing

Lucy Westbrooke, DipNurs, GradDipBus (Health Informatics)
Information Services
Auckland District Health Board, Greenlane Clinical Centre

Torunn Wibe, MNSc, RN
Researcher
Ullevål University Hospital, Senter for sykepleietjenesten, Medisinsk Divisjon

David Willock
Information Services
Queensland Health

Graham Wright, DN, RN, RMN, RNT, RNCT, MBCS, CITP
Professor, CHIRAD, School of Social Sciences
University College of Winchester

Table of Contents

Section I
Revolutionizing Nursing: Technology's Role

Section II
New Roles and Leadership Opportunities

SECTION III
Nursing Education and Information Technology

SECTION IV
Innovation Applied Through Informatics

SECTION V
The Electronic Health Record Initiatives Across the Globe

SECTION VI
The Near Future and Nursing

Dedications

This is for Sarah, Sam, and Jenny who enrich my life by keeping me in theirs, and as always—to my son, Kevin.

— Charlotte A. Weaver

To my extended family, who endlessly gave our shared time—especially son Jeremy, Jessica and granddaughters, Ashley, Aana, Skye & Storme Jade, and Edmond and Betty White, Sue, E. Clark, Craig, Lora & Randy, Loren & Wendy, Ann and families.

— Connie White Delaney

I would like to thank my colleagues and my wife, Marie-France, and my daughters, Delphine and Chloé, who have supported this added work.

— Patrick Weber

To my ever supportive husband, Peter Carr, and to our children and grandchildren, and also to my colleagues in Health Informatics, New Zealand.

— Robyn L.Carr

Acknowledgments

There have been many individuals and organizations who have worked behind the scenes to make this book possible, and we would like to recognize their contributions and support. The American Nurses Association, the American Medical Informatics Association, the International Medical Informatics Association, the Healthcare Information and Management Systems Society, and the European Federation for Medical Informatics, Nursing Working Group have all lent their support in encouraging this book's creation and dissemination across the international marketplace. We especially appreciate Neal Patterson, Chairman and Founder of Cerner Corporation, for his belief in the transformational importance of nursing in health care and to Trace Devanny and Paul Black for their unflinching support of nurses. We need to pay homage to the universities that have served as our academic homes—the University of Iowa, the University of Kansas, the University of Minnesota, and the University of Auckland.

To all our European colleagues who immediately accepted our invitation to participate in this exciting endeavor, we extend our special thanks for taking on the very difficult task of writing their chapters in English. We owe a big debt to HIMSS Vice President of Communications Fran Perveiler and HIMSS Senior Editor Nancy Vitucci for bravely taking on the first nursing book to be published by HIMSS and for partnering with us to produce a book in a timely way. And finally, to our developmental editor, Andrea Cimino, who kept us organized and on schedule and whose talented editing has contributed greatly to this finished product.

Charlotte A. Weaver
Connie White Delaney
Patrick Weber
Robyn L. Carr
Editors

Foreword

The introduction of clinical information systems to health care institutions has been a long, slow process. The fact that it has taken nearly 30 years for the industry to reach the tipping point in relation to adopting this technology is quite astonishing. Now, as we enter the twenty-first century, the introduction, implementation, and refinement of computer applications to patient care presents clinicians and administrators with an abundance of exciting opportunities to make significant improvements in patient safety and patient outcomes.

This volume, *Nursing and Informatics for the 21st Century,* is an extraordinary contribution to the growing body of literature in this important advance. It offers important insights and information useful to everyone involved in this work, from the novice to the most experienced and from the expert clinician to the expert information technology (IT) programmer.

Of particular importance is the explication of the leadership that nurses are giving to this technologic revolution taking place across the globe. This fact may prove surprising to some readers. It is, however, a logical and essential phenomenon, owing to the role that nurses play in their everyday practice.

First and foremost, nurses are, of course, clinical caregivers. Nowhere is that more evident than in inpatient settings. Not only do they render and/or oversee the personal services that patients receive, they are responsible for the large and growing number of therapeutic treatments that are adding to the complexity and cost of health care in every country.

Beyond the caregiver role, practicing nurses are responsible for integrating the services of virtually every other discipline and department that is in any way involved with care delivery. In this "integrator" role, they are charged with ensuring that the work of such diverse people as physicians, maintenance workers, porters, and pharmacists comes together in timely and appropriate ways. In other words, they weave together the threads that create the fabric that is patient care.

The combination, then, of caregiver and integrator experience provides nurses with a unique understanding of the ways in which health care organizations operate. Simply stated, nurses have first-hand knowledge of the structure, systems, and processes required in every setting, making their contributions to the introduction of clinical information technology applications essential to the success of any such endeavor.

This book is written primarily by and for nurses, but its readers should by no means be limited to members of that profession. It clearly contains a wealth of critical information, not only regarding what nurses need to know in order to function in this brave new electronic world but, perhaps more importantly, what nurses can and must contribute to ensure success for consumers and for the health care industry.

— Margaret L. McClure, RN, EdD, FAAN
Professor, College of Nursing and School of Medicine
New York University

Preface

This is a book that had to be written, and its imperative is linked to the explosion of electronic health record (EHR) national strategies occurring around the world. The impetus for turning to information technology (IT) in health care comes from governments' need to control spiraling health care costs and to assure value for money spent, even in the U.S. where health care is largely privately funded. Additionally, as the consumer public has become aware of the high level of error, waste, inefficiencies, and quality deficits in western medical systems broadly, governments have had to become accountable to tax payers for improving health care quality. Spurred by growing evidence that our western medical systems are marked by extensive variance in treatment approaches; surgical procedure rates; and outcomes and costs, governments, as the largest payers, began pushing for electronic medical record systems as a means to achieve standardization, safety, better efficiencies, and best practice.

Although not obvious at first, these trends are creating significant changes and opportunities for nursing. The rapid adoption of IT by health care systems is impacting nursing in a number of ways. The clinical transformation involved with bringing IT into the core clinical work processes of the health care team has required the full engagement of clinicians in multiple roles and at all levels of the organization. Nurses have been tapped to fill these roles more than any other discipline, which reflects their sheer numbers in the health care system, as well as the key role nurses play in achieving sustainable social and organizational change. The result has been the creation of new roles for nurses and career path options in leadership and explosive growth in the number of nurses working in informatics.

The EHR trend is happening simultaneously with nursing finally having achieved a standard nursing language. International standards for nursing terminology and nomenclature are now available in the marketplace with the release of ICNP® Version 1 (International Classification of Nursing Practice) and SNOMED CT.®[1,2] Together, standard nursing terminology and EHR systems deliver the enabling components needed by nursing to be able to name and examine their own practice. The components of EHR systems that provide this infrastructure include the ability to apply standard nomenclatures to care components, to provide structured clinical documentation with coded outcomes, and an ability to store all data because of the provision of a clinical data repository. These two forces, the EHR and availability of a standard nursing terminology, will enable nursing for the first time to make its practice visible, to show its contribution to patient outcomes, and to demonstrate what is uniquely nursing. Given the population size and longitudinal database represented in the clinical data repository of EHR systems, the science of nursing will be further supported by the opportunity to conduct population-based research and the option to use the most rigorous of quantitative methodologies in nursing research. Collaboration between nurse researchers and nurse leaders from service provider organizations becomes key in capitalizing on the opportunities that EHR systems afford to generate new nursing knowledge and the rapid application of that new knowledge back into practice.

The impetus for this book originated from discussions with nurse leaders from around the world at the 8th International Congress of Nursing Informatics (NI) in Rio de Janeiro in June 2003. The picture that emerged from these late night discussions was one of rapid adoption of EHR initiatives and of IT across the globe. It became apparent from these and following discussions that the national EHR initiatives were impacting nursing practice, science, and education internationally in profound ways. Change was occurring at a rapid pace internationally, and nursing was in the middle of this massive transformation. To delay in capturing this transition and the forces driving the changes meant that this turning point in nursing might be missed. For that reason, this book is an international look at nursing and the way in which IT is affecting practice, competencies required, roles, and opportunities.

Many of the nurse informatics leaders that participated in those late night informal "think tank" discussions at the NI 2003 Rio de Janeiro conference are contributors to this book. Although the focus of this book is informatics and the explosive change happening within nursing, this is not a nursing informatics book. The book title starts with "Nursing" because this body of work focuses on capturing the significant historical shift taking place within our profession today. Book contributions include recognized experts as well as innovators who rarely publish but who push the edge by using IT to bring new solutions to quality and efficiency challenges.

The book is organized into six sections, and its thirty-four chapters are richly peppered with thirty case studies from diverse international settings. Section I, entitled "Revolutionizing Nursing: Technology's Role," provides the opening framework for the book. In Chapter 1, Angela McBride gives a comprehensive overview of informatics in nursing practice that establishes the revolutionary impact on current trends in nursing. Other subjects covered include nursing knowledge, informatics competencies needed within all nursing roles, shifts in nursing education policy, the rise of consumerism, and the historical emergence of nursing informatics. Section II addresses the new roles and leadership opportunities being created for nurses in today's marketplace. This section also examines the leadership competencies required of nurse executives. Section III looks at the innovative work being done to use IT within nursing education. The contributions cover the use of virtual simulation laboratories to teach clinical skills, the embedding of core curriculum content into EHR clinical systems to teach nursing content and process, and multi-institution collaboration to leverage faculty and resources for informatics programs.

Section IV is devoted to covering the leading areas of innovation applied through informatics in the areas of evidence-based practice, nursing knowledge, and knowledge representation in clinical systems. Sermeus and colleagues present a multinational analysis of the impact of instituting diagnostic-related groupings systems and opportunities that this trend has created for inclusion of nursing information. Other leading edge subjects expand to include decision support and best practice, nursing management decision support, organizational analysis and modeling for decision support, quality improvement, and patient safety. Section V divides the globe into five geographic areas and systematically reviews the current state of nursing and IT across these geopolitical areas illustrated by case studies from seventeen countries.

Section VI closes the book by looking to the future. Subjects range from the promise of genomics for clinical practice and health services delivery to the growing emphasis on patient and family-centered care that extends beyond consumerism. Nursing's importance in any country can be assessed by the extent to which it is included in health policy and research funding. Brennan's chapter on the National Institutes of Health (NIH) Roadmap demonstrates that although progress is being made, there is still significant room for growth. The final chapter by Strachan, Delaney and Sensmeier critically examines the question of organizational affiliation and professional home for nurse informaticians. This closing chapter is a thoughtful review of the professional status of nurses within national and international informatics organizations and poses strategies for the future. During this first decade in the twenty-first century, it is clear that nursing is standing on a threshold looking out at tremendous opportunity for our science, practice, and profession. We hope this leaves each reader energized and inspired to step across that threshold and fully engage in seizing the opportunity that is now there for nursing.

Charlotte A. Weaver
Connie White Delaney
Patrick Weber
Robyn L. Carr
Editors

References

1. International Council of Nurses. *International Classification for Nursing Practice (ICNP®) Version 1.0.* Geneva, Switzerland, 2005.

2. SNOMED International. SNOMED CT® Mappings to NANDA, NIC, and NOC now licensed for free access through National Library of Medicine. News Release, January 25, 2005, available at: http://www.snomed.com/news/documents/012505_E_NursingMapsLicenseToNLM-Final._001.pdf. Accessed September 30, 2005.

Revolutionizing Nursing: Technology's Role

SECTION I

Introduction

Charlotte A. Weaver, PhD, RN

The six chapters that comprise Section I provide a powerful overview of the full impact of information technology (IT) on core aspects of nursing practice. This impact extends to clinical reasoning and to the nursing process: in the educational approach chosen for future nurses and in the skills and competencies needed for practitioners, researchers, and educators. A common theme across these six chapters is the various ways in which IT is creating new and more sophisticated dimensions in nursing, as well as opportunities for significant strengthening of nursing as a profession and for professional growth.

Angela McBride's opening chapter establishes the framework for the examination of IT's adoption within health care, a phenomenon that is revolutionizing nursing. McBride carefully builds the case for how profound and multidimensional these changes in nursing are and prepares the reader for the coming chapters that begin to plot out the exact nature of these changes. Pesut's chapter critically examines the nursing process model and presents the challenge that advances in nursing informatics will make possible for more effective nursing knowledge work than its current state. Pesut argues that technology and classification standards have positioned nursing to be at a third generation nursing process level. Pesut's model is based on outcomes and additional dimensions, e.g., the care context and patient's cultural context and participation in their care. Indeed, Pesut's position perfectly hands off to McDaniel and Stratton's following chapter on consumerism. McDaniel and Stratton present the business and practice opportunities that consumerism in health care hold for nurses. The authors highlight how this demand creates a need that nursing can fill as patients move from passive participants to full participants in their health care, a scenario in which accurate and timely health-related information becomes a highly valued commodity.

In Chapter 4, Dreher and Miller introduce the role of clinical nurse leader and the need for the professional nurse to be master's-level prepared. The authors emphasize that this role will require sophisticated informatics competencies, including the ability to support analysis of practice outcome data, knowledge generation, representation of clinical knowledge, and the use of clinical decision supports in clinical reasoning. While the proposal for the clinical nurse leader role as the entry level into professional nursing is controversial, Pesut's call for a higher level of abstract thinking, reasoning, and communications skills for nursing speaks in support of Dreher's and Miller's position.

In Chapter 5, Skiba, Carty and Nelson present a penetrating overview of the explosive growth in informatics education. The authors detail the informatics competencies needed in every position in the current health care environment. The educational demand for informatics skills and competencies touch all of nursing's domains across our health care systems. This means that health care organizations must develop strategies for educating their workforce, nurse executives must seek out expertise and leadership competencies to strategically lead the paperless and digital care system, and faculty must learn before they can teach the basic informatics competencies and skills required for the next generation of clinicians. Skiba and colleagues give us a thoughtful and thorough analysis of informatics courses and program expansion, as well as examining the existing gaps in education options to meet the demand. Section I concludes with Tallberg, Saba, and Carr as early leaders in our field, treating us to a historical review of nursing informatics' beginnings and its current position within nursing and informatics.

CHAPTER 1

Informatics and the Future of Nursing Practice

By Angela Barron McBride, PhD, RN, FAAN

Around the world, there is a major movement under way to make this the "Decade of Health Information Technology." Various governments are making billion-dollar investments to establish electronic health networks. On July 21, 2004, United States Secretary of Health and Human Services Tommy Thompson and Dr. David Brailer, the country's first health information technology coordinator, unveiled a strategic plan with goals for the adoption and diffusion of an electronic health record (EHR) that would aim for seamless continuity of care across settings/clinicians, maximize informed consumer choice, and improve public health through timely incident reporting.[1]

Although there is no aspect of nursing and patient care that will be untouched by the information revolution in process, most nurses are either oblivious to the enormity of the changes under way or feel unprepared for what is to come. What is true in the United States Department of Veterans Affairs' medical centers is probably true in most hospitals—information technology (IT) that enables computerized patient records and decision support is generally regarded as a positive development, particularly by administrators charged with facilitating system issues. However, frontline clinicians are more likely to view computers and new ways of doing things as troublesome barriers, adding to already-heavy workloads and interfering with existing work-flow patterns.[2]

Informatics—used in this chapter to encompass the broad and evolving knowledge base concerned with all aspects of information literacy, not just computer competence[3,4]—is still not perceived as fundamental to nursing practice, but rather as an add-on. Both the American Nurses Association's (ANA) *Scope and Standards of Practice*[5] and that organization's *Scope and Standards for Nurse Administrators*[6] list nursing fundamentals as the core activities of assessment, diagnosis, outcomes identification, planning, implementation, and evaluation—all of which can be transformed by IT. Yet, informatics is described in the former as a "role specialty," similar to education, research, quality initiatives, and case management. This conceptualization is pernicious because it obscures the extent to which IT is necessary to achieve both the aforementioned practice standards and the goals of education, research, quality initiatives, and case management.

Indeed, one can argue that nursing, particularly nursing administration, has long held goals—e.g., monitor the needs of vulnerable populations, document clinical problems, coordinate care, foster continuous quality improvement, utilize research findings, evaluate outcomes, integrate clinical and financial data in strategic planning—that were never fully achievable before the advent of twenty-first century IT. Although informatics certainly exists as a specialty that integrates computer and information sciences with nursing science, it is important to understand, too, how basic informatics is to the critical thinking and decision making that are fundamental to all nursing practice.[7]

The remainder of this chapter will elaborate on why nursing informatics isn't just for nurse informaticians anymore, much the way that strategic planning and cost-benefit analyses can no longer be considered the exclusive province of those with formal administrative titles. In this day and age, nurses at all levels and in all settings must be proactive and able to evaluate competing information. Nursing has long prided itself on understanding patients within their environments—describing the phenomena of nursing as the interactions between and among the nurse, patient, and environment that advance health. Yet the emphasis in education and practice remains on nurses as direct providers of care more than on nurses as coordinators of care within complex systems, when the latter is essential to realizing the former.

The "real" nurse is typically perceived as one who interacts on a one-to-one basis with patients and their families, always striving to meet their special needs. Although nurses provide routine care on a daily basis, they have been socialized to regard anything that is routine as suspect and not fully professional, because the *sine qua non* of professional practice has historically been to treat every patient as unique and pay devout attention to each individual's needs. But IT is shifting the emphasis away from the nurse striving always to achieve some version of clinical perfection and on to how the nurse must be supported by a work environment strongly committed to quality and safety, one in which patients can expect best practices.[8] And the support provided by the work environment will necessarily involve other nurses with specialized knowledge who may not be visible at the bedside but are essential to the successful care of the patient.

The Informatics Revolution

The Institute of Medicine's (IOM) various quality initiatives have each linked IT to the improvement of health care. The landmark report, *Crossing the Quality Chasm,* did not just emphasize the importance of IT in financial transactions and administrative processes, but noted[9] how crucial IT is to all aspects of clinical decision making, the delivery of population-based care, consumer education, professional development, and research. The 1st Annual Crossing the Quality Chasm Summit treated IT as a strategy essential to all reform and particularly important in expediting patient self-management in the chronically ill.[10] "Utilizing informatics" has been described as a core competency that all health care professionals will need in the twenty-first century.[11] And it is a competency important internationally[12] because IOM's quality initiatives have become priorities around the world.[13]

"Utilizing informatics" may be a core competency that all health care professionals will need sooner than later, but the majority of nurses lack IT skills. Many are still grappling with the word processing, e-mail, and bibliographic retrieval skills required just to complete online courses. Almost all nurses are unsure about meeting new expectations when the EHR is the norm and makes possible easier data retrieval to turn information into knowledge that guides practice. Core IT competencies have been identified at four levels of practice—beginning, experienced, specialist, and innovator—but these competencies have not been systematically incorporated by educational level (undergraduate and graduate) into curriculum changes, performance appraisals, and/or accreditation standards.[14] Nursing does not generally require students to use personal digital assistants (PDAs) the way their physician counterparts now do, although use of PDAs by nursing students is beginning to increase, particularly in nurse practitioner programs.[15,16]

Information literacy varies by year of graduation, with those who graduated before 1990 typically having weaker computer skills[17]—the same individuals who are likely to be in decision-making positions by virtue of their seniority. Because this group of veteran nurses is more likely to feel awkward and frustrated when new IT expectations are added to their existing portfolio of responsibilities, they may be less likely to embrace such changes themselves and to encourage others to do so. Nurses are less likely to make use of online evidence to support their work than are their physician counterparts.[18] Not only may they be constrained by lack of educational preparation but also by whether they think it is even their role to initiate information seeking related to patient care because they (and others around them) view physicians as the major decision makers.[19] All of these limiting factors are exacerbated by the fact that many nurses, unlike physicians and administrators, have limited on-the-job access to personal desktop computers and such features as e-mail, the Internet, and charting screens.[2]

Nursing schools have focused almost exclusively on using IT to expedite access to education rather than to prepare students for IT-enhanced practice. Nursing faculty have been pioneers in the development of distance learning—moving over the years from making didactic classes available via videotapes to two-way audio and video delivery to Web-based courses—but that is not the same thing as having the skills to integrate IT into their practicum courses.[20] Matters are complicated by the fact that nursing faculty and students typically have "guest" status as they rotate through a number of clinical and community agencies for their practicum experiences, so they may be unfamiliar with the IT systems in a particular institution or discouraged from using them. Perhaps for these reasons, the majority of nursing programs are not teaching information literacy skills or incorporating evidence-based practice into their curricula.[21]

In hospitals, there may be the perception that a few nurses with highly developed IT skills are enough for the institution to function when new systems are adopted, but that attitude overlooks the fact that nurses serve as the primary "interface" between IT systems and patients/families. Physicians and administrators may assign "primary responsibility for patient safety" to nurses,[22] but simultaneously omit the nursing viewpoint in the procurement, design, and implementation phases of IT systems that will affect future nursing practice. Nurse informaticians are prized, but they spend most of their time getting physicians and others to use new IT systems rather than working on the improvement of nursing practice.[23] Nurses regard this lack of IT investment in support of clinical nursing as a major issue in whether they regard their work lives as satisfying.[24]

Incorporating IT into practice and education is now at the same developmental stage as was research in previous decades. Research was once only incorporated into graduate research courses that actually had the word *research* in their titles. Now research is expected to be incorporated into all undergraduate and graduate courses because no aspect of nursing can be adequately discussed without reference to the classic studies that shaped what we now know. Nurses historically oversaw the implementation of physicians' research protocols, but did not focus on getting their own clinical questions answered.[25] Now journals and annuals are full of studies that support the scientific basis for nursing care of individuals across the life span during illness and recovery. In similar fashion, IT must now be incorporated into all undergraduate and graduate courses, not just informatics courses, and nurse informaticians must focus more on improving nursing care.

Quality Practice

The American Nurses Association (ANA) distinguishes between the aforementioned standards of nursing practice (assessment, diagnosis, outcomes identification, planning, implementation, and evaluation) and standards of professional practice, i.e., quality of practice, practice evaluation, education, collegiality, collaboration, ethics, research, resource utilization, and leadership.[5] The former emphasizes the critical thinking approach of the nursing process; the latter describes expectations for acting as a professional.

The IOM quality initiatives focus, in contrast, on six aims—safety, effectiveness, patient-centeredness, timeliness, efficiency, and equity—that are largely subsumed under quality of practice in the ANA's *Scope and Standards of Practice.* Both the ANA and the IOM statements expect the nurse to aim for quality, but there is a difference in how they approach the matter. In the former, quality practice is a standard each nurse must adhere to; indeed, the critical thinking approach of the nursing process is in service to quality. The IOM's quality initiatives, by contrast, move the emphasis away from the professional practice of individuals, believing that health care professionals can only achieve that desired level of practice when system supports are in place.

This shift in emphasis, occasioned as it first was by the IOM finding that most errors are the result of system failures, not individuals' mistakes,[26] should be a source of comfort to all nurses because this approach requires nurses to speak out when conditions are not safe. There is no one in the nursing profession who has not had the experience of being responsible for what was beyond one's personal control, and that situation only promotes a feeling of helplessness rather than encouraging competence. When the focus is on system supports, IT ceases to be primarily an avenue of technical innovation and becomes instead a shift in paradigm, with the nurse truly becoming a knowledge worker[27] who uses information to deliver best practices. One could be glib and say that nursing's decades-long emphasis on process had the unintended consequence of making nursing always seem to be in flux, never achieving outcomes. And there is some truth to that statement, because the focus on process rarely went so far as stipulating set outcomes. Consequently, the thousands of outcomes nurses actually achieved in working with their patients did not translate into aggregate data that others could easily see. Hopefully, that will dramatically improve as nurses come to view IT as in their best interests.

One would hope that nurses as a group would embrace IT with enthusiasm when they truly understand that the informatics revolution will make it possible for nurses to achieve their own goals, including the six aforementioned IOM aims. **Patient-centeredness** is the one aim that nurses excel at already, because they are constantly supporting patients and their families in their decision making; indeed, they would be more inclined to broaden the phrase to read **patient/family-centeredness.** IT has already enabled nurses to develop new ways of supporting patients and their families, e.g., teaching older adults to access patient education Web sites[28,29] and recommending asthma Web sites for parent education.[30] The Internet has been used to support family caregivers of cancer patients, assisting them in dealing with a roller coaster of physical, emotional, and psychological demands.[31] Nursing, with its definitional emphasis on helping patients and their families do what they would do unaided if they knew what to do, has used IT to promote patient/family self-management, e.g., e-mail discussion groups around back pain,[32] post-hospitalization recovery from coronary artery bypass graft surgery,[33] and continence health promotion.[34] Some nurses are working with engineers both to develop a personal robotic assistant for the homebound and to realize the possibilities of smart technology that can unobtrusively monitor changes in a person's activities of daily living at a distance, thus permitting senior patients to obtain watchful help without leaving their homes.[35]

Safety can be expedited by IT in many ways—from the use of bar coding around the administration of medications to wearing near-hands-free communication devices to stay in real-time communication with colleagues who can provide back-up assistance. IT makes possible seamlessness at points of transition, e.g., shift changes, moves between care settings or back to home, when mistakes or omissions are most likely to happen. Surveillance is a major nursing responsibility, and all sorts of event monitoring functions can be built with IT to alert the nurse to changes in physiologic status and other predictors of problems. IT also makes possible appropriate information sharing just before clinicians are about to make decisions, e.g., clinical systems that flash cautions and contraindications just before a procedure is undertaken.[36]

In our outcomes-oriented world, **effectiveness** has assumed new importance, if for no other reason than the fear that reimbursement policies will eventually be linked to the achievement of best practices. Quality improvement committees in every health care institution are tracking their progress using a range of indicators, e.g., Health Plan Employer Data and Information Set and Outcome and Assessment Information Set. IT makes possible online dissemination of constantly changing standards and policies, then permits benchmarking local outcomes against national averages for similar institutions.[37,38] Though current benchmarking focuses largely on whether services are provided, e.g., ordering fasting blood glucose and A1c tests for diabetic patients, the day is fast approaching when the emphasis will be on whether patients received, understood, and acted upon the information that might change these laboratory values and achieve the desired glucose control. The quality of nursing will eventually be determined by that linkage between processes and outcomes, which will be good news for those who believed all along that the nursing process was supposed to begin with assessment then proceed to evaluation (and not so good news for those in the field who have been content to deliver services removed from any consideration of the effectiveness of these services).

IT can facilitate **timeliness** in many ways, from improved scheduling of appointments and work schedules to ensuring that a unit's inventory of supplies is replenished automatically. IT permits continuous communication between patients and providers, thus eliminating much of the need for "just in case" (as opposed to "just in time") interventions. The Veterans Health Administration's new Care Coordination and My Health*e* Vet programs have eliminated routine clinic visits, focusing instead on seeing patients when actually needed.[39]

Efficiency is an aim that can be greatly enhanced by IT because so much time and money are wasted asking patients questions that they have answered many times before and repeating laboratory and imaging tests when results have been lost to the paper record.[40] IT makes possible targeted population-based interventions. Limited resources can thus be deployed strategically, e.g., using geographic information systems to provide care to the neediest or to target neighborhoods by zip code.[41]

Equity can be realized through IT in many ways, from providing some version of "telecare" to patients in rural settings to making sure that take-home information on discharge is printed in the patient's first language. Nurses have already provided end-of-life care over the lines via "telehospice."[42] Since IT programs offer the opportunity of mass customization, health information can be broadly disseminated yet tailored in terms of the patient's race, gender, age, and reading level. Nurses have already used these strategies successfully in cancer screenings.[43]

The enormity of the changes taking place challenges all of the health care professions. Nurses face the same problem that physicians do in realizing IOM's six aims because both professions have been socialized to think in terms of the person-to-person differences they can make in patients' lives, rather than how IT systems can support best practices. But nurses are more likely to be salaried employees of health care organizations using such systems, so they as a group are more likely to be comfortable with systems thinking and predisposed to work as part of a team, even though most of them would be inclined to agree that "all nursing practice, regardless of specialty, role, or setting, is fundamentally independent practice."[5] In context, the emphasis on independent practice is not a call for rugged individualism, but a reminder of the responsibilities each nurse bears in maintaining personal competence over a career lifetime. Nevertheless, the affirmation of nursing practice as independent practice (paralleling longstanding conceptualizations of medical practice as independent practice) signals how difficult it may prove for all concerned to harness so many individual impulses in service to the system changes ahead.

Achieving Nursing's Preferred Future

You can sound the clarion call, but change will not proceed apace unless it is viewed as a means of achieving what key players want. And one can reasonably argue that the informatics revolution in process has the potential to deliver what nursing has historically wished for as a profession. Nursing has long pursued goals that were never fully achievable before the advent of twenty-first century IT. Although nurse executives and nurse managers have long been charged with encouraging their staffs to be accountable for their practice, standardized measurements and outcomes (e.g., National Database of Nursing Quality Indicators) are only now becoming commonplace. Even when institutional data existed, they were typically focused not on nursing practice, but on physician interventions and financial matters because of their link to hospital reimbursement. Thus, nurses did not necessarily see themselves as central figures in the conversations about the importance of an EHR, nor did others see them that way.

Nurses have, however, begun to describe themselves in recent years as "knowledge workers"[27,44] in part because they want to buttress support for the importance of nursing research and in part because they want to counter stereotypical notions that all you need to be a good nurse is a caring heart, strong back, and gentle hands. But the move to describe themselves as knowledge workers sometimes sounded self-serving and did not capture the attention of others (e.g., physicians, administrators) before the IOM quality initiatives. In 2004, the IOM devoted an entire volume, *Keeping Patients Safe: Transforming the Work Environment of Nurses,* to the proposition that nurses must function as knowledge workers and that their work environments, therefore, must strive to display the hallmarks of a learning organization.[8] The report supports the importance of strong nurse leadership if quality and patient safety are to be realized and recommends additional education so nurses can meet new expectations, particularly around knowledge management and the design of work processes to reduce errors. Publication of this report, because it honors the work of nursing as essential to quality care and urges that the work environment of nurses be improved to support the nursing staff, was a watershed event.

Now the question is what will nurses do with this opportunity? After years of feeling underappreciated for their contributions, nurses are being seen as invaluable in areas that will only grow in importance as health care institutions make continuously strengthening patient safety part of their organizational cultures. Both the government's strategic plan for the development of the EHR and the various IOM reports also emphasize delivery of consumer-centric and information-rich health care—goals that dovetail nicely with nursing's self-definition as a profession. Even the systems orientation of the informatics revolution plays to nursing's strengths, because nurses are socialized to work collaboratively as members of teams and to think critically about processes likely to achieve the desired effect.

In many ways, this chapter is meant to be a major reframing. Instead of nurses' viewing the informatics revolution as an intrusion that gets in the way of one's real work with patients, it is important to appreciate the extent around to which the Decade of Information Technology can be a time when nursing fully comes into its own as a discipline and is perceived that way by others. Sure, students, faculty, and staff will have to learn new skills, but that has always been true of the field. This time, however, the new skills will only serve to reinforce the notion of nurses as knowledge workers exerting leadership in learning organizations.[45] The development of one integrated EHR means that what nurses contribute will be truly seen by all other health care providers. And the tele-care opportunities mean that nurses will not have to be limited by their shifts and place, as has so often been the experience of nurses working in traditional hospitals, but can begin to think and act all the more beyond the constraints of time, geography, and hierarchy. "Ask A Nurse" services have grown in recent times and are likely to expand further.

To embrace the informatics revolution is to exert leadership. The early leadership research was dominated by a preoccupation with relations-oriented behaviors (does the leader demonstrate caring and integrity?) and task-oriented behaviors (does the leader clarify tasks to be performed and monitor progress?). Now there is increasing emphasis on a third dimension, i.e., the way leaders initiate change and encourage organizational innovation.[46] And one of the most important components of organizational innovation in nursing and patient care is developing an informatics vision complete with goals.[47]

The American Association of Critical-Care Nurses recently published standards to promote healthy work environments.[48] That document reaffirmed that practice is driven by the needs of patients and their families, but noted that the quality of nursing practice and patient outcomes are inextricably linked to the quality of the work environment. It further identified six essential standards for a healthy work environment, with several demonstrating the extent to which informatics is important even when the word is not used. Skilled communication is listed as the first standard, and skilled communicators are described as having access to appropriate communication technologies and being proficient in their use. Another standard is effective decision making, which is achieved when data are transformed into meaningful information that guides decisions that can be subsequently evaluated for effectiveness. Yet another standard is authentic leadership, which is said to involve the design of systems.

Nursing has a long, proud history of innovation, dating back to Florence Nightingale's founding of public health statistics and design of military hospitals, both of which promoted healthy environments as a means of achieving quality nursing practice. Nurses today are similarly called to design the conditions of their practice. This time, information systems have replaced bricks and mortar, but Ms. Nightingale might be pleased to think that data continue to serve the transforming role in caregiving that her mortality and morbidity figures once did.

Acknowledgments

This chapter is an outcome of the author's experience in 2003–2004 as a Scholar-in-Residence at the IOM, made possible through collaboration among IOM, the American Academy of Nursing, and the American Nurses Foundation. Additional support was provided by a grant from the Independence Foundation and salaried leave from Indiana University-Purdue University at Indianapolis (IUPUI).

References

1. Thompson TG and Brailer DJ. *The Decade of Health Information Technology: Delivering Consumer-centric and Information-rich Health Care. Framework for Strategic Action.* Washington, DC: Department of Health and Human Services; 2004.

2. Lyons SS, Tripp-Reimer T, Sorofman BA, et al. Information technology for clinical guideline implementation: perceptions of multidisciplinary stakeholders. *J Am Med Inf Assoc.* 2005;12(1):64-71.

3. Kerfoot KM and Simpson R. Knowledge-driven care: powerful medicine. *Reflections Nurs Leadership.* 2002;28(3):22-24, 44.

4. Saranto K and Hovenga, EJS. Information literacy—what is it about? *Int J Med Inf.* 2004;73:503-513.

5. American Nurses Association. *Nursing: Scope and Standards of Practice.* Washington, DC: Nursesbooks.org; 2004.

6. American Nurses Association. *Scope and Standards for Nurse Administrators.* 2nd ed. Washington, DC: Nursesbooks.org; 2004.

7. American Nurses Association. *Scope and Standards of Nursing Informatics* Practice. Washington, DC: American Nurses Publishing; 2001.

8. Institute of Medicine. *Keeping Patients Safe: Transforming the Work Environment of Nurses.* Washington, DC: The National Academies Press; 2004.

9. Institute of Medicine. *Crossing the Quality Chasm: A New Health System for the 21st Century.* Washington, DC: National Academy Press; 2001.

10. Institute of Medicine. *The 1st Annual Crossing the Quality Chasm Summit: A Focus on Communities.* Washington, DC: The National Academies Press; 2004.

11. Institute of Medicine. *Health Professions Education: A Bridge to Quality.* Washington, DC: The National Academies Press; 2003.

12. Murphy J, Stramer K, Clamp S, Grubb P, Gosland J, Davis S. Health informatics education for clinicians and managers—what's holding up progress? *Int J Med Inf.* 2004;73:205-213.

13. Van de Castle B, Kim J, Pedreira MLG, Paiva A, Goossen W, Bates DW. Information technology and patient safety in nursing practice: an international perspective. *Int J Med Inf.* 2004;73:607-614.

14. Staggers N, Gassert CA, Curran C. Informatics competencies for nurses at four levels of practice. *J Nurs Ed.* 2001;40:303-316.

15. Huffstutler S, Wyatt TH, Wright CP. The use of handheld technology in nursing education. *Nurs Educ.* 2002;27:271-275.

16. Bakken S, Cook SS, Curtis L, et al. Promoting patient safety through informatics-based nursing education. *Int J Med Inf.* 2004;73:581-589.

17. Pravikoff D, Pierce S, Tanner A. Are nurses ready for evidence-based practice? *Am J Nurs.* 2003;103,5: 95-96.

18. McCannon M. O'Neal PV. Results of a national survey indicating information technology skills needed by nurses at time of entry into the work force. *J Nurs Ed.* 2003;42:337-340.

19. Gosling AS, Westbrook JI, Spencer R. Nurses' use of online clinical evidence. *J Adv Nurs.* 2004;47: 201-211.

20. Chastain AR. Are nursing faculty members ready to integrate information technology into the curriculum? *Nurs Ed Perspect.* 2002;23:187-190.

21. McNeil BJ, Elfrink VL, Bickford CJ, et al. Nursing information technology knowledge, skills, and preparation of student nurses, nursing faculty, and clinicians: a U.S. survey. *J Nurs Ed.* 2003;42:341-349.

22. Cook AF, Hoas H, Guttmannova K, Joyner JC. An error by any other name. *Am J Nurs.* 2004;104,6: 32-43.

23. Sensmeier J, West L, Horowitz JK. Survey reveals role, compensation of nurse informaticists. *CIN.* 2004;22:171, 178-81.

24. O'Neil E, Seago JA. Meeting the challenge of nursing and the nation's health. *J Am Med Assoc.* 2002;288:2040-2041.

25. McBride AB. Nursing and the informatics revolution. *Nurs Outlook.* 2005;53:183-191.

26. Institute of Medicine. *To Err is Human: Building a Safer Health System.* Washington, DC: National Academy Press; 2000.

27. Snyder-Halpern R, Corcoran-Perry S, Narayan S. Developing clinical practice environments supportive of the knowledge work of nurses. *CIN.* 2001;19(1):17-23.

28. Dauz E, Moore J, Smith CE, Puno F, Schaag H. Installing computers in older adults' homes and teaching them to access a patient education web site. *CIN.* 2004;22:266-272.

29. Nahm E-S, Preece J, Resnick B, Mills ME. Usability of health web sites for older adults. *CIN.* 2004;23:326-334.

30. Oermann MH, Gerich J, Ostosh L, Zaleski S. Evaluation of asthma websites for patient and parent education. *J Pediatr Nurs.* 2003;18:389-396.

31. Klemm P. and Wheeler E. Cancer caregivers online: hope, emotional roller coaster, and physical/emotional/psychological responses. *CIN.* 2005;23:38-45.

32. Lorig K, Laurent D, Deyo R, et al. Can a back pain e-mail discussion group improve health status and lower health costs? A randomized study. *Arch Intern Med.* 2002;162:792-796.

33. Brennan PF, Jones J, Moore SM, Visovsky C. A scalable technological solution to the challenges of posthospitalization recovery from CABG surgery. In: Nelson R and Ball MJ, eds. *Consumer Informatics: Applications and Strategies in Cyber Health Care.* New York: Springer-Verlag; 2004:33-39.

34. Boyington AR, Widemuth BM, Dougherty MC, Hall EP. Development of a computer-based system for continence health promotion. *Nurs Outlook.* 2004; 52:241-247.

35. Alwan M, Aversano T, Matthews JT, Rosen MJ. Technology in the pipeline to help older adults. *Public Policy and Aging Report.* 2004;14(1);14-15.

36. Ball M J, Weaver C, Abbott PA. Enabling technologies promise to revitalize the role of nursing in an era of patient safety. *Int J Med Inf.* 2003;69:29-38.

37. Bakken S, Cimino JJ, Hripcsak G. Promoting patient safety and enabling evidence-based practice through informatics. *Med Care.* 2004;42:II49-II56.

38. Brooten D, Youngblut JM, Kutcher J, Bobo C. Quality and the nursing workforce: APNs, patient outcomes and health care costs. *Nurs Outlook.* 2004;52:45-52.

39. Perlin JB, Roswell RH (2004). Why do we need technology for caregiving of older adults in the U.S.? *Public Policy and Aging Report.* 2004;14(1):22-24.

40. Cowden S, Johnson LC. A process for consolidation of redundant documentation forms. *CIN.* 2004;22: 90-93.

41. Riner ME, Cunningham CJ, Johnson A. Public health education and practice using geographic information system technology. *Public Health Nurs.* 2004; 21(1):57-65.

42. Whitten P, Doolittle G, Mackert M, Rush T. Telehospice: end-of-life care over the lines. *Nurs Manage.* 2003;34(11):36-39.

43. Champion V, Foster JL, Menon U. Tailoring interventions for health behavior change in breast cancer screening. *Cancer Practice.* 1997;5:283-288.

44. Sorrells-Jones J, Weaver D. Knowledge workers and knowledge-intense organizations. *J Nurs Adm.* 1999;29(7/8):12-18.

45. Mahoney R. Leadership and learning organisations. *The Learning Organisation.* 2000;7(5):241-244.

46. Yukl G, Gordon A, Taber T. A hierarchical taxonomy of leadership behavior: Integrating a half century of behavior research. *J Leadership and Organ Stud.* 2002;9:15-32.

47. McCartney PR. Clinical issues: leadership in nursing informatics. *JOGNN.* 2004;33:371-380.

48. American Association of Critical-Care Nurses. *AACN Standards for Establishing and Sustaining Healthy Work Environments: A Journey to Excellence.* Aliso Viejo, CA; 2005. Additional information available at http://www.aacn.org/AACN/pubpolcy.nsf/vwdoc/workenv. Accessed August 16, 2005.

CHAPTER 2

21st Century Nursing Knowledge Work: Reasoning into the Future

By Daniel J. Pesut, PhD, RN, APRN, BC, FAAN

The clinical thinking of nurses has changed over time, and the nature of clinical reasoning in nursing practice is likely to continue to change in the twenty-first century. Four trends supporting continued change and transformations are in the areas of (1) nursing informatics, (2) standardized nursing knowledge classification systems, (3) electronic health records (EHRs), and (4) more sophisticated data analysis techniques. As data on nursing care practices are captured and experience is gained, health services researchers will be able to analyze and evaluate nurse-sensitive patient care data and information in support of nursing knowledge work in the twenty-first century.

The purposes of this chapter are to:
1. Describe past and future generations of the nursing process that support clinical reasoning and the development of professional nursing expertise
2. Discuss how nursing informatics supports nursing knowledge work through the development of clinical reasoning and judgment skills
3. Explain how the outcome present state test (OPT) model of clinical reasoning is used with standardized nursing language to advance future nursing knowledge work
4. Explain how data mining techniques will affect nursing knowledge work in the future

Clinical Thinking in Nursing

The nursing process and the way nurses have represented clinical thinking have changed over time.[1] Think of your own professional history. Go back to a recent patient care situation you managed. How, specifically, did you think and reason about the nursing care needs of the client? Did you gather all the information about the client? If so, was the information "nursing-sensitive" or framed within the context (intensive care, home health, primary care clinic) of care in mind? Perhaps you based your reasoning on the medical or the patho-physiological condition of the patient.

What clinical vocabulary did you use to articulate nursing care issues, desired outcomes, and nursing interventions to achieve targeted outcomes? Did you translate the identified problem into a desired outcome? Did your clinical information system support or hinder your clinical thinking? How did the documentation system either structure or influence your clinical thinking? Did a theory guide your practice? Or was your thinking shaped by hospital and nursing policies and procedures, or by routines and rituals in your practice environment that developed over time?

Did the information system capture the nursing care provided to the patients? As you documented information in the patient record, did you understand where and how that information would be stored or used in the future? How has your own clinical thinking changed over time? How does your clinical thinking support your clinical judgments? How do you know when you make good clinical judgments? How would you explain the complexity of clinical thinking to someone else? What have you observed about the thinking and clinical reasoning patterns of students, mid-career colleagues, or older nurses? Are you ever curious to know how all the data collected on patients and their care might be analyzed for patterns that provide insights about future care practices?

Reasoning from the Past to the Future

In the U.S. since the 1950s, the nursing process has provided the structure for clinical thinking in nursing. Unlike other countries, the nursing process in the U.S. was designed to organize thinking to anticipate and quickly solve the problems patients encountered. Rituals, traditions, and standard operating procedures were replaced by clinical thinking grounded in problem solving.[2] The problem identification method stimulated educators to teach nursing process as a problem-solving method grounded in assessment. The first-generation nursing process (1950–1970) involved assessment, planning, intervention, and evaluation, along with structured clinical thinking through the lens of problem solving.[3] An assessment indicated a problem, and the solution or nursing care associated with the problem was determined and defined. Nursing actions, procedures, and interventions were developed and used in clinical settings.

As problem-solution patterns became apparent, a small group of nurses began to realize that the method was inefficient and ineffective. Certainly, classes of patient populations had similar nursing care needs. Around 1973, a group of nurses met in St. Louis, Missouri, at the first national conference for the classification of nursing diagnoses. The purpose of the conference was to initiate dialogue among practicing nurses about a standardized nomenclature to describe commonly occurring clinical problems. They called these standardized concepts *nursing diagnoses*.[4] A second-generation nursing process (1970–1990) evolved that explored the dimensions and processes of diagnosing and reasoning.[5] This required the evolution of the APIE model. The addition of diagnosis as an integral step in the traditional nursing process model resulted in the acronym *ADPIE* (assess, diagnose, plan, intervene, and evaluate)[6,7] to represent the "steps" of the nursing process.

Since 1973, great strides have been made in developing classifications of nursing knowledge. For example, the work of the North American Nursing Diagnosis Association (NANDA) at the time of this publication is in its sixth edition.[8] The Iowa Nursing Interventions Classification project (NIC)[9] and the Iowa Nursing Outcomes Classification Project (NOC)[10] have made major contributions to the systematic development and classification of nursing knowledge.

Through systematic research, nurses have developed taxonomies of labels, defining characteristics, activities, and indicators. They have organized nursing knowledge into domains and categories that give nursing a professional identity and that provide a structure to store common nursing language and knowledge. These taxonomies are coded so that financial information can be linked to nursing care services and other health care classification data systems. With many problems already identified, the nature of the nursing process evolved away from thinking about problems to solve and toward reasoning about relationships among problem-solution elements. Organizing and using nursing knowledge for the purposes of practice, education, and research continues to be a professional and lifelong learning responsibility.

Coding nursing diagnoses, interventions, and outcomes anticipated the possibility of EHRs that would enable the capture, storage, retrieval, and transformation of nursing care data. Advances in nursing informatics have set the stage for more effective and efficient nursing knowledge work. The clinical testing and evaluation of classification systems for practice constitute an ongoing professional responsibility. Consider relationships among different levels of nursing practice data and how these data might be used to advance nursing knowledge work. The Iowa NIC project model (see Figure 2-1) illustrates three levels of nursing practice data: the individual level; the unit or organization level; and the network, state, and country level.[11]

Of greatest importance to most clinicians is the individual-level data associated with patient care processes and outcomes. Knowledge in these systems contributes to clinical reasoning, decision making, judgment, and documentation of care delivered. At this level, practice data are organized to be relevant and useful in explaining client problems, nursing interventions, outcomes, and nurses' clinical decisions. Information about the client and the context is explained in terms of clinical knowledge that has been standardized in the form of classification systems or taxonomies. In fact, recent work has focused on harmonization of NANDA diagnoses, NIC interventions, and NOC outcomes[12] (see Table 2-1). When information at this level is collected and used according to a standardized system, it can be aggregated and used in a broader context at the unit or organizational level.

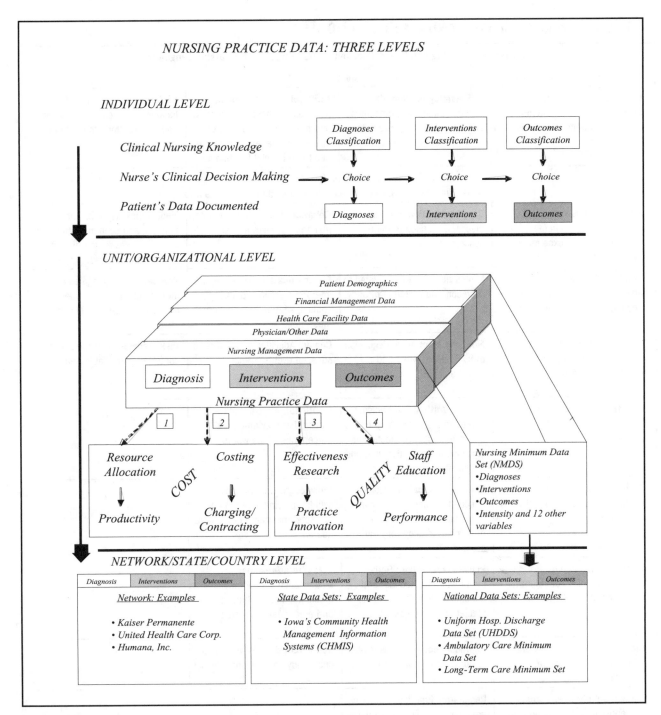

Figure 2-1. *Levels of Practice Data Diagram from the Iowa Nursing Interventions Classification (NIC) Project. (Source: Reprinted with permission from the Iowa Nursing Interventions Classifications Project © Iowa Intervention Project, 1997.)*

The work of managers and administrators who are most interested in the unit and organization level data is facilitated by standardized nursing knowledge classification systems. At the unit or organizational level, data about individual clients are combined into one system, which can be linked to other information systems, such as medical care data. At this level, analyses about common kinds of treatment can be performed according to four possible parameters: resources, costs, effectiveness, and education:

1. Data used for *resource allocation* result in measures of productivity.
2. Data related to *costs* provide information about charging and contracting.
3. Data to support *effectiveness* research have consequences for practice innovations.
4. Data about staff *performance* can be used for evaluation and planning.

Table 2-1. Harmonization of NANDA, NIC, and NOC[12]

Taxonomy of Nursing Practice: A Common Unified Structure for Nursing Language

Domains

I. Functional domain: Includes diagnoses, outcomes, and interventions to promote basic needs.	II. Physiological domain: Includes diagnoses, outcomes, and interventions to promote optimal biophysical health.	III. Psychosocial domain: Includes diagnoses, outcomes, and interventions to promote optimal mental and emotional health and social functioning.	IV. Environmental domain: Includes diagnoses, outcomes, and interventions to promote basic needs.

Classes:
Includes diagnoses, class outcomes, and interventions that pertain to:

Activity/exercise: Physical activity, including energy conservation and expenditure.	**Cardiac function:** Cardiac mechanisms used to maintain tissue profusion.	**Behavior:** Actions that promote, maintain, or restore health.	**Health care system:** Social, political, and economic structures and processes for the delivery of health care services.
Comfort: A sense of emotional, physical, and spiritual well-being and relative freedom from distress.	**Elimination:** Processes related to secretion and excretion of body wastes.	**Communication:** Receiving, interpreting, and expressing spoken, written, and nonverbal messages.	**Populations:** Aggregates of individuals or communities having characteristics in common.
Growth and development: Physical, emotional, and social growth and development milestones.	**Fluid and electrolyte:** Regulation of fluid, electrolytes, and acid base balance.	**Coping:** Adjusting or adapting to stressful events.	**Risk management:** Avoidance or control of identifiable health threats.
Nutrition: Processes related to taking in, assimilating, and using nutrients.	**Neurocognition:** Mechanisms related to the nervous system and neurocognitive functioning, including memory, thinking, and judgment.	**Emotional:** A mental state or feeling that may influence perceptions of the world.	
Self-care: Ability to accomplish basic and instrumental activities of daily living.	**Pharmacological function:** Effects (therapeutic and adverse) of medications or drugs and other pharmacologically active products.	**Knowledge:** Understanding and skill in applying information to promote, maintain, and restore health.	
Sexuality: Maintenance of modification of sexual identity and patterns.	**Physical regulation:** Body temperature, endocrine, and immune system responses to regulate cellular processes.	**Roles/relationships:** Maintenance and/or modification of expected social behaviors and emotional connectedness with others.	
Sleep/rest: The quantity and quality of sleep, rest, and relaxation patterns.	**Reproduction:** Processes related to human procreation and birth.	**Self-perception:** Awareness of one's body and personal identity.	
Values/beliefs: Ideas, goals, perceptions, spiritual, and other beliefs that influence choices of decisions.	**Respiratory function:** Ventilation adequate to maintain arterial blood gases within normal limits.		
	Sensation/perception: Intake and interception of information through the senses, including seeing, hearing, touching, tasting, and smelling.		
	Tissues integrity: Skin and mucous membrane protection to support secretion, excretion, and healing.		

Each institution defines and specifies the type of information most useful for documenting patterns and trends for the nursing service in the organization.

Administrators and researchers who are most interested in the network, state, and country level data find value in nursing knowledge classification systems. At this level, which represents the broadest scope of data about nursing practice, the nursing minimum data set (NMDS)[13] is an important contribution to the data management needs of many systems. The NMDS is a set of variables with uniform definitions and categories concerning the specific dimensions of nursing that meet the information needs of multiple data users in the macro health care system. Its purpose is to standardize information associated with the nursing care that patients receive in a variety of service settings. The data set contains three categories of elements: nursing care data, client data, and service data:

1. *Nursing care data* elements consist of (1) nursing diagnosis, (2) nursing intervention, (3) nursing outcome, and (4) intensity of nursing care.
2. *Client data* elements consist of (1) personal identification and (2) date of birth, sex, ethnicity, and residence.
3. *Service data* elements include (1) unique facility or service agency number, (2) unique health record of client, (3) unique number of principal registered nurse providers, (4) episode admission or encounter date, (5) discharge date, (6) disposition of client, and (7) expected payer.

The benefits of this kind of data set include the uniform collection of data that can be compared across a variety of parameters, the identification of trends related to client problems and the nursing care provided, and reliable data for evaluating quality assurance and costing nursing service. Data mining is also a valuable activity that can be developed with access to large data sets. Such databases can promote comparative research on nursing care, including relationships among nursing diagnoses, interventions, outcomes, and other clinical nursing research questions.

The development of the NMDS elements is a goal that supports nursing knowledge work, and many organizations and projects are devoted to that goal. Informed nurses are aware of these levels of practice data and realize that these data, taken together, describe and define the value-added nursing contribution to health care. The developments in nursing informatics and nursing knowledge classification systems support twenty-first century nursing knowledge work.[14] Clinical reasoning models that support the development of past and future knowledge work are needed if clinical thinking in nursing is to evolve into the twenty-first century.

The Outcome Present State Test Model of Clinical Reasoning

Robert Reich[15] suggests that twenty-first century knowledge workers need to develop four types of thinking skills:

1. *Abstraction*—the ability to discover patterns and meanings in data, information and knowledge, events, and circumstances
2. *Systems thinking*—an understanding of the complexity of cause-and-effect relationships between problems and solutions in a system
3. *Experimentation and testing*—the active analysis and evaluation of data, facts, and conclusions; interpretations; and knowledge of how to make judgments and interpretations from a set of facts, which requires curiosity and skepticism
4. *Collaboration and communication skills*—essential for negotiating and working in teams to find answers and to achieve outcomes

The outcome present state test (OPT) model of clinical reasoning is a concurrent information-processing model of clinical reasoning.[16] It is a third generation (2000–2010) nursing process model that provides a structure for clinical reasoning, including a focus on outcomes from systems thinking about relationships among nursing care problems associated with a specific client story. As relationships among nursing diagnoses are analyzed, framed, and developed, one discovers patterns and meanings in the data that define key aspects of a patient's nursing care needs. Building on the dynamic relationships among competing nursing care diagnoses leads to the identification of a key-stone issue, which is translated into a desired outcome. Outcome specification supports the development of clinical judgment skills.

The OPT model is illustrated in Figure 2-2. The model uses the facts associated with the situation's context and a client's story to support reflection and reasoning. Through consideration of the facts, nurses discover patterns and meanings in the data, information and knowledge, and circumstances associated with the client's story. Through clinical reasoning, the Web-like associations among client and nursing care needs are illustrated. Nurses examine the complex associations, as well as the cause-and-effect relationships, among interacting nursing diagnoses. Understanding the patterns of relationships helps to frame patient care needs and set the stage for outcome specification and decision making regarding interventions. Reflection and *concurrent* consideration of diagnoses, outcomes, and changes in client conditions lead to clinical judgments about the outcomes achieved. In this model, the clinical decision making is the choice of interventions to move clients from the present to the desired outcome states. Clinical judgments are formed as a result of comparative changes in client conditions through time, with desired outcome indicators.

Understanding and developing clinical judgments requires attention to four "C"s:

1. *Contrast* between a present and a desired state
2. A *criterion,* or clinical indicator, to specify the outcome achievement
3. *Concurrent* attention to and consideration for how the nursing intervention influences transitions to the future desired state from the client's presenting state
4. A *conclusion,* or opinion, about outcome achievement

Clinical reasoning involves observing and talking to oneself while thinking through all the elements of a complex, uncertain situation. The OPT model requires the use of executive cognitive processes, such as reflection (i.e., observing one's own thinking while thinking about client situations) and the intentional application of critical, metacognitive, creative systems and complexity thinking.[17,18]

Several questions that support reflection and the use of the OPT model are

1. What is the client's story? How are you framing this situation? What assumptions have you made?
2. How does the context of care influence the thinking and reasoning about this client?
3. Given the client's condition, what nursing diagnoses come to mind?
4. What evidence supports the diagnoses?
5. How are the diagnoses related to one another? How does each nursing diagnosis influence and affect the others associated with the client's condition?
6. Does one diagnosis represent a keystone issue?

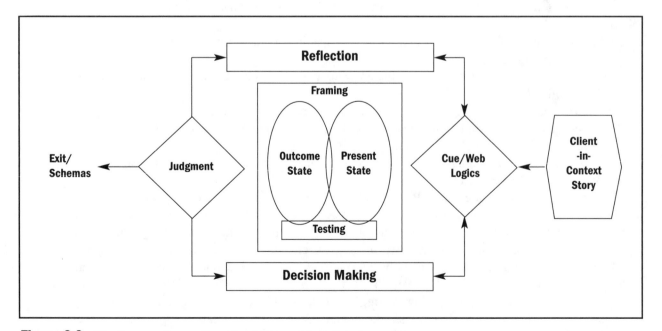

Figure 2-2. *The Outcome Present State Test (OPT) model of clinical reasoning.*

7. If attention is directed to the keystone issue, will other diagnoses be positively influenced or resolved?
8. Given the dynamic among the nursing diagnoses, how is the present state defined?
9. How can the present state be translated into a desired outcome?
10. Given the gap analysis between the desired outcome and present state, what nursing interventions will bridge the gap?
11. What clinical indicators, activities, information, or evidence is needed to achieve the desired outcome?
12. What are the four "C"s of clinical judgments in this case?
13. Does the situation need to be reframed to give it a different meaning based on the facts and judgment?
14. How does this experience strengthen my clinical thinking, reasoning, and development of professional nursing expertise?

Nursing Knowledge Work: Linking NANDA, NIC, and NOC

Consider how the OPT model provides a structure for linking nursing diagnoses, interventions, and outcomes. Given the structure of the model, nursing diagnoses lend themselves to present states, nursing outcomes lend themselves to desired outcome states, and nursing interventions are clinical decisions or choices among alternatives that move clients from their present states to the desired outcome states. The clinical indicators associated with outcome measures provide metrics for the testing and judgment phases of the OPT model's clinical reasoning processes.[19]

For example, consider the nursing diagnosis of anxiety. Based on the analysis of and reflection on a client's story, anxiety might be deemed the present state or a nursing diagnosis of concern. Anxiety control is the outcome. Several clinical indicators of anxiety control are listed in the NOC[20] system. Each of these indicators is scaled on a 1–5 metric that ranges from 1 (never demonstrated) to 5 (consistently demonstrated). For example, two such indicators are "reports adequate sleep" and "maintains concentration." The clinical indicators are exemplars of outcome criteria and provide evidence of outcome achievement. Scaling these indicators helps nurses measure the achievement of anxiety control.

Nursing interventions are clinical decisions or choices of interventions that may be used to facilitate the transition from present to desired state. The NIC[21] interventions of calming techniques, coping-enhancement anxiety reduction and decision-making support, and progressive muscle relaxation are all interventions that may or may not be appropriate, given the context and content of the client's story. One has to make clinical decisions about the appropriate choice of an intervention. Using the NOC clinical indicator scales provides evidence and a measure of outcome achievement. However, the meaning of the scale scores requires reflection and clinical judgment that, in turn, lead to additional clinical decisions, reframing, or the identification of a different priority for nursing diagnosis-outcome intervention.

Complexity and Twenty-First Century Nursing Knowledge Work

The beginning of twenty-first century nursing knowledge work is best exemplified in the work of Delaney and associates,[22-25] in data mining with standardized nursing knowledge classifications embedded in a hospital nursing information system. Given the kind of data mining techniques that have been tested and that continue to evolve, it is relatively easy to imagine future changes in the nursing process. Imagine what the next 10 to 20 years will be like, as hospitals and health care agencies incorporate standardized nursing language into information systems and electronic records. We might call developments over the next 10 years the fourth generation of the nursing process (2010–2020), organized around knowledge building. As data bases and systems are linked with a common nursing language system, it becomes possible to discover and data mine these repositories so that we can learn from the analysis of the patterns and relationships among nursing diagnoses, interventions, and outcomes.

As data accrue, we will likely begin to develop a fifth generation of nursing process (2020–2035), whose archetypes of care are empirically-based. As we refine these archetypes, we can learn the occurrence and epidemiology of nursing diagnoses, interventions, and outcomes for specific patient populations. We might also sort the data by the type of institution or level of primary, secondary, or tertiary care needs. As we gain more experience and understanding of which patterns are occurring, nurses can plan the care patients need more effectively and efficiently.

We might, in fact, move to another generation of nursing process (2035–2050). Given the data and tested prototypes of care, we could be able to develop predictive models of care that are based on the unique personal characteristics of the patient and that can be compared with empirical data derived from data aggregated from several institutions or from international databases of nursing knowledge. Simulations of patient care scenarios might, in fact, aid us in clinical reasoning, clinical decision making, and better clinical judgments. The evolution of these developments will focus nurses on the knowledge-management strategies that support their care practices.

Conclusion

As the health care industry shifts to an outcomes orientation and embraces electronic medical and health records, the nursing process and nurses' clinical reasoning are likely to change and evolve. Reflecting on the history of nursing process, one can pinpoint trends and transformations. These trends provide insights and an opportunity for discussion about modifications of the nursing process over time. Contemporary trends and forces suggest that another transformation of the process is needed. Contemporary nursing practice, with its focus on outcomes and on the complex analysis of multiple client conditions, requires critical, creative systems and complexity thinking. Nursing classification systems and taxonomies provide the clinical vocabulary for clinical reasoning in nursing.

Rather than "retro-fit" new knowledge into past linear problem-solving models, a different model of reasoning is needed. The OPT model provides structure for embracing the nursing knowledge work of the past thirty years. It is a structure that supports clinical thinking about relationships among nursing diagnoses, interventions, and outcomes. The continued evolution and development of nursing knowledge classification systems, as well as continued research into the dynamics of clinical reasoning, set the stage for further developments in nursing knowledge work.

Organized knowledge in nursing practice provides the foundation for the clinical vocabulary necessary in clinical reasoning and in building relationships among nursing knowledge elements. As information systems and electronic medical records provide ways for nurses to capture data related to diagnoses, interventions, and outcomes, there will certainly be ways to discover and mine the data associated with nursing knowledge that is embedded in health-related information technology systems. Such data mining activities contribute to our knowledge building and modeling, and support the development of empirical prototypes of care. The creation and evaluation of future empirically derived prototypes are likely to assist nurses making the value of nursing care explicit. As knowledge builds, we might very well arrive at a point where nursing knowledge captured in clinical information systems helps us craft individual plans of care that are empirically derived from clinical data supporting the value and differences that nursing makes. The nursing scholarship of the past thirty years, coupled with new models of reasoning and advances in technology and informatics, has provided the blueprints and architecture for twenty-first century nursing knowledge work.

References

1. Pesut DJ, Herman JA. OPT: transformation of nursing process for contemporary practice. *Nurs Outlook,* 1998;46(1):29-36.

2. Abdellah FG. *Patient Centered Approaches to Nursing.* New York: Macmillan; 1960.

3. Yura H, Walsh MB. *The Nursing Process: Assessment, Planning, Implementation and Evaluation.* 5th ed. Norwalk, CT: Appleton and Lange; 1988.

4. Gebbie KM, Lavin MA. *Classification of Nursing Diagnoses: Proceedings of the First National Conference.* St. Louis: Mosby Book Company; 1975.

5. Benner P, Tanner C, Chesla C. *Expertise in Nursing Practice.* New York: Springer Publishing Company; 1997.

6. American Nurses Association. *Standards of Nursing Practice.* Kansas City: American Nurses Association; 1973.

7. Pesut DJ, Herman JA. Metacognitive skills in diagnostic reasoning. *Nurs Diagn.* 1992:3(4):148-154.

8. NANDA. *Nursing Diagnoses: Definitions and Classification 2005–2006.* Philadelphia: North American Nursing Diagnosis Association; 2005.

9. McCloskey JC, Bulechek GM. *Nursing Intervention Classification.* 3rd ed. St. Louis: Mosby Book Company; 2000.

10. Iowa Outcomes Project. Johnson M, Maas M, eds. *Nursing Outcomes Classification (NOC).* St. Louis: Mosby Book Company; 1997.

11. Iowa Nursing Intervention Classification Project. Levels of practice data. *Image.* 1997;29(3):228.

12. Dochterman JM, Jones DA, eds. *Unifying Nursing Language: The Harmonization of NANDA, NIC and NOC.* Washington, DC: Nursebooks.org; 2003.

13. Werley H, Ryan P, Zorn C, Devine E. Why the nursing minimum data set? In: McClosky J, Grace HK, eds. *Current Issues in Nursing.* 4th ed. St. Louis: Mosby Book Company; 1994.

14. Pesut, D. Reflective clinical reasoning: the development of practical intelligence as a source of power. In: Linda H, Butcher H, Boese T. *Nursing in Contemporary Society: Issues, Trends, and Transitions to Practice.* Upper Saddle River, NJ: Prentice Hall; 2004.

15. Reich R. *The Work of Nations.* New York: Vintage Books; 1992.

16. Pesut DJ, Herman J. *Clinical Reasoning: The Art and Science of Critical and Creative Thinking.* Albany, NY: Delmar Publishers; 1999.

17. Kuiper RA, Pesut DJ. Promoting cognitive and metacognitive reflective reasoning skills in nursing practice: self-regulated learning theory. *J Adv Nurs.* 2004;45(4):381-391.

18. Kautz D, Kuiper R, Pesut D, Knight-Brown P, Daneker D. Promoting clinical reasoning in undergraduate nursing students: application and evaluation of the outcome present state test (OPT) model of clinical reasoning. *Intl J Nurs Scholarship.* 2005;2(1):1-21.

19. Johnson M, Bulechek G, Dochterman JM, Maas M, Moorehead S. *Nursing Diagnoses, Outcomes, and Interventions: NANDA, NOC, and NIC Linkages.* St. Louis: Mosby Book Company; 2001.

20. Iowa Outcomes Project. Johnson M, Maas M, Moorhead S, eds. *Nursing Outcomes Classification (NOC).* 2nd ed. St. Louis: Mosby Book Company; 2000.

21. McCloskey J, Bulechek G, eds. *Nursing Interventions Classification (NIC).* 3rd ed. St. Louis: Mosby Book Company; 2000.

22. Park M, Delaney C. Enhanced nursing care profile of older patients with dementia using nursing minimum data set (NMDS) and uniform hospital discharge data set (UHDDS) in an acute care setting. In: Marin H, Marques E, Hovenga E, Goossen W, eds. *Proceedings of the 8th International Congress in Nursing Informatics.* Rio de Janeiro, Brazil: E-Papers Services Editoirais, LTD; 2003:490-494.

23. Delaney C, Reed D, Clarke M. Describing patient problems and nursing treatment patterns using nursing minimum data sets (NMDS & NMMDS) and UHDDS repositories. In: Overhage JM, ed. *Converging Information, Technology, & Health Care: Proceedings of the American Medical Informatics Association 2000 Annual Meeting.* Philadelphia: Hanley & Belfus; 2000:176-179.

24. Delaney C, Ruiz M, Clarke M, Srinivasan P. Knowledge discovery in databases: data mining the NMDS. In: Saba V, Carr R, Sermeus W, Rocha P, eds. *One Step Beyond: The Evolution of Technology & Nursing: Proceedings of the 7th International Congress on Nursing Informatics.* Auckland, New Zealand: Adis International; 2000:61-65.

25. Clancy T, Delaney C, Morrison B, Gunn J. The benefits of standardized nursing languages in complex adaptive systems such as hospitals. *J Healthcare Information.* In press.

CHAPTER 3

Consumer Health Informatics: The Nature of Caring in the 21st Century

By Anna M. McDaniel, DNS, RN, FAAN; and Renee M. Stratton, MS

With the advent of the Internet and increased consumer access to technology, information to edu-cate consumers about their health is ubiquitous and the amount of health information available to the public increases exponentially every day. A recent Google search of Internet Web sites returned 660 million hits for the term health. *The consumer's role in health care has evolved from passive recipient to shared participant in decision making and ultimately to full responsibility for well-being, a transformation that has created an increased demand for health information. Information artifacts that encourage proper self-care and maintenance empower consumers to make choices that enhance personal health.[1,2] The nursing informatics community can play a vital role in helping to meet this demand by designing health information products that address consumers' needs and pref-erences for information.*

Consumer health informatics (CHI) is a branch of health informatics that analyzes information needs of consumers; develops, tests, and implements strategies to deliver health information to con-sumers; and integrates consumer preferences into health care information systems that promote shared health care decision making and support effective self-health action.[3,4] The emergence of CHI can be traced to the consumer advocacy movement that occurred in the U.S. during the 1970s. The focus on consumerism in the news media heralded an increased demand for accountability in the pro-vision of goods and services, including health care. In the 1980s, the self-help phenomenon became prominent, resulting in a vast increase in the amount of health information created for—and by—con-sumers. Access to the powerful information resources of the Internet dramatically increased in the 1990s. Other advances, such as "smart house" technology[5] and intelligent search systems[6] promise continued advancement of consumer health informatics into the twenty-first century.

Impact of Technology on Patient-Provider Relationships

Historically, the provider and patient relationship existed on a vertical plane, with physicians as the dominant entity.[7] The specialized knowledge and information that health care professionals pos-sessed had been inaccessible to the consumer, creating an information gap between patients and providers.[1] Through the advent of information technology (IT), this gap has narrowed, leading to a more equitable balance of power in the provider-patient relationship.[1,7] Consumers no longer rely exclusively on the provider for information about their health concerns. In fact, informed consumers who share in decision making with providers are more satisfied with care and are better able to cope with illness.[8] As consumer-centric health technologies continue to be developed, new roles for health care professionals with advanced knowledge of health behavior and informatics will emerge.

The degree of consumer autonomy over decision making in consumer health informatics can be conceptualized as a continuum (see Figure 3-1).

At the lowest level of consumer autonomy are CHI applications that facilitate data collection from consumers. For example, McDaniel et al[9] used interactive voice response technology to col-lect data on smoking status from patients prior to a primary care visit. Although "telehealth" sys-tems such as this one monitor patient progress, the consumer's role remains primarily passive. Access to personal medical information through electronic health records (EHRs) involves a some-what higher level of consumer participation. A recent Harris Interactive® poll found that only 13

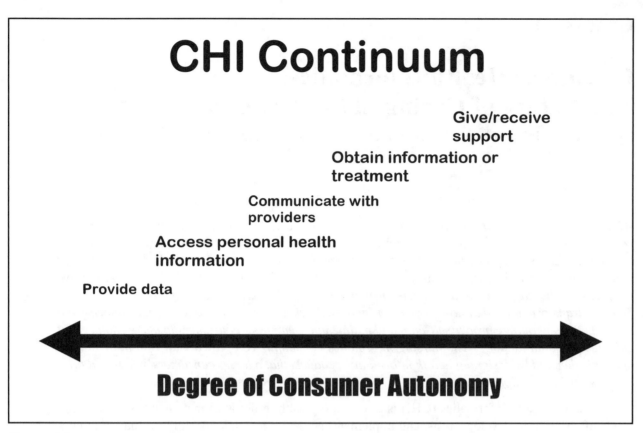

Figure 3-1. *CHI Continuum of Consumer Autonomy.*

percent of adults who maintain personal health records do so electronically, while 40 percent reported that they were likely to do so in the future.[10] A number of proprietary Web sites offer online services for individuals to assemble and store records such as results of tests, medical treatments, and prescriptions. Kim and Johnson[11] found limited functionality in a review of 11 Web sites with personal health records. Unsatisfactory methods for data entry, validation, and retrieval limited the site's usefulness for providing medical information to patients.

Patient-provider communication assumes a higher level of interaction and consumer autonomy than simply receiving and collating health history information. Although half of all Americans use e-mail,[12] it is relatively uncommon for consumers to communicate electronically with health care providers.[13,14] Providers generally avoid electronic communication with patients because of time constraints and lack of reimbursement.[1] Those providers who do communicate in this manner report benefits in terms of efficiency and within patient-provider relationships.[15]

A high degree of autonomy is required when a consumer searches for health information in response to an identified need. According to a 2005 Pew Internet and American Life Project report, approximately 95 million Americans have used the World Wide Web to search for health information.[16] Most e-health-seeking consumers, 91 percent, look for information about a physical illness, compared with only 13 percent who search for information about how to stay healthy.[17] Women are more likely to seek health information online than men.[13] Slightly more than half of all consumers, 57 percent, are seeking information for others.[13] In addition to increasing knowledge of health conditions, 70 percent of consumers report that the information found on the Internet influenced their personal health decisions.[13] Also, 50 percent of online consumers report that they asked their provider questions about treatment options or got a second opinion based on the information obtained on the Web.[13]

Virtual communities and online support groups represent the highest level of autonomy for consumers. More than 25,000 health-related support groups can be found on the Web.[18] Most of these groups are self-organized and have little oversight from health care professionals. A systematic review of studies evaluating the effects of online support groups found little evidence that these virtual communities had an impact on health or social outcomes.[18] In most of the studies reviewed, the peer support group was only part of a more complex investigator-designed informatics intervention. Furthermore, these studies represent a small fraction of online support groups.

Current Issues in Consumer Health Informatics

Privacy and Security

Despite increasing use of electronic sources for health information, many consumers are apprehensive about privacy.[10,17] Health care providers and institutions are also concerned with security issues related to Health Insurance Portability and Accountability Act compliance. The health care industry must walk a fine line between granting appropriate access to health information, ensuring security, and guaranteeing consumers' right to privacy. Masys et al.[19] tested a prototype system for sharing medical information with consumers over the Internet. No intrusion or attempts for unauthorized access were detected. Providers rated the usability of the system low because of the difficulty in using the complex system for secure logins. On the other hand, patients found the system easy to access.

Digital Divide

Unequal access and utilization of informatics technologies by all members of our society is a concern of the U.S. government.[20] Recent data suggest that the digital divide is narrowing. In the U.S. in 2002, 45 percent of African-Americans and 54 percent of Hispanics had Internet access, representing more than ten percentage points growth over 2000 figures.[21] This is good news, particulary because studies suggest that computerized support systems have the greatest benefits for individuals from underserved populations, many of whom are minorities.[22]

Unfortunately, the digital divide remains a very real problem for people with disabilities. In the U.S., only 38 percent of disabled individuals use the Internet, compared with 58 percent of all Americans.[21] Usability issues must be addressed to ensure that the disabled population can access the health information necessary for self-management. The National Cancer Institute has published evidence-based guidelines for Web design that incorporate recommendations for Web site usability by people with disabilities.[23] Other telehealth technologies, e.g., two-way video transmission, allow individuals with disabilities to maintain independence by removing the barriers of time and distance.

Quality of Information

Despite the widespread use of the Internet for health information, 86 percent of e-health consumers are concerned about the reliability of online sources.[17] A number of studies have examined the quality of consumer health information on the Web, and most were found to be deficient in terms of accuracy and completeness.[24] However, it is difficult to draw conclusions from these studies, as there are no uniform standards for assessing the quality of Web-based consumer information. Fallis and Fricke[25] examined published criterion for judging the quality of health information. Using conventional search engines to simulate the options available to the typical consumer, they examined 100 Web sites that gave health information on the treatment of fever in children. Only three of the published indicators correlated with accuracy of information on the sites.

Currently, the Web is an unregulated information environment. Indeed, anyone can purchase a domain name and publish information without regard to accuracy. Fallis and Fricke[25] have suggested the following methods to ensure the quality of online health information:

1. **Educate the consumer.** Nurses and other patient advocates should teach patients and families how to evaluate the reliability of online information sources.
2. **Encourage self-regulation and adherence to external standards.** Health informatics professionals should support the development of voluntary accreditation of sites by independent standards organizations, e.g., the Health on the Net Foundation.
3. **Pursue sanctions for fraudulent health information.** Although rare, when harm results from false or dangerous information, the informatics community should support whatever legal means necessary to hold those responsible liable.

Health Literacy and the Promise of CHI

The term *health literacy* is more than the ability to read health information. According to Bohlman et al,[26] "Health literacy is the degree to which individuals can obtain, process, and understand the basic health information and services they need to make appropriate health decisions." The Institute of Medicine estimates that 90 million Americans have difficulty understanding and using health information.[26] The thoughtful use of IT can overcome many of the barriers to health literacy, empowering all consumers to actively participate in health care decisions.

As demands on providers have intensified, the time spent with patients has become limited, which can decrease patient satisfaction and increase the patient's need for more information.[1] Terminology discrepancies can be barriers to health literacy for both the patient and provider, particularly when time is limited.[27] Discrepancy barriers can also prevent a patient from understanding the diagnosis and care recommendation, thereby lowering the level of active participation in the decision-making process and the development of a self-care plan. More importantly, patient-provider miscommunication can lead to negative (or even fatal) outcomes.[28]

Patients and providers can improve communication through increased terminology comprehension. The common communication bridge forged by patients and providers can promote meaningful dialogue and enhance patient understanding of care and treatment plans.[29] An innovative way to improve patient comprehension and understanding is through IT. IT reduces discrepancies between the consumer's learning style and the health professional's teaching strategies through the use of interactivity and multimedia elements.[30,31]

Another benefit of IT is the ability to deliver customized messages through targeting and tailoring techniques. Targeting addresses a specific population or domain. For example, smoking cessation maintenance messages target patients who have quit smoking. Tailoring further refines a message that is unique to a specific patient. Expanding upon the targeted messages example, cessation maintenance messages can be tailored to patients of a specific age. Patient attention and absorption resources are limited and vary by individual.[32] Message customization removes extraneous information, easing the patient's cognitive load.[31]

Summary

The IT revolution has created a new paradigm for health care. Previous limitations in technology, e.g., inadequate bandwidth, are quickly being overcome. Still, the informatics community faces many challenges to realize the vision of health care for all. A great need exists for appropriate knowledge management/discovery tools for consumers. New techniques in data mining and knowledge discovery may lead to the development of "learning" machines that will tailor information and adapt the interface to the user. Intelligent search strategies will overcome the problems consumers have in navigating the health information environment. Wireless technologies will allow communication and information exchange with consumers at any time or place. But many ask, "Is this really caring?"

Caring is the investment of one's resources in another to promote health.[33] What investments in CHI will the nurses of the twenty-first century make? First, the twenty-first century nurse must invest effort to understand the evolving capabilities of IT and learn how to integrate informatics applications into care. In addition, the nurse will need to invest intellectual capital to use existing and emerging technologies for knowledge development. Helping the consumer access and evaluate information will require investment of the nurse's knowledge and expertise. From these illustrations, it is clear that the nursing profession will remain at the forefront of caring and technology.

Escape from Nicotinia: A CHI Exemplar

Computer games are a common teaching strategy in public school settings but are seldom used for health education. Interactive computer gaming technology is uniquely suited to the delivery of smoking prevention education because information can be presented in an innovative, engaging manner that is familiar to children and adolescents. *Escape From Nicotinia* is a computer game designed to promote antismoking attitudes, enhance self-efficacy to resist peer pressure to smoke, and counteract the social forces encouraging smoking initiation in preadolescent girls.

The game uses narrative elements to engage players through role-playing and problem-solving modalities. In the storyline, the young female protagonist, Wendy Nevercoff, must rescue her friend, Cindy, who has been kidnapped by evil Joe Tobacco and is being held captive in the city of Nicotinia. Girls who play the game take on Wendy's role and must overcome challenges along six pathways. Each pathway was designed to influence the player's attitude about smoking and to impart knowledge of the health and social consequences of tobacco use. Before each challenge begins, players are approached by a Nicotinian, a strange-looking creature who offers them a cigarette. If a player accepts the cigarette, the game ends, and they must start the game again.

A pretest/posttest design checked the impact of the game on antismoking attitudes and beliefs. A non-probability sample (N = 34) of girls between the ages of eight and twelve years, who regularly attended a drop-in after-school program in two inner-city community centers, were recruited to test the game. After obtaining parental consent to participate, girls completed a pretest to assess attitudes and beliefs toward smoking. Following the four-week trial period, thirty-two girls completed the instrument a second time as well as a brief satisfaction survey.

Overall, antismoking attitudes and beliefs of the participants were significantly stronger following game play ($P = .016$). Knowledge of the consequences of smoking, as well as perceptions of smoking norms also improved significantly. Satisfaction with the game was high; the mean satisfaction rating was twenty-one out of a possible score of twenty-seven. Seventy-seven percent of participants agreed that the game was fun to play and that "playing computer games is a good way to learn about tobacco." The girls found the game engaging and enjoyed the multimedia aspects, but some participants felt the game was "too easy." There was a significant positive correlation between satisfaction with the game and posttest attitudes and beliefs ($r = .37$, $P = .043$).

References

1. Anderson JG, Rainey MR, Eysenbach G. The impact of cyber healthcare on the physician-patient relationship. *J Med Syst.* 2003;27(1):67-84.

2. Jones JM, Nyhof-Young J, Friedman A, Catton P. More than just a pamphlet: development of an innovative computer-based education program for cancer patients. *Patient Education and Counseling.* 2001; 44:271-281.

3. Eysenbach G. Consumer health informatics. *BMJ.* 2000;320:1713-1716.

4. Lewis D, Friedman C. Consumer health informatics. In: Ball MJ, Hannah KJ, Newbold SK, Douglas JV, eds. *Nursing Informatics: Where Caring and Technology Meet.* 3rd ed. New York; Springer-Verlag; 2002.

5. Stefanov DH, Bien Z, Bang WC. The smart house for older persons and persons with physical disabilities: structure, technology arrangements, and perspectives. *IEEE Transactions on Neural Systems & Rehabilitation Engineering.* 2004;12(2):228-250.

6. Gobel G, Andreatta S, Masser J, Pfeiffer KP. A MeSH based intelligent search intermediary for Consumer Health Information Systems. *Int J Med Inf.* 2001;64:2-3,241-51.

7. Dickerson SS, Brennan PF. The Internet as a catalyst for shifting power in provider-patient relationships. *Nurs Outlook.* 2002;50:195-203.

8. Kass-Bartlemes BL, Oritz E, Rutherford MK. Using informatics for better and safer health care. Research in Action Issue 6. AHRQ Pub. No. 02-0031. Rockville, MD: Agency for Healthcare Research and Quality; 2002.

9. McDaniel AM, Benson P, Roesener GH, Martindale J. An integrated computer-based system to support nicotine dependence treatment in primary care. *Nicotine and Tobacco Research.* 2005;7:S57-S66.

10. Taylor H. Two in five adults keep personal or family health records and almost everybody think this is a good idea. *Health Care News.* 2004;4(13):1-5. Available at: http://www.harrisinteractive.com/news/newsletters/healthnews/HI_HealthCareNews2004Vol 4_Iss13.pdf. Accessed June 15, 2005.

11. Kim MI, Johnson KB. Personal health records: evaluation of functionality and utility. *J Am Med Inf Assoc.* 2002;9;(2):171-180.

12. National Telecommunication and Information Administration. *Falling through the net: towards digital inclusion.* Washington, DC: U.S. Department of Commerce; 2000.

13. Fox S, Fallows D. Internet health resources: health searches and e-mail have become more commonplace, but there is room for improvement in searches and overall Internet success. *Pew Internet & American Life Project.* Available at: http://www.pewinternet.org/pdfs/PIP_Health_Report_July _2003.pdf. Accessed June 15, 2005.

14. Couchman GR, Forjuoh SN, Rascoe TG, et al. E-mail communications in primary care: what are patients' expectations for specific test results? *Int J Med Inf.* 2005;74(1):21-30.

15. Katz SJ, Moyer CA. The emerging role of online communication between patients and their providers. *J Gen Intern Med.* 2004;19(9):978-983.

16. Fox S. Health information online. *Pew Internet & American Life Project.* Available at: http://www.pewinternet.org/pdfs/PIP_Healthtopics_May05.pdf. Accessed June 15, 2005.

17. Fox S, Rainie L. The online health care revolution: how the Web helps Americans take better care of themselves. *Pew Internet & American Life Project.* Available at: http://www.pewinternet.org/pdfs/PIP_Health_Report_July_2003.pdf. Accessed June 15, 2005.

18. Eysenbach G, Powell J, Englesakis M, Rizo C, Stern A. Health related virtual communities and electronic support groups: systematic review of the effects of online peer to peer interactions. *BMJ.* 2004; 328;7449;1166.

19. Masys D, Baker D, Butros A, Cowles KE. Giving patients access to their medical records on the Internet: the PCASSO experience. *J Am Med Inf Assoc.* 2002;9:181-191.

20. National Telecommunication and Information Administration. *A nation online: how Americans are expanding their use of the Internet.* Washington, DC: U.S. Department of Commerce; 2002.

21. Lenhart A. The ever shifting Internet population: a new look at Internet access and the digital divide. *Pew Internet & American Life Project.* Available at: http://www.pewinternet.org/pdfs/PIP_Shifting_Net_Pop_Report.pdf . Accessed June 15, 2005.

22. Gustafson DH, et al. Effect of computer support on younger women with breast cancer. *J Gen Intern Med.* 2001;16:435-445.

23. National Cancer Institute. Research-based Web design and usability guidelines. Available at: www.usability.gov/guidelines/. Accessed June 15, 2005.

24. Eysenbach G, Powell J, Kuss O, Sa ER. Empirical studies assessing the quality of health information for consumers on the World Wide Web: a systematic review. *JAMA.* 2002;287(20):2691-2700.

25. Fallis D, Fricke M. Indicators of accuracy of consumer health information on the Internet. *JAMIA.* 2002;9:73-79.

26. Bohlman LN, Panzer AM, Kindig DA. *Health Literacy: A Prescription to End Confusion.* Washington, DC: The National Academies Press; 2004.

27. Zeng Q, Kogan S, Ash N, Greenes RA, Boxwala AA. Characteristics of consumer terminology for health information retrieval. *Methods Inf Med.* 2002;41: 289-298.

28. Campbell KE, Oliver DE, Spackman KA, Shortliffe EH. Representing thoughts, words, and things in the UMLS. *J Am Med Inf Assoc.* 1998;5:421-431.

29. Coiera E. Interaction design theory. *Int J Med Inf.* 2003;69:205-222.

30. Jones JM, Nyhof-Young J, Friedman A, Catton P. More than just a pamphlet: development of an innovative computer-based education program for cancer patients. *Patient Education and Counseling,* 2001; 44:271-281.

31. Mayer RE, Chandler P. When learning is just a click away: does simple user interaction foster deeper understanding of multimedia messages? *J Educ Psychol.* 2001; 92(2):390-397.

32. Coiera E. Information economics and the Internet. *J Am Med Inf Assoc.* 2000;7(3): 215-221.

33. McDaniel AM. The caring behavior checklist and the client perception of caring scale: measuring the caring process in nursing. In: Strickland OL, Dilorio C, eds. *Measuring Client Outcomes and Quality of Care. Measurement of Nursing Outcomes;* vol 2, 2nd ed. New York: Springer-Verlag; 2002.

CHAPTER 4

Information Technology: The Foundation for Educating Nurses as Clinical Leaders

By Melanie C. Dreher, PhD, RN, FAAN, and Judith Fitzgerald Miller, PhD, RN, FAAN

Serving as a wake-up call to the American public, To Err Is Human: Building a Safer Health System[1] *documented the grave and prevailing deficiency in quality that characterizes health care in the U.S.. As the first in a series of reports from the Institute of Medicine's (IOM's) quality initiative, the publication spoke to the serious need for improvement and reform. The second report,* Crossing the Quality Chasm: A New Health System for the 21st Century,[2] *offered a blueprint for such improvement. It urged all organizations, professional groups, policy makers, educators, and health care providers to engage in the organic change required to make health care safe, effective, timely, efficient, equitable, and patient-centered. It also called for the essential redesign of health professional education to prepare the numbers and the kinds of providers required to activate and grow a quality-centered health care system.*

Not surprisingly, the third report of the IOM Quality Initiative, *Health Professions Education: A Bridge to Quality,*[3] offered a strategy for redesigning the education of health professionals to promote and sustain a reformed and responsive health care system. The report identifies five core competencies for all health professions, notwithstanding their different orientations and theoretical underpinnings. According to the IOM, the health professional of the future must be able to (1) provide patient-centered care, (2) work in interdisciplinary teams, (3) employ evidence-based practice, (4) apply quality improvement, and fundamental to the preceding four, (5) make use of informatics. Indeed, all three reports acknowledged the critical role of information technology (IT) in the fundamental redesign of the U.S.' ailing health care system.

Academic Nursing Steps Up to the Challenge

Responding to the IOM's call for a safer, higher-quality health care system, the American Association of Colleges of Nursing (AACN) constituted the Task Force for Education and Regulation in 2000.[4] Acknowledging that the current and impending nursing shortages were integral to the quality issue, the Task Force examined the decreasing enrollments in baccalaureate nursing programs and health care quality deficiencies as two manifestations of a deeper structural problem in health care education and practice, both of which require equally penetrating solutions. The goals of the Task Force were to examine nursing education in relation to the IOM recommendations and to propose new models for educating professional nurses, who could contribute copiously in a redesigned health care system. The Task Force was joined in its deliberations by a panel of stakeholders who would use the services of these "new nurses." The stakeholders represented all levels of clients (individual, family, organization, community), as well as various venues of practice (hospitals, public health, long-term care, industry).

The outcome of two consecutive task forces (TFER I and TFER II) was a proposal to prepare nurses as advanced generalists, at the master's degree level, who would assume responsibilities of leadership at the point of care in a reformulated health care system. As "clinical nurse leaders" (CNLs), they would combine clinical knowledge and leadership skills to improve the health of clients (individuals, families, and/or communities) by engaging in a practice that is outcome-oriented, population-focused, evidence-based, intra- and interdisciplinary, and client-centered. They would not be prepared to be nurse managers or administrators; rather, they would function in care settings as direct providers, advocates, clinical decision makers, and coordinators of care. Essentially, these advanced generalists leaders would oversee the management and quality of health services as client and community advocates and as coordinators. Such nurses also would "care for" the environment in which they practiced, as well as for the client, creating a therapeutic context and a sustainable community in which an intra- and interprofessional health care team could maximize its potential.

At the same time that the AACN began its discussions of the preparation of such nurses, a similar movement was emerging related to specialty and advanced practice. Programs for a *doctorate of nursing practice* were being developed at the University of Kentucky (DNP) and Columbia University (DrNP) and quickly spread to other nursing schools and colleges. National-level task forces on the practice doctorate were established expeditiously in the AACN as well as in the National Organization of Nurse Practitioner Faculty (NONPF). As with the CNL at the generalist level, the dearth of leadership in nursing was the driving force behind initiatives aimed at the advanced and specialty level of practice.

Although a master's degree might have been appropriate at the early stages of specialty practice, the expansion of knowledge through nursing research has necessarily led to the increase in depth and length of specialty programs. In addition, advanced practice nurses began to identify that their clinically intensive curricula did not always prepare them for the leadership responsibilities inherent in specialty practice. With the addition of policy, fiscal, and organizational knowledge (including interprofessional concepts and evidence-based practice) to advanced clinical knowledge, doctor of nursing practice programs position nurses to be equal players in an interdisciplinary health care team. With clinical leadership education and credentials that are consistent with other health professions, advanced and specialty practice nurses are better prepared to increase their clinical effectiveness. Credentialing parity has the added advantage of attracting quality individuals to the nursing profession who seek the leadership opportunities and career advancement so apparent in other health professions.

As both the CNL and the DNP Task Forces began their work, it became readily apparent that the recommendations in *Crossing the Quality Chasm*[2] were already deeply embedded in the knowledge and values comprising the nursing paradigm. Virtually none of the five transprofessional core competencies identified in *Health Professions Education: A Bridge to Quality*[3] was new to professional nursing. Indeed, within the past decade, four-year nursing curricula have embraced each of these competencies, all of which can be found in the *Essentials of Baccalaureate Education,* published by the AACN in 1998.[5]

The provision of patient-centered care is a hallmark of professional nursing practice. As client advocates, well-educated nurses necessarily have assumed responsibility for coordinating care and integrating the recommendations of interdisciplinary teams. Likewise, the nursing profession has been a leader in the incorporation of evidence into practice, aided by the fact that most nursing is practiced in organizations capable of institutionalizing evidence in policies and protocols. The recent shift in nursing education and practice from process to outcomes has generated valuable criteria for evaluating both clinical and operational effectiveness. Moreover, nurses have always been activists in promoting the accessibility, effectiveness, and efficiency of the system to better serve the needs of all clients. Even informatics, admittedly the most recent addition to nursing's repertoire of skills, found its way into the 1998 *Essentials* document.

The Importance of Information Technology and Informatics Knowledge

Today, the case can easily be made that, although it is a relative latecomer to the skill set of most health professions, informatics is the most fundamental in that it enhances the performance of the other four IOM health profession competencies. The understanding and application of informatics facilitates and augments patient or client-centered care, interdisciplinary teamwork, quality improvement, and the incorporation of evidence into practice. The extensive application of informatics is a critical component of health care practice for all professions, especially for the nursing practice leaders needed to enhance the safety and the effectiveness of care.

Patient-Centered Care

Customizing the plan of care to the client's specific characteristics, needs, and desires is at the very core of nursing and a signature attribute of the health care system envisioned by the IOM. The electronic accessibility of information has made it possible for professional nurses not only to collect and use client-specific information in their care plan but also to share it, expeditiously, with other members of the health care team. In so doing, they[11] promote a system-wide understanding of the unique characteristics of clients and a coordinated team approach to the customization of individual care and community intervention." (Weaver, Delaney, Weber, Carr, 2006, p. 31)

The concept of patient-centered care also implies client self-management and participation in health-related decisions. Nursing practice leaders are expected to solicit and respect the client's perspective on the plan of care and to establish a climate of shared decision making,[6] whether the client is an individual, a school, or a whole state. Although inclusion of the client has always been a deep-seated nursing value, IT has created new possibilities for client-nurse partnerships. Viable self-management is dependent on having appropriate, accurate, and sufficient information, particularly in cases of uncertain and value-sensitive outcomes.[6] The personal health record is a critical aspect of patient-centered care.

Client education provides a good example of how IT can facilitate both the customization of intervention and the development of self-management capabilities. It is possible, for instance, to integrate electronic health record (EHR) data (e.g., age, gender, language, culture, educational level, energy level) with online information sources about a specific health topic to generate an electronic, client-specific teaching intervention.[7] Working with stroke victims and their caregivers, Hoffman et al[8] also describe computer-generated information tailored to the user's needs.

New generations of clients are increasingly comfortable with IT. For example, clients not only are willing but might even prefer to use e-mail to access laboratory results.[9] In the Couchman et al[9] study of 2,400 patients, e-mail was found to be a preferred mechanism to communicate with primary care physicians by 58.3 percent of the respondents.[9] Although patients were less willing to use e-mail to obtain the result of "high-stakes" tests such as brain CT scan, bone scan, mammogram, or prostate cancer screening,[9] there was nevertheless a high expectation for obtaining the results immediately via e-mail.

The IOM emphasis on self-management and health literacy[10] supports the role of both generalist and specialist clinical leaders in assisting clients to access electronic resources that expand their knowledge about effective health practices. Computer and telephonic technologies have been used to support many types of patients, i.e., family caregivers of persons with Alzheimer's disease.[11] Brennan[12] and others have demonstrated that laypersons can use these computer networks to make meaningful interpretations about health-related data. In the reformed health care system proposed by IOM, the role of the clinician leader will shift from teaching clients to guiding them to professional sources of information. It will also include validating the accuracy and appropriateness of Web-based information programs.[13]

Interdisciplinary Teams

Aging, chronicity, and the increasing complexity of contemporary health care require the coordination of multiple health professionals—working in multiple settings, at generalist and specialty levels—each of whom brings a particular expertise and perspective to solving the client's problem. Interdisciplinary teamwork offers an enormous potential for reducing errors, redundancy, and inappropriate care and for enhancing creative problem solving, safety, and effectiveness. The fulfillment of that potential depends, however, on how the members of the team interact and communicate. IT expands the continuity, coordination, and exchange among providers that are essential for safety and quality. It also promotes the efficient use of time and energy by establishing a standard common computational language and an interdisciplinary EHR as the foundation for communication and coordination.

Clinical leaders with master's degrees and doctorates will contribute to the content for the EHR so that it contains not only the traditional medical diagnosis and laboratory results but also nurse-sensitive information, e.g., current functional status, activities of daily living, ongoing care needs, family participation, spiritual history, client preferences, self-management goals, and similar information.[14]

Electronic reference information makes possible the use of uniform evidence-based care standards that can be implemented throughout a health system. At Intermountain Health Care, for example, more than 700 patient care documents and more than 1,000 other "information chunks" are accessible electronically.[15] These care standards reflect interdisciplinary collaboration and improved communication by all members of the health care team.

Evidence-Based Practice

Evidence regarding the most relevant phenomena to nursing practice (e.g., pain, hydration, mobility, elimination, skin integrity) is emerging in the nursing literature and making the nurse a more sophisticated provider. A major responsibility of clinical leadership at both generalist and specialty levels is the incorporation of such evidence into practice. Because nursing ordinarily is practiced in organizations, the introduction of evidence into practice has been facilitated by protocols and procedures that disseminate evidence institutionally. Today, electronic syntheses of evidence are readily available from various sources, e.g., the Cochrane Library, making the revision of policy and protocols faster and more accurate than ever before.[16]

A wide variety of handheld electronic and computer devices and personal digital assistants provide the means to access information at the point of care for immediate guidance and clinical decision support.[17] Examples of their use include checking for drug interactions, for treatment path, and for details about the pathophysiology and expected trajectory of an illness, for treatment path, and for national standards for incidence and prevalence of health problems. Additional support may be accessed with links to other relevant information and evidence. For example, once the care standards regarding the risk for falls are accessed electronically, the practitioner might see links to related information, e.g., medications that affect blood pressure.[15] As another example, systems that focus on drugs with topic maps are available.[18]

It is commonly thought that evidence is derived from research and then incorporated into practice. Informatics, however, provides a vehicle for systematically generating evidence from practice, by using technology to routinely document, retrieve, and analyze data regarding clinical progress, treatments, and outcomes, thereby using the data to transform information into knowledge. Informatics supports the synthesis of evidence, the review and implementation of practice guidelines, the revision of protocols, the provision of clinical information for the health team and consumers, clinical decision support, and consistent interdisciplinary communication. All of these benefits are central to a safe and high-quality health care system.

Quality Improvement

Perhaps the most recent trend of the past decade in nursing education and practice has been the gradual but perceptible shift in emphasis from process to outcomes. In a redesigned health care system, clinician and practice leaders will be evaluated on their demonstrated improvement in clinical, health, and operational outcomes. As the research reveals multiple ways of achieving quality outcomes, education for nurses who will be clinical and practice leaders focuses not on *how* to do something but rather on identifying the desired *outcomes,* along with the range of possibilities for achieving them effectively and efficiently. Nurses have been the most sensitive and often most vocal professionals concerning their clients' exposure to an unyielding health care system, characterized by long waits and brusque providers, not to mention lack of access.

The recent IOM reports[1-3,19] attest to the importance of informatics in ensuring safety and quality. Informatics is used to monitor patient progress (e.g., to view electronic reports of laboratory values data), to obtain decision support through information retrieval from library and other resources, to communicate with the health team, to assemble evidence for practice change, and to streamline work flow. Other examples of how IT can promote safety and decrease clinical errors are medication administration using bar codes, as well as computer access to information about drug interactions, therapeutic effects, and cautions.

Developments in "telehealth" have increased the health team's ability to assess and intervene at a distance, thus accelerating hospital discharge, avoiding costly trips by patients and providers, and eliminating waiting time for in-person clinic visits. Any number of physiologic parameters can be measured (e.g., weight, blood pressure, pulse, blood glucose, and heart sounds) and transmitted to a central monitoring station. Automated systems responsive to spoken dialogue have been developed.[20] The monitoring of data from the electronic record and the immediate access to laboratory values can provide trend data that enables practitioners, over time, to predict outcomes (including impending decline) and to make early interventions. Problems with illegibility, incomplete client data, the inability to find the patient record in the inpatient setting, and the poor organization of information are all prevented by the use of electronic client records.[21] Properly used, IT assists in reducing the length of hospital stay by facilitating the safety of client transitions to home or to other care facilities through the sharing of information and the determination of readiness.[19]

Summary

IT literacy is the set of knowledge and proficiencies needed to acquire, categorize, store, retrieve, and synthesize information competently.[22-24] In a redesigned health care system, IT clearly needs to be included in the preparation of nurses for leadership roles at the point of care and in specialty practice. As health advocates and managers, clinical and practice leaders in nursing must be able to

- Deploy IT to customize the care of clients
- Engage clients in self-management through access to health information
- Conduct routine evaluations of evidence in the policies and protocols governing practice and health intervention
- Engage the client as a full partner in care
- Integrate the work of the health care team
- Assess clinical practice and look for opportunities to improve health and clinical outcomes through decision support for care and operations

Further, in preparation for clinical leadership, practica in informatics should include opportunities to

- Design and implement care plans using electronic sources for decision support and for plan customization
- Review a policy and/or protocol using electronic synthesized evidence
- Incorporate innovation or evidence into interprofessional team practice using IT
- Diagnose and treat clients using IT
- Use system data sets to prepare reports about systems of care in direct care and community health, including high-cost and high-volume activities

Of all the health professionals, nurses are the best prepared to meet the challenges of contemporary and future health care, as envisioned in *Crossing the Quality Chasm*.[2] Chronic illness, geriatric care, and health problems that derive from socioeconomic dislocations are common challenges to nursing, as are health promotion and maintenance. Similarly, patient-provider partnerships, transparency in communication, and health management (as opposed to disease management) have long been part of the nursing arsenal. The inclusion of informatics as a fundamental component of nursing education and practice, truly helps nurses do what they already do—*better*. Informatics promotes and expands the promise and possibility of the nursing profession to assume a leadership role in the transformation of health care.

References

1. Institute of Medicine. *To Err Is Human: Building a Safer Health System.* Washington, DC: National Academies Press; 1999.
2. Institute of Medicine. *Crossing the Quality Chasm: A New Health System for the 21st Century.* Washington, DC: National Academies Press; 2001.
3. Institute of Medicine. *Health Professions Education: A Bridge to Quality.* Washington, DC: National Academies Press; 2003.
4. Long KA. Preparing nurses for the 21st century: re-envisioning nursing education and practice. *J Professional Nurs.* 2004;20:82-88.
5. American Association of Colleges of Nursing. *Essentials of Baccalaureate Education.* Washington, DC: American Association of Colleges of Nursing; 1998.
6. Ruland CM. Improving patient safety through informatics tools for shared decision making and risk communication. *Int J Med Inf.* 2004;73:551-557.
7. Doupi P, van der Lei J. Design and implementation considerations for a personalized patient education system in burn care. *Int J Med Inf.* 2005;74:151-157.
8. Hoffmann T, Russell T, McKenna K. Producing computer-generated tailored written information for stroke patients and their careers: system development and preliminary evaluation. *Int J Med Inf.* 2004; 73:751-758.
9. Couchman GR, Forjuoh SN, Rascoe TG, Reis MD, Koehler B, van Walsum KL. E-mail communications in primary care: what are patients' expectations for specific test results? *Int J Med Inf.* 2005;74:21-30.
10. Institute of Medicine. *Priority Areas for National Action: Transforming Health Care Quality.* Washington, DC: National Academies Press; 2003.
11. Mahoney DMF. Developing technology applications for intervention research: a case study. *Comput Nurs.* 2000;18(6):260-264.
12. Brennan PF, Moore SM, Smyth KA. The effects of a special computer network on caregivers of persons with Alzheimer's disease. *Nurs Res.* 1995;44(3):166-172.
13. Bernstam EV, Shelton DM, Walji M, Meric-Bernstam F. Instruments to assess the quality of health information on the World Wide Web: what can our patients actually use? *Int J Med Inf.* 2005;74:13-19.
14. Hellesø R, Lorensen M, Sorensen L. Challenging the information gap—the patient's transfer from hospital to home health care. *Int J Med Inf.* 2004;73:569-580.
15. Hougaard J. Developing evidence-based interdisciplinary care standards and implications for improving patient safety. *Int J Med Inf.* 2004;73:615-624.
16. Weaver C, Warren J, Delaney C. Bedside, bench and classroom: collaborative strategies to generate evidence-based knowledge for nursing practice. *Int J Med Inf.* In press.
17. Bakken S, Cook SS, Curtis L, et al. Promoting patient safety through informatics-based nursing education. *Int J Med Inf.* 2004;73:581-589.
18. Schweiger R, Brumhard M, Hoelzer S, Dudeck J. Implementing health care systems using XML standards. *Int J Med Inf.* 2005;74:267-277.
19. Institute of Medicine. *Keeping Patients Safe: Transforming the Work Environment of Nurses.* Washington, DC: National Academies Press; 2004.
20. Giorgino T, Azzini I, Rognoni C, et al. Automated spoken dialogue system for hypertensive patient home management. *Int J Med Inf.* 2005;74:159-167.
21. van der Meijden MJ, Tange HJ, Boiten J, Troost J, Hasman A. An experimental electronic patient record for stroke patients—part 1: situation analysis. *Int J Med Inf.* 2000; 58-59,111-125.
22. Saranto K, Hovenga EJS. Information literacy—what it is about? literature review of the concept and the context. *Int J Med Inf.* 2004;73:503-513.
23. Pravikoff D, Pierce S, Tanner A. Are nurses ready for evidence-based practice? *Am J Nurs.* 2003;103(5):95-96.
24. Tanner A, Pierce S, Pravikoff D. Readiness for evidence-based practice: information literacy needs of nurses in the United States. In: Fiesschi M, et al., eds. *MEDINFO* 2004. Amsterdam: ISO Press; 2004: 936-940.

CHAPTER 5

The Growth in Nursing Informatics Educational Programs to Meet Demands

By Diane J. Skiba, PhD, FAAN, FACMI; Barbara Carty, EdD, RN; and
Ramona Nelson, PhD, RN, BC

Information technology (IT) tools evolved along a path from automation to social collaboration. When IT was limited to mainframes and minicomputers, the focus was on the automation of routine tasks. As technology moved into the era of personal computers, the focus switched to individual productivity tools to augment human capacity. This shift moved IT from a number crunching to an "informatting" modality. The emergence of the Internet and the convergence of IT and communication tools provided the next transformation, to social collaboration. In this new era, IT tools foster communication, connectivity, and collaboration. The growth of technology in health care and the development of nursing informatics (NI) mirror this evolution. This is particularly evident as one examines the development of NI education from a global perspective.

Historical Perspective

In the 1970s, the first recommendations for the education of health care professionals in the field of informatics were introduced.[1] In those early days, courses on information processing, programming, and general applications in health care reflected a focus on automating the health care system. Computers in nursing courses first emerged in 1977[2] and fostered the development of computer literacy skills and a general understanding of computer applications in nursing practice, education, administration, and research. For many years, there were continuing education offerings and a handful of courses available. But initial efforts to educate health care professionals, including nurses, about IT applications in health care began with computer literacy. Nurses, like other health care professionals, needed first to understand what a computer is and how it could be used. Only when provided this foundation could they begin to use computer systems in health care.

In the 1980s the first books related to computers in nursing were published. A search of an electronic database that includes books in and out of print demonstrated that none of the books during this period used the term "informatics" but rather used terms such as "computer" and "nursing." In nursing education, the National League for Nursing spearheaded efforts in the development of computer education for nursing through the publication of two key resources: *Guidelines for Basic Computer Education in Nursing*[3] and *Preparing Nurses for Using Information Systems: Recommended Informatics Competencies.*[4] Also in this decade, the term "informatics" emerged, and the definition has evolved over time.[5] The emergence of a definition of NI[6] served as a foundation for the eventual development of two master's-level programs, one at the University of Maryland, College Park[7] and the other at the University of Utah, Salt Lake City.[8]

Throughout the 1990s, graduate NI programs began to take hold.[9] The curricula have varied from highly specialized applied clinical informatics to more generalized administrative and educational applications. To peruse the increasing number of programs in the U.S., Canada, and other countries, there are three excellent resources:

1. A list of educational opportunities from the Canadian Nursing Informatics Association: http://www.cnia.ca/education_links.htm
2. A list of educational opportunities from the American Medical Informatics Association (AMIA): http://www.amia.org/resource/acad&training/f1.html

3. A list of links courtesy of the International Medical Informatics Association (IMIA): http://www.imia.org/imia_lnks.html

From a global perspective, one has seen the rise of graduate informatics nursing programs in many countries. Of the courses or programs of study in nursing or health care informatics offered to nurses in various countries, this sampling, meant not to be inclusive, demonstrates that informatics is truly global. In the Netherlands, Goossen et al[10-12] described their seven-year experience starting in 1989, with the development of nursing information education at the Noordelijke Hogeschool Leeuwarden. Another example from the Netherlands is the work of Springer and colleagues[13,14] at the Hogenschool Holland. Many early efforts in Australia included assessing the learning needs of practicing nurses[15] and developing a core curriculum in NI.[16] In Brazil, NI began in the late 1980s with the introduction of courses into graduate education.[17] NI curricula are offered across four levels that correspond to undergraduate and graduate degrees. In Lebanon, Marini[18] described the development of an informatics course for undergraduate students. Faculty support was a necessary condition for success. She used the strength of the National League for Nursing Accreditation Standards to convince faculty to use computer technology as an integral element of the nursing curriculum.[19] A survey of nursing schools in Korea indicated that computer courses were offered since 1984 in most schools. The first NI course was offered in 1994 and is now offered in 20 percent of the nursing schools. There are also five schools that offer nursing informatics courses at the graduate level.

In Finland, Saranto and Leino-Kilpi[20] conducted a three-round Delphi study to identify the computer literacy skills needed to teach nurses about IT. Expert panels consisting of practicing nurses, nursing educators, nursing students, and consumers were part of the study. Several content areas emerged. Computer skills included understanding the basic components of the computer, knowing how to use a computer, and resolving error situations. Nurses should also be able to use hospital information and patient monitoring systems, know about system security, and recognize the obstacles and prerequisites of automated data processing.

Informatics Competencies

In 1997, the National Advisory Council on Nurse Education and Practice convened a national NI working group to create a National Informatics Agenda for Nursing Education and Practice.[21] This agenda identified five prioritized areas, as shown in Table 5-1.

Core informatics skills for nursing students and practicing nurses included
1. Basic computing skills (word processing, e-mail, spreadsheets, presentation graphics, databases, bibliographic retrieval, and Internet skills)
2. Use of clinical information systems
3. Implementation of policies related to privacy, confidentiality, and security
4. Use of decision-making tools to support clinical practice
5. Information management
6. Use of standard nomenclatures for nursing's language and content on emerging technologies

Many informatics specialists are practicing in the field that "lacked the knowledge of informatics theory and principles required to develop technology solutions." There was a call for support of spe-

Table 5-1. National Informatics Agenda for Nursing Education and Practice[21]

1.	Educate nursing students and practicing nurses in core informatics content
2.	Prepare nurses with specialized skills in informatics
3.	Enhance nursing practice and education through informatics projects
4.	Prepare nursing faculty in informatics
5.	Increase collaborative efforts in nursing informatics

cialized areas "(language nomenclatures, consumer health informatics, shared decision-making tools, distance learning strategies, and human computer interface design) within informatics programs."[21]

As an outgrowth of this national agenda,[21] several nursing studies were conducted in an attempt to address the informatics core competencies, which were specific for nursing students, practicing nurses, and informatics specialists. One major study sought to identify informatics competencies for nurses at four levels of practice, as described below.[22]

- **Beginning Nurse:** Fundamental information management and computer skills; use existing systems and available information in their practice
- **Experienced Nurse:** Highly skilled in computer and information management skills to support their particular practice. They use existing systems but offer suggestions for improvements.
- **Informatics Specialist:** Bachelor of science degree or above prepared nurses who possess additional knowledge and skills in the areas of computer science, information science, and nursing science.
- **Informatics Innovators:** Informatics specialists who are prepared to conduct informatics research and generate new knowledge and theory in the discipline[22]

This study, using a three-round Delphi method, identified 281 valid competencies, clustered into three major concepts: computer skills, informatics knowledge, and informatics skills. *Computer skills,* defined as "proficiency in the use of computer hardware and software,"[22] were equivalent to computer literacy or IT skills. *Informatics knowledge* represented the "theoretical and conceptual basis for the specialty,"[22] whereas *informatics skills* were considered "the use of methods, tools, and techniques particular to informatics."[22]

For the *beginning nurse,* the competencies were mainly centered on computer skills (i.e., the ability to use applications), such as using desktop software, working with a clinical information system, or conducting a literature search. Some informatics knowledge was required, such as recognizing the importance of nursing data for practice and the impact of computers on practice, as well as attaining knowledge of privacy and security issues, and familiarity with the basic components of a computer system.

For *experienced nurses,* computer skills and informatics knowledge were more balanced. Informatics knowledge included supporting efforts toward the use of a structured nursing language, as well as describing applications that would support nurses in various practice roles and in research. The experienced nurse also had a few informatics skills related to evaluating health information on the Internet, assisting patients with the use of databases to make informed decisions, participating in the selection process of an information system, and acting as an advocate for system users.

For the *informatics specialist,* there were numerous computer skills and informatics knowledge competencies. The computer skills expanded to include project management and quality improvement processes. Their informatics knowledge and skills likewise expanded to include the competencies associated with an information system's life cycle (planning, system analysis, design and development, implementation, and evaluation), impact (social, legal, ethical, and policy issues), data structures (databases, taxonomies), and usability. Additional informatics skills were related to fiscal management, programming, and the roles that specialists incorporate into their practices.

For the *informatics innovator,* there were the additional competencies related to evaluation, research, and the development of practice or educational systems. The following Web site lists the competencies: http://www.nurs.utah.edu/informatics/competencies.htm.

Other articles began to appear that specifically highlighted the informatics competencies of different nursing roles. Building on the previous work,[22] Bickford[23] identified informatics competencies of nurse managers, and Curran[24] did the same for nurse practitioners. For nurse managers who are considered experienced nurses, their "leadership role influences the attitudes of other nurses toward computer use for nursing practice, acts as an advocate of system users, markets the system or applications to others and participates in the selection and implementation of systems."[23] For nurse practitioners, Curran[24] selected most of the thirty-two competencies for the experienced nurse. She also added fourteen new competencies associated with the knowledge and skills related to evidence-based practice (EBP). An example of a new competency is "uses applications to aggregate and analyze data for forecasting, accreditation, clinician value, nurse-sensitive outcomes, evidence-based practice and quality improvement."

For several years, many focused on computer literacy skills for nurses, but with the widespread use of the Internet and increased attention to evidence-based practice, information literacy skills began to dominate the literature. An international literature review by Saranto and Hovenga[25] revealed that "information literacy was an ambiguous term", and in some instances there was overlap in competencies across the concepts of computer literacy, information literacy, and informatics awareness.[25] They conclude that there is a "general consensus that information literacy and information technology literacy are a foundational educational outcome for all health professionals."[25] In the U.S., Tanner, Pierce, and Pravikoff[26] conducted the National Nurse Information Literacy for Evidence-Based Practice Study, which assessed a large randomized, stratified sample of practicing registered nurses for their perceived level of information literacy skill, knowledge, and competency. Their findings documented "significant gaps in nurses' information literacy skills and their abilities to appraise research. Further gaps are identified related to their utilization of research. Most nurses are not ready for evidence-based practice."[26]

The International Medical Informatics Association (IMIA) Working Group 1[27]: Health and Medical Informatics Education developed a set of recommendations for informatics education. These recommendations served as a framework for the development of courses, course tracks, or specialty programs. They supported international activities in the education of health and medical informatics specialists, and they encouraged future educational developments in various countries. The recommendations are described as a three-dimensional framework including (1) professionals in health care (nurses, physicians, and specialists), (2) type of specialization (IT users, specialists), and (3) degree levels (bachelor's, master's, doctoral).[27] As stated in the report, these recommendations are based on a variety of reports from several countries, including the National Nursing Agenda for Nursing Education and Practice.[21] The recommendations provide learning outcomes for all health care professionals in their role as IT users (using information processing methodology and information and communication technologies) at the bachelor's level and for specialists at presumably the graduate level. The knowledge and skills are classified into three domain areas: (1) methodology and technology for the processing of data, information, and knowledge; (2) medicine, health and biosciences, and health system organization; and (3) informatics/computer science, mathematics, and biometry. For the health care professional as an IT user, there should be two European Credit Transfer System credits and for the specialists, there should be sixty credits. For specialist programs for nurses, it is recommended that 67 percent of the credits be in the methodology and technology domain, 25 percent in the informatics and computer science domain, and the remaining 8 percent in the medicine and health domain.

A leader in the development of health informatics education standards, the United Kingdom outlined the core content for health informatics in clinical education in their document, *Learning to Manage Health Information*. The eight core areas were (1) communication, (2) knowledge management, (3) data quality and management, (4) confidentiality and security, (5) secondary use of clinical data and information, (6) clinical and service audit, (7) working clinical systems, and (8) "telemedicine" and "telecare." In the National Health Service in England, the European Computer Driving License (ECDL) was adopted as the reference standard for basic IT skills in 2001. The ECDL was established in 1988 by the Finnish Computer Society and was quickly adopted as a national standard in IT competency in Finland. A 2004 national study[28] examined the progress of ensuring that health care professionals have the necessary knowledge of, skills in, and attitudes toward health care informatics. The results of this survey indicated that progress was slower than expected. Few new clinicians have been exposed to the eight core content areas. "Nearly all prequalified courses (nursing and medicine) make some provision for teaching IT skills."[28] Although there were endorsements for a core curriculum, few educational providers had heard of the ECDL. When comparing medical and nursing programs, "there were marked differences in terms of how much coverage was given to the different core areas."[28] One of the barriers identified in the study was the "lack of understanding of health informatics and how often it was equated with IT skills."[28]

The Canadian Nursing Informatics Association[29] conducted a national study to assess the nursing informatics opportunities for undergraduates, the preparedness of faculty, and the information and communication technology infrastructure support available for these educational opportunities. With more than 95 percent of the schools of nursing participating, the survey identified many interesting findings that were then presented and discussed by referent groups. First, "there is a need to have concurrent education and capacity building of educators, clinicians and students."[29] Although many schools had informatics in the curriculum, there was a need to identify core competencies and outcomes. Many schools expressed the need for more information and communication infrastructure and associated personnel. A series of recommendations were generated for a variety of associations to work on nursing informatics educational opportunities and corresponding infrastructure.

In Australia, a 2004 report by Conrick et al described "a strategy for the development of NI and the building blocks for EHRs in Australia.[30] It provides clear direction for government on the educational and information needs of nursing, and the engagement of nurses across all practice settings." The report recommended that a national approach to the development of competencies and their integration into all nursing curricula is necessary. The International Computer Driver's License (ICDL) should be a beginning standard. It is recommended that undergraduate nursing students need basic computer literacy skills as a minimum entry standard.

Nursing Informatics Working Group: Think Tank

In 2004, the Nursing Informatics Working Group (NI-WG) of the American Medical Informatics Association (AMIA)[31] recognized the need to identify the diverse existing graduate content and established the Think Tank on Nursing Informatics Education. Its charge was to evaluate the status of graduate curricula in NI. With the growth of informatics programs both nationally and internationally, it was deemed an appropriate time to reflect on the nature and scope of graduate preparation in informatics. The purpose of this examination was to reach consensus on the necessary requirements of a master's-level informatics degree program that reflects the American Nurses Association's[32] *Scope and Standards of Nursing Informatics Practice*.

The think tank's review included four specific stages. First, there was a cursory review of the current curriculum of NI programs. Second, a brainstorming session was held to identify key concepts in an informatics curriculum. Third, a small group of the think tank reviewed the literature and examined current models of informatics education, including but not limited to the IMIA informatics scientific map on content, the NI standards and scope of practice, and the identified AMIA (Education Working Group) core competencies. The final stage consisted of a series of conference calls to reach consensus on a model and final review of a draft document.

The review identified eight single-focused informatics specialty programs and six combined programs with informatics united with health and/or community systems. All programs offered both full- and part-time study. Only a few programs were totally available online. The average number of credits for the completion of a master's degree was forty credits (SD = 3.75) with the lowest being thirty-six and the highest being forty-five. The number of credits allocated for required informatics courses, not including practicum credits, ranged from seven to twenty-seven credits with the average being 13.87 credits (SD = 6.21). The number of credit hours allocated to practicum ranged from three to six, with an average of 3.76 (SD = 1.16). The number of clinical hours was different across institutions and ranged from approximately 135 hours to 600 hours. All programs stated that preceptors must have a minimum of a master's degree or higher and must currently be working in the field. There were exceptions in two programs that targeted rural and underserved areas where there might not be master's-prepared individuals. Certification in NI was listed as desirable but not required by one school.

The programs had between one and twenty-two faculty associated with informatics. The faculty had appointments in nursing, medicine, library science, or business schools, and adjunct appointments, as well as other supporting faculty. Faculty appointments were defined as having academic rank (assistant, associate, and professor) and being either tenured or in the tenure track. Adjunct or supporting faculty included preceptors, clinical faculty, and visiting faculty. Fifty percent of the schools had three or more faculty appointments in nursing. The remaining half had only one or two faculty appointments. Of the faculty appointments, 50 percent of the schools had at least one tenured faculty member. The need for more faculty prepared with a specialization in informatics was strikingly obvious.

Despite several attempts, no consensus was reached on a single model to underlie an informatics curriculum. A model was deemed premature at this time. So, a narrative organization of the concepts, themes, and content was selected to represent the Think Tank's work. Four major constructs emerged: (1) data-information-knowledge, (2) decision support, (3) knowledge representation, and (4) human computer interaction. Context (including the cultural, economic, social, and physical aspects of internal and external environments) also surfaced as an important construct. Informatics practices (embodied knowledge or skill sets that are learned and perfected over time) also became apparent as a result of the review process. These practices included information management, database management, and systems and project management. The results of our emerging themes are consistent with content areas generated by the American College of Medical Informatics's white paper on training future informaticians and the Education Working Group of the American Medical Informatics Association. The NI-WG Think Tank Education Task Force report is available on their Web site: http://www.amia.org/working/ni/main.html.

Implications of Nursing Informatics Programs

In the midst of the rapid proliferation of IT—of devices to capture, store, and retrieve ever greater amounts of health care information—NI education is at a crossroad. Forces within and outside the profession are impelling those in NI education to produce qualified individuals who can use systems, apply knowledge to the analysis of computer data, and research and design systems for advanced applications. Major roadblocks to the development of specialists are the dearth not only of faculty in general, but specifically, of faculty qualified to teach informatics, and the limited number of academic programs available to credential and prepare informatics specialists.[31,33,34] The demand for qualified specialists in informatics will continue to grow. The creation of a National Center for Information Technology Leadership (http://www.citl.org/), whose major focus is the expansion of the electronic medical record and the interoperability of clinical data to facilitate health care reform, promises to be a major force in informatics.

How is the nursing profession addressing the issues of market demands, availability, and educational preparation? In the past decade, a number of initiatives including collaborative ventures, education programs, and business partnerships have evolved in an attempt to address the issue of NI practice and educational preparation. These initiatives will continue to promote interaction, collaboration, and joint projects among informaticians in health care. The next sections examine the implications of the growth of NI on the preparation of informatics specialists, the practicing nurse, and newly graduating nurses.

The Informatics Specialist Role

The scope and standards of informatics practice[35,36] were the initial attempts to define the practice of informatics as a specialty within nursing. Following this, in 1995, the first credentialing examination in NI was offered in the United States. In 2004, the American Nurses Association published a revised document on the scope and standards of NI practice.[32] The document identified NI as a discipline-specific practice within the broader domain of health informatics and reiterated the elements of data, information, and knowledge as part of the metastructure of NI. It also clearly identified the informatics nurse specialist as a "registered nurse who is educationally prepared at least on the master's degree level."[32]

Given the newness of the specialty, how are the academic programs configured to provide informatics education and preparation on a graduate level? Recent work by the AMIA NI-WG[31] indicated that fourteen of the graduate programs supported either a single-focused informatics specialty or a combined program with a concentration or minor in informatics. What is clearly encouraging about this work is the attempt to examine graduate NI content on a national level and establish a baseline on which to guide future curriculum development and accreditation standards.

The preparation of the informatics nurse specialist in a graduate education program is essential. The domain was supported as early as 1996 as a specialty possessing the characteristics essential to a specialty: (1) a differentiated practice, (2) a defined research program, (3) educational programs, and (4) a credentialing mechanism.[37] In subsequent years, the educational domain of informatics has expanded to incorporate sophisticated areas of study and research, including but not limited to decision support, knowledge representation, and human computer interaction.[31] These areas of study presuppose a knowledge of sciences, including information, cognition, and computer science, as well as some basic knowledge of linguistics in the area of knowledge representation.

As the research work of the nurse informatician expands, it will enrich the body of nursing science, provide for the inclusion of the domain in sophisticated computer systems, and promote collaboration with other disciplines in the expanding field of health informatics. The work and professional knowledge of the master's-prepared expert will lay the groundwork for advanced research in informatics and provide opportunities to collaborate and pursue research and projects on a doctoral level.

Informatics is positioned to transform health care. NI is positioned to develop innovative models of care and collaboration that incorporate cognition, social change theory, usability models in clinical system development, consumer informatics, and education.

Informatics and the Practicing Nurse

IT has dramatically changed communication and interaction in society; in the next decade, it will also transform health care through integrated networks, sophisticated information systems, and interactive communications. The emergence of systems that connect providers, consumers, and organizations and that allow for the sharing of data and information will result in dynamic models of care and collaboration. Health care providers will be required to interact with these systems and use them in the delivery of care in all settings.

How are practitioners being prepared to work in this dynamic interactive society? Surveys have indicated a vital need to infuse informatics competencies into the faculty development curriculum as well as into student education.[34] In addition, nurses in practice need to develop basic-to-expert computer and information management skills.[22,24] The expertise and knowledge needed by practicing nurses are directly related to their areas of practice and to their levels of nursing expertise. For example, nurse practitioners in a primary care setting are required to manage large amounts of data and information, issue reports to regulatory agencies, and provide data for reimbursement. They should also possess the skills and knowledge needed to capture and manipulate data for tracking, trending, and decision making related to the patient population. Communication systems that promote patient and consumer interactions should also be part of their practice. These skill sets are different from those of nurse managers in a critical care unit, who are responsible for collating large amounts of rich clinical data and promoting immediate access to evidence-based systems by staff for informed clinical decision making.

Customizing information systems and access based on settings, expertise, and level of practice is a challenge to the informatics specialist as well as to nurses in general practice. Establishing clinical dyads that support collaboration between the informatics nurse specialist and the practicing nurse can promote exciting models of care that will optimize the use of IT and benefit patient outcomes.

Nurses must take individual responsibility to promote their knowledge and skills in the use of IT in order to consider themselves minimally competent to practice in an information-intensive profession. There has been a proliferation of venues for them to support the development of their information management knowledge and skills and to promote their continuing professional development in informatics.[38,39] These venues take the form of workshops, seminars, conferences, professional journals, networking, and special interest groups.

Informatics: From Student to Practicing Nurse

An area that deserves special attention is the informatics preparation of the novice nurse. Nelson[40] has proposed an undergraduate model of informatics that incorporates computer literacy, information literacy, and basic NI. Possessing these skills and knowledge provides the beginning practitioner with the core competencies needed to practice in any area of nursing. Reinforcing them in the practice setting is essential to maintaining professional competence. Promoting access to information and knowledge sources at the point of care is essential to safe practice; this may require a change in the practice culture. Studies have indicated that nurses often do not have access to interactive knowledge sources to inform best practice.[26,41]

Other strategies to promote basic informatics skills are innovative models of collaboration between vendors and clinical agencies. All learning laboratories should have bedside terminals and offer access to a simulated EHR. Nurses who are educated in such a culture that promotes and supports access to information and knowledge will expect it as a normal condition of their practice. They will incorporate interactive tools and understand the value of accessing and manipulating clinical data and information.[42] They will bring these skills and expectations to the clinical arena and work synergistically with clinicians and nurse practitioners.

Professional Roles and Responsibilities in Informatics

One of the difficulties in identifying the scope of a new specialty is that the roles and functions vary from setting to setting. This is particularly so in an industry that is rapidly adopting technology faster than the clinicians can develop the expertise to work with it. A review of the literature therefore supports a myriad of roles and responsibilities for nurse informaticians. A recent Web survey of 537 nurses in informatics practice indicated that only 10 percent of those surveyed had a formal nursing informatics degree and less than 2 percent were pursuing one.[43] The authors reported that one-third of respondents had a master's degree in nursing and 14 percent had a master's degree in business administration. These data illustrate that nurses are being hired at a rapid rate in IT, specifically for the implementation of clinical information systems. More importantly, these data support the need for additional informatics programs and the importance of promulgating a model that differentiates advanced or master's-level informatics practice.

The variety in educational preparation is mirrored in the diversity of the roles and responsibilities of nurses in the undifferentiated field of clinical informatics. Although the majority of nurses work in hospitals, frequent employment sites also include vendors, health systems, and consultants. Willson et al[44] reported that the clinical setting was a commonly cited environment for nurse informaticians. In addition, the titles and responsibilities are also varied, with clinical analyst, application specialist, and informatics nurse or clinical information specialist being the most common. The specific responsibilities vary and include project management, system implementation, screen designer and developer, and product manager.

What does the variation in education, responsibilities, and role definition tell us about the field of NI? It is clearly amorphous, ill defined, and open to interpretation. It is safe to say that nurses will continue to be hired as the market demands and that the theories and models of NI may or may not be represented.

Summary

NI is a new specialty. It is unique in that the rapid advances of technology are placing demands on a workforce that may or may not be qualified to meet the demands. There are questions regarding the availability not only of current informatics education programs but also of prepared informatics specialists with advanced knowledge of informatics models and theories. Clearly the market in many instances is driving the practice.

The challenge is to forge collaborative coalitions among industry, clinical, and academic settings to support responsible, informed, and innovative models that promote the needs of all stakeholders. Emerging and documented theories and models of informatics, as well as the demands of practice, should inform the education and research of informatics. This is the work of all informatics professionals, and it holds great promise for dramatic changes in health care in the next decade.

References

1. Anderson J, Gremy F, Pages J. *Education in Informatics of Health Professionals.* New York: American Elsevier Company; 1974.
2. Ronald JS. Computers and undergraduate nursing education: a report on an experimental introductory course. *J Nurs Ed.* 1979;18(9):4-9.
3. Ronald JS, Skiba DJ. *Guidelines for Basic Computer Education in Nursing.* New York: National League for Nursing; 1987.
4. Petersen HR, Gerdin-Jelger H. *Preparing Nurses for Using Information Systems: Recommended Informatics Competencies.* New York: National League for Nursing; 1988.
5. Staggers N, Thompson C. The evolution of definition for nursing informatics: a critical appraisal and revised definition. *J Am Med Inf Assoc.* 2002; 9(3):255-261.
6. Graves J, Corcoran S. The study of nursing informatics. Image: *The Journal of Nursing Scholarship.* 1989;21:227-231.
7. Heller BR, Damrosch SP, Romano CA, McCarthy MR. Graduate specialization in nursing informatics. *Comput Nurs.* 1989;7(2):68-77.
8. Graves JR, Amos LK, Huether S, Lange LL, Thompson CB. Description of a graduate program in clinical nursing informatics. *Comput Nurs.* 1995;13(2):60-70.
9. Carty, B. Nursing informatics: graduate education. In: Carty B, ed. *Nursing Informatics Education for Practice.* New York: Springer; 2000.
10. Goossen WTF, Jeuring G, Dassen TWN. Seven years experience in nursing informatics education: Part 1. *Inf Tech Nurs.* September 1996;8(3):8-10.
11. Goossen WTF, Jeuring G, Dassen TWN. Seven years experience in nursing informatics education: the courses. *Inf Tech Nurs.* December 1996;8(4):12-14.
12. Goossen WTF, Jeuring G, Dassen TWN. Seven years experience in nursing informatics education: changes over the years (third article in a series). *Inf Tech Nurs.* 1997;9(1):9-11.
13. van Aalst EH, Springer H. The training of the informatics nurse: an intermediary between the discipline of nursing and the developers of information systems. In: Greenes RA, Peterson HE, Protti DJ, eds. *Proceedings of the 8th World Congress on Medical Informatics. International Medical Informatics Association.* Edmonton, Canada: HealthCare Computing & Communications Canada, Inc.; 1995.
14. Skiba D, Springer H. Computer-mediated learning experiences spanning the globe: a pilot study between schools of nursing in the USA and the Netherlands. In: Greenes RA, Peterson HE, Protti DJ, eds. *Proceedings of the 8th World Congress on Medical Informatics. International Medical Informatics Association.* Edmonton, Canada: HealthCare Computing & Communications Canada, Inc.; 1995.
15. Carter BE, Axford RL. Assessment of computer learning needs and priorities of registered nurses practicing in hospitals. *Comput Nurs.* 1993; 11(3):122-126.
16. Axford R, McGuiness B. Nursing informatics core curriculum: perspectives for consideration and debate. *Informatics in Healthcare Australia.* 1994;3(1):5-10.
17. Marin HF. Nursing informatics in Brazil: a Brazilian experience. *Comput Info Nurs.* 1998;16(6):327-332.
18. Marini SD. Introduction of nursing informatics in the nursing baccalaureate program at the American University of Beirut. *Comput Info Nurs.* 2000; 18(5):240-247.
19. Park H. Nursing informatics in Korea. *Comput Info Nurs.* 2002;20(3):101-107.
20. Saranto K, Leino-Kilpi H. Computer literacy in nursing: developing the information technology syllabus in nursing education. *J Adv Nurs.* 1997;25:377-385.
21. National Advisory Council on Nurse Education and Practice. *A National Informatics Agenda for Nursing Education.* Washington, DC: Department of Health & Human Services, Health Services Resources Administration; 1997:23,385.
22. Staggers N, Gassert C, Curran C. A Delphi study to determine informatics competencies for nurses at four practice levels. *Nurs Res.* 2002;51(6):383-390.
23. Bickford C. Informatics competencies for nurse managers and their staffs. *Seminars for Nurse Managers.* 2002;10(2):110-113.
24. Curran C. Informatics competencies for nurse practitioners. *AACN Clinical Issues.* 2003;14(3):320-330.
25. Saranto K, Hovenga E. Information literacy—what is it about? literature review of the concept and the context. *Intl J Med Info.* 2004;73:503-513.
26. Tanner A, Pierce S, Pravikoff D. Readiness for evidence-based practice: information literacy needs of nurses in the United States. In: Fieschi M, Colera E, Li Y-C, eds. *Proceedings of the 8th World Congress on Medical Informatics.* International Medical Informatics Association: OmniPress; 2004:939.
27. International Medical Informatics Association Working Group 1: Health and Medical Informatics Education. *Recommendations of the IMIA on Education in Health and Medical Informatics.* 2000. Available at http://www.imia.org/endorsed.html. Retrieved on February 27, 2005:267.
28. Murphy J, Stramer K, Clamp S, Grubb P, Gosland J, Davis S. Health informatics education for clinicians and managers—what's holding up progress? *Intl J Med Info.* 2004;73:205-213.
29. Clarke H. Educating tomorrow's nurses: where's nursing informatics? Office of Health and the Information Highway, Health Canada. 2003. Available at the Canadian Nursing Informatics Association site: http://www.cnia.ca/education.htm. Accessed February 27, 2005:5.

30. Conrick M, Hovenga E, Cook R, Laracuente T, Morgan T. *A Framework for Nursing Informatics in Australia: A Strategic Paper.* Health Informatics Society of Australia - Nursing Informatics Australia, Melbourne: Department of Health and Ageing; 2004.

31. American Medical Informatics Association's Nursing Informatics Working Group: Think tank on nursing informatics education. Educational Think Tank Report; 2004.

32. American Nurses Association. *Scope and Standards of Nursing Informatics Practice.* Washington, DC: American Nurses Publishing; 2001:12.

33. American Association of Colleges of Nursing. Faculty shortages in baccalaureate and graduate nursing programs: scope of the problem and strategies for expanding the supply. 2003. Available at http://www.aacn.nche.edu/publications.htm. Accessed February 27, 2005.

34. McNeil B, Elfrink V, Bickford C, et al. Nursing information technology knowledge, skills, and preparation of student nurses, nursing faculty, and clinicians: a U.S. survey. *J Nurs Ed.* 2003;42(6):341-349.

35. American Nurses Association. *Nursing Informatics Standards of Practice.* Washington, DC: American Nurses Publishing; 1995.

36. American Nurses Association. *Scope of Practice for Nursing Informatics.* Washington, DC: American Nurses Publishing; 1994.

37. Panniers T, Gassert C. Standards of practice and preparation for certification. In: Mills M, Romano C, Heller B, eds. *Information Management in Nursing and Health Care.* Philadelphia: Springhouse Publishing; 1996.

38. Smith K, Bickford C. Lifelong learning, professional development, and informatics certification. *Comput Nurs.* 2004;22(3):171-181.

39. Newbold S. Nursing informatics organizations: virtual and otherwise. *Computers in Nursing.* 2003;21(3):275-281.

40. Nelson R. Core informatics: content for an undergraduate curriculum. In: Carty B, ed. *Nursing Informatics Education for Practice.* New York: Springer; 2000.

41. Pravikoff D, Pierce S, Tanner A. Are nurses ready for evidence-based practice: a study suggests that greater support is needed. *Am J Nurs.* 2003;103(5):95-96.

42. Connors H, Weaver C, Warren J, Miller K. An academic-business partnership for advancing clinical informatics. *Nurs Ed Perspect.* 2002;23(5):228-233.

43. Sensmeier J, Horowitz J. Survey reveals role, compensation of nurse informaticists. *Comput Nurs.* 2004;22(3):172-177.

44. Willson D, Bjornstad G, Lussier J, et al. Nursing informatics: career opportunities. In: Carty B, ed. *Nursing Informatics Education for Practice.* New York: Springer; 2000.

CHAPTER 6

The International Emergence of Nursing Informatics

By Marianne Tallberg, PhD, RN, MA, PHN; Virginia K. Saba, EdD, RN, FAAN, FACMI; and Robyn L. Carr, RGON

Nursing informatics (NI) commenced as an integral part of medical informatics, which emerged in the 1960s as the computer industry began to grow. The name, informatics, *emanates from the French word* informatique, *or the study of information. In 1960, the International Federation for Information Processing was established. In 1968, the International Federation for Information Processing formed its Technical Committee (TC4) to address the medical uses of automation. Later, in 1980, TC4 was officially named the International Medical Informatics Association (IMIA), and eight years later IMIA became a separate association.[1] In 1979, the Canadian Organization for the Advancement of Computers in Health became a founding member of TC4/IMIA, and Dr. David Shires, the Canadian IMIA representative, became president in 1980.*

Meanwhile in the U.S., the first Symposium on Computer Applications in Medical Care (SCAMC) took place in 1977. Every year, SCAMC attracted an increasing number of participants—including nurses. SCAMC along with the American Association of Medical Systems and Informatics (AAMSI) and the American College of Medical Informatics (ACMI), the forerunner of the American Medical Informatics Association (AMIA), formed in 1990.

Early Literature

In the 1960s, inspired by information on automation from the U.S., the World Health Organization (WHO) arranged for three seminars on automatic data processing in health care, but nurses were not invited to attend until the one held in 1971.[2] Also during the 1960s, the *American Journal of Nursing* published the first articles on automation. In 1965, "Automating Nursing's Paperwork" appeared, followed by "Automating Nurses' Notes" in 1966; both were among the first articles written by nurses. Also, at the American Nurses Association (ANA) biannual conference in 1967, one of the first papers on automation, "A Head Nurse's Viewpoint of Automation," was presented.[3] A search for references in the International Nursing Index for 1966 (its first year), using the terms "automatic data processing" and "computers," yielded twelve references involving the U.S., the United Kingdom, and Sweden. Enlarging the search with other terms ("monitoring," "automation," and "programmed instruction") produced a total search result of fifty-eight references, many of which were not only from other European countries, but also from Canada, Korea, and Japan.[4]

Early Conferences

During the same period, there was an early interest in bringing the computer into hospitals. Nurses in countries such as Sweden, the United Kingdom, Canada, and the U.S. were becoming active and interested in the new technology. They began working as intermediaries between the health care staff and computer specialists, and, as a result, the role of the nurse informatician was born. Also around this time, the term *nursing informatics* was coined. The first nursing invitational conference focusing on computers and nursing was held in Fairfax, Virginia, United States, in 1973. It was conducted by the National League for Nursing (NLN), coordinated by Goldie Levenson, and sponsored by the

Division of Nursing, U.S. Public Health Service (PHS). Coordinated by Saba, the conference focused on "Management Information Systems for Public/Community Health Agencies."[5] The NLN and PHS also conducted five workshops on the same topic between 1974 and 1975 and concluded the series with another national conference in 1976.

The first international conference in which nurses participated was the inaugural IMIA conference (Medinfo), held in 1974 in Stockholm. A handful of nurses presented papers describing informatics from a nursing perspective.[2] Then in 1977, the first Research Conference on Nursing Information Systems took place in Chicago, Illinois, U.S.. Other conferences were conducted to discuss the impact of computers on health care. They were sponsored by governmental organizations, continuing education departments, schools of nursing, hospitals, and/or developers of computer systems.

Early Organizations

During the 1970s, an increasing stream of papers primarily addressing hospital applications, computerizing nursing notes, and care plans appeared in nursing journals. In 1976, the European Federation of Medical Informatics was initiated and began to arrange the Medical Information Europe conferences. Further, beginning in April 1978, nurse's experiences and visions about electronic data processing impact on nursing were presented at a meeting arranged by the Nordic Nurses Association in Stockholm – Lindingö, Sweden, April 1–2. The issue was discussed in the various Nordic countries' nursing journals.[2] Over the decade, the topic of the impact that computerization could have on the nurse's role in health care became popular.[2] However, many nurses did not really understand what computerization was all about and, in general, had negative attitudes regardless of their country of practice.

Working Group Eight

In the late 1970s, many countries that had established national organizations focusing on medical informatics either joined or became affiliated with IMIA. The Medinfo conferences sponsored by IMIA continued to occur every three years. In 1980, at the Medinfo conference in Tokyo, Japan, Kathryn Hannah and Maureen Scholes conducted the first nursing workshop at a Medinfo conference. But the real breakthrough came in 1982, when an enthusiastic group, with Scholes as the leading nurse, arranged a symposium. The Impact of Computers on Nursing symposium, in London, drew 550 participants. The conference was followed by an invitational workshop consisting of fifty-nine persons—mostly nurses. All the attendees had some knowledge of computers in nursing practice, administration, education, or research and all had been invited to continue discussions in Harrogate, United Kingdom. One product of this workshop was a request to the IMIA general conference for the establishment of a working group on NI under the initial chairmanship of Scholes. At the 1983 Medinfo Conference held in Amsterdam, a full-day nursing seminar, organized by Elly Pluyter-Wenting, was conducted. Approximately 200 enthusiastic participants attended, representing thirteen countries. The first meeting of IMIA Nursing Working Group Eight (WG8) took place there, during which Scholes continued as chair, Hannah was nominated and elected vice-chairman, and Elly Pluyter-Wenting became secretary.[2]

In 1985 the second nursing informatics conference, Nurses' Uses of Computers and Information Science, sponsored by WG8 and the Canadian Nurses Association, was held in Calgary, Canada. That conference focused on computer ethics and the interaction of nursing with other disciplines and was followed by an invitational symposium. The conference established the format for subsequent WG8 conferences, which are held every three years and followed by an invitational symposium that produces documentation advancing the theoretical framework for developing nursing informatics.[6] The Medinfo held in Washington, DC, U.S. in 1986 included many nursing papers, which were well integrated into the scientific program.

WG8 was also invited to arrange a "nursing day" at the Medical Informatics Europe '87 conference in Rome, Italy. The high number of attendees contributed to the huge success of the day.

Yolande Elsig, the Swiss nurse member of WG8, was one of the keynote speakers during the conference. The third WG8 conference, Where Caring and Technology Meet, was held in Dublin, Ireland, with approximately 1,000 participants from twenty-three countries. Now, for the first time, an open call for papers was initiated. In his opening address, John Naisbitt, a well known futurist, formulated ten mega-trends for nursing and health care. He acknowledged the wellness business as a part of the health care fabric. "People will search for quality of life, the privatization of health care will be a fact in the post welfare state, and we will experience an increase in corporate health care activism." He has been right.[7] The invitational post conference at Killarny focused on decision support systems for all aspects of nursing.[8]

Educational Efforts

The conferences and the formation of organizations led to the introduction of informatics in schools of nursing. In 1977, the State University of New York at Buffalo, New York, U.S., initiated the first undergraduate academic course on computers and nursing.[5] Schools of nursing conducted workshops to educate nurses about this new specialty. Related articles were appearing in journals, papers were being presented at national and international conferences, and books were being published on nursing and computers. The new specialty advanced from nursing automation, to computers in nursing, to NI.

The first NI textbook was published in 1980.[9] In 1984, the first NI journal (*Computers in Nursing*), published by Lippincott Williams & Wilkins and edited by its founder Gary Hales, targeted the growing number of nurses interested in computers and nursing. The same year and periodically until 1993, Christine Bolwell commenced to evaluate computer software through the *Directory of Educational Software for Nursing.*[10,5]

A special WG8 conference, held in 1987, focused on developing computer literacy for nursing, and A Special Task Force on Education was offered as an open symposium in Stockholm, Sweden. The symposium was followed by a working conference in the Djurö archipelago, which resulted in a book identifying the competency levels for nurses in informatics.[11] It was considered the primer for the educational competencies of nurses in this emerging field. The University of Maryland started, in 1990, a summer school to enhance informatics knowledge for nurses. At about the same time the idea took on a following in Europe.

In the 1990s, EDUCTRA and its successor, IT-EDUCTRA supported two projects proposed by the Commission of European Communities.[12,13] One project sought to train health professionals in the use of computers and telecommunication, the other to teach health sciences by means of "telematics." The Nightingale Project, directed by Professor John Mantas[14] and funded by the European Union, focused on the planning and implementation of strategy in training nurses in the use and application of health care information systems. The Nightingale Project conducted several conferences and workshops in different European countries and published many books to serve as resources.

Professional Organizations

The American Nurses Association

In 1984, the American Nurses Association (ANA) initiated its Council on Computer Applications in Nursing (CCAN), which provided professional leadership in promoting computer technology in nursing in the United States. The CCAN conducted workshops, published several newsletters and monographs, developed a software directory, and generated other materials critical to advancing the field. It conducted a demonstration theatre and software exchange at all ANA conferences and gave several awards for excellence in the field. The CCAN also described the conceptual framework of NI as the interrelationship among nursing data, information, and knowledge for the users of the system and defined NI as the relationship among computer science, information science, and nursing science.[5]

In 1990, the CCAN was renamed the Steering Committee on Databases to Support Nursing Practice. Mandated to establish data standards for ANA nursing practice, it marked the initial effort to discuss the need for standardizing nursing terminology for the computerized systems that document patient care. Also, in 1990, the ANA House of Delegates recognized the Nursing Minimum Data Set (NMDS) developed by Harriet Werley. The NMDS consists of 16 data elements, four of which focus on nursing diagnoses, interventions, outcomes, and intensity; the remaining 12 on demographic data. These minimum data elements were deemed essential for the documentation of nursing care in both paper-based and computer-based patient records.[15]

The NMDS was considered the umbrella for the four classification schemes that the committee "recognized" in 1991–1992: (1) the North American Nursing Diagnoses Taxonomy 1 of Nursing Diagnoses, which was initiated in the 1970s; (2) the Visiting Nurse Association (VNA) of the Omaha System developed by the VNA of Omaha, Nebraska, which focused on community health documentation; (3) Saba's Home Health Care Classification System (currently renamed Clinical Care Classification System), which was developed through research to assess, document, code, and classify nursing diagnoses, interventions, and outcomes; and (4) the University of Iowa Nursing Intervention Classifications, which was developed by consensus to document nursing interventions. These classifications were subsequently integrated into the Unified Medical Language System of the National Library of Medicine, allowing online searches for nursing terms. Also in 1991, the ANA recognized NI as a new nursing specialty. Since then, the ANA has approved nine more nursing-related classification schemes.[5] The ANA has also initiated a certification program for nurses to be credentialed as a NI expert.

International Council of Nurses

In 1988, the ANA submitted to the WHO the NANDA Taxonomy I for inclusion into ICD-10, which was being developed. However, because of a lack of consensus from other WHO countries, the project was taken over by the International Council of Nurses (ICN) in 1988, and the development of the International Classification of Clinical Nursing Practice (ICNP) was initiated. Not until 1996 was the alpha version of ICNP published. Since then, the classification has advanced to a beta version that was published in 1999. During this period, the ICNP was translated into many languages and tested to determine its usefulness as a classification for documenting patient care.[16] The ICNP is developing as a "unifying framework," with strong input from IMIA-NI members. The ICNP® Version 1 was launched at the ICN 23rd Quadrennial Congress in Taiwan in May 2005.

Informatics at the National Level

Already in the 1970s, British nurses met to discuss the impact of computers—especially on nursing. Their meetings were the forerunners of today's British Computer Society Nursing Group. Holland was also among the countries with early energetic nurses. In many countries, nurses were active members in their national medical informatics associations. In Canada, the Canadian Organization for the Advancement of Computers in Health Nursing Special Interest Group was established in 1990 under the leadership of Kathryn Hannah but was disbanded in 1999. However, in 2001, Lynn Nagle established a new organization called the Canadian Nursing Informatics Association. Sweden experienced the same pattern, with an active group between 1987 and 1995 and in 2004, a new association formed for NI as a subgroup to the Swedish Nurses Association.

In 1984, Australia appointed Evelyn Hovenga as its representative to IMIA WG8. But it was not until 1985 that Australian nurses organized themselves to promote informatics. Currently, NI is the work of a special interest group within the Health Informatics Society of Australia, which came into existence in 1993. Nursing Informatics New Zealand was started in 1991, the first health-related informatics organization in New Zealand. It later joined with the New Zealand Health Informatics Foundation, founded in 1993, to form the current Health Informatics New Zealand, which is a strong, active group keeping health IT current with consideration of national needs and international trends. In 1994, Robyn Carr was appointed the New Zealand representative on IMIA-NI. Pacific Asia is now strongly represented. Other established NI groups are in Israel (1999), South Africa (2003), and Slovenia (2004).

International Projects

Several European efforts have focused on the uses of computers in nursing. In the RICHE project for an open hospital information system supported by the Commission of the European Communities (CEC), a nursing panel led by Elly Pluyter-Wenting evaluated the nurse care plan as part of the electronic patient record (EPR). Specifically, the TELENURSE project, directed by Randy Mortensen and Gunnar Nielsen and conducted by the Danish Institute,[17] was created to support the design and development of the ICNP project. The Wellbeing, Integrity, Prevention & Safety (VIPS) model, developed in Sweden by Margareta Ehnfors in 1997, addresses the structure of nursing care in patient records and serves as a standardized framework for nursing documentation.[18] Another project of international interest is the Integration of a Reference Terminology Model for Nursing, a standard designed to accommodate the various nursing terminologies and classifications currently used. The proposal for the model was submitted in 2000 on behalf on the IMIA Nursing Informatics Special Interest Group (IMIA-NI) and the International Council of Nurses (ICN) to the U.S. Tag Working Group Three, who in turn approved it while submitting it to the International Standards Organization (ISO) Technical Committee 215. After many meetings and discussions, it was approved in 2003. This was the first international nursing standard ever passed and has great significance in ISO member countries that generally implement approved ISO standards.[19] Currently the ICN is implementing a Web site to list all research and testing materials covering the research and its applications for a five-year period.

The Growth of Nursing Informatics

The IMIA-NI Conferences 1991–2003

Looking at the trends in topics for papers submitted to the NI conferences, we can see increases in the interest for language and classifications. The increase was 4 percent from 1988 to the Nurses Managing Information in Health Care conference in Melbourne, Australia in 1991. By the Texas, U.S. conference (Nursing in a Technological Era) in 1994, the increase was another 3 percent. This was topped at the Stockholm, Sweden conference (The Impact of Nursing Knowledge on Health Care Informatics) in 1997, where 19 percent of the papers had this focus, constituting an increase of 9 percent.

Since the first conference, nurses have clearly shown their recognition of the necessity of education in informatics. During the two latest conferences (One Step Beyond: The Evolution of Technology and Nursing in Auckland, New Zealand, 2000 and E-health for All: Designing Nursing Agenda for the Future in Rio de Janeiro, Brazil, 2003), part of the attention has been on the usability of the Internet for teaching purposes, for both students and patients. On the whole, nurses have presented a broad view on different aspects of NI, the knowledge has advanced and matured, and the focus has become more customer-centered. The conference titles also show a growing confidence in the development of the singular speciality.[2]

The Development of NI Working Groups

In the middle of the 1990s, the IMIA-NI General Assembly decided on the establishment of working groups for different purposes. Covering a number of disciplines that permit greater in-depth input and analysis, the groups function mostly by e-mail, while providing the opportunity for their worldwide membership to meet at specific times at conferences. Interested people can join by contacting a group's chair and by obtaining details of the groups from the Web address: http://www.imia.org/ni/index.html.

The Twenty-First Century

The current millennium is already offering a fresh view of NI. As a new professional specialty, the field is now part of nursing practice and of the nursing profession in many advanced countries. The vendors of IT systems are embracing the experience of nurses, both in the development of their products and in the implementation of their systems. Based on all previous work in the field, NI will soon be an integral component of nursing practice and patient care.

The new century will bring further advances in the integration of IT into the health care industry and into nursing. Professional organizations will continue to support and promote the field. Nursing educators will continue integrating IT and NI into their curricula, and nursing researchers will utilize IT in conducting studies on subsequent improvements in nursing practice. The credentialed NI experts will be educated and trained to be knowledgeable in the field.

The nursing profession has never before been so information-reliant—a fact recognized throughout this book—or so interfaced with education and the health record in an environment of reliability, accessibility, and technological accuracy. Nurses at both academic and practicing levels will publish more books and articles and present more papers at national and international conferences and workshops. Nursing Web sites will continue to improve, not only providing information on patient care conditions, but also offering support groups to counsel patients with specific disease conditions.

In this exciting new century of rapid advances, major NI conference themes are already recognizing that technology and nursing are coming together to provide e-health for all, thus generating a workable and positive agenda for the future. These new opportunities are recognized throughout this book, bringing with them a challenge for IMIA-NI to harness the power and direction of IT to widen the horizons for nurses targeting improved patient care.

References

1. Collen MF. *A History of Medical Informatics in the United States: 1950 to 1990.* Washington, DC: Philadelphia: Hanley Belfus; 1995.
2. Scholes M, Tallberg M, Pluyter-Wenting E, eds. *International Nursing Informatics: A History of the First Forty Years 1960–2000.* Swindon: The British Computer Society; 2000.
3. Bryant Y. Bibliography. In: M Scholes, Y Bryant, Barber B, eds. *The Impact of Computers on Nursing.* Amsterdam, Holland: North-Holland; 1983:563-578.
4. *International Nursing Index.* New York: American Journal of Nursing Company; 1966.
5. Saba VK, McCormick KA. Historical perspectives of nursing and computers. In: *Essentials of Computer for Nurses.* 2nd ed. New York: McGraw-Hill; 1996.
6. Hannah KJ, Guillemin WJ, Conklin DN, eds. *Nursing Uses of Computers and Information Science.* Amsterdam, Holland; 1985.
7. Naisbitt, J. Nursing and computers. Keynote presentation at: WG8 Conference, Where Caring and Technology Meet; June 20 1998; Dublin, Ireland.
8. Ozbolt JG, Vandewa D, Hannah KJ, eds. *Decision Support Systems in Nursing. Including Proceedings from the Third International Symposium on Nursing Use of Computers and Information Workshop: June 24–27, 1988: Killarney, Ireland.* St. Louis: Mosby Co.; 1990.
9. Zielstorff R, ed. *Computers in Nursing.* Wakefield, MA: Nursing Resources; 1980.
10. Bolwell C. *Directory of Educational Software for Nurses* (Pub. #4–2278). New York: National League for Nursing Press; 1984-1993.
11. Peterson HE, Gerdin-Jelger U, eds. *Preparing Nurses for Using Information Systems: Recommended Informatics Competencies. Proceedings of the Working Group Eight Task Force on Education; June 10–13, 1987; Djurö, Sweden.* New York: National League for Nursing; 1988.
12. Hasman A, Albert A, Wainwright P, Klar R, Sosa M, eds. *Education and Training in Health Informatics in Europe. State of the Art–Guidelines–Applications.* Amsterdam, Holland: IOS Press.
13. Hasman A. Education and training in health informatics. The IT Eductra Project. In: Gerdin U, Tallberg M, Wainwright P, eds. *Nursing Informatics '97: The Impact of Nursing Knowledge on Health Care Informatics.* Amersterdam, Holland: IOS Press; 1997.
14. Mantas J, ed. *Health Telematics Education.* Amsterdam, Holland: IOS Press; 1997.
15. Werley H, Lang NM. *Identification of the Nursing Minimum Data Set.* New York: Springer; 1988.
16. International Council of Nurses. ICNP: *International Classification of Nursing Practice: Beta.* Geneva, Switzerland: ICN; 1999.
17. TELENURSE: Telematics Applications for Nurses. Summary Description. Telematics for Health Care European Commission DG XIII; 1995.

18. Ehnfors M. Nursing information in patient records. Towards uniform key words for documentation of nursing practice. In: Grobe SJ, Pluyter-Wenting ESP, eds. *Nursing Informatics: An International Overview for Nursing in a Technological Era. Proceedings of the Fifth International Conference on Nursing Use of Computers and Information Science, San Antonio, Texas, USA, June 17–22, 1994.* Amsterdam, Holland: Elsevier;1994.

19. Saba VK, Carr R, Sermeus W, Rocha P. *ISO One Step Beyond: The Evolution of Technology & Nursing. 7th International Congress Nursing Informatics Proceedings.* Auckland, New Zealand: Adis International Limited; 2000.

SECTION II

New Roles and Leadership Opportunities

Section II

Introduction

Charlotte A. Weaver, PhD, RN

As the health care industry has turned to bringing automation into the core of clinical care delivery, the demand for clinicians to assist in this transformation has caused an explosion in the number of nurses assuming informatics roles. Section II documents the industry's demands on nursing to fill these various roles and examines the leadership opportunities that these demands are creating at the highest organizational levels.

Section II includes ten chapters that are supported through six case studies. The lead off chapter by Knecht and colleagues maps out the new leadership competencies required of nurse executives whose organizations undertake moving to an electronic health record system. The accompanying three case studies by Hertzler, Ambrosini, and Reck provide rich descriptions and practical hands-on lessons learned from these nurse executives who have successfully led their organizations through transformation and adoption. Weaver and Walker describe the role of the chief clinical informatics officer that is occurring at corporate levels of large integrated delivery systems (IDNs). These IDNs usually cover multiple states, wide ranges in size and type of hospitals and health systems, and number from 30 to 100 organizations. The theme of new leadership opportunities is carried through in Nagle's look at the increasingly common occurrence of "nurse in the chief information officer role," and Croft's case study maps out the career path and skills needed to make this role transition.

It is not often that the inside operations of corporations are exposed to public view. In their description of the information technology industry's corporate chief nurse officer role, Weaver, Cato and Latimer give us a look at the industry's efforts to mirror the clinical executive leader roles of health care organizations and the business drivers behind this role. Nurse leadership in health policy, standards, and health care at a national government level are addressed by Vande Walle and colleagues from Belgium, Moorer and Rick from the Veterans Health Administration, and also Warren on standards in the United States.

All sides of health care are involved in this phenomenon of dependence on nurses in translator roles between clinicians and technology staff. The extreme expression of this dependence is represented in Murphy and Gugerty's examination of nurses as project managers over complex clinical information system implementations. Creating a win-win outcome for health care systems involves close collaboration between the nurse informatics leader and skilled project managers, as shown in the accompanying case study by Fry and Willock.

Section II closes with Sensmeier's analysis of the rapid growth in nurses seeking professional affiliation as newcomers into their roles and the field. Sensmeier reports on the surprise of finding that of the 580+ nurses attending the first Healthcare Information and Management Systems Society (HIMSS) Nursing Informatics (NI) Symposium in 2004, more than one-third of those nurse attendees were attending their first HIMSS meeting and indicated that they had been in their role for under one year. This growth continued into 2005 with over 650 nurses attending the NI Symposium event. Sensmeier examines changes in the health care industry driving this explosive growth in clinical nurses who are being recruited into informatics roles within their organizations, and titles her chapter, "Every Organization Needs Them: Nurse Informaticians." It is a fitting close to this section on new roles, career paths, and leadership opportunities.

CHAPTER 7

Clinical Transformation and Nursing Executive Leadership

By Karen Knecht, BSN, RN; Roy L. Simpson, RN, C, FNAP, FAAN; and Charlotte A. Weaver, PhD, RN

Most of the industrialized world is on a committed march toward achieving an electronic health record (EHR).[1-3] Across the globe, health care organizations are focused on implementing integrated clinical information systems (CIS) that make up an EHR, and this will continue for the foreseeable future.[4] Driving the adoption of such extensive information technology (IT) in care delivery is a quest for better quality at lower costs.[5-8] EHR systems hold the potential for all clinical and administrative processes to be fully automated and integrated.[4] Because the clinical solution components within an EHR system go to the core of care delivery work processes, these system implementations bring about clinical transformation. Given the existing operational role of the chief nurse executive (CNE), who is responsible for all patient care services, the magnitude of these transformational efforts will significantly elevate the CNE's influence in health care organizations.

This chapter describes the new skills and role functions that the CNE will be called on to demonstrate in leading these types of initiatives. It also presents a rationale for proactive engagement on the part of the CNE and provides a roadmap to help CNEs guide the clinical transformation.

Transformational Impact of the EHR

Virtually every major health care provider organization is currently engaged in or is about to start a process to implement an integrated CIS in pursuit of the EHR vision.[1-3,9] An integrated CIS is a set of applications from a single vendor that provides the core functions of results reporting, intelligent orders management, and clinical documentation (including care planning and electronic medication management). It is part of a larger IT strategy that includes integration with other clinical applications and provides the foundation for an EHR.[4,10] Countries including the U.S. are moving toward implementing EHR systems because of an urgent need to control health care costs.[1,6,11-13] Increasingly, besieged health care provider organizations are under pressure to deliver improved outcomes with a shrinking bottom line; as a result, IT is being recognized as an essential business strategy for the operational survival of health care organizations.[14]

Although studies have shown genuine, realizable benefits from these clinical systems, they have also revealed their complexity and their potential for harm when not applied appropriately.[15,16] Because an EHR system introduces high levels of automation and computerization into every clinician's practice, it may easily be the largest, most intricate project ever undertaken by a health care organization. Therefore, its components are typically implemented in stages and over an extended period of time.

An EHR system touches almost every aspect of the health care provider organization. Its implementation involves many users, particularly nurses and physicians. It affects how users will communicate and interact with patients and with other members of the health care team, and it significantly changes how health care providers process, synthesize, and interact with data.

The selection and implementation of software systems have traditionally been the domain of hospital IT departments. However, an EHR is not just a technology project; it is also a strategic business and clinical initiative that requires the full participation of the executive team. The CNE is increasingly being called on for leadership to ensure that the EHR system is designed in a way that will yield clinical transformation.[17-19] Health care organizations are best positioned to realize the full potential of their investment in an EHR when they can treat its implementation for what it represents: organizational and clinical transformation at the deepest level,[20] involving substantial change in the form, nature, and function of how work is carried out and enabled by IT.[21]

New Role Dimensions for the CNE

Although the American Nurses Association's (ANA's) standards for nursing administrators require that direct care providers be involved in the selection, implementation, and analysis of outcomes of information technology,[22] the role of the CNE in clinical system implementations is much greater. It requires more than monitoring proposals and participating in IT strategic planning. The CNE's informatics leadership in EHR initiatives is about "owning" a vision of IT's potential uses in nursing. Whether this potential involves work flow modification, quality improvement, enhanced patient and family care, or some other goal, its actualization requires a vision that is clear, attainable, and aimed at meeting the specific needs of nursing for each unique organization. As the primary voice and advocate for nursing within an organization, the CNE is clearly the most appropriate person to formulate, promulgate, and administrate that vision. And therein lies the CNE's power.

An EHR initiative requires multimillion dollar expenditures over several years. Its implementation can be successful only when there is a well-defined road map based on strong guiding principles for the management of organizational change. The road map must be developed and carried out by the organization's executive clinical leadership. Although this role is often shared between the chief medical officer (CMO) and the CNE, it is the CNE who has operational control over resources and budgets for the patient care departments and staff that will be most affected. Work flow redesign often changes practice standards, practice scope, and has ramifications for regulatory requirements. The CNE will also have to balance the competing needs of salary costs for additional resources and capital to support the organization's long-range vision and goals. For all of these reasons, the nurse executive's direct oversight and participation is essential. The CNE ensures timely and appropriate decision making and prevents delays in the work team's process.

As the executive clinical leader for the EHR implementation, the CNE does not need IT knowledge or technical expertise. Technical expertise can reside in the nurse informatician or other informaticians on the CNE's team. Rather, the CNE must provide the vision for how the technology is used to gain patient safety and efficiency benefits. In redesigning work processes, the CNE must evaluate proposed changes within a larger context. The CNE's responsibility for patient care services confers the authority for validating that the newly designed work processes facilitate communication and support efficiencies across the entire care team. Other key leadership functions that can be done most effectively by the CNE include guiding the organization to consensus with regard to standards and outcome measures and mentoring managers through the implementation process. The skill sets needed by the CNE to manage these complex transformation initiatives are all in the leadership realm.[23,24] They include being a visionary risk taker and an inspiring and effective communicator, one who can build consensus while making hard decisions, who can create effective cross-organizational work teams, who uses power effectively, and demonstrates courage and tenacity.[24-27]

The CNE's Road Map for Transformation

At the core of the transformational effort is changing how people work on a daily basis through the optimization of technology. The three key areas of organizational and clinical transformation that require the CNE's leadership and active involvement are:

1. Creating and executing an effective project organization
2. Planning, designing, and deploying new processes and technology to improve patient safety, streamline work flow; ensure standard practice, enable best practice, and define measures and care process outcomes
3. Ensuring the management of organizational change

Creating and Executing the Project Organization

At the onset of a project of this magnitude, a well-defined organization should be established. Although detailing the project structure, committees, roles, and resources are tasks that normally fall to the project manager on an information services (IS) team, it is the CNE who is responsible for identifying the best individuals to fill the roles and for assigning resources. The executive team must approve the project structure, resources, and budget, and appoint executives, physicians, and managers to the various committees.

The project team reports to a multidisciplinary executive steering committee, which must include, at a minimum, a senior physician, a nurse executive, and a hospital administration representative. The executive steering committee is charged with facilitating and assuming active accountability for strategic decisions, as well as with allocating the capital funding and resources to achieve the project's goals.

Multidisciplinary Work Teams and Project Teams

A factor critical to the success of an EHR clinical system initiative is the extensive and consistent use of multidisciplinary teams that work under the direction of the executive steering committee and are coordinated by the project management office. The project management office is that segment of the IT department that carries responsibility for managing the detailed development of the project plan, resources, tasks, and timeline. Much has been written about successful cross-organizational implementations in which work teams have been used extensively.[28,29] The importance of teamwork and strong multidisciplinary collaboration is also reflected in magnet hospitals' experience with EHR implementations. Magnet hospitals are those health care organizations that were first recognized in the 1980s for their ability to attract and hold nursing staff, and these qualities of nursing excellence have been formalized in the "Magnet Hospital" program under the auspices of the American Academy of Nursing.[30,31] Health care organizations pursuing Magnet Hospital status appear to gain advantages for successful clinical system implementations. One group of investigators attributed this phenomenon to the magnet characteristics of strong team communication, self-governance, and support for the optimization of nursing practice.[32]

A massive amount of teamwork is needed to accomplish organizational and clinical transformation. In addition to redesigning work processes, the work teams also do much of the validation and detailed decision making. Each work team is led by a member of the IS project team and is composed of subject-matter experts from relevant clinical and operational areas of the organization. The work teams give final approval to all screen designs, screen flows, and associated data definitions; ensure that the designs provide clinically relevant, accurate views of patient information; and make recommendations for work process changes.

Work teams are the "glue" of an implementation project because they bring in the expertise of the frontline staff and end users. They are needed long after the initial design phase has been completed, through the conversion and postconversion phases. They also may provide input on the resolution of issues or on changes needed for the implementation strategy or the educational plan. To ensure that frontline staff and domain expertise are readily available for problem solving, it is important that work teams be accessible throughout the implementation's life cycle. Flexibility of access may have scheduling ramifications, and, given nursing shortages, this can be a contentious area, which is another reason why the CNE's involvement is crucial.

Several types of clinical and nursing resources are required for the multiple roles of the work and project teams involved in a clinical system implementation. The two sets of end-user experts needed in work groups are the domain experts, who represent the work flow and operations of a given department or clinical unit, and the clinicians giving direct care, who participate as subject-matter experts. These experts are needed to explain and validate the clinical care processes to the IS staff who will design the system and develop the specific software solutions. Subject-matter experts provide clinical, operational, and content expertise needed to describe current work process and to guide the designing and building of new work processes. Domain experts are knowledgeable about a given clinical area, department, or discipline. Other important clinical and nursing resources include educators, trainers, and "super users," who provide support during go-live activities.[33,34]

Within the IS department, dedicated project teams carry out the system building and implementation work of the project, including analysis, design, building, testing, training, and deployment of the system. These full-time resources include clinical and systems analysts, who may be formally trained in nursing informatics (NI) and who work in close collaboration with the IT department. The informatics nurse director or analyst often leads the system and process analysis work teams and serves as a liaison to the IS project team. This role entails reviewing system design and content and gaining validation from the subject-matter and domain experts. Clinical informaticians draw on their clinical expertise to ensure that the technology solutions will support the newly designed work processes. The IS team's efforts must be guided and validated by the multidisciplinary work teams to ensure that the new system works for end users.

The effectiveness of the work and project teams and the success of the overall project are directly related to the skills and leadership abilities of the clinical and nursing personnel who lead the transformational activities. A major responsibility of the CNE is to ensure that the right resources are assigned with dedicated time to do the project work and that the project team is effective and sufficiently staffed to get the work done. Under resourcing key work groups is a common occurrence in clinical system implementations and tends to happen when the CNE is not directly involved and informed of the processes and work effort required to do the design work. Given that clinical implementations can be lengthy endeavors with different stages of work intensity over the life of the project, some changes in resource assignments (including individuals, team leads, or numbers of staff) usually are required to keep the project organization optimally tuned and moving forward.

Use Meeting Facilitators

To derive good designs and to resolve issues, it is important that work and project team meetings be efficient and well-run. Because of the project's complexity, it is desirable for the CNE to have the option of using trained facilitators for the major planning and design sessions to help build consensus and to promote timely decision making. When outside consultants are not available, members of the project team could serve as facilitators. Anyone serving in this role should be trained in meeting facilitation methodologies, including scheduling and coordinating, maintaining discipline, producing agendas, presenting pertinent data, promoting decision making, capturing issues and next steps, recording minutes, and serving as the key point person for work team members.[28]

Planning, Designing, and Deploying New Processes and Technology

The key to successful clinical transformation is the integration of process redesign with the standard system implementation life cycle. The top bar in Figure 7-1 shows the IT life cycle for a system implementation. The successful execution of these phases filters down, reflecting parallel planning for cultural and organizational changes, including adoption of new work and business processes, management structures, and role change. Although the figure portrays the life cycle as sequential and linear, in reality the transformation and cultural change may involve iterative moves between planning, validation, piloting, and reassessing as an organization gains experience in shifting from partially automated operations to those that are entirely paperless.

Planning through Strategic Decision Making

The fundamentals of selecting the appropriate core CIS have been well described.[35] However, the most important decisions for planning are made after the vendor is selected. New processes must be designed around core clinical system capabilities. Organizations may find that there is no perfect match for their needs among the EHR systems in the current marketplace; the key is to choose the best match available and then maximize the functional potential of the system to attain the greatest value possible.

Planning for and designing new processes in accordance with technological capabilities is a major component of the transformational effort, and it requires a structured, well-planned framework for change. Applying new technology to current work processes inevitably results in some degree of chaos and confusion. Role functions are altered, some functions disappear while others

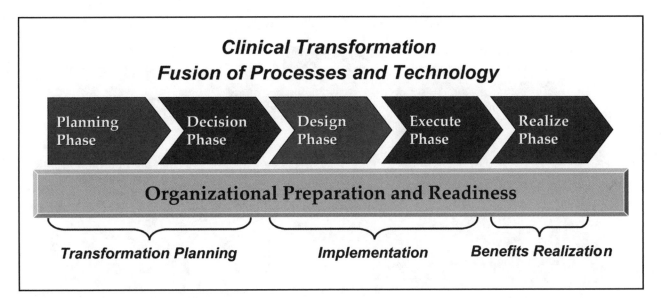

Figure 7-1. *Integrating Process Redesign with the Standard System Implementation Life Cycle.*

are added, departmental tasks are reallocated among staff, and poor practices that were previously hidden may now be exposed. The framework that has been used most successfully by organizations to navigate these choppy waters is one of evaluating proposed changes in the context of whether they are in the best interests of the patient.

For credibility, the framework for defining and realizing the EHR vision should be established at the executive level and arbitrated at the executive steering committee level when necessary. This responsibility should not be delegated to middle management. Key issues that must be addressed are related to which processes will change and how standardization and content will be managed to support the new processes.

Figure 7-2 uses the example of nursing's dietary referral process to show the levels of decision making across the project governance structure. Decision making flows from the executive steering committee to the work teams. Once the high-level strategies are established, the tactical work to create the new processes can be carried out at the management and staff levels.

Key Considerations

When making strategic decisions that revolve around process changes, effects on compliance to regulatory requirements; the interdisciplinary nature of the care process, resources, costs, and time, as well as the organization's threshold for change, must all be considered. Additionally, a focused planning and decision making effort is needed to ensure that there are an adequate number of devices for data input and printing. Clinicians will not tolerate having to wait for access to a computer to do their work, and adoption of the new work processes will be quickly undermined when devices are not available. Nurses are experts at designing workarounds and reverting to former work processes when system availability is compromised. These challenges commonly arise in relation to printer failure, an insufficient number of devices, devices that are ergonomically unacceptable, slow system response time, and frequent downtime. Many organizations moving to electronic work processes determine the number of devices needed by the number of pens required for paper-based operations. Because each clinician and staff member needs a pen to do their work, this translates into one device per individual. Regardless of the benchmark, having an appropriate number of devices is critical to ensuring the optimization of work processes using new technologies.[36]

Documentation standardization and content management across disciplines and departments are major opportunities supported by the EHR. The more standardization, the greater the potential for gains in efficiencies and quality of documentation. Standardization also allows more effective management and monitoring of process improvements and quality outcomes. Organizations that have not grappled with standardizing practices and processes need to give this careful consideration.[37,38]

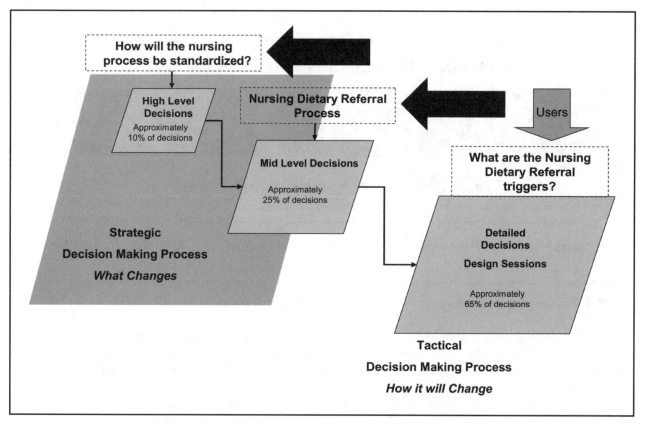

Figure 7-2. *Levels of Decision Making Across the Project Governance Structure.*

The case studies that follow Chapter 7 give vivid examples of how three CNEs (from a rural community hospital, a metropolitan teaching medical center, and a large integrated health care delivery network) navigated the complexities of documentation standardization and cultural transformation in their organizations. What these case studies bring to life is how difficult it would be to achieve full transformational benefits without executive leadership and direction for standardizing process and content across the organization.

Designing for a World with EHRs

Once the framework for change has been established, the work of designing the EHR must be carried out in coordination and collaboration with the clinical system design. This requires special attention by the CNE because it is easy for the effort to become IT-driven.

The system must be built to fit the new work processes. To ensure that interpretation gaps do not occur between the design specified by the clinicians and the IT staff who are building the system, close clinician–IS collaboration must continue through the building and testing phases. The CNE relies on the work teams to validate that the system will support the new processes. It is extremely valuable for the CNE, when possible, to participate in the testing of the integrated system. Roles and responsibilities as well as policies and procedures must be refined and new ones created. This content must be interwoven with the educational materials so that users being trained on the new system can learn processes rather than just functions.

Successful Implementation

As with system building, implementation often becomes geared toward system preparation while organizational readiness and preparation of the user community are overlooked. This is more likely to happen when implementation is delayed. Therefore, at the beginning of the project and approximately six weeks prior to the conversion date, a formal organizational preconversion assessment (described in detail below) should be made to thoroughly evaluate readiness and risk. Preparation of the user community should begin early in the process and should occur through multiple media. Communication strategy is part of transformation planning and implementation strategy (as discussed below). Super users, who are trained in both the application and the new processes, can provide the core support for the go-live.

Managing Transformational Organizational Change

Clinical transformation means major social and cultural change for an organization. In the health care industry, the experience and skills needed to effect such major transformation are still in their infancy.[21] What is known is that EHR system implementations are difficult and complex, requiring committed focus and energy on the part of an executive team and its board. The organization's financial investment is so large and the stakes so high that the initiative represents a "bet your business" commitment. The need to obtain major operational and quality improvements can be a "bet your job" proposition for the executive team.

The following section discusses the strategic components for managing transformational organizational change. These include collaboration and communication, accountability and governance, learning and training, and measuring and monitoring. Although the CNE does not bear total responsibility for managing organizational readiness and system adoption, it is helpful to have these supportive guidelines established at the start and carried throughout the life cycle of the transformation.[19-21]

Collaboration and Communication

Because organizational and clinical transformation touches all departments and disciplines, there is a need to involve all management levels in collaborative decision making. The user community (supporters as well as dissenters) must be represented on work teams and serve on key committees for consensus building, acceptance, and adoption to happen. The CNE is in a strategic position to work across all levels and disciplines to ensure widespread organizational involvement.

Early in the project's planning phase, a well-defined communication strategy for all phases of the initiative should be developed. Messaging can take the form of newsletters, signage, and formal and informal meetings, and it can range from a succinct one-minute elevator speech to a formal presentation. Regardless of its duration, a message must convey a clear description of what is being done, why it is happening, and what it means for the employee and for patient care. CNEs should mentor their department and unit managers so that those individuals can deliver the same messages and answer the same questions when staff challenge why they are being asked to make changes. Messages should be tailored to the board, senior executives, management, and even the community at large. "Over-communication" need not be a concern; it is impossible to provide too much information.

Accountability and Governance

Active accountability and controls for decision making must be established by the highest levels of the organization at the beginning of the project. The CNE should review the project governance structure to validate that the decision reporting function carries accountability at each level of work assigned. Projects of this magnitude must be guided, supported, understood—and sometimes fought for—throughout an organization. They require sophisticated, multitiered governance and physician participation, with active accountability practiced for the smallest project team to the corporate board. The CNE is a critical member of the executive leadership team, with responsibility for ensuring adequate and appropriate clinical and nursing representation at all levels of the project governance structure.

Learning and Training

Large, complex initiatives require learning and training. Learning is focused on educating the organization about changes that are going to occur, their rationale, and how technology will enable them. Training should concentrate on showing users how their daily work will be carried out with the new system (process focus)—*not* on how buttons and tabs work on the new CIS (functional focus). Both education and learning must address all levels of the organization and must be customized to the unique needs of each segment of the user community.

Measuring and Monitoring

It is important to establish baseline measures prior to system conversion. Defining such measures so that they can be quantified and related back to project goals allows for tracking both benefits achieved and process improvements. The CNE should regularly review outcome measures to assess short-term and long-term benefits and to direct ongoing refinement of process changes. It may also be helpful to compare results with industry benchmarks in order to determine the organization's standing in a broader context.

Ensuring Organizational Readiness and Preparation

Organizational readiness is critical to ensuring that the transformation gets a strong foothold. Providing a structured set of communications and educational activities will ensure that hospital management, physicians, and staff understand what will change with the introduction of the new CIS. They should also build on the new system, its associated policies and procedures, and the roles and responsibilities that support the new processes. The role of the CNE is to provide status updates in the context of the executive steering committee and to plan and execute remediation strategies for alignment as needed. The project management team develops the organizational readiness and preparation plan, defines resource requirements, and creates the communication plan. The CNE and the leadership team are jointly responsible for funding and obtaining resources and for ensuring that each component of the plan is executed.

During early project activities, an initial assessment should be conducted to provide a foundation for developing the organizational readiness plan. This assessment should include the following components:

1. **Governance transition:** The governance structure moves its focus to organizational and go-live readiness and preparation. Key activities include designating a go-live facilitator who will oversee all project activities and report to the go-live committee; ensuring that new policies, procedures, roles, and responsibilities are incorporated into training materials; and identifying and committing resources for go-live support, including super users and trainers.

2. **Organizational readiness plan:** Based on the organizational readiness assessment, a risk mitigation plan is developed. This plan will be incorporated into process transformation meetings and the communication and education plans.

3. **Communication plan:** This plan focuses on upcoming key project events and major process changes that will affect the organization. It is directed at five organizational levels: administrators, directors and managers, physicians, end users, and super users.

4. **Process transformation meetings:** These meetings are conducted with the three major care provider groups: physicians, departmental personnel including nursing, and interdisciplinary staff.

5. **Downtime procedures:** Training users what to do when the system goes down is critical to reassuring them that their work processes will not be compromised.

6. **Education plan:** This plan focuses on current users, new hires, temporary staff, and student users.

7. **Super user preparation:** Super users are staff members who provide core support for go-live. They are well-versed in the operational side of the organization, having received additional system and process training on supporting end users.

8. **Security administration:** A well-defined process that complies with the current requirements of the Health Insurance Portability and Accountability Act (HIPAA) should be put in place to support "24/7" users.

9. **Command center:** A command center should be set up to provide resources and skills to end users for their go-live needs.

10. **Go-live plan:** This plan focuses on risks and develops associated risk mitigation strategies for a successful go-live. Key activities include conducting a go-live readiness assessment; develop-

ing an issues management process; creating a facility go-live checklist, including an overall schedule of go-live events and a specific user schedule of such events; and holding a "go forward or delay" decision day with senior executive leadership.

11. **Post go-live:** Once the system is live, there will be system and process refinements. A good rule of thumb is that 80 percent of work flow processes will be right, 10 percent wrong, and 10 percent just missed. After the refinements are complete, the key metrics identified at the start of the project should be collected, then compared and contrasted with baseline metrics and evaluated in light of strategic project goals. The collection and reporting of metrics should be ongoing.

Summary

Organizational and clinical transformation is a significant effort undertaken by health care organizations that commit to implementing an EHR system. These systems hold dramatic potential for improving care delivery and the nursing's practice environment. Importantly, they also elevate the organizational role of the CNE.

CNEs must be front and center in guiding their organizations through the massive transformation enabled by EHR systems. This change in their role is filled with both challenges and opportunities. The challenges come from the new knowledge and skills required to effectively guide and mentor transformational projects that involve the life cycle of system implementation; this expertise is not usually a part of a CNE's formal education or prior job experience. The opportunities stem from the critical role that the CNE plays in helping to deliver massive transformation and the quality and cost improvements that drive the organization's investment in EHR.

The ability to succeed in such an undertaking is the most sought after skill in the marketplace today. CNEs who can achieve substantial improvements with the implementation of an EHR system will have positioned themselves as powers on the executive team and will have access to career path opportunities within the organization and in the broader marketplace. In this new world, CNEs help transform health care organizations through visionary leadership, active decision making, and execution of a well-developed road map that is enabled, not led, by technology.

References

1. Thompson TG, Brailer DJ. *The Decade of Health Information Technology: Delivering Consumer-Centric and Information-Rich Health Care. Framework for Strategic Action.* Washington, DC; Department of Health and Human Services; 2004.

2. Commonwealth of Australia. Clinical information project. Available at: http://www.healthconnect.gov.au/building/Building.htm#CIP. Accessed January 12, 2005.

3. NHS Executive. Information for health: an information strategy for the modern NHS; 1998. Available at: www.nhsia.nhs.uk/def/pages/info4health/1.asp. Accessed February 25, 2005.

4. Committee on Data Standards for Patient Safety, Institute of Medicine. *Key Capabilities of an Electronic Health Record System.* Washington, DC: National Academic Press; 2003. Available at: www.nap.edu.

5. Menadue J. *Breaking the Commonwealth/State Impasse in Health.* Sydney: Whitlam Institute, University of Western Sydney; 2004.

6. Goldsmith J, Blumenthal D, Rishel W. Federal health information policy: a case of arrested development. *Health Aff.* 2003;22:45-55.

7. Business Round Table. BRT-sponsored initiative focuses on patient safety. Press release, January 26, 2000. Available at: www.brtable.org/press.cfm/375.

8. NHS Information Authority. NSF Information Strategies, February 2005. Available at: http://www.nhsia.nhs.uk.nsf. Accessed June 11, 2005.

9. Healthcare Information and Management Systems Society. 16th Annual HIMSS Leadership Survey. Available at: www.HIMSS.org. Accessed June 11, 2005.

10. Dick RS, Steen EB, Detmer DE, eds. *The Computer-Based Patient Record. An Essential Technology for Health Care.* Institute of Medicine. Washington, DC: National Academy Press; 1997.

11. *Information Technology: Benefits Realized for Selected Health Care Functions.* GAO-04-224. A Report to the Ranking Minority Member, Committee on Health, Education, Labor and Pensions, U.S. Senate; October 2003. Washington, DC: General Accounting Office; 2003.

12. Heffler S, Smith S, Keehan S, et al. U.S. health spending projections for 2004-2014. *Health Aff.* 2005;24: 356-361. Available at: http://content.healthaffairs.org/cgi/content/full/hlthaff.w5.74v1. Accessed June 3, 2005.

13. Broder C. Leavitt is starting to turn healthcare IT gears. *Healthcare IT News,* 2005; July: 4-6. Available at: www.HealthcareITNews.com. Accessed July 11, 2005.

14. American Hospital Association. *AHA White Paper: The State of Hospitals' Financial Health 2002.* Chicago: American Hospital Association; 2002.

15. Koppel R, Metlay JP, Cohen A, et al. Role of computerized physician order entry systems in facilitating medication errors. *JAMA.* 2005;293:1197-1203.

16. Ash JS, Berg M, Coiera E. Some unintended consequences of information technology in health care: the nature of patient care information system-related errors. *J Am Med Inform Assoc.* 2004;11:104-112.

17. Nahn R, Poston I. Measurement of the effects of an integrated, point-of-care computer system on quality of nursing documentation and patient satisfaction. *Comput Nurs.* 2003;18:220-229.

18. McCartney PR. Clinical issues: leadership in nursing informatics. *JOGNN/NAACOG.* 2004;33:371-380.

19. Smith C. New technology continues to invade healthcare: what are the strategic implications/outcomes? *Nurs Adm Q.* 2004;28:92-97.

20. Lorenzi NM, Riley RT. Informatics in healthcare: managing organizational change. In: Ball MJ, Weaver CA, Kiel JM, eds. *Healthcare Information Management Systems: Cases, Strategies, and Solutions.* New York: Springer-Verlag; 2004:81-93.

21. Rose JS. IT: transition fundamentals in care transformation. In: Ball MJ, Weaver CA, Kiel JM, eds. *Healthcare Information Management Systems: Cases, Strategies, and Solutions.* New York: Springer-Verlag; 2004:145-160.

22. American Nurses Association. *ANA Scope and Standards of Nursing Informatics Practice.* Washington, DC: ANA Press; 2001:vii.

23. Hinton WP, Elberson K. Collaboration: leadership in a global technological environment. *Online J Issues Nurs.* 2004;10:6-10.

24. Katzenbach JR. *Real Change Leaders: How You Can Create Growth and High Performance at Your Company.* New York: McKinsey; 1995.

25. Johnson T. Executive synergy: the artful balance of vision, strategy, and innovation. *Nurse Leader.* 2004;3:23-25.

26. Gardner J. *On Leadership.* New York: Free Press; 1993.

27. Hirschoff A, ed. *Ensuring IT Success: Components of Effective Implementation in Nursing Practice. Nursing Executive Center Practice Brief.* Washington, DC: Advisory Board Company; 2001.

28. Scholtes P. *The Team Handbook: How to Use Teams to Improve Quality.* Joiner Associates; 1992. Available at :http://www.joiner.com/prod.ttha.cfm. Accessed September 30, 2005.

29. Morey JC. Error reduction and performance improvement in the emergency department through formal teamwork training: evaluation results of the MedTeams Project. *Health Serv Res.* 2002;37:1553-1581.

30. McClure ML, Poulin MA, Sovie MD, Wandelt MA. *Magnet Hospitals: Attraction and Retention of Professional Nurses.* Kansas City, MO: American Academy of Nursing, 1983.

31. McClure ML, Hinshaw AS. *Magnet Hospitals Revisited: Attraction and Retention of Professional Nurses.* Washington, DC: American Academy of Nursing, 2002.

32. Kirkley D, Johnson AP, Anderson M. Technology support of nursing excellence: the Magnet connection. *Nurs Econs.* 2004;22:94-98.

33. Schuerenbuerg BK. Nurses' new duty: caring for IT. *Health Data Management.* April 1, 2005. Available at: http://www.healthdatamanagement.com/html.current/pastissue.cfm.

34. Zytkowski ME. Nursing informatics: the key to unlocking contemporary nursing practice. *AACN Clin Issues.* 2003;3:271-281.

35. Gunasekaran S, Garet D. Managing the IT strategic planning process. In: Ball MJ, Weaver CA, Kiel JM, eds. *Healthcare Information Management Systems: Cases, Strategies, and Solutions.* New York: Springer-Verlag; 2004:22-34.

36. Biohealthmatics. *Mobile and wireless computing.* Available at: http://www.biohealthmatics.com/technologies/emergtech/mobilecomputing.aspx. Accessed May 2005.

37. Averil CB, Zielstorff R, Delaney C, Cary B, Ferrell MJ. Setting standards in nursing data sets in information systems. *Proc AMIA Symp.* Philadelphia: Hanley & Belfus; 1998:745-749.

38. Lunney M, Delaney C, Duffy N, Moorhead S, Welton J. Advocating for standardized nursing languages in electronic health records. *JONA.* 2003;35(1):235-241.

Case Study 7A

Informatics Leadership:
What Chief Nurse Executives Need to Know
Barbara Hertzler, MS, RN

Why the Nurse Executive's Role is at the Table

At some point in the near future, most nurse executives will be faced with the challenge of moving their organization from using a paper medical record to an electronic health record (EHR) system. This commitment requires significant financial and clinical investment. For organizations that truly understand the clinical transformation required to support this investment, the chief nurse executive (CNE), in collaboration with the chief medical officer (CMO), will assume natural leadership roles.

The most important point in this case study is that a CNE does not require technological expertise or formal informatics knowledge to be an effective change agent; such expertise lies with information services (IS) staff and others. CNEs are best served by surrounding themselves with experts, including a nurse informatician whose function is to translate between the clinical and technological worlds.

The CNE's role in clinical transformation is to define the clinical vision and to put in place the infrastructure and processes to make that vision a reality. Leading the transformation strategy requires presence and leadership at the executive table. Clinical leadership is key to ensuring value for staff and improving outcomes with clinical system investments. IS staff cannot effectively lead these projects; they lack sufficient understanding of clinical processes to assess the impact that system design has on clinical operations. Project decisions must be guided by clinicians if the redesigned processes are to be safe and efficient while delivering value to patients and staff. This organizational transformation requires active participation and persistence by clinical leadership and continual clarification throughout the build-to-test phases of the project. The only way to guard against IS-led decisions creeping into the end product is for clinical leadership to be clearly accountable for decision making. This means they must be actively engaged from the point of system selection through go-live conversion and into the system-sustainability phase.

Differentiating Between the CNE and Nurse Informatician Roles

The total financial investment for a new clinical information system can easily exceed $80 million for a medium-size hospital. The costs include internal resources; network infrastructure; training; ongoing system sustainability; and hardware, software, and professional services provided by vendors. Because of the massive financial investment and extensive resources required across the organization, executive leaders need to be involved in the key project decision making. Typically, the CNE has the formal authority and autonomy to allocate and reallocate funds and resources as needed throughout the entire life cycle of the project. When this responsibility is delegated to second-tier leaders, such as nurse informaticians or IS staff, the CNE may be tempted to back away from difficult or contentious decisions. Despite the fact that such an initiative is so all-consuming, that the cost is so enormous, and that the failure risk is so high, the CNE must not hand off system leadership to anyone else.

The Role of the Corporate CNE at Trinity Health System

Trinity Health was formed in May 2000 with the consolidation of Holy Cross Health System and Mercy Health Services. Headquartered in Novi, Michigan, Trinity Health comprises 25 member organizations that span seven states and encompass 45 hospitals, 384 outpatient clinics and facilities, several long-term care facilities, home health/hospice programs, and senior housing communities.

Almost immediately upon the formation of Trinity Health, the system-wide leadership developed an information technology (IT) strategy. Their goal was to consolidate clinical systems into a single software supplier platform to gain a standardized EHR system. This strategic initiative, named Project Genesis, called for integrating a host of IT systems, ranging from some that were nonexistent and outdated to others that were well-entrenched and viable. It also required integrating two different nursing cultures: one with an existing corporate CNE role (Mercy Health) and one lacking that role (Holy Cross).

Recruitment for the position of senior vice president of patient care services/CNE took place at the beginning of the merger process. The national search committee specified that the preferred final candidate should have CNE experience, at both the hospital and system levels, with responsibility for overseeing nursing practice and clinical operations. I was selected for this position, whereupon I vacated my role as Mercy Hospital corporate CNE and moved quickly to assume my new responsibilities, which coincided with the beginning of the IT strategy roll out.

At the outset, the Trinity corporate CNE was expected to be a key change leader, working with all nurse executives of Trinity Health member organizations in the design and implementation of Project Genesis. My prior operational experience gave me credibility and helped me build strong working relationships with the nurse executives at the regional member organization level.

Trinity Health's solution for achieving a common culture centered around the goals of Project Genesis and included empowering the Trinity corporate-level CNE with responsibility for nursing and ancillary clinical documentation across the system. In conjunction with the CMO, the CNE was charged with creating system-wide teams, developing a common vision, and devising high-level strategies for clinical transformation and system implementation. The creation of a united front of clinical executive leadership was imperative for successful clinical transformation. The CNE-CMO partnership was also an important model for collaborative relationship between these positions at the local health care organization level.

Defining Nursing's Vision

The urgency associated with planning for Project Genesis also helped contribute to the development of a nursing vision and strategic plan to ensure the delivery of high-quality, evidence-based nursing care. During the first six months of my tenure, my main priority was to build relationships among local member organizations and to establish the high level of trust that would be needed to carry out Project Genesis. This entailed becoming familiar with each site and holding face-to-face meetings with nurse executives and their organizational leaders.

To promote a deeper understanding of the current environment, each hospital CNE conducted round-the-clock town-hall-type meetings to obtain feedback from nursing staff. The valuable information gained led to the identification of system-wide themes centering on clinical work flow and relationships, nurse satisfaction, and evidence-based practice. These themes served as the basis for developing Trinity Health's nursing vision and became the guiding principles for Project Genesis system design.

Message from Frontline Nurses

An important theme that emerged from the town-hall meetings was frustration about the inability to understand the impact of nursing care on patient outcomes. Nurses in particular expressed a lack of fulfillment from their work because they could not always quantify the impact of their care on patient improvement. They were hopeful that the adoption of a new clinical information system (CIS) would make it possible for them to better understand their contribution.

Another theme that was expressed was the perception that nursing documentation was burdensome and conflicted with bedside care. Additionally, clinicians noted concern about the unavailability of information to facilitate good clinical decision making. Clearly, Trinity Health nurses knew what a CIS needed to support the delivery of reliable, evidence-based care. The system requirements that they specified were (1) support to reduce documentation time, (2) sufficient information for good clinical decision making, and (3) availability of data to measure the impact of care on patient outcomes.

The town-hall-meeting data provided direction for Project Genesis. Identified needs included

1. Technical support at the bedside, with a clinical decision rules engine to provide reminders and alerts that promote best practice
2. Evidence-based professional guidelines embedded into order sets and documentation tools
3. Examination of the relationship between interventions and patient outcomes to generate best-practice knowledge across Trinity Health

Table 7A-1. Trinity Nursing Plan

Strategic Goals	Trinity Nursing Plan	IT implications/potential
Improve performance to benchmark levels	**Creating Future Innovative Models of Care** Trinity Core Clinical Practice Model	Trinity Health staffing models with defined principles and measures of effectiveness
	Trinity-sponsored innovative models of care demonstration project	Online clinical documentation based on evidence-based practice guidelines and care paths
Develop and maintain an outstanding workforce	**Cultivating Healthy Work Environments** Collaborative physician nurse programs	Multidisciplinary clinical practice guidelines
	Empowerment and accountability model development	Shared leadership strategies that engage nursing in clinical decision making
	Nursing career pathways	
	Intra-system employment opportunities	
	Benefit and compensation improvements	Technology to support aging nurse population
	Support to older workers	
	Improving provider supply and nursing performance Delineation of Trinity Health identity for nursing with associated recruitment and retention materials	Online BSN and MSN completion programs Online refresher programs to support the return of inactive nurses
	Legislative advocacy position for nursing	Online learning support for frontline clinical leadership with core competencies for all Trinity clinical leaders
	Developing Effective Leadership Role competencies for clinical leaders	
		Frontline leadership curriculum development
Advance and support industry-leading innovation	**Trinity Health sponsored demonstration initiatives** System-wide care improvement teams developing evidence-based tool kits	Hardwiring EBP guidelines into online clinical documentation
	Rapid replication of innovative models	Rules and alerts that support compliance with regulator standards

4. Common language to support multidisciplinary communication, collaboration, and standardization.
5. Improved working conditions to address the nursing shortage.

The identification of these needs led to the delineation of guiding principles of redesign and became the basis of Project Genesis' clinical transformation strategy.

During the current-state-analysis phase of Project Genesis, it became increasingly evident that patient-care delivery models, staffing models, and clinical roles required significant redesign to support the transformation vision. On the basis of this knowledge and of data from the nursing balanced score card, a plan for nursing services across Trinity Health was developed (see Table 7A-1). This plan served as a road map for Trinity Health patient-care executives over a three-year period and supported Project Genesis' strategic goals for improving nursing practice and clinical care, including

1. Top-quartile performance for RN vacancies, turnover, and satisfaction
2. Development of an outstanding workforce, with an increase in the number of nurses with BSN and MSN degrees
3. Recognition as an industry benchmark for the design of innovative models of care
4. Recognition for excellence in nursing leadership, practice, and professional development

It was quickly realized that implementation of the new CIS would be an important vehicle for achieving Trinity Health's strategic vision

Governance Structure and Ownership of Vision

The Trinity Health nursing plan was formally presented to and adopted by the Trinity Health Clinical Leadership Council (CLC) prior to redesign and transformation planning. The CLC comprises key patient care and medical staff executives across Trinity Health and is co-chaired by the corporate CNE and CMO.

The CLC took an active role in further defining the assumptions of the plan for clinical transformation, including clinical documentation standardization, evidence-based practice innovations, point-of-care applications, and provider order entry standards (see Table 7A-2). In collaboration with corporate communications staff, the CLC also assumed responsibility for a communications strategy for Project Genesis. Components of the communications plan are described in Table 7A-3. Broad ownership of the project's vision, tactics, approach, and communication was crucial to system-wide adoption across all 25 member organizations.

The CLC continues to play a vital role in providing review and ownership of all strategic clinical decisions for Project Genesis. It meets face-to-face quarterly and by teleconference monthly. Keeping the communication channels open between the system-wide project governance teams and the member organizations has been key to continuing deepening acceptance and ownership of the new system.

As with any CIS implementation, the bulk of the work in Project Genesis was accomplished through taskforce teams. At the convening of each taskforce, it was important that the CNE make a personal connection with the group. This opened lines of communication and made it clear that the CNE was available to respond quickly to unresolved issues.

To ensure ongoing decision making and improvement, three executive leadership governance groups were initiated:

- **The Clinical Executive Oversight Group (CEOG)**—This group holds a monthly meeting, co-chaired by the CNE and CMO and with representation from clinical and informatics leadership across Trinity Health. This group's role is to address unresolved issues, make recommendations for enhancements, and provide a forum for member organizations to make customization requests.
- **The Clinical Rules Oversight Group (CROG)**—This group holds a monthly meeting, co-chaired by the CMO and attended by hospital CMOs, CNEs, and pharmacists across Trinity Health. The group's role is to focus on the development of clinical rules and alerts.
- **The Chief Information Oversight Group (CIOG)**—This group holds a monthly meeting, co-chaired by the CNE and IS leadership, with representation from member organization CNEs and practicing clinicians. The group's role is to respond to requests for new documentation tools and to the need for revisions and updates to existing forms.

Communications Planning

An internal Trinity Health document described Project Genesis as "a management challenge of a magnitude and scope unlike any organization has previously experienced." The challenge facing the management team was communicated as follows: "To elevate the core systems implementation from what has been primarily thought of as an information services project to what is, in every respect, a change management challenge for all of Trinity's management, staff, and physicians." This change management challenge is being accomplished one member organization at a time, with significant leadership from the corporate team and member organization leaders. Trinity Health has described the progression as a "diffusion process leading to the eventual adoption of desired behaviors."

To guide the process, Trinity Health established a comprehensive corporate communications strategy (see Table 7A-3), divided into three phases:

- Development of awareness and interest
- Evaluation, trial, and adoption
- Reinforcement and post-go-live evaluation

This corporate-level strategy has been implemented through member-organization-customized communication plans and tool-kits. The goal of the member-organization-specific plans is to prepare each organization to understand and undergo clinical transformation relative to its unique environment, requirements, and needs.

Table 7A-2. Example of System Clinical Transformation Assumptions and Local MO Decisions

	Organizational Assumptions	MO Decisions
Order Entry	Computerized physician order entry (CPOE) is used for all inpatients.	
	Care/order sets are developed by MO clinical staff and medical staff departments. (Involves pharmacists, laboratory and appropriate disciplines.)	Determine which care/order sets will be designed and utilized
	Care/order sets support ease of order entry for the physicians and other clinical staff.	
	Care/order sets are developed based on research, patient safety and clinical accreditation standards.	Establish policy to define use of verbal orders
	Verbal orders are limited and restricted to emergent situations or situations where physicians do not have access to remote computer devices.	
	RNs and pharmacists input medication orders as defined in MO-specific protocols, policies and/or medical staff rules and regulations.	Identify outpatient areas that will use CPOE
	RNs or other licensed clinicians accept and enter other written or verbal orders as defined in MO-specific policies, medical staff rules and regulations or state law.	
	RNs or other licensed clinicians accept and enter other written or verbal orders at sites where CPOE is not available (e.g., outpatient diagnostic testing, outpatient therapy, ambulatory surgery, preadmission testing, etc.).	
	Clerks enter written orders (except medications) during the transition period to full CPOE.	Set parameters of transition period
	In the event an order generates an "alert" or "reminder" during order entry, the clerk contacts an RN or physician for completion of that order.	
Clinical Decision Support	Each MO guides the build of clinical decision support through existing committees and clinician representation on the Clinical Rules Oversight Group.	Identify representative to system Clinical Rules Oversight Group and Clinical Information Oversight Group
	IT dept. builds the selected rules, alerts and reminders to specificity that limits inappropriate activation of an alert.	Identify rules, alerts and reminders to be used in the MO
	Rules that provide evidence-based clinical decision making and support patient safety and professional standards of practice are available and defined from multiple established sources.	
Medication Documentation	Documentation of medication administration is completed online using the eMAR (electronic medication administration record), which is the single source of truth for all inpatients.	Determine whether to use the eMAR for outpatients
	For safety reasons, printing of the eMAR is strongly discouraged and is prohibited in the process of preparation and administration of medications.	
	Medications ordered for patients going to an inpatient bed upon transfer from a clinical area that is not using CPOE must be input prior to transfer from the area.	Determine where—on paper or in the eMAR—staff in the non-CPOE area should document first doses of inpatient medications

continued on next page

Table 7A-2. *continued*

Clinical Documentation	Where automated forms are available, all clinical documentation should be done online.	Determine:
		Which current forms will be replaced by automated forms
	Authentication of clinical documentation is done electronically.	Which paper forms will need to be revised
	Evidence-based nursing interventions are defined as a care activity provided or delivered to the patient rather than defined as a device or item (e.g., "medication administration" vs. "medication"; "incision site care" vs. "dressing").	Which forms must be added to fill functionality gaps
	Interdisciplinary care planning may be completed online or via paper forms during transition phase.	
	Dictation, consults and test results are available for review within the electronic medical record and are acknowledged and/or authenticated online.	Determine how care planning will be done after implementation and until PowerPlan is available
	Physician progress notes are recorded on paper and remain in the hardcopy medical record.	

From Implementation to Operation:
Life Cycle of a Clinical Information System

The readiness-and-implementation framework for Project Genesis is a seven-stage process. Although the scope, process flow, clinical documentation, terminology, and order sets have been standardized for all of Trinity Health, each site's implementation began with a current-state analysis to document local work processes and then moved into future-state design using prior agreed-on best practices. Representatives from each local member organization worked with the taskforce teams to translate current into future state. After considering each member organization's current business processes, the taskforce teams defined the unique decisions that each site was required to consider. This process is illustrated in Table 7A-2, which delineates member organizations' localization decisions against each clinical transformation assumption. Once the design and process-flow decisions were completed, the final validation step was to communicate the plan, project, and process changes to all affected parties.

Since November 2002, we have successfully implemented the new CIS at six member organizations:

- **Mercy Hospital,** a 104-bed acute-care hospital with 15 nonacute-care beds, in Port Huron, Michigan
- **Mercy General Health Partners,** a 208-bed acute-care hospital with 14 nonacute-care beds, in Muskegon, Michigan
- **Saint Mary's Health Care,** a 230-bed acute-care hospital with 94 nonacute-care beds, in Grand Rapids, Michigan
- **Battle Creek Health System,** a 172-bed acute-care hospital with 211 nonacute-care beds, in Battle Creek, Michigan
- **St. Joseph's Mercy of Macomb,** a 273-bed acute-care hospital with 120 nonacute-care beds, in Macomb County, Michigan
- **Mercy Medical Center,** a 194-bed acute-care hospital with 75 nonacute-care beds, in Mason City, Iowa

Although Trinity Health planned to employ the predefined seven-step readiness process at each member organization, it soon became clear that lessons learned from each site's implementation would inform, and perhaps lead to modifications in, subsequent implementations. The site of the initial implementation was a rural hospital, chosen for its small size, limited complexity, and eager senior leadership. The readiness process began in November 2002; implementation was scheduled for May 2003. However, in the course of the first implementation, Trinity Health identified a need for more post-go-live support for system sustainability. The scope of the implementation included clinical documentation at point-of-care, results viewing, pharmacy, e-MAR documentation (electronic medication administration record), and provider order entry. It represented a first in the industry; there were no preexisting road maps to follow. The magnitude of the cultural and organizational change caused by the implementation required ongoing support well into three months postconversion. This reality, coupled with planned product upgrades, delayed implementation at the second site. As the complexity of the clinical environment increased, Trinity Health adjusted the imple-

Table 7A-3. Example of a Communications Plan

Task	Description	Objectives	Deliverable
Determine communications vehicle forums and responsibilities	**WHO** the audience and the messenger should be **HOW** communications will be delivered (e.g., via meetings, message boards, displays) **WHEN** communications should begin and how often it should occur **WHERE** communications about the project should be delivered (i.e., the forum)	To ensure availability of useful and timely information To support appropriate audiences in their journeys through the phases of change	MO communications plan
Develop member organization specific communications tools	Vehicles to include (among others): • PowerPoint presentations at regularly scheduled meetings • Message/story board displays in public areas of the facilities • Banners to announce milestones • Contests to fuel interest	To identify and/or create vehicles by which to disseminate/implement the MO communications plan	MO communications tools
Deliver awareness communications (12–15 months prior to go-live)	Designed to create awareness and interest via high-level presentations to • MO Board of Directors • MO physician leadership and staff • MO executive management • MO departmental management • MO staff	To build awareness and foster understanding of the project by delivering key messages to MO's affected groups	Implementation of communications tools and tactics
Deliver evaluation and adoption communications (9 months prior to go-live)	During this phase, the member organization audiences will learn how to use the system and specific activities they will be involved in during the months prior to go-live.	To provide detailed information that promotes understanding and adoption of the upcoming implementation	Implementation of communications tools and tactics

mentation schedule to provide adequate time for incorporating new insights about learning tools, to customize these tools for each site, and to ensure site stability before moving to the next implementation.

Going forward, Trinity Health is focused on creating as paperless an environment as possible. By providing ongoing training and encouraging staff to use the system rather than reverting to manual processes, the organization is working hard to bring automation to the bedside for real-time use.

Summary

Over the course of six CIS implementations, Trinity Health clinical leadership has learned numerous logistical, technological, and operational lessons. However, the key insights that will help other nurse executives to take on similar implementations are universal and not defined by a specific type of health care system, facility, or country. It is important not to fear or be intimidated by the technology. The guiding question should be, "What does the system need to do to deliver value to my staff and to improve patient care?" Frontline staff can clearly communicate the barriers and frustrations that they encounter with the current care delivery system. If your vision and guiding principles for system transformation target the concerns and obstacles identified by your frontline nurses, you will have a system that delivers value to clinicians and patients.

In today's marketplace, new clinical systems that build the necessary components for an EHR bring massive change to processes and roles. These implementations truly bring about clinical transformations, complete with change management implications and requirements. They ought not be viewed as IT projects. Executive clinical leadership is essential when the organization is to receive full value from the investment it has made. The value of a system lies not in its ability to automate current practices but rather in its potential to help an organization become more effective and efficient.

Given the scope of the Trinity Health clinical system implementations, the sequential timing of interdependent tasks and milestones was critical. Project management by a skilled person with formal project-management education and credentialing was key. But equally important was communication of the project plan to the clinical executive leadership team, so that interdependencies could be appropriately resourced and sequenced. The bottom line: an effective project-management plan is one that is manageable.

When it comes to clinical transformation in acute-care settings, successful, lasting change is also about winning the hearts and minds of nurses. Nurses account for approximately 90 percent of the production processes in hospitals. When the nursing organization adopts an innovation, the rest of the care-team members, including physicians, will be brought into the transformation.

Successful change management requires a change agent. As keeper of the clinical vision and guardian of nursing's interests, the CNE is the most appropriate change agent for nursing, providing both the leadership and the power to translate the clinical vision into the reality of improved practice and care.

Case Study 7B

Chief Nursing Officer's Role in IT and the Delivery of Care

Rebecca Ambrosini, MSN, RN

Information Technology: New Hope for the Future of Clinical Care

In the not-too-distant past, doctors and nurses relied on intellect and empathy, as well as a few simple surgical procedures and medications, to treat their patients. Today, patient care is supported by an extraordinary array of sophisticated machines, procedures, and pharmaceuticals, along with an armada of highly skilled specialists. But these advancements in technology and health care introduce challenges that health leaders must manage to deliver safe, efficient, and effective care. At Uniontown Hospital in Pennsylvania, expert nurse leaders, armed with sophisticated information technology (IT) systems, drove the clinical process changes required to optimize outcomes in today's remarkably progressive yet increasingly complex environment.

As with most organizations, Uniontown's transformation of care delivery needed to meet the expectations of its community and workforce. That effort required aggressive process and work flow redesign; improved information availability; grounded decision support based on relevant, time-sensitive information; and the adoption of evidence-based practice guidelines.

Yet this approach is not always the norm. Traditionally, patient care in most hospitals evolved by adding on to old processes and manipulating or forcing modified processes to fit with new technology and new goals for patient outcomes. Many years of well-intended incremental quick fixes usually resulted in a clinical maze of dangerous curves, system failures, and dead ends. In many respects, system expansion was treated the same as facility expansion: repair, renovate, and expand what is in hand, an expensive and resource-intensive approach. Given the opportunity, however, many hospitals are learning that it is best to demolish the old structure and build anew. This realization can also be applied to the realm of clinical IT, in which a similar opportunity exists to demolish antiquated systems and replace them with a more fully integrated, contemporary architecture.

Implementation of an advanced clinical information system (CIS) and the attendant transformation of care processes require a governance structure that engages clinical stakeholders, assures timely and focused decision making, and establishes clear accountability. The transformation journey will completely disrupt every aspect of care and the work of all clinical providers. The outcome of the chaos can either be a positive care transformation with an improved clinical culture, or the complete meltdown of care delivery, resulting in a dissatisfied staff, turnover, and possible patient harm.

Uniontown Hospital faced all of these challenges in addition to others, some common and some unique. Unique to Uniontown were physician shortages as a result of a statewide liability crisis, recruitment concerns, and low reimbursement levels for Medicare and Medicaid patients. And similar to other organizations, Uniontown also faced the challenges of growing regulatory requirements, the high cost of clinical technology for service enhancement, and an aging facility. Uniontown decided that a comprehensive, patient-centered clinical information system could positively affect many of these issues. The next step was to develop a mission and vision for the project.

Uniontown's Clinical Information System: Its Mission and Vision

Professional nurses spend more time in direct patient care than any other health care professional and traditionally are responsible for ensuring that patients receive the care they require regardless of any system failures. This role of integrator has grown burdensome because the frequent failure of insufficient systems compromises the quality of patient care and of the work environment. With this in mind, Uniontown adopted the following clinical information mission: to improve patient outcomes, ease staff lives, and support efficient use of resources at the point of care. Uniontown envisioned an electronic health record (EHR) as the foundation for all clinical functionality—it would support clinical decision making and increase patient safety by providing access to complete patient information to all clinicians at the point-of-care. To achieve these goals, the chief nursing officer (CNO) and chief information officer (CIO) established the following strategies to guide care transformation, including

1. Develop and own the expert-driven clinical information system with support from IT specialists
2. Prioritize system design based on the degree of impact on patient safety initiatives
3. Redesign clinical processes to realize the maximum value and benefits of the clinical information system solution
4. Provide abundant point-of-care access to the system and to patient information
5. Enlist robust executive leadership for change management
6. Reallocate time saved in process, documentation, and technology efficiencies to improve patient care services
7. Offer extensive training to ensure that all are successful in achieving the required competencies. Leave no one behind

Project Initiation and Governance

Uniontown's CIS initiative represented a bold, comprehensive, all-encompassing strategy for realizing profound transformation. To be successful, however, it was imperative that Uniontown engage a single clinical technology partner with proven solutions reflecting best practice. Uniontown wanted a uniform platform and a rapid implementation strategy. Cerner Corporation, Kansas City, Missouri, fit the bill, and together Uniontown and Cerner committed to implementing nineteen clinical applications in just nine months.

Although choosing the correct technology partner was important, success would depend on more than clinical automation. True success could only be achieved when Uniontown leaders paid particular attention to the staff whose work flow processes would have to change to create a new clinical culture. Although it would cause the discomfort that accompanies any profound change and a significant consumption of human and financial resources, Uniontown realized that an integrated clinical IT solution was the best path not only to improved care, but also to a more satisfying work environment. But this journey of hope would change everything for the two groups served by nurse leaders: patients and clinical caregivers. Given the enormity of this change, it was apparent that nurse executive sponsorship would not be enough to get the job done; the CNO would have to be the shepherd, guiding clinical professionals past obstacles to a focused, achievable, and measurable vision. The CNO had to take ownership, full responsibility, and accountability, for every aspect of the clinical IT implementation.

To complement the CNO's executive leadership role, Uniontown established three teams: the Clinical Implementation Team, the Process and Work Redesign Team, and the Training and Education Team. The governance structure set the foundation and direction for the initiative and established the role and responsibility of each team.

The Clinical Implementation Team consisted of the CNO, several expert clinical department managers, an exceptional staff nurse, and a clinical IT analyst ad hoc. The team was charged with the responsibility of making all design functionality decisions, which technology experts then incorporated into applications. The pressures of a rapid build and implementation demanded timely decision making. This meant that dozens of clinical leaders and hundreds of direct caregivers were relying on the team's competencies and decision-making skills. It was therefore critical that the team's decisions were accurate and based on best practices because the build would drive the process redesign and begin to guide the clinical culture. The team had to consider process implications and process redesign opportunities. Because of the critical nature of the team's responsibility, it was imperative that the CNO actively participate in the team's work. As CNO, I dedicated myself to being present at every step of the journey. My role was not to make the decisions, but rather to empower the team to make aggressive decisions. We did not want to replicate current care delivery processes or slow progress by asking too many other groups to consider the team's decisions. With support and empowerment, the team's decisions drove the system design rapidly toward the predicted outcomes.

The Clinical Implementation Team was also responsible for transferring knowledge to the Process and Work Redesign and Training and Education teams so they could achieve their goals. Lastly, the Clinical Implementation Team, with the help of the Process and Work Redesign Team, was responsible for application and integration testing, as well as measuring success following implementation.

The Process and Work Redesign Team was responsible for leading process redesign across all disciplines and departments, facilitating the work flow framework, and transferring process and work flow knowledge to the Training and Education Team. This team, which consisted of several expert clinical department managers and the CNO, was asked to align processes with system design and to synchronize implementation of the new processes with the system implementation. Again, my participation on and empowerment of the team were imperative. Process redesign required experienced leaders to facilitate, negotiate, and gain the timely consensus of all key stakeholders.

The decision to base the system design on best practice added to the team's challenges. Essentially, we were communicating to our staff that the way we had always practiced would probably change forever. Although the resulting improved care outcomes were intuitively appealing, concern still loomed in the hearts of clinical providers. Professional nurses, as well as other clinicians, have very set, routine ways in which they do their work. At Uniontown, time management had become a key to surviving the increased workloads caused by cost efficiency pressures, care complexities, and system failures. In addition to staff perception that work flow must not be disrupted, 48 percent of Uniontown Hospital employees had worked with the old processes from ten to thirty-five years. Although the staff did not like the old care delivery system and associated system failures, they felt comfortable with it. Every clinician was going to wake up on implementation day to face new care processes, with the familiar, paper-based information access and documentation routine replaced by a computer.

To address these issues and put the staff at ease, the Process and Work Redesign Team conducted point-of-care provider focus groups to define the current work flow for each process and associated process failures. This gave the staff incentive to take ownership, helping to develop enthusiasm for the new processes, which would be more powerful and eliminate process failures. Ultimately, as a result of these focus groups, staff could see the value of technology and best practice.

The Training and Education Team was made up of clinical directors and educators who had the responsibility of designing the numerous course curricula, including material preparation and course schedules, as well as identifying and training "super users," a core group fully trained in all solutions. More than 750 employees received 20,000 hours of training in a six- to eight-week period prior to go live. The team's philosophy was to provide classroom training that would incorporate the new technology with the new processes and work flow. They also ensured that individuals had scheduled practice time away from the clinical setting, during which trainees were monitored and supported by super users. Every employee successfully completed all requirements and competencies prior to go-live.

The Critical Nature of the CNO Role

Transforming the clinical culture involved a conscious decision to abandon the leadership paradigm of control, power, and knowing what is best for others. Although it may be tempting to control or manage such a far-reaching initiative as this, everyone at Uniontown Hospital was better served by a more participatory approach on my part.

The leadership ideas of stewardship, empowerment, and partnership carry with them the promise of creating the passion, spirit, and commitment required for success. Filled with anticipation of great change and fear of chaos, staff began to search for strong leadership, someone who would accept ownership and responsibility for providing a safe, secure environment. Ironically, profound and lasting change depends on the degree of ownership and responsibility each employee feels for the success of a venture, as opposed to management taking all of the ownership and responsibility. The challenge then for the CNO is to create a clinical culture that he or she and others in the organization can believe in and to do it as an offering rather than a demand; in other words, to make a commitment to a larger vision and to demonstrate that commitment by example. This requires the CNO to be deeply accountable for the outcomes without acting to define the purpose of others, as well as to understand that those closest to the work have better knowledge of the work and will therefore make more informed decisions.

A strategy to transcend control and caretaking does not appear to be congruent with the CNO's accountability and responsibility for care transformation, yet it is essential for success. Control creates low risk-taking, which is at odds with asking people to break the rules and take chances. Caretaking, or believing you know what is best for others, denotes self-interest and mistrust, a disastrous image to project during a time that requires significant trust. The alternative to power and caretaking is partnership, which carries with it the intention to redistribute power and balance responsibility. Partnership is a way for accountability to be exchanged in both directions. To initiate this new approach, the CNO needs to give permission for staff to break the rules; but giving permission and setting the expectation that the rules must be broken for valuable change is insufficient. The CNO and other leaders must provide constant encouragement and rewards to create a safe environment. A culture of partnership promotes shared responsibility; staff feels empowered and is willing to work toward common goals. Partnership allows everyone to explore the rewards of autonomy with the CNO in the room for support and encouragement.

The fundamental question for a CNO to ask is What strategy will best create the passion and commitment needed in employees to achieve common goals? Each CNO will need to assess the organization's culture, strengths, weaknesses, and readiness for change to design strategies that will create a workplace that evokes commitment.

Fortunately, at Uniontown Hospital, the development of competent, team-oriented, risk-taking nursing and clinical leaders had been under way for many years. Being a learning organization with strong business initiatives that put patient outcomes at the center clearly gave us the advantage of having a foundation on which to advance transformation. Building on that trust and credibility to create the vision was my first and most important strategy as CNO.

That vision had to be articulated consistently to large and small groups, but more importantly to individuals. Each person needed to hear the hope of the vision and to understand exactly what it would mean to him or her, including how it would affect that person's work and goals for patient care. This could not be accomplished with long meetings or philosophical discussions, so the Clinical Management Team created an "elevator talk." The goal was to articulate the clear connection between the vision and achievement of concrete results in the amount of time it took to ride an elevator from the main floor to the top floor. For example, there was deep frustration about access to the paper chart. There could be as many as ten people who needed access to the information in the paper chart at the same time, but, of course, only one would succeed in having such access. The constant power struggle for the paper chart would be eliminated with an EHR system, which would enable multiple care providers to access the same information at the same time. This sounds like a simple message, but it had a profound impact on creating the foundation for commitment to clinical automation. As CNO, I created and articulated many such messages to staff every day.

One of the most challenging yet rewarding roles of the CNO is that of guiding the integration of clinical processes and work across care providers and clinical departments. Traditionally, clinical departments functioned in silos and rarely recognized the interdependence of their work, thus producing fragmented processes and frustration when outcomes were not achieved. Paying particular attention to the interdependence of clinical groups is vital to achieving full value of integration and thus performance achievement. To do this, you must build personal relationships with those involved and understand the work of all. In my case, constant communication helped produce a broad understanding of everyone's work and enabled me to connect people who could help each other, leading to numerous win-win situations.

Finally, the pursuit of perfection, so basic to our work in patient care, can get in the way of a rapid implementation strategy, which was key to providing as much functionality as possible to improve performance immediately. Helping everyone to understand that we were on a journey and would eventually reach perfection was critical to moving steadily forward, getting the technology into the hands of providers so they could begin to experience the improvement in both their work lives and their patient care.

Conclusion

The implementation of a CIS at Uniontown Hospital has dramatically improved patient outcomes, work process, and the lives of care providers. It became the catalyst for radical reform and motivated an army of care providers to form new relationships for the purpose of improving care and easing peoples' lives. The rapid system design and process redesign based on best practice and evidence-based guidelines, while challenging, gave us a superior foundation with immediate, measurable improvements. We have experienced remarkable adaptation to the technology, as well as to the process and work redesign by clinical care providers. Our challenge now is to keep up with the insatiable hunger for more.

When the staff and leadership are faced with complex process or care issues, they turn first to clinical technology for resolutions. This successful paradigm shift was largely a result of the incredible commitment by Uniontown leadership to create a safe environment that embraced change, fostered partnerships, and respected point-of-care clinical decision making. We have made significant progress on our journey of care transformation and have experienced the hope that it brings. We are confident the journey will only get more exciting and much more rewarding.

Case Study 7C

Clinical Transformation at Penn State Milton S. Hershey Medical Center

Donna L. Reck, MSN, RN, BC

Founded in 1963, Penn State Milton S. Hershey Medical Center (HMC) is one of the leading teaching and research hospitals in the U.S. The 479-bed academic health center is a provider of high-level, patient-focused medical care. HMC admits nearly 26,000 patients, accepts nearly 800,000 outpatient visits, receives more than 45,000 emergency department visits, and performs approximately 20,000 surgical procedures annually. The campus also includes Penn State College of Medicine (COM) and Penn State Children's Hospital, the region's only hospital for children.

In the early 1990s, HMC experienced increasing external pressure to introduce technology into the patient care arena. Coupled with the needs to increase efficiency, eliminate redundancy, and remain competitive, it was essential to bring technology to the clinicians. Following a review of the clinical system, a needs assessment, and an evaluation of vendor offerings, we established long-term goals for the automation of clinical work flow, including implementing a computerized provider order entry (CPOE) application.

Organized for Success

The organization of the COM and HMC provided an important foundation for successful transformation of care delivery. The governance is unified by the fact that the chief executive officer (CEO) of HMC is also the senior vice-president for Health Affairs at Penn State University and also dean of its college of medicine. The various interdependent missions of the academic health center are thereby linked. Because of this linkage, we were able to achieve a high level of coordination among the teams (Clinical, Academic, Research, Physical Resources, Finance, Human Resources, Strategic Relations, and Information Resources) (see Figure 7C-1).

By 1995, we were committed to the use of information technology (IT) as a tool to improve patient safety and quality care, increase efficiency and patient satisfaction, recruit and retain talented clinicians, and maintain employee satisfaction. The critical, multidimensional role the chief nursing officer (CNO) would play became clear as we took the first step toward achieving this vision by providing clinicians with access to results reporting, and as the comprehensive initiative (see Table 7C-1) began to unfold.

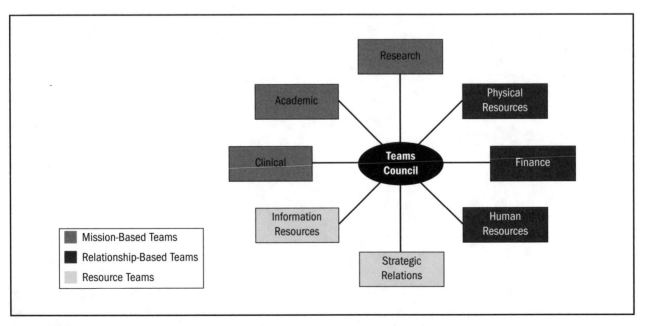

Figure 7C-1. *Unified Campus Teams Structure.*

Table 7C-1. Phases of Initiative to Automate Clinical Workflow.

Solution Profile

- Selected Cerner in 1995
- Early Millennium adopter
- - PowerChart

- Enterprise Agreement Q12003

- In Production
  - PowerChart M2003.01
  - InBox for Edit and Sign for all physicians

- Other Systems
  - Misys for Clin Labs
  - IDX for RIS PACS
  - Lawson for financials and materials management

	Phase 1	Phase 2	Phase 3
	FY04	**FY05**	**FY06**
	Pharmacy	Surgery	Medical Records
	Clinical Documentation	Anesthesia	Cardiology
	Transcription/Deficiency	Access Mgmt	Pathways
	MR Publish	Ambulatory	Physician Doc
	CPOE with meds	Critical Care	Outpatient Pharmacy
	ED Triage and Tracking	Positive Patient Identification	Personal Health Record

PENNSTATE
Milton S. Hershey Medical Center
College of Medicine

We are World Class

Clinical Transformation and the CNO Role

We experienced marked success and satisfaction as we steadily expanded the breadth of results reporting over the next few years, including the introduction to online edits and signature of key clinical documents. Recognizing the interdependent roles of every member of the care team and the interlocking work flows that unify care across the continuum, we committed to install CPOE in 2003. With this decision, we embarked on a process of selecting a vendor that would help us achieve the full integration of solutions we needed to meet our goals.

The CNO played a critical role in this vendor selection. Each stakeholder assembled a team of clinicians from each discipline to assist in evaluating different vendors and their products from that discipline's perspective. The nursing team identified six objectives to assist in evaluating the different vendors: (1) to provide clinical decision support and decrease clinical errors, (2) to deploy a clinical database that could easily be accessed by all care providers for orders and retrieval of information, (3) to build a system that was flexible, integrated, and familiar enough for the staff to easily adjust their workload, (4) to allow multidisciplinary subject matter experts to design the screens, (5) to create a tool for the recruitment and retention of nurses, and (6) to standardize documentation throughout the institution. The team participated in vendor presentations, site visits, vendor demonstrations, and evaluations. The final step was providing a specific vendor recommendation to the CNO.

Supporting the unified campus team's structure and our organization's values of respect, trust, teamwork, and collaboration, the executive stakeholders (the chief operating officer, chief financial officer, chief medical officer (CMO), chief information officer, and the CNO) selected the vendor that would ultimately support HMC's strategic vision. To accurately represent the nursing perspective, especially its differing opinions pertaining to care delivery, and to serve as an advocate for the 26,000 inpatients and 800,000 outpatients served annually, it was critical for the CNO to be knowledgeable and articulate, and able to understand the issues as well as the concerns of the nurses.

Executive Sponsorship

The executive team met with the clinical information system (CIS) project management team weekly to review progress, discuss barriers, and address other issues facing the organization, as well as make recommendations and appropriate high-level decisions. The meetings were an effective way to provide rigor and discipline to the process and to keep everyone on track.

To achieve the overall project goals, it was important that the CIS project be clinically driven by nurses and physicians, who would ultimately ensure the successful adoption of this technology in the delivery of patient care. The particular importance of design decisions regarding patient flow placed the CNO and CMO in the critical role of leading the transformation of care delivery. The dedicated time and active engagement of these executives demonstrated to the project team and to the organization that this ambitious clinical transformation was important to the overall success of the enterprise. The clinical leadership on this project helped to align the organization and its initiatives (see Figure 7C-2).

The project structure below the executive oversight team was critical to success. Lead nurses and physicians served as champions to ensure that clinical processes and care of the patient drove project decisions. These knowledgeable, credible individuals dedicated substantial time to the project, during which they engaged other clinicians across each operational unit and specialty area. One important aspect of the clinical champion role was to design a system using currently available software that would be based on the desired future state of care delivery. The clinical champions provided sponsorship through process leadership. They identified current work flow, defined the future state, and developed specific order sets to support the new work flow design. They were the clinical experts guiding the transformation and shaping how care would be different in the future.

The clinical leaders also helped define how best to configure the system for use in our organization. Under the guidance of the CNO and CMO, they directed specific groups responsible for various parts of the project. The CNO was the executive sponsor of the clinical documentation team and the Emergency Department triage and tracking team. The CMO sponsored the CPOE, medication management, and clinical decision support teams. The CNO and CMO met weekly with their teams, helping to resolve issues, holding the teams accountable for timelines, sharing information, challenging team decisions, providing guidance, and supporting the team through difficult decisions. They developed a detailed understanding of the technology and collaborated with the teams about delivering care with the new capabilities—keeping what was best for patients, and, secondarily what was best for clinicians, at the forefront of the decision-making process.

Lessons Learned

We have come a long way, completing all of Phase 1 (FY '04) and beginning Phase 2 (FY '06). However, we still have additional solutions to implement over the next several years to complete our fully integrated system. We have identified several strategies that will assist us in implementing future solutions.

Recruit Active Executive Leadership

Create an executive oversight group to identify the importance of the project to the organization. In addition, appoint clinical executives to lead specific project groups. Having the clinical executives engaged sends a strong message about the organization's commitment to improving patient care. Executives can help provide structure and accountability, resolve issues, remove barriers, share information, and integrate the health care team. Executive participation also communicates the importance of transformation, which is the key to a successful CIS implementation.

Partner with the CMO

It is essential for the CNO and CMO to be partners in the redesign and transformation of care delivery. They are the role models for the organization and the clinicians who, in a clinically driven system, will use this technology as a tool to care for patients. The CNO leadership role is critical to having an equally balanced team and incorporating technology as part of the operational day-to-day life of clinicians. It is essential for nurses, physicians, pharmacists, and other clinicians to make collaborative decisions about the flow of patient care and to have an understanding and appreciation of each other's practice. This is critical to a clinical transformation project's success.

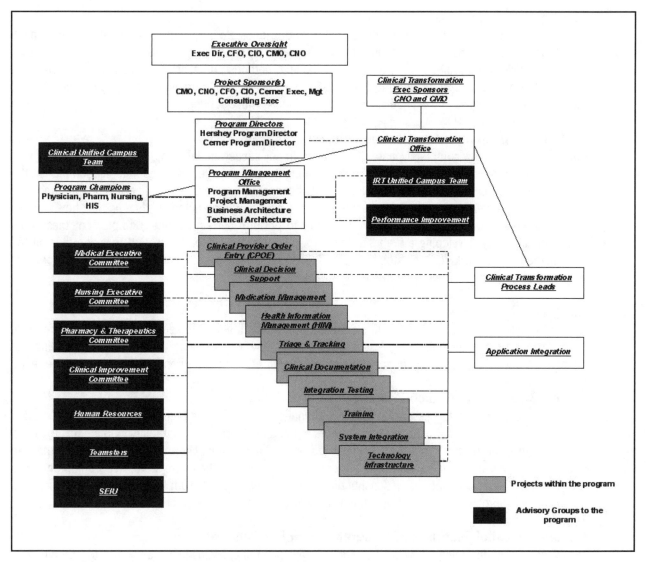

Figure 7C-2. *Clinical Leadership on Workflow Transformation Project.*

Engage the Clinicians

Involve clinicians early and at every step in the design. It is critically important to hand pick clinicians who will be assigned to the project full time, as it is a clinical system, not an IT system. They are the project's clinical leaders and must be respected for their clinical knowledge and ability to "get things done and done right" in the organization.

Develop Super Users

Consider developing at least 20 percent of your users into "super users," or trained clinicians who serve as role models, leaders, and content experts. They should be available in every clinical area. Super users can assist with order set and work flow design, guide policy development, and participate in design sessions with integrated teams. They also can participate in integration testing, which provides a forum for each discipline to walk through the new work processes to identify issues early in the implementation process. This provides a way to get all the good ideas on the table, encourage discussion, and identify the best changes to make in the transformation effort.

The super users are also the first and best line of support during go-live. Making sure that a super user is present in each clinical department/unit on each shift will provide support and reassurance to clinicians as they interact with the system for the first time.

Identify Training Needs

It is important to identify the training needs of staff and to dedicate sufficient staff and space for training. Staff training must be mandatory; holding staff accountable for attending the session or sessions reinforces the importance of the project. Using a variety of training methods and sessions is very helpful. Offering a combination of mixed sessions and more focused classes for individual groups within the organization, as well as pocket resources and manuals, are critical for successful adoption.

Participate in Continuous Communication

Communicating clearly, completely, and often is a key in any successful large implementation. Working with a member from the strategic relations or public relations department, develop a communication plan at the very beginning. Identify the key stakeholders and the strategies necessary to keep them updated and engaged, using a variety of methods. Project leaders can send out brief, helpful hints regarding how to make minor revisions following implementation or on how to perform certain actions. Complement these brief communications by developing a Web site that provides additional information and that contains all the training materials needed for "one-stop shopping." Reinforce all messages through active use of super users to keep the lines of communication open.

Integrate the Team

It is important to frequently bring the different work flow teams together to keep the project on track. Have weekly discussions regarding design issues, new work flow and practice patterns, team building, an improved product, and greater understanding of the complexities and interdependencies of the care team.

Create Structure and Accountability

One measure of project success is the ability to manage a timeline. It is helpful to use tools that provide detailed tracking and that add structure to the work of the team, create accountability, and identify the need for any course correction. This use of tools can be particularly helpful when venturing into areas that are new to the organization, such as developing order sets and mapping the future state. Reporting progress to the executive leadership team using "dashboards," i.e., one-page charts with key measures and outcomes showing weekly progress, reinforces the importance of tracking progress on critical tasks.

Conduct Parallel Testing and Integrated Proof-of-Concept

The excitement of designing a new CIS for patient care is one thing; seeing how it all comes together in practice is another. It is exceedingly important to conduct both parallel and integration testing. In the design phase, we imagine how we would like to organize the work flow. Integration testing is a laboratory evaluation of how well our theoretical design works in a controlled environment. Parallel testing takes us one step closer to reality by applying the new tools to a relatively small sample of unscripted clinical activity. When testing the efficiency of new work flows, here are some relevant questions to consider:

1. Are the new work flows efficient?
2. Can clinicians adjust to the new flows?
3. Do the work flows facilitate the coordination of care that is required?
4. Does the new system improve communications among care providers?

It is important to realize that no matter how many rounds of integrated testing are performed, it is the parallel testing and the test driving of the system that provide the greatest insight into the future delivery of care.

Celebrate the Successes

Each step and milestone has countless hours of hard work behind it. Remember to capture and celebrate the moments along the way. It is not just about the destination, it is also about the journey. Take time to recognize, reward, and reflect on a job well done!

Conclusion

Penn State Hershey Medical Center is committed to utilizing technology as a tool to improve patient safety and quality care, increase efficiency and patient satisfaction, recruit and retain talented and dedicated clinicians, and maintain employee satisfaction. The transformation of our care delivery is enabled by IT. The visible champions leading this change and counting on its success are the clinicians, as led by the CNO and the CMO.

CHAPTER 8

Nurses in Chief Information Officer Positions

By Lynn M. Nagle, PhD, RN

An increasing number of nurses are assuming the role of chief information officer (CIO) in health care organizations. This trend is emerging within the health sector in tandem with significant investment into information and communication technology solutions to support clinical care delivery.

Over the past two decades, the focus on information and communication technologies (ICTs) has been slowly building within the health sector. Although the delivery of health services has always been data intensive, the tools to effectively transform data into information to support clinical and management decision making have been lacking. Notwithstanding the rapidly evolving sophistication of technology, the development and acquisition of adequate software and hardware solutions for health care has been a slow process. Despite advances in the use of ICTs in other industries, heretofore there has been limited demand from the health sector for comprehensive, integrated clinical solutions. Although many health care organizations adopted financial and departmental systems (e.g., laboratory, nursing workload measurement) early on, it is only recently that integrated clinical information systems (CIS) have become a strategic focus for most.

In the past, most organizations typically would have recruited a technology expert (e.g., director of information technology) to set up and manage ICT strategy. With limited focus on implementing tools to support the processes of clinical care delivery, this role seemed sufficient at the time. However, nurses' engagement in information technology (IT) initiatives has been steadily increasing over the past three decades. In most health care settings, nurses involved in ICT projects typically have reported to a director of information services, most often an individual with technical expertise. Few organizations created regular full-time positions for nurse informatics specialists. Indeed only a small number have recognized the need to establish these positions beyond the usual temporary assignments that are project driven. Even fewer settings have established a nursing or clinical informatics program. And although nurse authors have advocated for the development of a nurse informatics specialist or nurse informatician role in health care settings,[1,2] few have written about the trend of nurses filling the most senior-level IT positions, such as chief information/informatics officer (CIO).[3]

In recent years, the focus on ICTs has intensified within health care organizations as upper management, care providers, payors, and consumers are recognizing the value of technology solutions that support (1) individual and population health information management, (2) organizational strategy, (3) operational efficiency, (4) clinical care delivery, and (5) quality improvement. For example, the design and deployment of CIS have matured to the extent that computerized provider order entry (CPOE) with embedded decision support is currently a leading initiative in many facilities. On a wider scale, many countries are deploying regional ICT solutions to integrate health information across jurisdictions and sectors. Globally, there is a veritable obsession within the health care industry to achieve the ultimate "holy grail" of a longitudinal, computerized health record for all citizens. Indeed it appears that there is currently an unprecedented concentration on ICTs as the solution needed to transform health care across the globe.

Beyond the systems implemented to support clinical care, information outputs have become a key corporate resource in monitoring performance metrics, assuring accountability, and securing competitive advantage. The considerable investment in ICT solutions has led to the creation of a senior-level position responsible for IT and information management (IM), typically the CIO. Incorporating this role into the executive management team has become commonplace in most industries and supports the strategic positioning of ICT initiatives.[4,5]

Outside of health care, CIOs are members of the executive team, deploying real business skills and strategic insight that can benefit the entire corporation.[5] The role of CIO has evolved in direct proportion to the greater emphasis placed on knowledge of core business processes rather than on in-depth knowledge of technology.[6] Similarly, because health care organizations obsess about the ability of ICTs to support clinical care and comprehensive IM, they commonly fill health care CIO roles with individuals who have a broad knowledge of technology and a deep understanding of clinical care delivery. Increasingly, they fill them with clinicians, including nurses.

An Emerging Trend

Nurses have a comprehensive view of the continuum of care and an appreciation of the contributions made by the multidisciplinary care team. An understanding of the processes of health care delivery brings an invaluable perspective to the identification, implementation, and evaluation of ICT solutions to support clinical care, as well as to the development and selection of appropriate tools to support clinical practice. Nurses in these roles consider themselves to be "bilingual," i.e., fluent in the languages of clinical care and technology.

Nurses' training and complex work processes are solid preparation for successfully leading major scale projects.[3] In addition, nurses with effective problem-solving abilities, and planning skills, as well as the capacity for multitasking, are particularly well-tooled to engage in strategy development and project management. Nursing education programs typically incorporate basic communication skills to prepare nurses for engaging with patients and colleagues. Many nurses with an interest in developing informatics expertise seek additional learning opportunities to advance their knowledge of ICTs. Historically, opportunities for nurses and other clinicians to advance their ICT acumen with direct relevance to health care settings have been limited. To date, few basic nursing education programs have integrated core informatics competencies into their curricula,[7,8] and a very limited number of institutions offer graduate and postgraduate study. However, as the number of nurses with advanced preparation in health informatics increases, we may see an influx of individuals bringing both clinical and technical knowledge to key leadership positions.

Today's health care organization is challenged by the organizational transformation and change management required to successfully implement ICTs. Successful deployment of clinical ICTs is highly dependent on the effective engagement of clinicians for the entire life cycle of a project. Most importantly, it is vital to involve clinicians in key decisions associated with the selection of an ICT solution, redesign of work flow processes, and implementation strategies to ensure long-term buy-in and adoption. The presence of a clinician participating in strategy development discussions has been shown to lend credibility to the project and to secure the confidence of the end users from the outset.[3,9]

Education and Skills

In identifying the need for the traditional requirements of the CIO role to change to support the needs of organizations, Huggins remarked,[10] "We've moved beyond the days when technical experience was the predominant qualification for the job. Now the CIO must be many things to many people, and one of the most important attributes he or she must bring to the job is leadership." He further advocates that the greatest strength of a CIO will be his or her capacity to effectively communicate, both verbally and in writing.

In a 2003 multi-industry survey of CIOs, the top three personal skills deemed most pivotal to one's success included (a) effective communication skills, (b) strategic thinking and planning, and (c) understanding of business processes and operations. The attribute identified as least critical across many types of industry was "technical proficiency."[4] Determined to focus on the central business of health care delivery, many organizations have moved to outsource technology services as much as possible.[11] The purchase of services for help desk, desktop, server, network, and "telephony" support is becoming commonplace in many organizations. This shift provides yet another reason for clinical grounding to outweigh the importance of technology expertise as an essential CIO attribute.

Nevertheless, those aspiring to the CIO role should develop a number of key skills and an understanding of IT and IM basics. Hersher[11] describes the evolution of the CIO role and provides a good synthesis of the hard and soft skills required, including being a visionary, an effective change agent, and a risk taker. Other essential skills, such as strategic planning, contract negotiation, and performance measurement, are usually developed through experience and mentoring beyond that provided in basic education programs. Legislative and reporting requirements, although varied among countries and jurisdictions, are also core knowledge to bring to the oversight of systems policies and procedures. Finally, the clinician CIO brings what is probably the most important perspective to bear on IT and IM strategies: how health care services are delivered and managed.

Many CIOs have acquired IT skills through technical training opportunities, such as seminars, workshops, and certificate and degree programs. They learn IM principles from generic business education or health administration programs, although few combine IT and IM principles and then apply both to the health care arena. Most nurses who have assumed the role of CIO or director of clinical informatics have acquired their knowledge and skills through a variety of educational experiences.

With the ever-increasing demand for health informatics expertise, formal education programs have been established in many countries, but remain few in number. For example, in 2002, a Canadian health informatics education summit[12] projected a severe shortfall of health informaticians within that country over the next five to ten years. Although conferences, seminars, and workshops offer opportunities for networking and focused study, more intensive training programs are needed to hone clinical informatics leaders. Without further development of health informatics programs and related faculty, the lack of such expertise and leadership will make the delivery of "e-health" agendas difficult and unduly protracted.

Positioning for Success—The Challenges

When first assuming the CIO role, individuals are often told in jest that the acronym CIO stands for "career is over." From the perspective of other industries, the CIO position is typically viewed as one of short tenure and limited success. A 2003 survey of IT executives found that 59 percent of the multisector respondents (n = 539) had been in their current position for fewer than five years.[4] The failure of ICT strategies often results in significant negative outcomes for a business, including the loss of substantial investments; such inadequate or failed solutions ultimately lead to the CIO's dismissal.

Increasingly, corporations, including health entities, are viewing IT and IM as key corporate resources. The CIO focus has shifted from securing IT staffing and specific technologies to assuring that the ICT initiatives are strategically aligned within the corporation. Health care organizations are slowly beginning to realize the need to invest more in this area. CIOs are continually challenged to cut costs, increase productivity, and identify revenue opportunities.[4] Whereas other industries (e.g., banking) typically invest upwards of 10 percent of their operating dollars in IM and IT, health care organizations in North America average between 1.5 percent to 3 percent.[13] Many have advocated for a marked increase in this allocation to successfully deliver on the e-health agenda. Most CIOs would still identify the scarcity of resources, both human and financial, as a major impediment to the advancement of ICT strategy.

Other common barriers to CIO effectiveness have been identified as (a) conflicting business priorities, (b) competing capital projects, (c) lack of alignment of IT strategy with organizational goals, (d) lack of time for strategic thinking and planning, (e) difficulty demonstrating the return on investment for IT, (f) lack of key skill sets, and (g) ineffective communication with and engagement of end users.[4] As in other industries, the health care CIO's focus needs to be on "partnering with business units and aligning IT strategy with corporate strategy"[4] to increase operational efficiency, reduce costs, improve patient satisfaction and clinical outcomes, and drive the adoption of innovative solutions.

Factors key to a successful CIO have been identified as follows:
1. Being a member of the senior management team
2. Involving leaders and users at all phases of IT and IM initiatives
3. Having an executive or steering committee to oversee IT investment decisions[4]

As a CIO for approximately seven years, I have experienced many of the previously described challenges and more. A key philosophy that has served as the foundation of successful initiatives throughout my tenure has been adopting a participative approach with all stakeholders. Designating clinician champions as part of any clinical system project is the single most effective strategy to ensure adoption of ICT solutions. In addition, making sure that your senior colleagues understand the goals and ultimate benefits to be gained from ICT investments will help to secure their support in the allocation of capital dollars, the assignment of clinical experts, and the endorsement of your overall strategy. In the past, senior executives left IT strategy to the technical experts; today, with the focus on organizational transformation, everyone has a vested interest in the supporting technologies. Being a clinician brought a certain degree of credibility to my work, but it also meant that I had to prove my technological abilities.

Realizing the Benefits

The "bilingual" CIO is positioned to effectively align the IT, IM, and clinical experts to achieve optimal solutions. My journey to becoming CIO of a large teaching hospital began many years before being hired into my position. However, thoughts of becoming a CIO had never been paramount in my career plans; my path to the role was somewhat serendipitous. I wanted to be a nursing leader in the field of health informatics and influence ICT directions within my own organization. In addition, I saw an opportunity to contribute to the informatics education of nurses. Hence, included in my plans was the creation of a graduate course in nursing informatics (NI) at the University of Toronto, Ontario. Little did I know what was in store for me in the years ahead!

In the mid-1980s, my affinity for informatics drove me to attend as many informatics-related conferences and workshops as possible. Professional meetings and forums were and continue to be pivotal to learning about the field, offering opportunities to network and to stay abreast of emerging ICT solutions. During the course of my doctoral studies, I deliberately selected elective courses that would enhance the breadth and depth of my technical knowledge. Such academic credentials lend standing to individuals seeking senior-level positions in any organization. Academic preparation, publications, and participation in professional forums all add credibility when presenting oneself as a candidate for the CIO role.

If you were to examine the scope of accountabilities and portfolios among health care CIOs, it is likely that you would find a great deal of variation in how the role is executed, especially among nurse CIOs. In my experience, one of the most common questions asked of the nurse CIO is how did you ever get from nurse to CIO? The following is an abridged version of my own evolvement to the role of CIO at Mount Sinai.

To expand my experience with system selection, design, implementation, and evaluation, I took the opportunity to lead informatics initiatives within the hospital's nursing department. This opportunity allowed me to work closely with a seasoned director of IT, who taught me important business skills such as contract negotiation. My role evolved from director of nursing with NI responsibilities added to my clinical portfolio, to managing director of clinical utilization, which included responsibility for health records and utilization management, and eventually to CIO. The CIO role added responsibility for all ICTs, including voice and data. In 2004, my role evolved to senior vice president, technology and knowledge management with the additions of quality and performance measurement, library services, registration services, and corporate privacy. The integration of IT and IM led to the logical blending of responsibilities assigned to my position by corporate.

The CIO Role at Mount Sinai Hospital

At Mount Sinai Hospital in Toronto, Canada, the informatics team comprises a combination of IT and clinical experts. Both groups report to the CIO via a director of ICT and a director of clinical informatics (a nurse). The ICT group brings a wealth of experience with backgrounds in programming; database management; application support; computer training; telephony; and desktop, network, and server management. The core ICT services are, however, largely outsourced to a service provider. The primary role of the ICT team is not only to support the clinical informatics team, but to also ensure alignment of IT strategy with IM strategy. The clinical informatics team includes medical, nursing, pharmacy, laboratory, allied health, and diagnostic imaging experts. With few exceptions, these individuals have been temporarily reassigned from their primary work environment to support execution of the CIS strategy. Most of these individuals bring no core technical expertise to their new assignments, but they quickly learn what they need to know. They teach the ICT team about the processes of care and the "how and why" of technology solutions that will work in clinical care environments. Policy development and approval occurs through collaboration between these teams and other organizational stakeholder groups.

The program is further enhanced by close alignment of the quality and performance measurement (QPM) program, which is accountable for the dissemination of performance metrics and benchmark data (e.g., organizational efficiency and growth, patient safety and satisfaction, and outcomes) throughout the organization using a balanced scorecard methodology. The director of QPM (a nurse) also reports directly to the CIO and provides a link between quality improvement opportunities and IT strategies. The other informatics business units—health records management, privacy, library and registration services—are woven, as appropriate, into the initiatives of the portfolio. Each of these groups is expected to serve the organization with a prevailing philosophy of collaboration and end-user engagement in decisions and future directions. Having the IT and IM strategy leaders report to a single senior-level position ensures that both efforts are well-aligned.

Lessons Learned

On a personal level, assuming the role of CIO was a daring but exciting career shift. Becoming reasonably fluent in the language of technology has been a challenging extension of previous clinical training and experience. Converging the two knowledge bases to affect significant change in the management of health information has been incredibly rewarding. But there have also been many tough decisions and rethinking of strategy along the way and, of course, some lessons learned that are worth sharing.

Managing the Environment

First of all, accept that the technology is the easy part. Changing people's perspectives and work processes is by far the most difficult aspect of the CIO's role. Working in another role (preferably a senior position) within an organization affords you insights into organizational culture and operations that can be beneficial in the execution of your role. Know your user community, understand the politics, and identify the decision leaders; they will make or break you. Have a clear vision and a strategic plan that can be easily articulated throughout the organization. Ideally, invite key stakeholders to participate in the development of an IT strategy; they will be more likely to assume ownership and shared responsibility for its successful execution.

Designing Successful Teams

Make sure that the rest of the senior team is behind you, especially the chief executive officer (CEO). Find enthusiastic, resilient clinical leaders who can relate to the end-user community, and try to have a representative group of disciplines involved. Identifying and recruiting effective project managers and leaders is key; the talents of your team make you look good. Bringing technical and clinical expertise together avoids the all-too-frequent disconnect between users and solutions. Communicate your achievements, milestone events, and priorities widely within the organization, but also profile your teams' success stories in publications and at conferences. Many ICT projects span several years, so staff appreciation, encouragement, and recognition are critical to sustaining interest and commitment to the end.

Knowing Your Vendors

Look to other CIO colleagues to share experiences, advice, and ideas; having a forum to regularly discuss shared issues can be extremely helpful to all. These discussions can be remarkably helpful for learning about particular vendor solutions. Managing the ICT vendor world is yet another dimension of the role to be mastered. The novice CIO can be easily led astray by vendor assurances that their product(s) can absolutely do everything being asked and more. Many a CIO has been wooed into "bleeding-edge" rather than leading-edge technology solutions; always keep the adage "buyer beware" in mind. Similarly, given the current pace of technology changes, try to avoid immediate obsolescence, and thoroughly research potential ICT options. You will likely have scarce dollars to begin with, so invest them wisely. If you are a risk taker, up to a major challenge, enjoy large-scale projects, and see the inherent benefit of clinical CIO leadership, then the role is worth considering.

Considering the Role of CIO?

In contemplating the role of CIO, the nurse needs to consider a number of potential challenges: (1) acquiring sufficient breadth and depth of technical expertise to manage voice and data systems and large-scale projects, (2) earning the confidence of all constituents from the board of directors to end users, (3) developing a strategy that is aligned with the corporate vision and priorities, (4) optimizing constrained ICT investments, and (5) creating a culture that embraces technology as a means, not an end. Nurses are well-suited to the CIO role, given their comprehensive understanding of the health system.

Regardless of skill and credibility, nurses need to acquire some core expertise related to the architecture of IT to succeed in this role. Although the nurse CIO need not be an expert in every aspect of technology, he or she needs to understand the basic components and to stay informed about emerging ICTs. There are a multitude of educational offerings to facilitate learning in this area: seminars, workshops, and certificate programs focus on specific components, such as voice and data networks. Perhaps more difficult to acquire but equally essential are skills associated with the development of an IT vision and strategy, the art of contract negotiation, and the ability to lead organizational transformations. The theoretical elements can be gleaned from most basic business or health administration programs, but the real learning needs to happen on the ground. Developing these skills need not be a matter of trial and error; try to identify possible mentors who can coach you in these areas. Finally, the most important skill to be nurtured is the ability to communicate with frontline staff, team colleagues, the board of directors, and the vendor community. Ultimately, look for opportunities to engage patients in dialogue about technology solutions that may make their navigation of the health system easier. At times, their insights are most enlightening in the development of strategy.

Given the ubiquitous nature of technology today, it is likely that the CIO role will shift even further away from technology such that in the future, the position of chief knowledge officer (CKO) may supplant the CIO of today. Others suggest that in the future the CIO role will become more of an implementation function than a strategy function.[14] It is not too soon to consider whether the required skill sets for CIOs will suffice for the CKO role of the future. As the balance eventually shifts away from IT to IM (and it will), nurses trained as knowledge agents may be even better positioned for senior roles of the future.

The answer to the question, how many nurse CIOs are out there? is as yet unknown. Anecdotally, there are more than one might think, but no one has yet quantified this as a definitive trend. There are many reasons why nurses make excellent CIO candidates. If not as CIO, there is certainly a tremendous demand for leadership in clinical informatics. Are you up to the challenge?

References

1. Lange LL. Informatics nurse specialist: Roles in health care organizations. *Nurs Adm Q* 1997;21:1-10.
2. Romano CA, Heller B. Nursing informatics: A model curriculum for an emerging role. *Nurs Educator* 1990;15:16-19.
3. Nagle LM. Nurses carpe diem. In: McArthur J, Carr R, Westbrooke L, Honey M, and Bakken S, eds. *One Step Beyond: The Evolution of Technology and Nursing, 7th* [on CD-ROM]. International Congress for Nursing Informatics, Auckland, New Zealand; May 2000.
4. Cosgrove-Ware L. The survey: What you have to say. *CIO Magazine,* April 1, 2003, 67-70.
5. Ciulla J. Step up and lead: Today the CIO role can be as big as you want it to be. *CIO* 2002;15,17:1.
6. Overby E, Varon E. The six best practices: What leading CIOs do. *CIO Magazine,* April 1, 2003, 74-80.

7. Nagle LM, Clarke HF. Assessing informatics in Canadian schools of nursing. In: Fieschi M, Coiera E, and Yu-Chuan JL, eds. *Proceedings 11th World Congress on Medical Informatics* [on CD-ROM]. San Francisco; 2004.

8. McNeil BJ, Elfrink VL, Pierce ST. Preparing student nurses, faculty and clinicians for 21st century informatics practice: Findings from a national survey of nursing education programs in the United States. In: Fieschi M, Coiera E, and Yu-Chuan JL, eds. *Proceedings 11th World Congress on Medical Informatics,* San Francisco; 2004.

9. Nagle LM, Ormston D. Transforming silos into an integrated enterprise. In: Marin H De F, Marques EP, Hovenga E, Goossen W, eds. *Proceedings 8th International Congress in Nursing Informatics,* Rio de Janeiro, Brazil; 2003.

10. Huggins GW. The changing face of the CIO. *CIO Canada* 1999;7:38-40.

11. Hersher B. The Role of the CIO: The Evolution Continues. In: Ball M, Weaver C, and Kiel JM, eds. *Healthcare Information Management Systems: Cases, Strategies, and Solutions.* 3rd ed. New York: Springer Verlag; 2004:161-172.

12. Office of Health Information Highway and University of Victoria. *OHIH-UVic Summit: Final Summary Report.* Toronto, Ontario: May 13-14, 2002 (unpublished report).

13. Sensmeier J. Transformational technology. *Int Rev Patient Care* 2005:114-115.

14. Prince CJ. Will the CIO role be obsolete? *Chief Executive* 1999;146:64-68.

Case Study 8A

Moving from Clinical Nurse to Information Technology Leader

Cheryl R. Croft, BSPA, RN, FCCJ

Introduction

Had anyone predicted 10 years ago that I would be working as the chair of information services (IS) for Mayo Clinic Jacksonville, Florida, I would not have believed them. The nursing profession offers great flexibility, but chief information officer? It is a role I did not expect to find myself in, and the opportunity brought with it many questions. What character traits would I need? How would I prepare for such a dramatic change and transition? The following case study explores my progression from care delivery nurse to information technology (IT) leader.

The Organization

A highly progressive organization, the Mayo Clinic Jacksonville afforded me the opportunity to apply my nursing experience to an important strategic goal. Mayo Clinic Jacksonville opened in 1986 as a tertiary care center. Most of the physicians who work there are specialists with in-depth knowledge of specific diseases and new treatment and research breakthroughs. Mayo uses a team approach to provide diagnosis, treatment, and surgery, giving patients access to a broad range of many different specialists as needed. This integrated system allows us to thoroughly evaluate and treat complex medical problems in one location. Patients who require hospitalization are admitted to nearby St. Luke's Hospital, a Mayo Clinic hospital with 289 private rooms.

Mayo Clinic Jacksonville employs approximately 5,000 individuals, including staff physicians, scientists, fellows, residents, predoctoral students, and support staff. We serve approximately 80,000 patients per year in the clinic setting and average approximately 14,000 inpatient admissions annually. For more than a decade, Mayo Clinic Jacksonville has shown a powerful commitment to embracing IT for inpatient and outpatient clinical practice. The organization views IT not only as a means to drive the paper chart from our environment, but also as an opportunity to re-engineer processes to maximize safety, productivity, and quality of care.

I started at Mayo Clinic Jacksonville 14 years ago. My first role in IS was clinical operations manager in 1995. I became the chair of IS in March of 2000. During my 10-year tenure in IS, I have participated in or directed more than two dozen enterprise and departmental system implementations of varying scopes and complexity, as depicted in Table 8A-1.

The Role

In my role as chair of IS, I am responsible for establishing the overall strategy for implementation of systems, computer operations, systems administration, and systems support for Mayo Clinic Jacksonville's automated environment. I engage in strategic planning for hardware, software, networks, and communications. Such planning requires working collaboratively with physicians, division/department chairs, administrative colleagues, and our allied health staff. My extensive clinical background combined with my more recently developed IT knowledge enable me to serve as an effective liaison between our clinical and technical teams. I understand and represent the needs and requirements of both unique groups and lead them toward shared success.

Background/History

I graduated from Florida Junior College in Jacksonville with an associate's degree in nursing in 1977. Over the next three years, I worked in medical-surgical nursing at two different hospitals. From this experience base, my nursing career progressed rapidly to the administrative aspect of nursing. I fulfilled roles as charge nurse, assistant head nurse, head nurse, nurse manager, and nursing operations coordinator over the next

Table 8A-1. System Implementations Completed from 1995–2005

Person Management	OB	Encoder
Common Data Repository	Registration/Patient Accounting	Tumor Registry
Order Management	Outpatient Billing	Templated Documentation
Scheduling	Radiology Information Management	Surgical Scheduling
Laboratory	Master Patient Index	Critical Care
Medical Records	Ophthalmology	Revision Level Conversions
Pharmacy	Human Resource	Year 2000 Compliance Testing
Ambulatory ordering	Chart Deficiency	Disaster Recovery Planning and Disaster Recovery Planning and Testing

four years. Each role increased my breadth of knowledge in hospital operations and in health care in general. I had the opportunity to work on the design of a nursing acuity system prototype, which was my first experience with flowcharting and systems design. I also continued my education at multiple institutions throughout this timeframe and benefited greatly from mentoring by the vice president of nursing.

In 1985, I took the opportunity to manage a fourteen-physician primary care practice that was part of a multispecialty group medical practice. The primary care practice was to act as a "feeder" for the specialty practice. This role allowed me to broaden my exposure to additional areas of health care operations, e.g., medical records, registration, laboratory, radiology, and materials management. It also introduced me to the power of automation, specifically, the use of IS to support operations and billing processes, e.g., registration, billing, dictation, transcription, and laboratory.

Four years later, I was offered the position of personnel director for both the primary and the multispecialty practices. Until then, personnel had been outsourced to the local hospital, but the practices wanted to bring this capability in-house. Because I was to be a one-person department for a time, I received permission to purchase computer hardware and software to assist in the setup of the joint personnel department. From my recent operational experiences, I had begun to realize the value of IT to increase the efficiency and accuracy of routine functions. I purchased two workstations, two printers, and three software programs: a word processing program, a database management program, and a desktop publishing program. With these I created an applicant tracking program; recruitment, acceptance, and rejection letters; and the templates for advertisements in our local paper. I taught myself to perform these functions, realizing that automation was key to effectively executing the many tasks for which I alone was responsible. Without these tools, I could not have delivered the services required of this newly developed department.

My operational focus expanded to include the coordination of satellite facilities, nursing, laboratory, radiology, patient accounts, and medical records. Importantly, I led my first selection and implementation process, in this case for a new patient accounting system. Yet, as enriching as these opportunities were, I longed to return to acute care nursing. In the face of rising business uncertainty within the physician practice group, I decided to make a career change.

I accepted a nurse recruiter position for Mayo/St. Luke's Hospital in 1991 and moved into a nurse manager position for the postoperative surgical service in 1992. This position transitioned into director of patient care, in which I oversaw surgical services, the progressive care unit, dialysis, and coordination of the unit secretary staff. During these many transitions, I continued to contribute to many automation projects, e.g., radiology system implementations and material management system upgrades. I also completed my degree (BSPA) at St. Joseph's College, Windham, Maine, with an emphasis on health care administration.

The Nursing Automation Challenge

I was highly vocal about the inefficiency afflicting our unit secretaries, who had to enter orders into five different computer systems while managing a desk in a busy nursing unit. The sentiment earned me the role of project manager for the implementation of a common ordering system. While serving in this role and in addition to my existing assignments, I was offered a position in the IS department by administration; they wanted me to bridge the gap between the clinical and technical staffs regarding automation of health care issues. At first I declined the offer, as I was very happy in my current position and felt extremely fortunate to have made the transition back to clinical nursing. I was concerned that accepting this new position would mean leaving clinical nursing for good. After the third such offer, I decided to become clinical operational applications manager for a period of one year. It was a difficult year of transition, and I faced an exceedingly steep learning curve. I mourned the loss of clinical nursing—it took a year to reconcile my emotions and appreciate the contributions I could make as a nurse in translating health care automation into valuable tools for patients, clinicians, and the organization. My final transition into informatics came with the recognition that my clinical experience would play a crucial role as I applied myself to IT initiatives that would benefit nursing and patient care. That was nine years ago. The position continued to evolve; I became director of clinical and business applications, leveraging the successful implementation strategies and collaborative practice models employed in the clinical areas to the business areas. I was then asked to consolidate the applications and technical services as chair of IS. I was flattered to be selected to lead efforts to automate clinical practice and to drive the vision for the transformation of care delivery in our practice.

Character Traits

Throughout the various roles and career transitions I have experienced, several personal traits have consistently served me well. These include a visible willingness to consider and accept change, solid organizational skills, unwavering perseverance, an ongoing desire to learn new skills and expand my knowledge base, and the ability to evaluate and redesign processes, as well as to effectively communicate the reasons for and benefits of such change to a variety of audiences. Also instrumental was my strong belief that automation represents the future of health care. I saw how IT could enhance patient safety and care and that the accompanying data collection would become a powerful source to influence education, research, and outcomes.

Opportunities/Strategies for Learning

I certainly came into the chair position at a distinct disadvantage. I had only taken a couple of basic computer courses in college and had only written a few lines of code. Initially, I encountered some resistance from IS staff who felt that only technically educated and trained people should be eligible for the position. Yet today, I credit my staff of very technically competent individuals for my IS education. They responded willingly every time I requested an explanation of hardware configuration requirements, capacity concerns, interface specifications, or application functionalities. To deepen my knowledge, I read numerous white papers on HL7, HTML, portable devices, bar coding, and platform comparisons. Application manuals also offered a wealth of information. It soon became apparent to me that much of what I was learning could be applied to multiple systems and applications.

Despite being hesitant about my entry into unfamiliar and uncharted territory, I had confidence in the clinical value I would deliver. Fortunately, my previous experiences with IT served me well during this time. These experiences provided a foundation to work from and helped me to connect the dots in this puzzling new world. A key strategy for me as a manager over diverse technical teams was to use a collaborative approach, especially in the context of a health care organization that is embarking on major, complex automation projects. I held many meetings to discuss options and arrive at a consensus with my team. I soon realized that I needed to expand this collaborative approach beyond the IS department. My clinical expertise and tenure with the organization enabled me to envision and implement both the structure and processes needed to support automation, bridging the technical and clinical areas to achieve successful implementations. Realizing that we needed our users to partner with us if solutions were going to meet the needs of the institution and map to the users' work flows, we established multidisciplinary implementation teams. We also offered the same educational programs to our user community as we did to the IS staff. For instance, to increase project management skills in our institution, we developed a curriculum and contracted for educational services to teach staff project management using our standardized tool sets. The inclusion of our user partners in these educational opportunities helped make automation a reachable institutional goal.

One resource that helped me in my IT journey is *A Peacock in the Land of Penguins,* by Ken Blanchard et al.[1] This book provided important insights into the issues of diversity, creativity, and innovation in the workplace. Another book that had a profound effect, providing the vision for how to structure and operate the IS department, is *The Information Paradox,* by John Thorp and DMR's Center for Strategic Leadership.[2] The authors observe, "Those who understand where and how to apply information technology in order to drive value will be the winners in the emerging knowledge economy."

Certainly this is what automating health care is all about: Information as the focus. The systems are merely a delivery mechanism. The questions I have continually asked myself are the following: How do we use information to enhance patient care? How do we apply information to improve decision making? How do we deliver information to clinicians so that they can personalize their approach and their choices? And how can we measure the value of automation for our institution and prove the value proposition in changing our clinical and hospital practice to an IT-supported practice? Simply automating current processes does not take full advantage of all IT has to offer. I realized that we required a more comprehensive process redesign to successfully apply IT to health care. This created more challenge and more change. Health care processes are complex but are also teeming with opportunities to realize quality and efficiency improvements. As an IT leader with substantial clinical expertise, I encourage you to take advantage of all opportunities for quality improvement training. You will be surprised at the commonalities among the tool sets and the opportunities they provide to improve work flow.

Chief Information Officer

Why me in such a role? Certainly serendipity played a part in my success. On-the-job training and participation in multiple high-profile projects brought my skills to the attention of administration. Flexibility in my career path afforded me many opportunities to increase my knowledge of health care and my knowledge of how to transition between inpatient and outpatient practices. A systems orientation and the ability to analyze process have been critical to my success. Nursing was a great training ground for my current role because the ability to multitask, prioritize, and handle crisis situations is a critical skill set for IS professionals. Understanding the needs of your user community is tremendously helpful when undertaking the challenge of health care automation. My clinical experience and understanding of health care processes also aided the development of constructive relationships with clinical departments, easing the transition to new work flows and processes.

Recommendations

If you wish to pursue a career in IT, seize the opportunity to work on any automation implementation that you can. Seek out knowledge. There is a wealth of material on project management, new technologies, and implementation experiences available in periodicals, books, and on the Internet. Another book I have found helpful is *Crucial Conversations,*[3] which offers practical tips on improving your communications when the stakes are high. Additional strategies to assist with communication and learning are: (1) partner with your colleagues to learn about their areas of expertise, (2) take advantage of the certification programs now available for electronic health records and project management, (3) develop your management and leadership skills throughout the transition, and (4) identify mentors who can assist you with applying these skills in real situations.

These resources and my mentors have been invaluable during my transition from clinician to an organizational IT leader. My role is a demanding one, yet I find great satisfaction in balancing the responsibility to sustain operations with the drive to transform the future of care delivery in our organization. As I told my CEO when he complimented my transition, you can apply the nursing process to any situation and succeed!

References

1. Thorp J, DMR's Center for Strategic Leadership. *The Information Paradox: Realizing the Business Benefits of Information Technology.* Canada: McGraw-Hill Ryerson Limited; 1998.

2. Hateley BJ, Schmidt W. *A Peacock in the Land of Penguins.* USA: Berrett-Koehler Publishers, Inc.; 1995.

3. Patterson K, Grenny J, McMillan R, Switzler A. *Crucial Conversations.* USA: McGraw-Hill; 2002.

CHAPTER 9

The Newest CXO Role: The Clinical IT Strategist

By Charlotte A. Weaver, PhD, RN, and Amy Walker, MS, RN

Increasingly, health care organizations are placing nurses in executive-level positions as members of the chief executive team. In particular, the role of an executive-level nurse informatician has emerged within the health care information technology (HCIT) industry and health care organizations over the last five years.* Although the actual title varies, in large, integrated delivery network (IDN) organizations and global HCIT companies, the most common are chief nurse information officer (CNIO) and chief clinical information officer (CCIO).[1] These executive-level nurse informaticians tend to have extensive information technology (IT) job experience, advanced graduate degrees, and formal credentials in informatics. Within IDN and HCIT companies, these CNIO/CCIOs are driving IT strategies, serving as a liaison between clinical leadership and the IT segment, and overseeing process redesigns and system implementations.

The complexity of health care work processes becomes more evident as health care organizations and governments worldwide adopt electronic health record (EHR) clinical systems and move toward filmless and paperless operations.[2] Care delivery has evolved over the past 150 years on a cottage industry business model. Technology and science advances of the past century have been added to this cottage industry structure without transformation; new practices have simply been layered onto old.[3] The mixture of new roles and specializations with outdated traditions has made health care the most complex and difficult industry to automate. Indeed, health care represents the last major industry to move to automation.[4]

As health care organizations around the world march toward EHR implementation, new clinical informatics roles are emerging to help bridge the cultural differences between the clinical and IT engineering worlds. Clinicians think and work in a nonsequential, multitasking mode, using work processes that often are nonlinear, convoluted, and highly varied.[5] In contrast, engineers and programmers tend to design systems utilizing work processes that are sequential, linear, logical, and singularly tracked. Designing according to the 80/20 rule, meaning that the most common work flow process variations are covered but not exceptions, is unacceptable. In healthcare, the "rare" or "almost never" exception often carries significant patient safety, or ease-of-use ramifications. Nor is it easy for IT professionals to gain an insider's understanding or sufficient domain expertise through observation or work flow analysis in order to design IT solutions that work for clinicians. The health care industry is not the banking industry. The highly variable permutations in work-flow order and steps, personnel, and decision tree branching may remain invisible if left to nonclinicians to discover and understand. It is exactly this complexity of health care work processes that has made it extremely difficult for IT companies to successfully build information systems that fit clinicians' work flow and that deliver value.

The HCIT industry has delivered clinical systems for more than 40 years, but it is only in the past few years that clinical information systems (CIS) have reached sufficient maturity to enable EHR adoption in the marketplace.[3,6,7] As paper-based, manual operations give way to automation, both health care organizations and the IT industry seek out clinicians to provide the domain expertise required. Within care-provider organizations, large numbers of nurses have been recruited to help

---

* Rosemary Kennedy was promoted to this role in 2004 at Siemens Medical Solutions (rosemary.kennedy@siemens.com); Joan Sullivan has held this position at Bay State Health System since 2002 (joan.sullivan@bhs.org).

manage the massive organizational transformation that clinical IT implementations incur, as well as to correctly define and implement reengineered processes for all disciplines, not just nursing. In addition, nurses have worked for decades with HCIT software companies as members of application development teams.

The significant difference with the new leadership roles currently evolving within service organizations and HCIT companies is that nurse informaticians are leading teams, defining strategies and priorities, and participating at the executive level to help set business directions. These functions may be shared with a chief medical officer (CMO) or a chief medical informatics officer (CMIO), a partnership characterized by collegiality and strong teamwork. This dual clinical leadership also mirrors the optimum role relationship needed between a health care organization's chief nursing officer (CNO) and CMO in the context of CIS' implementations. In the case history presented in this chapter, the IDN organization created a corporate level team that included a CMO, an information services' medical director, and a CCIO to engage their clinical leader counterparts across numerous member health care organizations.

Why Nurses?

On the health care organization side, these informatics nurse leaders are filling a demand for an executive to effectively lead at a strategic level and to oversee the operational management of the deployment of advanced clinical and financial information technologies. What's behind this phenomenon? Leading-edge administrators define EHR clinical automation initiatives as "clinical transformation projects" that result in major cultural and process changes. These chief executive officers (CEOs) direct their clinical executives to take ownership of EHR implementations, as well as the redesign process such change entails.[8] At a minimum, EHR implementations disrupt the way people work, think, and communicate across teams, as well as with patients and their families.[9] As important as the technology piece of these projects is, the people, culture, and planning for major change represent more than 80 percent of the work necessary for adoption to occur.[10]

EHR projects are essentially clinical process transformation initiatives and, because of this, CNOs are increasingly given executive responsibility for implementation outcomes. Unlike a CMO, who has minimal operational or budget duties, a CNO has the heaviest operational work span of any member of the executive team. Additionally, in the U.S., CNOs are often responsible for all care delivery departments, including emergency, operating room, pharmacy, laboratory, respiratory therapy, physical therapy, and clinical nutrition. Consequently, nursing administration becomes a catalyst in driving the vision and hard work that goes into process redesign. Realistically, however, most CNOs' first encounter with IT may be in the context of the organization's decision to undertake an EHR implementation. A driver for the CNIO role is the need for a senior advisor who can support the nurse executive's ability to engage and lead these major clinical transformations. Fundamentally, the CNIO represents a nurse who knows both the operational world of health care delivery and the technical world of HCIT. In most health care organizations, the CNIO is a liaison between IS and nursing administration and functions as a close guide and resource to an organization's CNO.

The need for a clinician to serve as a translator between IT and the clinical component at the strategic executive level reflects the industry's maturity in recognizing the cultural complexity of these change initiatives. And as we have seen from the Healthcare Information and Management Systems Society (HIMSS) Nursing Informatics Survey 2004,[1] nurses are filling a myriad of roles in support of IT adoption. These trends are happening mostly as IT advances into the acute-care sector. In contrast to ambulatory care, transformation in acute-care settings is all about nursing. Winning nurses over for any new change is key for organizational adoption and for meaningful transformation. In the acute-care space, we have seen this lesson play out with physician-focused computerized provider order entry (CPOE) projects that did not include nurses in redesign and system use.[11,12]

There is, however, another dimension behind current thought that explains why nurses have been tapped to fill clinical informatics roles over other professionals. As a discipline, nursing fosters team players who value communication and who work by consensus.[13] In addition, nurses carry role functions that are unique in the health care field. Hospitals are complex social organizations that require agents who can cross boundaries and departments to make care delivery happen. Margaret McClure, past president of the American Academy of Nursing and the long-standing nurse leader behind the magnet hospital initiative, describes this function of nursing as being the organization's "integrators."[14] Nurses have long described this function as "nursing the system," (i.e., doing what must be done to prevent gaps in care during "hand off" of patients, such as channeling information to other members of the care-delivery team). Nurses learn the integrator role early in their careers as they gain familiarity with the subcultures and production work processes of other departments. Nurses develop the job skills (particularly communication skills), domain expertise, and flexibility to work harmoniously as generalists in multidisciplinary teams. Combined, their skills, experience, and knowledge make nurses valuable participants in the IT projects that transform the very core of care delivery.

The fact that nurses are being tapped to fill the CNIO/CCIO role rather than professionals from other disciplines, such as pharmacists or physicians, also broadly reflects the advancement of nurses into upper management positions. Prior to 1970, nurses rarely held positions on the executive management team beyond the nursing organization. When they did, nurses held such titles as "nursing director" rather than vice president or CNO. Nurses gained access to executive-level opportunities when nursing education evolved from apprentice-style, hospital-based nursing schools to university-oriented settings. The advanced degrees and university-based education for nurses that started in the 1960s provided the skills necessary for them to advance into a broad array of management positions. Those leadership roles helped launch the career opportunities of the current generation of nurses who hold CEO, chief operating officer and other corporate officer positions including the corporate level of large, IDN health care systems. The position of CNIO/CCIO reflects the advancement of nurses into strategic leadership positions and the preference for placing nurses in clinical informatics roles over those in other disciplines.

A CCIO Case History at Adventist Health System

This case history explores how nurse Amy Walker achieved the position of CCIO at Adventist Health System-Information Services (AHS-IS).

AHS is the largest, not-for-profit, Protestant health care organization in the U.S. with thirty-eight hospitals in ten states. Employing a staff of 44,000 and 6,634 physicians, and having total revenues of approximately $4.1 billion, AHS serves nearly four million patients annually. The AHS corporate office and data center are located in central Florida. The AHS system has three IT entities that service their hospital organization: Florida Hospital (seven sites), Centura Health (four sites), and AHS Information Services (twenty-seven sites). The hospital facilities serviced by AHS-IS are divided geographically into seven regions.

Amy Walker's Career Path to CCIO

My career path to the CCIO position has been paved with luck, strategy, perseverance, and the help of mentors. On many occasions, I have simply been at the right place at the right time. At those times, I seized the opportunity to take on new challenges and solve difficult organizational problems. I have consistently moved out of my work comfort zone to assume new responsibilities. Fortunately, mentors have taken the time to provide counseling, constructive feedback on my work performance and new opportunities. Not all of my mentors have been nurses. In fact, many of those who helped me the most in my career have not been in the health care profession.

Nursing Background

Newly graduated with a BSN in 1981, I was fortunate to find and assume a position in a coronary care unit. I spent the next several years in the critical care area as a staff nurse and earned my critical care registered nurse certification. I moved on to a number of other clinical positions in frontline patient care, education, nursing supervision, and management. I ended the direct care phase of my nursing career as a medical-surgical, orthopedic, and neurology nurse manager. During my five years as a nurse manager, I worked closely with the vice president of patient care services who mentored me and, years later, supported my candidacy for CCIO. I owe this nurse leader a great deal.

Informatics Background

After nearly ten years in clinical nursing, I began looking for a new challenge. The University of Maryland at Baltimore had a program in nursing informatics (NI). Students in this program were referred to as "pioneers," and this appealed to me. Although I had only used a computer to place orders and retrieve results at the hospital, I enrolled for a masters of science in NI. It took nearly five years to complete the program, while attending school year-round and working full time at Washington Adventist Hospital. I finished the program in 1993.

The NI curriculum included classes in leadership, IT project management, systems design and analysis, database structure and design, research, and other core technology courses. Upon graduation, I accepted an application analyst position with a health care IT vendor. I left the nurse manager position at my hospital, thus marking my transition from direct patient care into informatics. This was a hard step to take, but I wanted to work in the field of informatics and my hospital had no such positions.

IT Experience

As an application analyst, I worked on development and support teams, design completion, testing, and support of clinical and nonclinical applications. I also built a knowledge base on project management of software development. The knowledge base included all of the tasks and tools involved in ensuring that quality software was shipped to clients. The experience I gained in this position allowed me to learn the real world of systems analysis and solution development for the marketplace. I had the opportunity to lead the development of design specifications for an integrated transcription system. I learned to outline current work processes and to translate them into new work processes using IT. In informatics, this skill set is referred to as "current to future state work flow analysis." Although the transcription system design was a small project, it taught me the life cycle steps required to deliver a quality application, as well as how to manage work to meet software delivery deadlines. It was this product development experience that gave me the knowledge and skills to work with vendors' development and engineering teams, capture design specifications, estimate scope of work, plan for code installs, and hold the conversations needed to get the right functionality and work flow from clinical solutions for our AHS staff and clinicians.

IT Education

Within six months of taking the application analyst position, I returned to school for the additional technical knowledge needed to lead software development projects. In my position, I produced detailed external design documentation that an engineer converted to programming specifications. Although my master's degree had taught me project management and database and systems design, I wanted more knowledge and proficiency in systems architecture and programming. I felt that this knowledge would enable me to more effectively interact with the technical members of my teams. I enrolled at a local university and took evening classes in systems analysis and design, programming, telecommunications and networks, operating systems, and computer languages. I enjoyed these classes and found it stimulating to be in IT classes with people outside of the health care industry.

Project Management Experience

After nearly one year as an application analyst, I began to wish for additional responsibilities, a new challenge, and greater client contact. When a colleague phoned with a new opportunity, I decided to move. The phone call came from a friend I had worked with at a large IT firm during my practicum in graduate school. The friend was now a principal at a firm specializing in health care IT consulting for military clients. Several positions were available for a project that involved defining requirements for the military's next-generation computer-based patient record. I assumed the role of project manager and gained valuable experience in managing a large team in a consulting environment with deadline-driven hard deliverables.

Implementation Experience

At project completion, my growing network of colleagues and professional friends helped me immediately move into a manager position within a large health care IT vendor. Over the following four years, the positions I held included implementation project manager, project executive, and strategic account manager. In these roles, I learned the sales and implementation side of the IT business, as well as what it means to work for a publicly traded company. I gravitated toward work in implementations; it was in this role that I had accountability for functional and technical teams creating integrated clinical and financial solutions. I realized that leading project teams and implementations was what I wanted to do within informatics.

In 2001, a colleague recruited me to interview with AHS-IS for the position of director of clinical informatics. This position was responsible for leading the implementation projects across their IDN. I moved to this new opportunity because it represented career growth and advancement in the area of informatics that I love—the implementation of clinical systems that transform organizations.

Becoming CCIO

The Importance of Networking

I cannot overemphasize the importance of networking in building your career. Friends, colleagues, and friends-of-friends use networks to get recommendations for potential job candidates. Most of my job opportunities happened because colleagues contacted me offering introductions and connections for new positions and career advancement. For those just starting this journey, take the time to build relationships with your fellow students and colleagues in professional organizations. They will open doors for you throughout your career, as they have for me.

Initially my role at AHS-IS was director of clinical informatics, and I was charged with implementing the initial modules of a clinical documentation system. But in late 2001, the AHS corporate executive leadership determined that it needed to contract for all the required modules of an advanced clinical information system before proceeding with implementing the first site. The outcome of this evaluation process, with decision making that included CEOs and CNOs from across the company, was the conclusion that having an integrated clinical information system that could fully support the advanced clinical systems required in the future, including CPOE with evidence-based clinical pathways, was strategically important. The system selection process concluded in July 2002. As a result of this development, I was charged with the responsibility of implementing the advanced clinical information system. The EHR project was named "iConnect" to communicate its role as a connector between health care providers and patients.

After negotiating the contract, I began guiding the enterprise design and implementation at the first hospital selected for prototype implementation. As this chapter goes to print, the third hospital is preparing to convert to the standardized, enterprise build for the iConnect system, validating its ability to accommodate the size and organizational variation across the AHS health care organizations. In December 2004, I was promoted to the CCIO position at AHS-IS, and the following is an overview of my role in AHS's EHR journey.

Adventist Health System's EHR Journey

The primary strategic goal driving AHS's decision to invest in an enterprise-wide, standard EHR system was a commitment to improve quality of care and patient safety, following release of the 2000 Institute of Medicine (IOM) report on the quality of the U.S. health care system. The corporate executive leadership team set other strategic objectives to improve work flow, efficiencies, and care delivery, as well as the patient experience.

Executive Sponsors and Governance Structure

The AHS team appointed to serve as the iConnect executive governance committee started as a hands-on group, meeting weekly beginning in September 2002. The executive team members selected to champion iConnect have invested large amounts of time, energy, and effort over the past three years to meet the project's aggressive objectives. They remain committed to implementing the iConnect system.

The governance team consists of the following executives:

Executive Sponsor:	Senior Vice President of IS
Physician Sponsors:	Medical Director of IS
	Vice President, Chief Medical Information Officer
Project Director:	CCIO
Divisional CIO:	AHS-IS CIO
Vendor Representative:	Project Executive

The AHS corporate chief financial officer (CFO) has been a strong, consistent supporter of the iConnect project. The CFO provided strategic guidance and an immediate escalation path for issue resolution and decision making when required. This was a crucial element in AHS' ability to move quickly and accomplish so much in such a short period.

Project Phasing and Roll Out Approach

AHS made the decision to do a big-bang implementation, rolling out a standard-build enterprise design of the iConnect system to all twenty-seven AHS-IS hospital organizations over a five-year period. AHS, which contracted for seventeen applications on a single database architecture, worked with its software supplier to rapidly design and build the system. Driving this strategy was the need to implement a large number of hospitals while keeping costs down and realizing rapid benefits. "Big bang" meant that all applications and changes in work flow and functionalities would go-live simultaneously at the given hospital. The first three hospital sites chosen for conversion would test multifacility functionality, scalability, and the breadth of clinical applications. These initial sites would validate the enterprise build, providing proof-of-concept. The rapid rollout of the remaining twenty-four AHS organizations is scheduled for completion in twenty-one months.

Design Approach

The AHS-IS design approach required that subject matter experts from all seven regions would develop the corporate model for each of the ten application groups. The application groupings were as follows: Registration, Scheduling, Orders, Clinical Documentation, Pharmacy, Health Information Management/Document Scanning, Radiology, Surgical Services, Emergency Department, and Charge Services. That model consisted of a standard design and build for the integrated database, screens, tables/files, forms, flow sheets, and reports. A corporate clinical informatics project manager was assigned to each application group. Teams were careful not to work in silos; to avoid that scenario, an integration project architect was assigned to ensure that issues were sorted appropriately across the applications. The framework for the AHS enterprise-wide standard iConnect model was to use industry best practices and standards whenever available. At times, this proved a challenge because a best practice or standard had to be aligned with the vendor's functionality. As a consequence, the AHS design team, with assistance from the software supplier, had to define the "best practice" for iConnect in five months.

To mitigate the risks of a big-bang design and implementation approach, the project leadership team added a proof-of-concept milestone and a well-planned change management plan. The proof-of-concept process will take place after the third hospital goes live. Table 9-1 lists the iConnect application groupings.

Table 9-1. iConnect's Applications and Features

Application Groupings	Features
Integrated Clinical Repository with Rules Engine	
Patient Access	• Master patient index • Registration, Admission, Discharge, Transfers and Eligibility Management
Order Management	• All orderables, including clinical • Results reviewing • Order sets
Comprehensive Clinical Documentation and Care Planning	• Clinical charting for all services, to include 185 forms • Nursing, cardiopulmonary, rehabilitative care, social work, pastoral care, online forms and flow sheets • Critical care (CC) flow sheets with automatic capture of ventilator and CC monitor data • Task and open order management • Clinical pathways • Electronic medication administration throughout the hospital
Pharmacy	• Inpatient pharmacy, order entry, and rules • Pharmacy documentation • Adverse drug event alerts
Enterprise Scheduling	• Surgery, selected inpatient, and outpatient ancillary appointments
Surgical Services	• Peri-, intra-, and postoperative documentation • Preference card management
Health Information Management	• Coding • Digital imaging for all paper documents • Document deficiency tracking • Physician electronic signature
Radiology Management and Mammography	• Interface to Picture Archive Central System (PACS) • Radiology transcription and electronic signature
Emergency Department	• Tracking board, triage, and Emergency Department documentation
Personal Digital Assistant for Physicians	• Results and transcription review

Choosing Initial Activation Sites

The three hospitals chosen for initial activation were selected based on specific criteria. The first (Hospital A) has an exceptionally strong leadership team that was keen to be first. The second site (Hospital B) has a satellite campus, and the third (Hospital C) is a larger facility with full specialty services and teaching programs.

First Activation

Hospital A is a 215-bed, full-service community health system offering comprehensive medical services. The hospital employs 1,400 staff and provides care in more than thirty specialties. Hospital A went live in January 2004, with a major code upgrade in April 2004. The upgrade was necessary so that AHS would have multi-facility logic going forward with the rollout. The leadership at this organization has always been supportive of the project. Particularly, the CNO maintained a positive can-do attitude throughout the entire implementation. The project could not have been successful without her support.

Second Activation

Hospital B is a two-campus facility with 300 beds. It is a medical-surgical hospital with significant business in behavioral and rehabilitative patients. Hospital B went live in April 2005, with two additional applications added to the initial scope of the enterprise model: an integrated laboratory system and structured physician documentation in the emergency department. Other planned scope additions include CPOE (as a pilot at one campus) and clinical pathways with evidence-based practice content.

Third Activation
Hospital C, a 386-bed acute-care facility, went live in the third quarter 2005, with the following additions to the initial enterprise model:
• Emergency department prescription writing (pilot)
• Intensive Care Unit (ICU) with outcomes and reporting
• Neonatal ICU (NICU) and obstetrics flow sheets
• Labor and Delivery, NICU, and Post Anesthesia Care Unit bedside device integration
    Hospital C also converted to the IDN billing system.

Project Structure and Management
Standard project management methodologies provided the necessary structure and tools needed to orchestrate the project. These included detailed team member roles and responsibilities, policies and procedures for agendas and minutes, issue tracking and resolution, escalation protocols, design document templates, detailed project plans, status reporting procedures, and standards for database design. The CCIO coordinated development of the project structure and management tools and oversaw all project management activities. A corporate application team of approximately 30 staff from AHS-IS's clinical informatics team within the CIS department reported to the CCIO. Without this high-performance team's dedication to AHS and its mission, the iConnect project would never have been successful.

In addition to the corporate CIS team, each hospital has an IS team, CIS hospital director and, importantly, a clinical informatics director. The CIS hospital director leads and manages project events at the hospital level. In addition, a consultant was engaged to focus on the detailed operations of the rollout, so the CCIO could direct her energies to interacting with the leadership team at the facility, continuing to build consensus for the AHS clinical model, and planning for future enhancements.

System Build and Testing Approach
AHS based its implementation approach on outsourcing the system build to the software supplier partner. This strategy leveraged AHS resources and enabled a rapid design and build. However, the corporate AHS-CIS team performed all the testing, including the rounds of integration testing that accompanied issue resolution and new code implementation.

Change Management and Organizational Readiness
It was imperative that on go-live, users understood the new work processes and could competently use the new system. To ensure user acceptance and organizational readiness, the project leadership team planned several critical events. These included (a) staff involvement with system design, (b) work flow mapping (existing and future), (c) end-user validation of the build, (d) scenario role-playing, (e) parallel testing, (f) milestone sign-offs, (g) proof-of-concept review sessions, (h) mandatory user practice sessions, and (i) setting competency requirements.

Activation
Thus far, the big-bang approach has worked for AHS. For the second hospital (Hospital B), the cutover from the paper and manual systems took place in an impressive seven days, after which the command center closed and the project implementation team moved on to issue resolution and a system upgrade. AHS attributes this success to the following:
• A no-failure attitude at all organizational levels
• A strong hospital leadership
• Internally driven change

- Excellent support by all team members
- Strong partnership with software supplier
- Disciplined project management structure and methodologies

Closing Thoughts on the CNIO/CCIO Role

Considering the skill sets needed by a CNIO/CCIO, first among those is the ability to establish credibility with and ultimately win the confidence of all the players at the executive table. This is achieved in part by working well with people, motivating those around you, and competently delivering on technology initiatives. The CCIO should be an integrator of people, processes, and systems, resulting in strong coalitions across health care disciplines at all organizational levels. Therefore, the CCIO must have financial, clinical, project management, and IT expertise.

The CCIO needs the financial acumen to evaluate sales agreements, understand contract law and legal language, and negotiate deals. Other important financial skills include revenue cycle management, charge capture, and patient accounting fundamentals. As a formulator and driver of IT strategy, the CCIO may represent major change and disruption to other members of the clinical leadership team. Knowing the principles of managing social change and the elements that evoke resistance to change are crucial tools. The CCIO is an important supporter and resource to an organization's clinical leaders, who must maintain a shared positive outlook during the implementation of advanced clinical technologies. As the clinical champion, the CCIO must remain optimistic throughout the project and keep the vision in front of the team. Team morale rests on the CCIO's shoulders.

Finally, the level of technical knowledge the CCIO needs requires formal education in informatics and project management, as well as deep job experience. Bright, masterful nurses and nurse managers often are recruited into informatics without the benefit of needed formal education. The result is that these talented nurses are often kept at the team or middle-management level because they have not acquired the knowledge and skills needed to advance and to be successful at the executive level. The most powerful preparation an experienced clinical nurse can have as he or she attempts to land this role is a formal education in informatics enhanced by job experience. One without the other creates performance vulnerabilities and leadership deficits.

In conclusion, advanced integrated clinical information systems, such as AHS's EHR, are becoming simpler to implement largely because nurses are driving these implementations and removing the roadblocks having to do with organizational change management. Nurses are designing, building, perfecting, and optimizing advanced clinical information systems. The CNIO/CCIO—a nurse with the appropriate skills—will remain a driving force to successfully deploy these technologies and achieve user acceptance. We encourage nurses to strive toward this career goal.

References

1. Sensmeier J, West L, Horowitz JK. Survey reveals role, compensation of nurse informaticists. *Computers In Nursing.* 2004;22:171,178-181.
2. Wachter RM. The end of the beginning: patient safety five years after "To Err Is Human." *Health Affairs.* 2004.
3. Goldsmith J. *Digital Medicine. Implications for Healthcare Leaders.* Chicago: Health Administration Press; 2003.
4. Dick RS, Steen EB, Detmer DE, eds. *The Computer-based Patient Record. An Essential Technology for Health Care.* Washington, DC: National Academy Press; 1997.
5. Page A, ed. Institute of Medicine. *Keeping Patients Safe. Transforming the Work Environment of Nurses.* Washington, DC: National Academy Press; 2004.
6. Institute of Medicine. *Crossing the Quality Chasm. A New Health System for the 21st Century.* Washington, DC: National Academy Press; 2001.
7. *Information Technology: Benefits Realized for Selected Health Care Functions.* GAO-04-224. A Report to the Ranking Minority Member, Committee on Health, Education, Labor and Pensions, U.S. Senate. October 2003.
8. McCartney PR. Clinical issues: leadership in nursing informatics. *JOGNN.* 2004;33:371-380.
9. Lorenzi NM, Riley RT. Informatics in healthcare: managing organizational change. In: Ball MJ, Weaver CA, Kiel JM, eds. *Healthcare Information Management Systems: Cases, Strategies, and Solutions.* New York: Springer; 2004:81-93.

10. Rose JS. IT: transition fundamentals in care transformation. In: Ball MJ, Weaver CA, Kiel JM, eds. *Healthcare Information Management Systems: Cases, Strategies, and Solutions.* New York: Springer; 2004:145-160.

11. Koppel R, Metlay JP, Cohen A, et al. Role of computerized physician order entry systems in facilitating medication errors. *JAMA.* 2005;293(10):1197-1203.

12. Ash JS, Berg M, Coiera E. Some unintended consequences of information technology in health care: The nature of patient care information system–related errors. *J Am. Med. Informatics Assoc.* 2004;11(2):104-112.

13. Donahue MP. Nursing: *The Finest Art.* 2nd ed. St. Louis: Mosby; 1996.

14. McClure ML. Differentiated nursing practice: concepts and considerations. *Nurs Outlook.* 1991;39(3):106-110.

Case Study 9A

Nursing and IT:
The Auckland District Health Board Experience

Doon Hassett, BBS, BN, GradDip Bus (Health Informatics), and Kara Hamilton, RGON

Introduction

This case study describes how the Auckland District Health Board (ADHB) in New Zealand put technology into practice. In relating this story, we will explore the challenges and rewards of this journey and the lessons learned, as well as provide our recommendations to others. A central theme in this case study is the role of nurses and the origin of their recruitment to this information technology (IT) initiative. We will also examine the evolution of the organization's focus from IT itself to the more valuable objective of informatics adoption.

Geography: Where We Are and What We Do

New Zealand is made up of three islands in the South Pacific and is similar in size to Britain, Japan, or Colorado. Auckland, with a population of just over one million, is the largest city and is situated near the top of the North Island. In New Zealand, as elsewhere in the world, health care faces challenges such as escalating costs, new technologies, and nursing shortages. New Zealand has a government-financed, public health care system. Health policy and funding are administered by the central government in Wellington. Elections in New Zealand occur every three years, and as such, government policy, naming conventions, organizational structures, and reporting lines have the potential to change. During the sixteen years we have worked in New Zealand, the health system has had four major restructures, each reflecting basic change in health care funding. These philosophies have ranged from full government funding to user charges, with health organizations competing for each health dollar. The current government administration allocates health funding based on selected-population targets.

The ADHB is both a provider and a funder of public hospitals and health services for the central Auckland region. Of the current twenty-one district health boards in New Zealand, ADHB is the largest public health care provider. ADHB employs approximately 7,500 staff across the hospital facilities and community services; has approximately two million patient contacts annually; provides primary, secondary, and tertiary services to the central Auckland region; and provides quaternary services to the entire country.

Early Days for IT in Health

The first computers were introduced into the four ADHB hospitals in 1988 and were only used by the administrative staff to record health events into the patient administration system (PAS). PAS was a basic, transaction-based system that recorded inpatient and outpatient activity. Clinical input into PAS was limited to senior nursing staff and involved the updating of patient condition codes. Senior staff nurses on the ward found the data input, which was a series of numeric codes, to be highly unfriendly to use. Nurses learned to use the system by developing a crib sheet which was taped to the desk. The numeric code, "17", for example, meant that the patient was on ward leave. Several years later, the children's hospital persuaded the Information Services (IS) Department to build an inpatient system that better met its needs. In 1996, the Children's Hospital Inpatient Systems (CHiPs) went live, although the incumbent PAS system was still used for outpatient activity.

In 1997, PAS was discovered not to be Y2K compatible. A decision was made to replace PAS with CHiPs throughout the organization and that an outpatient scheduling system would be bought "off the shelf." The ADHB conducted a system selection process and identified McKesson's outpatient scheduling system, called Pathways Healthcare Scheduling System (PHS), as the top-rated choice.

At this time, we were unit nurse manager and clinical charge nurse over a busy cardiothoracic surgical ward at Green Lane Hospital. We both were active users of a ward PC; therefore, we were considered "IT experts." Subsequently, the Auckland Hospital general manager invited us to join a review team going to the U.S. to assess HBOC's PHS scheduling system. We promptly agreed.

PHS was adopted as the preferred outpatient management system and that, together with CHiPs, comprised the new systems to be rolled out to the four ADHB hospitals.

Our move to nursing informatics (NI) as a career path came with the invitation by Green Lane hospital's general manager to join the implementation project team. Specifically, our role was to liaise with the specialties and to customize the outpatient scheduling system design and build to fit the work flow needs of the different end users.

The ADHB organization carefully developed the project teams for the inpatient and outpatient system implementations to ensure buy-in and end-user adoption. To do this, the organization selected a representative from each hospital who was well-known and had deep organizational knowledge and extensive networks across all strata of the hospital. We saw this offer to join the project team as an ideal opportunity to develop our skills, to profile nursing, and to make a positive change. We left our nurse manager roles, and moved into the PHS project team as Green Lane Hospital representatives in 1998.

The Project Team

Two project teams were formed: one would implement CHiPs and the other PHS. Each team had a project manager reporting to a project director, who in turn reported to a steering committee. The IS department worked in an integration role while also assisting with the required networking and wiring.

The CHiPs team consisted of eight external developers, a training team consisting of four staff (working over both projects), and two hospital representatives, one from Women's Health and the other from Auckland Hospital. The hospital representatives were responsible for application configuration, testing, and troubleshooting, as well as their obligations as hospital representatives. Our PHS implementation team also had representatives from Children's Hospital and radiology, three PHS vendor staff, and a report writer. As the Green Lane representatives, our duties included not only the application configuration and "builds" in PHS, but also ensuring that reporting (organizational and ministerial) as well as any Green Lane–specific needs were met.

Because the Children's Hospital already had CHiPs, it was chosen as the project site for the initial PHS rollout. Until this time, ADHB was largely paper-based, so initially there was a significant lack of computer skills throughout the organization. Enormous effort went into training all staff.

The systems were then rolled out to the other three hospitals with both project teams and key IS staff assisting on go-live days. The project was completed within sixteen months, and the year 2000 came and went without a hitch. At the end of the project, the hospitals' management team realizing the importance of good communication links with the IS department, created new roles. These roles reported through the hospitals and were responsible for hospital representation on all things IT. They were also responsible for the ongoing configuration of the new applications. Again, as a result of having been on the project from the beginning, we were viewed by the ADHB as being in an ideal position to develop this role for Green Lane Hospital.

The Information Services Representative Role

As the use of computers within the health care setting has grown, so too has the demand for clinical IT systems and solutions. The demand is predominately driven by clinicians who require health funding reporting detail, research data collection, roster solutions, trends analyses (both national and international), and more.

In the early stages of computer technology options, the specialty and the IT departments would meet to collaborate on projects and to discuss clinical and service requirements. However, both parties had a fundamental lack of understanding of what the other did or could do. Consequently, systems were developed that did not meet clinical requirements. To address this gap, the initial IS representative role was created. Clinicians and hospital management recognized the need for a champion to liaise with the IT department, serve as interpreters for clinicians' input, and communicate their needs to the IT department. At Green Lane, the role reported directly to the hospital general manager. Several years later, the role was incorporated into the IT department. At this stage, the IS service representative role was formalized in a job description with an expanded scope. Job criteria included being an articulate communicator, being objective and assertive, and having proven experience in a health care discipline, clinical credibility, and corporate knowledge. We transitioned into these new roles based on our prior experience and performance in the system selection and on the implementation teams. We became nurse informaticians through a bit of serendipity and most certainly through on-the-job training.

New Hospital and Organizational Restructure

In 2003 a new hospital was opened. This nine-level, 710-bed acute care hospital encompasses 70,500 square meters (the biggest footprint in the southern hemisphere) and combined the acute services of Auckland, Green Lane, and National Women's Hospitals. It was built adjacent to (and linked with) Auckland Hospital and Children's Hospital. Construction was largely completed by mid-2003, and the majority of the services had transferred to their new locations by 2004.

Massive Changes to Organization

The amalgamation of hospitals, with their different processes and quirks, into one autonomous facility resulted in significant change and stress for all. Process redesign, with corresponding changes to roles, responsibilities, and reporting lines, coupled with the actual physical move, resulted in extensive staff redundancies.

A new project team, called the Change Program, was established primarily to take responsibility for the new processes. The Change Program team was divided into various subteams who were briefed to determine, align, and implement the best practice and procedures in all aspects of the hospital. This team was outside the IT department, and although they collaborated regarding changes to system configuration, there was little interaction between the two groups regarding process changes.

Accomplishments

Since 1998 ADHB has moved from an organization with very limited computing ability to one in which approximately 5,000 PCs are used. Computers and their applications are now an essential part of patient management. A variety of departmental and service management systems have been installed, e.g., maternity and theater systems. New functionality to CHiPs and new clinical information systems have also been installed. Nurses now use electronic whiteboards to manage patient allocations and condition codes, order diets, and more. Clinicians now view and approve laboratory results, radiology images, reports, and patient correspondence online, and with the introduction of the electronic discharge summary, general practitioners now get a patient summary e-mailed to them as their patient is discharged from the hospital. Patients' old clinical records are scanned and made available to authorized users anywhere in the organization, although current patient notes remain paper-based.

As nurse informaticians, we have assisted in the implementation of all of the previously discussed new systems. Having a comprehensive understanding of organizational work flow has been invaluable to ensuring the successful implementation of software.

Next Steps

The three health boards in the Auckland region no longer work in their separate operational worlds. They now collaborate before buying or adapting software whenever possible to achieve the maximum benefit for all. Regional collaboration means that the health of all Aucklanders can be improved by increased efficiency of communication and integration of systems across the region.

ADHB currently has three major IT projects to focus on in 2005. A new pharmacy system has been approved, and a new referrals system for both external and internal referrals is under way, as is a new clinical database project.

Lessons Learned

Throughout the last seven years, extensive and ongoing change has meant that numerous lessons have been learned. Our greatest challenge was not the systems, but rather the people involved in the change.

Although some embrace change, the unrelenting amount and scope of change that has been undertaken in recent years has brought with it confusion, resistance, and fear. The sheer speed of this change has been astounding and, for some, at times, overwhelming. Within the last seven years, ADHB has gone from being entirely paper-based to an almost entirely computer-based organization. Correspondingly, this has led to a lag in the skill set needed to accompany it.

Although lack of computer literacy remains an issue, the degree of literacy has improved dramatically. In 1998 the majority of staff at ADHB needed to be taught how to use a mouse and negotiate a Microsoft Windows environment. Although this is no longer the case, there remain pockets of the workforce who loath to take up computers. Sadly, nurses are one of these pockets. Although the younger generation of nurses, having used computers during their training, is now more computer savvy, the older generation is still somewhat reluctant to use them. The introduction of clinical systems is improving this situation, but we still have a long way to go.

People are the most important part of any IT project. Stakeholders and champions must be identified early to increase the chances of successful implementation. Communication with all parties must be continuous, honest, and open. All assumptions, misconceptions, and grievances should be aired and agreement over scope, priorities, and needs obtained. Project costing, especially in training and the ongoing post implementation support, should not be underestimated. For IT projects to be successful, a coordinated, paced approach must be undertaken, with change management and process redesign incorporated into the project.

Recommendations

The main pitfalls in IT projects happen around communication, clinical buy-in, process redesign, and stress management. Accurate and timely communication is essential and not just with the people immediately involved in the process but with the wider community as well. Working groups and reference groups are relatively easy to convene at the start of a project, although ongoing input and energy may be needed to ensure that they continue to feel part of the project. We found that, although the hospital newsletter is an important vehicle to spread project objectives, facts, and figures, the main positives (and negatives) of projects often were already known well before the newsletter was printed. Targeting the main communicators in each department to ensure they had the facts early prevented a lot of misconception and misunderstandings.

Gaining clinical buy-in and finding departmental clinical champions are necessary steps for any project to succeed. The project must be perceived to deliver benefits to the clinicians and/or patients. Without clinical buy-in and clinical champions within the departments, the project will falter and may fail. Process redesign needs to occur in conjunction with the roll out of the new application, not as an addendum to it. For any project to be successful, work flow issues, local specialty idiosyncrasies, and internal and external reporting paths need to be taken into account. These processes need to be adaptable enough that individual service quirks can be accommodated, if necessary, but standardized so that the process is transparent, logical, and improves service delivery. Lastly, the amount of stress that occurs for people when change is happening should never be underestimated. Stress can be significantly reduced with good, open communication and robust support mechanisms.

The nurse informatician, whatever the actual title, plays an important role in assessing risk, need, and symptoms of distress and in defining strategies and plans for effective interventions. This is basic nursing. But in the IT role, the nurse is assessing individuals, teams, departments, and the organization, and designing plans for interventions that range from one-on-one communications to organization-wide interventions. In this sense, in order for nurse informaticians to be effective guides and change agents within the organization, they must stay positive and optimistic throughout the duration of the implementation life cycle, which sometimes can be prolonged and bumpy.

CHAPTER 10

Developing National Health Information Policy: Contributions of an Informatics Nurse Specialist

By Judith J. Warren, PhD, RN, BC, FAAN, FACMI

National governments play a crucial role in determining health care policy and the types of information to be used in establishing such policy and in allocating resources. In the U.S., the Department of Health and Human Services (HHS) is the "government's principal agency for protecting the health of all Americans and providing essential human services, especially for those who are least able to help themselves."[1] Collecting, analyzing, and disseminating health-related information is a vital responsibility, which has led HHS to play a major role in setting standards for health data and parameters for health information privacy. HHS is also responsible for the development of regulations to implement health-related legislation; for example, the Health Insurance Portability and Accountability Act of 1996 (HIPAA) and the Medicare Prescription Drug, Improvement, and Modernization Act of 2003 (MMA), both of which have profound implications and requirements for the use of health data and information systems.

To assist HHS with these responsibilities, the National Committee on Vital and Health Statistics (NCVHS) was created as the "statutory public advisory body on health data, statistics, and national health information policy."[2] This highly influential committee consists of eighteen individuals from the private sector, sixteen who are appointed by the Secretary of HHS and two who are appointed by the U.S. Congress.[3] In January 2004, the Secretary of HHS appointed the first nurse to this committee.

This chapter offers reflections on the committee's influence in health care data and information systems, the development of skills necessary to qualify for an appointment to the committee, and the contributions of the nursing perspective.

As outlined in Table 10-1, NCVHS serves as a forum that brings together the public and private sectors over concerns regarding health data and information systems. The committee develops its agenda on the basis of requests that originate with HHS. All committee meetings are open to the public and are broadcast over the Internet. Although only invited individuals may provide testimony at the meeting, the committee provides open microphone time for others to present their perspectives, and the committee also accepts mailed comments. This public forum is critical to gaining consensus for the recommendations that NCVHS initiates. Through the consensus process, NCVHS supports the evolution of a shared national health information infrastructure that promotes the availability of valid, credible, timely, and comparable health data. This process of inclusion creates a foundation for successful work. Another function of the committee is to provide scientific and technical guidance concerning the use of health statistics, information systems, and related services.

To accomplish these tasks, only individuals with specific skill sets are selected to serve on the committee. Prospective members must have distinguished themselves in at least one of the following fields: health statistics, electronic interchange of health care information, privacy and security of electronic information, population-based public health, purchasing or financing of health care services, integrated computerized health information systems, health services research, consumer interests related to health information, health data standards, epidemiology, and the provision of health care services.

The committee has three subcommittees: Populations, Privacy and Confidentiality, and Standards and Security. Complementing the subcommittees' efforts are two work groups: Quality and National Healthcare Information Infrastructure.

Table 10-1. The Specific Functions of the NCVHS

- Monitor the nation's health data needs and current approaches to meeting those needs; identify emerging health data issues, including methodologies and technologies of information systems, databases, and networking that could improve the ability to meet those needs.

- Identify strategies and opportunities to achieve long-term consensus on common health data standards that will promote (i) the availability of valid, credible, and timely health information, and (ii) multiple uses of data collected once; recommend actions the federal government can take to promote such a consensus.

- Make recommendations regarding health terminology, definitions, classifications, and guidelines.

- Study and identify privacy, security, and access measures to protect individually identifiable health information in an environment of electronic networking and multiple uses of data.

- Identify strategies and opportunities for evolution from single-purpose, narrowly focused, categorical health data collection strategies to more multi-purpose, integrated, shared data collection strategies.

- Identify statistical, information system and network design issues bearing on health and health services data which are of national or international interest; identify strategies and opportunities to facilitate interoperability and networking.

- Advise the Department on health data collection needs and strategies; review and monitor the Department's data and information systems to identify needs, opportunities, and problems; consider the likely effects of emerging health information technologies on the Department's data and systems, and impact of the Department's information policies and systems on the development of emerging technologies.

- Stimulate the study of health data and information systems issues by other organizations and agencies, whenever possible.

- Review and comment on findings and proposals developed by other organizations and agencies with respect to health data and information systems and make recommendations for their adoption or implementation.

- Study the issues related to the adoption of uniform data standards for patient medical record information and the electronic interchange of such information.

Source: NCVHS Charter, 2004.[3]

The full committee meets approximately four times a year, whereas the subcommittees and work groups meet independently. Members self-select to serve on the subcommittees and to participate in the work groups on the basis of their expertise and interests.

Because NCVHS has an enormous impact on health care programs and policies in the U.S., many individuals and organizations seek to become members. However, there is no representation for such major organizations as the American Medical Association (AMA), the American Nurses Association (ANA), or the American Medical Informatics Association (AMIA). The charge of NCVHS is critical and requires high levels of expertise; therefore, individuals are selected without regard to associated organizations.

Committee members are often asked, "How did you get chosen for appointment by the committee?" To be selected, an individual must possess not only the necessary skills and expertise but also a reputation for personal integrity and leadership. Often, the next question then is, "What can I do to gain the required expertise and reputation to become an appointee?" The following case study of the first nurse member of NCVHS illustrates how one might accomplish this goal.

An Informatics Nurse's Path to
Becoming a National Health Policy Advisor

Informatics nurses are uniquely positioned in health care. They usually begin their careers as staff nurses, thus becoming experts on the experiences and needs of patients, the flow of work and information within organizations, and the collaboration required to work effectively on multidisciplinary teams. Later, they develop new skills in informatics and systems thinking. Informatics nurses master data analysis, data quality, data retrieval, data sharing, and logical querying. They learn how data entered once can be used many times on behalf of patients, the health care team, and the health care organization. Knowledge and skills are acquired on the job, through continuing education, and in graduate programs.

Informatics Expertise

I gained my initial expertise by serving on a medical records' committee and by designing documentation forms. Later, I was co-chair of an electronic health record (EHR) implementation team, which developed and executed a multidisciplinary problem list. I then taught nursing informatics (NI) as a faculty member at a state university. Although, through this experience, I earned recognition as a local expert, I did not yet have enough perspective to function as a national policy advisor.

To gain that perspective, i.e., learn about the "big picture" issues, trends, and innovations, I became active in two national professional organizations, the ANA and AMIA. Both have major initiatives and efforts focused on national policies and regulations concerning health data and information systems.

In the ANA, I served on the Steering Committee for Databases Supporting Nursing Practice, and, as chair, I helped the committee to evolve into the Committee for Nursing Practice Information Infrastructure. Working with leaders in the field, participating in collaborative projects, and representing the ANA perspective, I began to understand the national requirements of health care information and the role of nursing in that domain. I also honed my skills in public speaking, leadership, negotiation, and teamwork.

In AMIA, I volunteered for several projects of the Nursing Informatics Working Group (NIWG). Again, I had opportunities to refine my informatics and leadership skills and to build my reputation. As a result, I was elected to the board of directors, through which I learned considerably more about the issues and concerns of health care informatics, not just those of NI. I also quickly realized that my role was one of advocacy for the patient and the clinician.

My involvement in both of these organizations helped to familiarize me with nursing and informatics issues at the national level. By investing in myself—participating in the organizations and volunteering for projects—I gained expertise in identifying problems and issues, articulating their essentials, and leading efforts to find solutions. I also acquired a national reputation for my informatics expertise and leadership.

But was I ready to serve as a national health policy advisor? The answer was "no."

Standards Development Expertise

Because a key function of NCVHS is to recommend health data standards, knowledge, and expertise in developing health care informatics standards is required of some prospective NCVHS members. This expertise is sought when identifying potential appointees because a key function of NCVHS is to recommend health data standards. Standards are needed to promote interoperability of data and information and to ensure privacy, confidentiality, and security. In the past, the committee has recommended standards for transactionss[4] and messages.[5,6] It monitors these and other standards to guarantee that they meet user requirements.[7,8] It is essential that NCVHS members know not only how standards are developed and adopted but also their scopes and domains, so that they can determine which standards are ready for widespread adoption or for inclusion in federal regulations. Another function of NCVHS is to facilitate cooperation between various standards development organizations, so members may also understand how standards development organizations relate to each other.

My expertise in standards development was acquired through working with Health Level Seven (HL7). First, I had to gain technical skills in information modeling, because the evolution of the Reference Information Model—the basis for HL7 message standards—is derived from object modeling and specifies the use of Unified Modeling Language. As I studied the Reference Information Model, I learned more about information models and how an abstract model can assist one in understanding the complexity of health care information. I also gained confidence in working with people from different backgrounds and perspectives—clinicians, information technologists, as well as individuals from other countries—to achieve the kind of understanding and consensus that leads to successful standards formation. Finally, I developed the knowledge and skills for facilitating work within HL7, becoming one of the few nurses to fill the role of co-chair on a technical committee. I learned how to express information in messages in a way that the perspectives of all members of the health care team were included and to ensure that quality patient care was delivered.

But was all of that enough expertise to function as a national health policy advisor? The answer was "no."

Terminology Development Expertise

Another important area of knowledge and expertise sought by NCVHS has to do with the development of health care terminologies, because a key function of NCVHS is to recommend code sets, or standardized terminologies. Both HIPAA and MMA have requirements for specifying code sets in legislation and regulations. NCVHS members must know the leading terminologies that are in use and understand how the characteristics of good terminology apply to each.[9] As with standards, members must learn not only how terminologies are developed and adopted but also their scopes and domains as well so they can determine which terminologies are ready for widespread adoption or for inclusion in federal regulations. They must also understand how different terminologies relate to each other, so that they can facilitate cooperation between terminology developers. Additionally, they must grasp the interrelationships between health care informatics standards and standardized terminologies.

Three activities helped me to acquire expertise in terminology development. Early in my career, I was introduced to the North American Nursing Diagnosis Association (NANDA), the nursing diagnoses system for care planning.[10,11] I learned how to use the NANDA diagnoses to document the accountability of nurses and the contributions of nursing to patient care.[12] After attending a NANDA conference, I volunteered to be a member of the Taxonomy Committee. I subsequently served on the board of directors and as president of NANDA. In these roles, I presented papers and consulted with various people and organizations. These activities improved my speaking skills and further enhanced my reputation as an expert in nursing languages. No other experience has better helped in my understanding of the nature and uniqueness of nursing, and it has contributed to all my other activities. It has also enabled me to articulate my understanding of others, especially non-nurses. This is the power of language!

Next, I served as the ANA liaison to the Systematized Nomenclature of Medicine (SNOMED®) international editorial board.[13] This required me to learn new technical skills to represent nursing in the development of a multidisciplinary terminology optimized for use in an EHR.[14] Areas that I mastered included terminology modeling; knowledge representation and concept coding approaches; multiaxial, hierarchical, and multiple inheritances structures; semantics and syntax; and searching strategies. As I assisted in integrating more nursing content into the SNOMED® Clinical Terms (CT), I learned how to structure knowledge and to make concepts less ambiguous, so that any health care discipline could use the terminology to represent patient data. I also gained an understanding of the relationships among concepts used in health care and of the ways that metaconcepts, such as diagnoses, procedures, findings, and goals, are represented. We made the conscious decision to create SNOMED® CT as a patient-centered terminology, not a discipline-centered one.

Finally, I participated in a research team that tested the International Standards Organization terminology model used for nursing diagnoses.[15] This study looked at both informatics standards and standardized terminologies. The intersections between the Reference Information Model and International Standards Organization terminology models, informatics standards, and terminologies became explicit and increased my understanding of how they worked together to provide interoperability for health care data.

But was this enough expertise to function as a national health policy advisor? The answer was "no."

Leadership Expertise

Strong leadership expertise is required to distinguish yourself in any of the following fields: health statistics, electronic interchange of health care information, privacy and security of electronic information, population-based public health, purchasing or financing health care services, integrated computerized health information systems, health services research, consumer interests in health information, health data standards, epidemiology, and the provision of health services. To be recognized and to function at the national level, you must develop leadership skills in four domains.

First, you must be able to work in and lead multidisciplinary teams. This requires a deep understanding and valuing of your voice and the voices of others. This ability to know a voice requires recognition of different perspectives and cultures. You must also know how what you do relates to what other team members do, and you must be able to express the relationships of "doing" in a way that demonstrates why the team cannot succeed without all of its members. The most important skill is the ability to listen to others as they articulate their perspectives. Additionally, you must be able to validate your understanding of what others have communicated about their perspectives and work to create win-win solutions. This strategy may necessitate creating space in the solution for your own perspective because a good solution must contain all voices of the team. The team may need help in recognizing the need for all voices and in knowing when all voices are present.

Second, your goal of participating in health policy and regulation development at the national level must be focused on enhancing patient care, not nursing care. You must advocate for patients, not nurses. This may sound odd, but, in fact, the nursing perspective often is one of patient advocacy. Nursing care contributes to positive patient outcomes and should only be discussed in those terms. Discipline-specific needs should be discussed only when talking about staffing issues. This does not mean you should abandon supporting nursing; it simply means that the focus should be on the patient. Discussions about nursing should occur in professional venues.

Third, you need strong interpersonal skills and a high level of personal integrity. The importance of your ability to get along well with others and to behave in a socially acceptable way cannot be overemphasized. When joining a new team, determine the formal and informal rules of behavior. Do not be so eager to demonstrate your knowledge that you inadvertently reveal a lack of preparedness (such as not having read the right documents or not knowing how documents were developed) or that you imply that the work of the team was inferior (because it did not have the benefit of your brilliance in contributing to prior work). First and foremost, be courteous and show respect for others. Remember too, that your reputation contributed to your selection. Continue to behave with the highest integrity, thereby engendering and maintaining trust.

Finally, verbal and nonverbal communication skills are invaluable. Learn to write well. Master the art of summarization and synthesis of complex topics. Learn to speak well. Speak positively; negative messages reflect back on you. Dress for success. Above all, send the right message, and send it in the right way.

But is that enough expertise to function as a national health policy advisor? The answer is finally "yes."

Serving on the NCVHS

Serving on the NCVHS has been a tremendous experience. I have had an opportunity to influence health care policy and HHS regulations that are designed to implement federal legislation. I chose to become a member of the subcommittee on Standards and Security as my skills were best suited for its work.[16]

Most of the work in 2004 has concerned making recommendations for implementing e-prescribing. Although the MMA has specified standards and code sets for physicians engaging in e-prescribing, I was able to influence a change in wording (from *physician* to *prescriber*) in the legislation. I could not have done this had I not understood my voice and the voices of other team members. This effort became a win-win solution and was adopted by HHS.

Participating in policy development at the national level requires that you "sit at the table." This phrase hearkens back to the days of monarchies, when being invited to sit at the king's table meant you were able to engage in conversation with both him and his advisors, thus having the chance to influence royal decrees that guided government actions. Not much has changed since that time, although the king has been replaced with executives of government agencies and national advisory committees. For the voice of nursing to be heard, nurses also need a seat "at the table." Participation is by invitation only and is based on whether an individual (not a group or organization) has valuable expertise, a reputation of past performance in similar groups, and the ability to "play" well with others.

You can develop that expertise and reputation by investing in yourself and volunteering to work on projects that will challenge you. To continue the "at the table" metaphor: show up, display good table manners, know how to use the knife and fork, refrain from attacking or name-calling, acknowledge your host—and *no whining!*

This is an exciting time to be in health care informatics. We have an opportunity to help create a health care information system that will reduce medical errors and support quality patient care. But to make a difference, you must have knowledge, skills, and an opportunity to influence innovation and change. We have such an opportunity—but only when we, as individuals, are in a position to contribute and collaborate. We must be "at the table."

References

1. U.S. Department of Health and Human Services. What we do. Available at: http://www.hhs.gov/about/whatwedo.html. Accessed February 28, 2005.
2. National Committee on Vital and Health Statistics. Available at: http://www.ncvhs.hhs.gov. Accessed February 28, 2005.
3. National Committee on Vital and Health Statistics. Charter 2004. Available at: http://www.ncvhs.hhs.gov/charter06.pdf. Accessed February 28, 2005.
4. Accredited Standards Committee X12. 2004. Available at: http://www.x12.org. Accessed February 28, 2005.
5. Health Level Seven. 1997. Available at: http://www.hl7.org. Accessed February 28, 2005.
6. National Council for Prescription Drug Programs. 1977. Available at: http://www.ncpdp.org. Accessed February 28, 2005.
7. International Organization for Standardization. 1946. Available at: http://www.iso.ch. Accessed February 28, 2005.
8. ASTM International. 1996. Available at: http://www.astm.org. Accessed February 28, 2005.
9. Cimino JJ. Desiderata for controlled medical vocabularies in the twenty-first century. *Methods Inf Med.* 1998;37:394-403.
10. NANDA International. 2005. Available at: http://www.nanda.org. Accessed February 28, 2005.
11. NANDA International. *Nursing Diagnoses: Definitions and Classification, 2005-2006.* Philadelphia: NANDA; 2005.
12. Warren JJ. Accountability and nursing diagnosis. *J Nurs Adm.* 1983;13:3437.
13. SNOMED International. 2004. Available at: http://www.snomed.org. Accessed February 28, 2005.
14. Henry SB, Warren JJ, Lange L, Button P. A review of major nursing vocabularies and the extent to which they have the characteristics required for implementation in computer-based systems. *J Am Med Inf Assn.* 1998;5:321-328.
15. Bakken S, Warren JJ, Lundberg C, et al. An evaluation of the usefulness of two terminology models for integrating nursing diagnosis concepts into SNOMED Clinical Terms. *Int J Med Inform.* 2002; 68:71-77.
16. National Committee on Vital and Health Statistics, Subcommittee on Standards and Security. 2004. Available at: http://www.ncvhs.hhs.gov/sssmemb.htm. Accessed February 28, 2005.

CHAPTER 11

Nurses in IT Policy: Belgium's Information Communication Technology Strategies

By Eric Vande Walle, MS, BN, BInformatics; Marc Glorieux, MSc, RN; and Walter Sermeus, PhD, RN

In the mid-1980s, a few nursing pioneers in Belgium and the Netherlands took the initiative to organize Nursing Informatics Conferences.[1] Names that are indelibly connected with these conferences include Denis Vandewal, Tonny Gypen, Elly Pluyter-Wenting, Georges Evers, Josette Jones-Wouters, and Arie Hasman, all who have played important roles in the development of nursing informatics (NI) in the International Medical Informatics Association (IMIA) and other organizations. The yearly conferences contributed significantly to nurses' participation in the development of hospital information systems in Flanders and the Netherlands. The conferences initiated the new role of "systems nurse," which was later renamed "information systems nurse" and then "informatics nurse." Because automating the information and data flow around the primary care process was so complex, hospitals needed nurses who had informatics degrees. The last of these conferences occurred in 1990. Since then, various organizations have continued the initiatives started by these early pioneers. This case study provides an overview of the initiatives and policies developed by the professional nursing associations, universities, and government.

Professional Nursing Organization Initiatives

The professional nursing organizations in Belgium (representing both the Dutch and French speaking regions) took the initiative to enhance the role of nurses using information and communication technologies. In the Dutch speaking region, the National Professional Association of Catholic Flemish Nurses and Midwives (NVKVV) began offering informatics courses in 1989 and established a working group on nursing informatics (NI) in 1992. In the French speaking region, nursing organizations supported an independent initiative called SIXI (Soins Infirmiers & Informatique; see its Web site, www.sixi.be) in 1987. This case study focuses on the Dutch speaking initiatives, which have addressed training and education, research, and practical support.

Training and Education

Since 1989, the Continuing Education Centre of the NVKVV organized an advanced education program for informatics nurses. This program originally concentrated on nursing, system development, and the use of informatics technology to manage the care process. Today's training consists of a two-year study certificate program that covers theory about patient records; coaching methods for change processes communication; analysis and development techniques; market research; security (technology and policy); legal issues; contract negotiation; privacy legislation; professional confidentiality and privacy; data management; standards in health care; statistics; and epidemiology. The last semester consists of an internship with a company or institution. After obtaining the certificate, an informatics nurse has the knowledge and skills required to support a nursing department's care process automation policy. The program also aims to build bridges between the end user and the informatics department or software supplier. Since its start, 86 participants have graduated. Table 11-1 lists the kinds of positions filled by the 2005 informatics nurse graduates. They are working in various domains where their responsibilities may include the following:

1. Coordinating between internal and external developers/suppliers
2. Implementating applications for electronic scheduling, appointment planning, electronic nursing/patient records, and medication management (on the ward/in the pharmacy)
3. Supporting tasks, including help desk, maintenance of in-house applications, and support of groupware

Research

To increase the limited number of nursing applications available, in 1994 the NVKVV's Working Group of Informatics Nurses developed a list of requirements for automating the primary patient care process. It was titled "Technical Specifications of a Comprehensive Nursing Information System."[2] All the Dutch speaking hospitals were invited to participate in this project. Some forty participants from twenty-three Flemish hospitals helped to write the plan. They formulated four main domains of the project, with a separate project group for each: nursing records, procedure book,[3] medication management, and personnel planning. The working group's subsequent report contained both the clinical and the technical specifications of a comprehensive nursing information system.[4] Since its release, several software companies started developing nursing care applications, with a few providers basing their work on the requirements outlined in this document.

In 2000, the Working Group of Informatics Nurses received a two-year research grant from the Belgium federal government to develop a minimal electronic nursing record to address the need for standardization. An increasing number of hospitals, as they started working with several software suppliers, confronted difficulties transferring data from one application to another, e.g., between software for intensive care and that used as a medical record system, and then to yet another program for nurses. Remarkably, these applications were mostly stand-alone and incompatible with one another, and thus offered little of the surplus value of an automated electronic health record (EHR). Hospitals felt the absence of standards even more sharply during transfers of patients from one health care sector to another. The working group study aimed to spur the development of a usable exchange data set for electronic communication between nurses of different sectors. The data set outlined a general framework for the development of a comprehensive electronic nursing patient record.[5] As a result of the study, a minimal electronic nursing record became the common denominator for nursing records in acute care hospitals, psychiatric hospitals, homes for the aged, and in community nursing settings (see Figure 11-1).

A new project originated from this study, which was also financed by the Belgium federal authorities. From the start, the Belgian NI community envisaged a far-reaching electronic information exchange among nurses of different health care departments. It would also refine and complete the data set from the first project, the minimal electronic nursing record. This resulted in the Electronic Nursing Records Communication (ENRC) in 2002,[6] a data set that is both an admission document for one department and a discharge document for another (see Figure 11-2).

Table 11-1. Roles Taken by Graduates of the Advanced Education Program for Informatics Nurses in 2005 (n = 22)

	Frequency	Percentage
Informatics Nurse	12	54.55
Head Nurse	3	13.64
Nursing Director	2	9.09
Nurse	2	9.09
Other	2	9.09
Project Assistant	1	4.54
Total	22	100.00

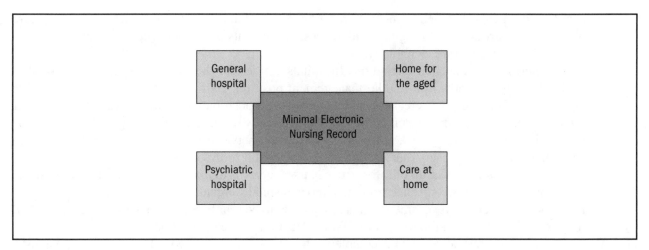

Figure 11-1. *Health Care Sectors Covered by the MENR.*

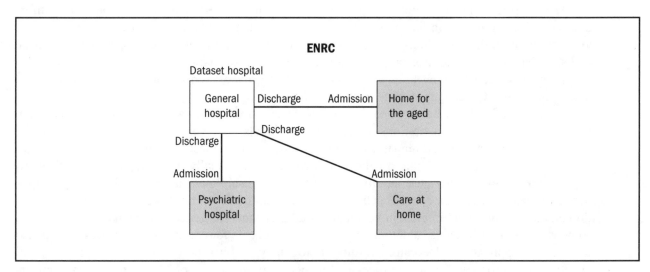

Figure 11-2. *Structure of the Electronic Nursing Records Communications (ENRC).*

Test results showed that nurses were reasonably satisfied with the workability and surplus value of the ENRC. However, although the information sender (the general hospital) was also usually quite satisfied with the discharge form, the receiver was usually less satisfied with the received document. The research group learned that it must integrate the expectations and needs of the receivers when setting up a discharge document, whether for the receiving department or sector.

The Belgium government also asked the research group to test the ENRC's compatibility with the federal quality assurance requirements (BIOMED). One priority was to improve the quality of nursing care documentation for hospitalizations. The project showed that ENRC, by providing good admission and discharge data, improved the quality of nursing assessment data and therefore enhanced the quality of the entire nursing record. To an important degree, the ENRC has standardized nursing records and electronic communication across all departments. What remains is for the Belgium federal government to resolve the technical details, e.g., software requirements, and to establish security policies for working with ENRC.

Support to Practice

Since 1995, the Working Group of Informatics Nurses has organized a yearly conference on automation and health care, providing a forum for the exchange of experiences with automation projects. Hospital experts share their efforts to develop patient records within the general framework of their hospital's information system. Homes for the aged, psychiatric institutions, and community care facilities also participate. During the conferences, participants discuss concepts, models, and existing software and hardware technology.

An increasing number of institutions (hospitals, homes for the aged, etc.) hire an informatics nurse who usually works in a middle management position, coordinating the automation of care applications. Other hospitals create a middle management position within the nursing department or in the informatics department, sometimes reporting directly to the general manager. Regardless, the informatics nurse's primary task is to serve as a liaison between the information technology (IT) department and the end users (nurses, doctors, allied health professionals).

One of the Working Group of Informatics Nurses' goals is to make the role of informatics nurse a recognized role that becomes incorporated into a hospital's organizational chart. The role of informatics nurse must meet government standards in order to be reimbursed. The working group worked in close cooperation with the Ministry of Public Health to develop a proposal for regulation.

The role of informatics nurse is complementary to the role of "medical informatics specialist," which has a legal basis in Belgian hospitals. In this context, the informatics nurse oversees the integration of nursing records into the hospital information system.

The informatics nurse supports the general policy of the health care institution concerning information and communication technology (ICT). She or he supports operational processes and provides strategic information; encourages communication among the end users, computer scientists, and suppliers involved; advises on policy concerning ICT projects; outlines adequate ICT training programs; gives advice about ICT security policy in the broadest sense; and is involved in contract negotiations and ICT budget management.

The effect of ICTs on Belgian health care varies according to the size and characteristics of each institution. For instance, institutions for elderly individuals have very minimal automation of the care process. Apart from administrative applications, most of these institutions have a software package for care planning and medication management, usually from a software company. Psychiatric hospitals widely use automation, with a multidisciplinary approach. The multidisciplinary automated patient record reflects this attitude. In community nursing we see advanced automation and also widespread interest in personal digital assistants. In general hospitals, the situation is somewhat different. They use automation on quite a large scale for administrative processes and also for medical applications (laboratory results, radiography, result server), usually from commercial vendors. But automation for care processes (medical and nursing records) is limited. Only university hospitals have succeeded in implementing care applications on a large scale, usually by developing their own applications.

Unfortunately, the nursing record is not often the first priority, and consequently it succeeds only with great difficulty or not at all. In the nonteaching acute care hospitals, the development of automated care applications often leads to "island automation." Only a limited number of hospitals succeed in automating the care process by developing their own system, or by implementing IT systems for supporting patient care throughout the whole institution with private means.

Most software suppliers still lack a broad array of nursing applications, with the exception of the Administratief Centrum Caritas (ACC). When the Working Group of Nursing Informatics presented its requirement package in 1994, this company was the first to show its willingness to develop the different applications for nurses in several institutions. The electronic nursing record, medication and appointment management modules, and procedure book are now operational in several institutions.

The Working Group of Informatics Nurses, inspired by its own information requirement package and by the list of demands from the federal working group's "nursing record" (1996), established criteria for a more objective evaluation of software. The criteria feature detailed questions about the available functions of software packages for nursing units, e.g., nurse management and input of patient administration data, procedure book, nursing care record, case history and care planning, medication management, paramedic records, and assessment and treatment planning.

University Initiatives

Of all the Belgian universities, the Catholic University of Leuven has always played the most prominent role in developing NI in Belgium. The NIC conferences at the end of the 1980s started as a joint initiative of the Catholic University of Leuven and the University of Maastricht. Later, the Working Group of Informatics Nurses and the professional nursing associations took over the initiative.

The research at the Catholic University of Leuven mainly focused on the development of the nursing minimum data set and on international projects, such as TELENURSE,[7] NIGHTINGALE[8] and WISECARE,[9] funded by the European Union (EU) in its fourth framework program (1994–1998). These projects are described in detail below.

TELENURSE[7] started as a concerted action on "telematics" (an EU-term denoting the combination of telecommunications and informatics) for nursing in November 1994 (then called TELENURSING), led by Mrs. R. Mortensen from the Danish Institute of Health and Nursing Research. It resulted in the EU-funded project TELENURSE in 1996. The aim was to promote an international classification for nursing practice (ICNP) and a clinical nursing minimum data set (NMDS) in electronic health care records to counter the lack of uniform comparative descriptive data on hospital nursing and its cost effectiveness. The main role of the Catholic University of Leuven was to develop the list of requirements for the NMDS.

NIGHTINGALE[8] is the acronym for Nursing Informatics, Generic High Level Training in Informatics for Nurses, General Applications for Learning and Education, an EU-funded project led by Professor J. Mantas, University of Athens. NIGHTINGALE seeks to boost telematics training for nurses in Europe through the use of information systems and in coordination with other health sector training initiatives. A professional nursing users group advised on presenting the project at workshops and conferences. NIGHTINGALE eventually produced courseware material, a multimedia software package, and an NI handbook.

WISECARE[9] was the acronym for Workflow Information Systems for European Nursing Care. The EU provided funding from 1997 until 1999, and the Catholic University of Leuven led the project. The goal was to systematically exploit clinical nursing data stored in EHRs for clinical and resource management to shift from isolated knowledge to knowledge sharing for the purpose of improving patient care. The project focused on symptom management for oncology patients across Europe. It continued as WISECARE+, by support of the Royal Marsden Hospital and the European Oncology Nursing Society. Professor N. Kearney, University of Stirling, now leads the project.

The main NI research effort is a development of the Belgian nursing minimum data set (B-NMDS) (1985–2004). It defines a nursing minimum data registration as "systematic registration of the smallest number possible of unequivocally coded data, with respect to or for the purpose of nursing practice, making information available to the largest group possible of users according to a broad range of information requirements."[10]

The registration in Belgium is regulated by the "Royal Decree of 14 August 1987 concerning the rules according to which certain statistical data items must be communicated to the Minister of Public Health." This Royal Decree stipulates that from 1988, all general hospitals are legally bound to register these data items and hand them to the authorities.

This registration of an NMDS includes five kinds of data: general data about the institution, patient data, a specific set of twenty-three nursing care interventions, data on activities of daily living, and nursing staff data. Registration takes place in all Belgian general hospitals for all hospitalized patients four times a year during a fifteen-day period (the first fifteen days of March, June, September, and December). From 1988 to 2005, a unique representative sample of twenty million nursing records from Belgian hospitals was collected. The data set is mainly used to calculate the yearly hospital budget since 1994. Approximately 15 percent of the budgets for surgical, medical, pediatric, and intensive care departments is based on the B-NMDS.

It is obvious that the B-NMDS, which dates back to 1985, needs updating. Health care, and more specifically nursing care, changed during those years. New techniques and procedures have been introduced, with a great emphasis on evidence-based nursing care and quality indicators. The role of nurse now includes patient teacher/adviser/counselor to help the patient become independent as quickly and easily as possible. Health care organizations now take a more process-oriented, integrated, interdependent, cross-institutional care pathway approach. Nursing terminology and classification systems have developed internationally. In various other countries, NMDSs have been introduced.

On July 1, 2002, the Belgian Ministry of Social Affairs, Public Health, and Environment commissioned two universities (the Catholic University of Leuven and the University of Liège) to update the B-NMDS.[11] The plan is for the B-NMDS-2 to be operational by 2007.

Informatics Education

Between 1994 and 1995 ERASMUS, an EU-initiative for collaborating universities in Europe, worked with the University of Athens to offer a master's course in Health Informatics, organized by the University of Athens, which included the topic of NI. Since 2004, the master's degree in Healthcare Management and Policy at the Catholic University of Leuven offers a major in health care informatics. The Universities of Brussels, Ghent, and Antwerp also offer this major.

Belgian Government Initiatives

Obviously, the government has played a crucial role in the development of NI in Belgium. Mrs. A. Simoens-Desmet, Belgium's top nursing officer for more than 20 years, contributed greatly to these achievements.

In 1999, the government launched the Telematics Standardisation Commission for Health Care[12] to advise the Minister of Public Health on issues about telematics in health care. Nurses are members of this commission. Professor F. Roger-France was president of the Commission from 1999 until 2004, when Professor G. De Moor succeeded him. The Commission enacted several initiatives for a comprehensive policy in health care telematics, including

1. In 1999, regulatory requirements for the medical record were established (RD May 3, 1999).
2. In 2001, an electronic signature and certification law was passed (Law July 9, 2001).
3. Also in 2001, a general structure for the electronic exchange of health care data was approved.
4. In 2002, accreditation of software requirements for general practitioners was established.

The Commission has also launched several research projects, including

- To provide recommendations and quality criteria for hospital information systems
- To implement Kind Messages for Electronic Health Care Record Belgian Implementation Standard
- To develop a European emergency health card
- To launch regional health care networks (the real future of health care informatics and telematics).
- To approve ENRC
- To develop criteria for safe health on the World Wide Web
- To finance projects to enhance communication between general practitioners and hospitals (forty-six projects in 2003)

Conclusions

The development of NI in Belgium is a result of the unique collaboration among government, professional nursing organizations, and universities. The government has invested large sums in the development of nursing minimum data sets, EHRs, communication standards, etc. The universities have been reliable partners in conducting this research and in advising government, health care professionals, and health care institutions on how to realize change. The professional nursing organizations offer training, education, and support to guide implementation in the various health care settings. All of the Belgian NI pioneers can be proud of how much their initiatives have achieved.

References

1. Vande Walle E. Verpleegkunde en informatica: historiek. *Verpleegkunde & Vroedkunde zakboekje.* Diegem: Kluwer Editorial; 2000: 31-40.

2. Maertens R, Goossens M, Gadeyne P, et al. Informatiebehoeftenpakket voor een geautomatiseerd verpleegkundig informatiesysteem. *Project automatisering Vlaamse ziekenhuizen.* Brussels; 1994.

3. Vande Walle E. The computerized procedure book: a tool for nursing practice. How to link with patient records? In: *Proceedings of the European Health Records Conference.* Maastricht; 1995.

4. Vande Walle E, Gadeyne P, Ven T. Ziekenhuisinformatiesystemen. *Verpleegkunde & Vroedkunde zakboekje.* Diegem; Kluwer Editorial, themagedeelte; 2000:131-178.

5. Vande Walle E, Glorieux M. *Minimale dataset elektronisch verpleegdossier.* 2001. Available at: http://www.health.fgov.be/telematics/symposium/v2000.

6. Werkgroep informatiesysteemverpleegkundigen. *Het ENRC: Electronic Nursing Records Communication.* 2002. Available at:
   http://www.health.fgov.be/telematics/symposium/v2001,
   http://www.health.fgov.be/telematics/symposium/v2002,
   http://www.health.fgov.be/telematics/symposium/v2003,
   and http://www.health.fgov.be/telematics/enrc.

7. Mortensen R. ed. *Telenurse in Europe.* Amsterdam: IOS-Press; 1997.

8. Mantas J, Hasman A. *Handbook Nursing Informatics.* Amsterdam: IOS-Press; 2002.

9. Sermeus W, Kearney N, Kinnunen J, et al., eds. *WISE-CARE Workflow Information Systems for European Nursing Care.* Amsterdam: IOS-Press; 2000.

10. Sermeus W, Delesie L, Van Landuyt J, et al. *The Nursing Minimum Data Set in Belgium: A Basic Tool for Tomorrow's Health Care Management.* Brussels/Leuven: Ministerie van Volksgezondheid en Leefmilieu & Centrum voor Ziekenhuiswetenschap; 1994.

11. Sermeus W, Van den Heede K, Michiels D, et al. Revising the Belgian Nursing Minimum Dataset: from concept to implementation. *Intl J Med Info.* In press.

12. Health Telematics Commission. Available at: http://www.health.fgov.be/telematics/. Accessed April 17, 2005.

CHAPTER 12

Nursing Informatics Roles within the Veterans Health Administration Experience

By Oyweda Moorer, MSN candidate, RN, BC, and Cathy Rick, MSN, RN, CNAA, FACHE

Along with privilege comes pride in working for the largest integrated health care system in the United States of America. The Department of Veterans Affairs (VA) has been serving our nation's heroes since 1862. President Abraham Lincoln's charge to the VA gave rise to our mission: "To Serve Those Who Have Borne the Battle and Their Widows and Orphans." The Veterans Health Administration (VHA) of the VA was authorized in 1930 to provide health care to those who have defended our country's freedom.[1] Today more than six million veterans are enrolled for VHA care, and of these, more than four million currently receive VHA care. Today, the VHA comprises 158 medical centers, 858 community-based clinics, 133 nursing home care centers, and home care programs with an average daily census of more than 17,000. The VHA expects the number of participants in the home care program to double by 2006.[2]

The VHA integrated health care system spans across each U.S. state and territory. Twenty-two Veterans Integrated Service Networks (VISN) provide regional management and service coordination to veterans. Each VISN develops appropriate regional initiatives that comply with national strategic goals and ensure organizational stewardship with a system wide perspective.[2]

The 58,000 VHA nurses are the backbone of the VA health care team, influencing every aspect of patient care. The interdisciplinary health care team relies on nursing staff to provide expert assessment, care planning and coordination, disease management, health promotion and maintenance, and treatment of complex acute and chronic conditions. VA nurses take pride in developing, testing, and implementing innovative practices to ensure safe, effective, and efficient quality care. This chapter highlights the VA's innovations in information systems, in particular the contributions of nursing informaticians.

The role of nurse informatician evolved over a twenty-year period at the VHA, starting as a liaison to the informatics departments at local facilities. Today, the VHA nurse informatician is a practicing expert engaged in software and systems design, development, and implementation. Fueled by the increasing use of new clinical technologies, the role of VHA nurses with information technology (IT) responsibilities changed in response, becoming more central to the VHA IT program's success. VHA was the first health care system to acknowledge the nursing informatician role in a professional practice model. This role in VHA was developed in the mid-1980s and now, some 20 years later, physicians and staff wonder how they could possibly function without the support. In addition to providing support to VA clinicians, VHA nurse informaticians contribute to academic programs as instructors and preceptors, helping to create the next generation of nurse informaticians.

The Evolution of IT at the VA

Before the 1980s, IT focused on capturing and managing health care business processes. When the VHA implemented the Decentralized Hospital Computer Program (DHCP) in the early 1980s, it reflected a new focus on clinical applications. By the mid-1990s, DHCP became known as the Veteran's Health Information Systems and Technology (VistA). The VistA system consists of more than ninety separate business operations including health data systems for registration, enrollment, and eligibility; provider systems; management and financial systems; and education systems.[1] Two main features of VistA are the Computerized Patient Record System (CPRS) and the Bar Code Medication Administration System (BCMA). Both facilitate improvement in health care delivery, patient outcomes, and patient safety. VistA has sparked national and international interest; numerous other health care organizations in the U.S. and abroad have adopted it.

CPRS

The VHA implemented CPRS in the mid-1990s. Unlike earlier VHA applications, CPRS is a patient-centered rather than a department-centered system. It makes patient information more accessible across settings and among clinicians and supports clinical work processes, record access, and patient safety. The application supports and integrates an array of programs e.g., order entry, digital imaging, laboratory orders/results, progress notes, and more (see Figure 12-1). A key aspect to the CPRS is its ability to develop templates when needed to meet patient care needs that are unique or specific to a particular facility or program. Another key feature is its ability to alert clinicians to a number of patient care needs e.g., immunizations, routine laboratory tests, patient risks, and clinical guidelines used in performance improvement. Nurse informaticians played a pivotal role in its implementation and supported clinical staff by helping to develop localized templates.[3]

BCMA

The VHA implemented BCMA during the fall of 1999 and all of 2000. The computerized system, as shown in Figure 12-2, ensures that patients receive the correct medication in the correct dose at the correct time and visually alerts staff when proper parameters are not met. A nurse uses a bar code

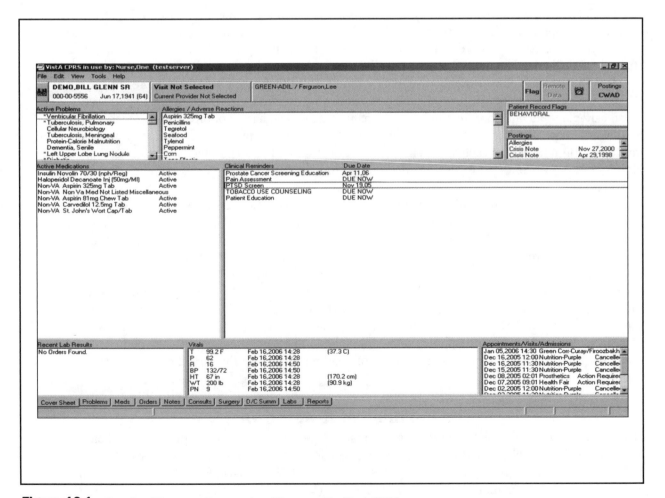

Figure 12-1. *Sample of Programs Supported and Integrated by VistA CPRS.*

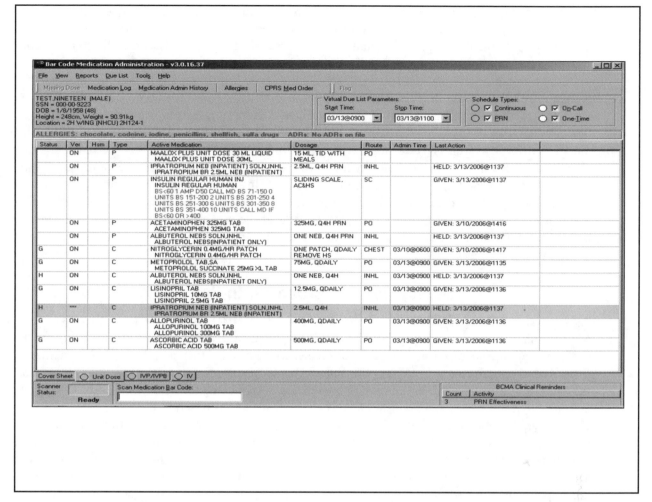

Figure 12-2. *BCMA Screen Overview: Unit Dose Tab.*

scanner to identify patients by their bar-coded identity bracelet before scanning the bar code label on their medications. As each patient's wristband and medication is scanned, BCMA validates the medication and updates the medication administration history. The BCMA system is directly tied to the order entry and pharmacy applications. The bar code scanners are wireless, and the electronic record, designed in a similar format as a paper medication administration record, sits on a laptop computer attached to a medication cart.[4]

The Future of VistA

VistA continues to evolve and will soon become known as Health*e*Vet, which will be more integrative than its predecessor. Development and implementation of Health*e*Vet began in the fall of 2004 with the implementation of MyHealth*e*Vet, which is a patient-interactive component of Health*e*Vet. To promote patient participation in health care decisions, MyHealth*e*Vet provides patients with access to certain parts of their medical record, for example, to refill prescriptions, view appointments, and contribute information to the health history. Nurses have played an integral role in the development, implementation, and management of these applications.

The Evolution of Nursing Informatics at the VA

Following deployment of DHCP in the early 1980s, nurses' roles in developing and implementing IT expanded. The VHA established a nurse liaison role to help informatics departments at local facilities to train nursing staff in the new technology. Focusing on clinical processes supporting health care delivery, each department e.g., nursing, radiology, laboratory, appointed teams to develop content for applications. Nurse teams developed administrative and clinical content e.g., admission assessment, care plans, nursing staff demographics, and more. The nurse liaison, as a consultant to the developers of nursing applications, helped maintain applications, develop procedures, orient new nursing staff, and train staff in new technologies. The nurse liaison became known as the Nursing Automated Data Processing Coordinator.

VHA, with the implementation of DHCP, trained a cadre of nurses to support nursing applications. As early as 1985, ADPs were responsible for training all nursing staff on the use of the computer (hardware), as well as navigating the program applications (software). Over the years, this role gained additional titles, reflecting facility program complexity and increased areas of responsibility. Today, most VHA facilities employ nurse informaticians. In some small VHA facilities, nurse informaticians may perform dual roles, whereas large, complex facilities may employ several nurse informaticians. To obtain a description of the current role of the nurse informatician and to gauge the level of support of the role as perceived by nursing staff and nursing management, surveys were sent out to nursing staff at VA field facilities.

Survey Reveals Broad Definition and
Complexity of VA Nurse Informatician Role

VHA nursing staff were surveyed to gather demographic data to better understand staff perceptions of the nurse informatician role during the implementation of the CPRS and the BCMA systems. To foster broad dissemination to informatics nurses, nurse managers, and nurse executives at all 157 facilities, an electronic link was e-mailed connecting respondents to a custom Web-based survey. Two forms of the survey were constructed. The survey questions posed to the nurse informaticians were related to education and work background, the levels of technical and educational support they provide, the role they played in CPRS and BCMA implementation, and perceptions of their current role. Survey questions presented to the staff nurses, nurse managers, and nurse executives centered around their views of nurse informaticians' levels of technical and educational support provided during implementation and ongoing upgrades of CPRS and BCMA and their perceptions about the roles of the nurse informaticians.

E-mails were sent directly to the VHA Nursing Clinical Informatics workgroup, containing twenty-three nurse informaticians. In addition, an e-mail was sent to each nurse executive, instructing them to participate in the survey and requesting that they forward the survey links to nurse informaticians, staff nurses, and nurse managers within their facilities. Survey distribution was conducted in this manner to provide anonymity for staff nurses, in support of labor management partnerships. Because of this distribution method and the fact that the survey site did not register the number of individuals who may have logged onto the site but did not complete the survey or save their answers, the total number of staff who received notice of the survey is unknown. At the time of the survey, VHA employed approximately 31,022 staff nurses, 1,913 nurse managers, and 125 nurse executives. Nurse informaticians are not captured as a separate job category, nor are they listed in any national database, therefore exact numbers in VHA were unavailable for this survey. Survey responses received for each category totaled 121 staff nurses, 111 nurse managers, 50 nurse executives, and 98 nurse informaticians.5

All respondents were registered nurses with an average of five years as an informatics nurse and an average of five years in their current positions. In addition, 48 percent held a master's degree, 37 percent held a bachelor's degree, 11 percent held an associate's degree, 4 percent held a high school diploma, and 1 percent held a doctorate. Asked about specific informatics education, 34 percent planned to seek a degree in nursing informatics (NI), and 9 percent were certified in NI by the American Nurses Credentialing Center (ANCC). In terms of technical responsibilities, 43 percent of respondents support multidisciplinary teams, whereas 32 percent provide technical support to nursing staff only. Regarding educational responsibilities, 42 percent provide educational support to teams, whereas 39 percent provide educational support only to nurses (see Table 12-1).

Table 12-1. VA Nursing Staff Perceptions Regarding Levels of Technical & Educational Support Provided by VA Nurse Informatics

What is the scope of Technical Responsibility of Informatics Nurses in the VA system?

	Respondent Category			
	Inf RN N=98	Staff RN N=121	Mgr RN N=111	NE RN N=50
Provide technical support for **NURSING** staff only	32%	16%	11%	10%
Provide technical support for **MEDICAL** staff only	0%	1%	3%	0%
Provide technical support for **NURSING & MEDICAL** staff	9%	21%	26%	20%
Provide technical support for **MULTIDISCIPLINARY TEAMS**	43%	48%	53%	57%
Other:				
*[Provide technical support for **All of the Above**]*	9%	0%	n/a	n/a
*[Provide technical support **CLINICAL/ADMINISTRATIVE**]*	5%	1%	n/a	n/a
*[Reports Minimal technical support for **NURSING** staff]*	n/a	3%	5%	4%
[Reports unawareness of informatics role and/or nurses in their facility]		7%	n/a	n/a
Miscellaneous responses	1%	3%	3%	8%

What is the scope of Educational Responsibility of Informatics Nurses in the VA system?

	Respondent Category			
	Inf RN	Staff RN	Mgr RN	NE RN
Provide educational support for **NURSING** staff only	39%	18%	13%	10%
Provide educational support for **MEDICAL** staff only	0%	0%	1%	2%
Provide educational support for **NURSING & MEDICAL** staff	9%	21%	21%	22%
Provide educational support for **MULTIDISCIPLINARY TEAMS**	42%	48%	50%	59%
Other:				
*[Provide technical support for **All of the Above**]*	6%	0%	n/a	6%
*[Provide technical support **CLINICAL/ADMINISTRATIVE**]*	4%	1%	n/a	n/a
*[Reports Minimal technical support for **NURSING** staff]*	n/a	5%	7%	n/a
[Reports unawareness of informatics role and/or nurses in their facility]	n/a	7%	n/a	n/a
Miscellaneous responses	0%	1%	6%	6%

Inf RN=Informatics Registered Nurses (RN); Mgr RN=Nurse Managers; NE=Nurse Executives

The respondents held more than twenty titles as a group, including the most prevalent—clinical applications coordinator (41 percent) and nursing automated data processing applications coordinator (26 percent). A sizeable group, 27 percent, fell under the heading "other." Six percent were NI coordinators. Of note, one respondent was a chief information/informatics officer (CIO), with thirteen years of practice as an informatics nurse and eight years in the CIO position. This person has a master's degree in nursing education and is ANCC-certified in NI.

The Nurse Informatician Response

The survey asked respondents to identify their roles from a list compiled mostly from the American Nurses Association's *Scope and Standards of Nursing Informatics Practice:* consultant, educator, project manager, researcher, policy developer, decision support staff, and outcomes manager.[6] Additional roles were added, including change agent, facilitator, process improvement coordinator,

Table 12-2. Self-Described Roles* in Computerized Patient Record System (CPRS) & Bar Code Medication Administration (BCMA) Implementation In VA System

ROLES	CPRS Percent	BCMA Percent
Educator	91%	84%
Facilitator	63%	73%
Advocate	59%	68%
Change Agent	58%	65%
Consultant	55%	63%
Leader	45%	59%
Process Improvement Coordinator	42%	54%
Project Manager	41%	51%
Policy Developer	30%	51%
Outcomes Manager	22%	32%
Decision Support Coordinator	20%	26%
Product Developer	17%	23%
Researcher	14%	22%
Other (e.g., *Software enhancer/tester, technical support, champion*)	9%	9%

Roles are ranked from highest to lowest by the frequency of nurse informaticians selecting that choice when asked to define their implementation role.

* Question posed to VA Nurse Informaticians (n=98)

and leader. The top five roles were educator, facilitator, advocate, change agent, and consultant. The role of educator topped the list for both the CPRS and BCMA implementations (see Table 12-2).

The survey also asked staff to describe the top five current nurse informatician roles. The result was educator, consultant, change agent, facilitator, and advocate (see Table 12-3). These were almost identical to the roles identified in the CPRS and BCMA implementations.

Nursing Staff and Nursing Management Response

More than one hundred staff nurses, fifty nurse executives, and more than one hundred nurse managers responded to the survey. They identified their perceptions of the current role of nurse informatician and of the ideal informatics role to support nursing practice. Staff nurses prioritized the top five roles as educator, consultant, facilitator, advocate, and policy developer. Nurse managers chose consultant, educator, facilitator, policy developer, and advocate as the top five. Nurse executives identified them as educator, consultant, facilitator, project manager, and change agent. Staff nurses listed three additional roles as well: template builder, procurement specialist, and committee representative (see Table 12-3).

When nurse informaticians answered the question about ideal roles to support nursing practice, they selected product developer as number one. In contrast, staff nurses and nurse executives selected process improvement coordinator, and nurse managers selected educator.

VHA nurses in all categories believe that IT should be advanced to improve patient care and to support the practice of nursing. Nursing will benefit as a result. Survey group members in all categories viewed the general role of nurse informatician as essential to support nursing practice. All

Table 12-3. VA Nursing Staff Descriptions of Nurse Informaticians' Current Roles

What is the current role of Informatics Nurses in the VA system?			
[Roles are ranked from highest to lowest by number of nurses who selected that choice]			
Informatics RNs	**Staff RNs**	**Nurse Managers**	**Nurse Executives**
Educator	Educator	Consultant	Educator
Consultant	Consultant	Educator	Consultant
Change Agent	Facilitator	Facilitator	Facilitator
Facilitator	Advocate	Policy Developer	Project Manager
Advocate	Policy Developer	Advocate	Change Agent
Leader	Process Improvement Coordinator	Change Agent	Advocate
Policy Developer	Leader	Project Manager	Policy Developer
Project Manager	Product Developer	Process Improvement Coordinator	Product Developer
Process Improvement Coordinator	Change Agent	Leader	Process Improvement Coordinator
Outcomes Manager	Project Manager	Product Developer	Leader
Researcher	Decision Support Coordinator	Researcher	Outcomes Manager
Decision Support Coordinator	*Other*	Decision Support Coordinator	Decision Support Coordinator
Product Developer	Researcher	Outcomes Manager	*Other*
Other	Outcomes Manager	*Other*	Researcher

Other Roles [Informatics RNs]:
Troubleshooter, policy & process developer @ server level, information security officer

Other Roles [from Staff RNs]:
Fourteen respondents reported lack of understanding of the role; other roles included template builder, procurement specialist, committee representative

Other Roles [from Nurse Managers]:
Three respondents reported lack of understanding of the role; five reported lack of support; other roles included problem solver

Other Roles [from Nurse Executives]:
Several reported the absence of RNs in the informatics roles

survey participants noted how important it is for the nurse informaticians to be able to work with teams across disciplines and to develop standards that facilitate work processes. They view the role as key to the growth and success of performance improvement programs, data management, and integration of IT with the nursing process. As one survey respondent stated, "Without their support and leadership in our organization, nursing knowledge and performance will surely suffer."

Improving Patient Care and Safety

To focus system-wide attention on improving care and enhancing patient safety, the VHA developed a national performance measurement system, based on sets of clinical guidelines, to measure organizational performance in meeting patient care practice standards. Performance measures use best evidence to relate specific practice to desired patient outcomes. Electronic documentation of diagnosis and treatment provides the database for extracting indicators of health care needs and measuring actual care provided. This database supports facility-specific performance improvements that allow comparison to regional and national practice across the VHA system.

Nurse informaticians played a pivotal role in implementing this system. Creating templates for data extraction from the electronic record (CPRS) was key to the ability to benchmark clinical performance and compare information across the entire VHA system. In addition to creating templates to support VHA's performance measurement system, nurse informaticians were instrumental in developing clinical reminders, educating nursing and medical staff, and working with quality improvement offices to design dashboards for clinical and operational information display.

CPRS has proven to be one of the most important elements to improving patient care and safety. The sophisticated CPRS includes prompts and reminders to enhance care at the bedside. These advances in information management (IM) provide the entire health care team with real-time support for evidence-based practice at the point of care. The ability to trend data over time and to create charts or graphs relating data elements to each other enhances nurses' ability to draw well-informed conclusions regarding disease management and treatment options. Nurses are able to present a more comprehensive summary of patients' conditions to the multidisciplinary team as treatment plans are developed and modified. The electronic record and bar code medication administration tools augment safety initiatives by providing quick access to multidisciplinary perspectives. Team members easily navigate from each other's progress notes to diagnostic reports and the patient's health history, including primary and specialty care previously received in ambulatory, hospital, and/or long-term care settings at any VA facility. Nursing staff rely on nurse informaticians to train them in current applications and to help them increase their proficiencies in using these advanced IM tools.

The Future of Nursing Information Technology and Nurse Informaticians at the VA

New nursing programs will emerge because the VHA now has the technology to support improvement in patient care and safety. One such program that is currently under development at twelve VA sites is the VA Nursing Outcomes Database (VANOD). This is a nursing quality indicator database linking nursing practice with patient outcomes. It is evidence-based and will allow benchmarking and comparison at the local, regional, and national levels. The database will examine relationships between nursing-sensitive patient outcomes and structural elements. The VHA technology enables the nurse informatician at each site to extract administrative and clinical data from various files and patient records and to assemble them into reports for comparison among VA facilities nationally. VANOD will facilitate best practice and patient care improvement. As this is piloted, nurse informaticians at each site are coordinating informatics support, creating templates, and developing reminders to extract data elements for specific quality indicators. They will also work with researchers, IT staff, and nursing staff to develop training materials and procedure manuals. It is anticipated that the nurse informatician will be the project manager for implementing this initiative.

The nurse informatician role will become more complex. In addition to training clinicians regarding IT, they will need to develop programs to educate patients and families. They will need to share knowledge with community health care organizations through publications, research, programs, and Internet presentations. Nurses with master's degrees in NI will need to build bridges between the academic and practice environments, sharing knowledge and skills and mentoring new master's-prepared informatics nurses. They will need expanded skills in human factor analysis, and they will be responsible for promoting evidence-based practice in informatics.

Summary

The role of nurse informatician in the VHA has evolved over the years from educator to a much more complex role. As the work environment has become more technologically demanding, nurses at all levels of the VHA consider the role essential to nursing practice and patient care. Nurse informaticians are visible on a daily basis to staff nurses, troubleshooting problems that arise. They provide leadership to the informatics program across disciplines, supporting the entire health care team. Informatics nurses participate in the research of health systems, nursing practice studies, product design, and development. National support for research that advances technology and nurses' participation in applications and systems development, are encouraging signs that these goals can be reached. As technology continues to advance, the role of nurse informatician will continue to change.

Acknowledgement

Special acknowledgement to Rebecca Kellen, RN, BSN, MS, Clinical and Data Nurse Specialist in the Office of Nursing Services, Department of Veterans Affairs, Washington, DC, for her contribution in developing content for this chapter.

References

1. Department of Veterans Affairs. *Strategic Document, VISION 2020.* Washington, DC: Department of Veterans Affairs; 2003.

2. Department of Veterans Affairs. *Veterans Health Administration Quarterly Report.* Washington, DC: Department of Veterans Affairs; 2004.

3. Department of Veterans Affairs. *Computerized Patient Record System Fact Sheet.* Washington, DC: Department of Veterans Affairs; 2004.

4. Department of Veterans Affairs. *Bar Code Medication Administration Fact Sheet.* Washington, DC: Department of Veterans Affairs; 2004.

5. Department of Veterans Affairs, Veterans' Integrated Service Network Support Service Center (VSSC). *OnBoard Employees Report, Human Resources Data Mart (HRDM).* Available at: https://vaww.fcdm.med.va.gov/pas/en/src/Proclarity.asp. Accessed August 18, 2005.

6. American Nurses Association. *Scope and Standards of Nursing Informatics Practice.* Washington, DC: American Nurses Publishing; 2002.

CHAPTER 13

Nursing within Wall Street: A Close Look at the Corporate Chief Nurse Officer Role

By Charlotte A. Weaver, PhD, RN; James A. Cato, MSN, MHS, EdD (candidate), RN, CRNA; and Gail E. Latimer, MSN, RN

This chapter is an up-close, insiders' view of the role of the chief nurse officer (CNO) in the health care information technology (HCIT) industry. The authors, shown in Figure 13-1, belong to the first generation of CNOs to fill this role, and they represent the three major global software suppliers that were the first in the industry to create and fill the CNO position. This new role in nursing has its roots in the explosion of information technology (IT) and its impact on clinical care delivery and on nursing as a discipline, practice, and profession. It is not accidental that, within a four-year period, these corporate, publicly-traded IT businesses have responded to marketplace drivers to define the CNO role as imperative and critical to their business success. The authors have collaborated to identify role similarities, trends, and differences so as to leverage the lessons learned for the benefit of those who will follow in their footsteps. The fact that nurses from three major competitors in the HCIT industry are working collaboratively on this project is a testament to nurses' ability to see a higher goal—that is, what is in the best interest of our profession and ultimately our patients and their families.

Marketplace Drivers for the Industry's Adoption of the CNO Role

All three of the authors' employers have offered nursing solutions as part of their clinical systems for fifteen years or longer. So why create a CNO position now? Although the HCIT industry has been offering rudimentary clinical solutions for physicians and nurses since the late 1960s, the effort to truly automate core clinical processes did not get serious until the late 1990s. Out-of-control costs and shockingly poor quality drove organizations and governments to focus on building an electronic health record (EHR) infrastructure. Throughout the 1990s, however, the initial investments went into physician solutions, e.g., order entry, and ambulatory practices. This strategy did not deliver the expected results because of poor adoption of the systems in acute care and the creation of vertical "silos," i.e., various teams working in isolation of one another. For instance, by emphasizing ambulatory care or the general practitioner's office, the systems would create a partial EHR per single practitioner, inaccessible and non-sharable with other parts of the health system. Internationally, health policy makers quickly came to define a need for an EHR that would break out of the silos and work effectively across the care continuum. The EHR strategy became a widespread IT strategy in health care by 2000.

With this focus, nursing became a front-and-center player throughout the HCIT industry. Excluding physician office practice, nursing encompasses 90 percent of the production processes in acute care, home care, and long-term care. In these settings, *cultural transformation starts with nursing.* With the emphasis shifting to bringing IT into the core delivery processes in acute care, the HCIT industry realized that, without nursing on board, both initial sales and the reference sites needed to support future sales were at risk. In this economic climate, nursing suddenly mattered.

An Explosion in Demand: Nurses Needed in Every Informatics Role

The U.S., with approximately 2.8 million nurses, is an example of the need to keep nurses in the decision-making loop. Given that nurses do more than 90 percent of the production work processes

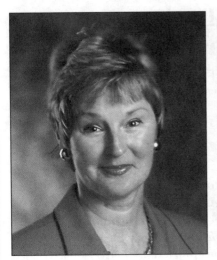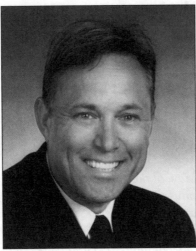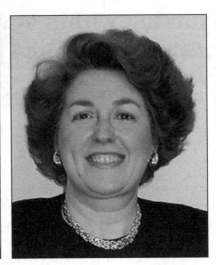

Figure 13-1. *Chapter authors Charlotte A. Weaver, James A. Cato, and Gail E. Latimer.*

in acute care, it is easy to see that they are the largest user group of a clinical information system. Systems adoption will not happen without them. As health care organizations began to commit to EHR initiatives, nurses were not only at the table in the evaluation and selection process but often cast the deciding vote.

Yet, as nurses looked critically at the systems, they found them lacking. By the late 1990s, the marketplace was demanding flexible and functionally robust clinical systems to support the complexity of clinicians' work flow in acute care. This was an industry first! Never before in the history of the HCIT industry have the work processes of nurses and the acute care team been primary drivers—either in buying decisions or in industries' prioritization for their research and development departments. With this shift in the marketplace, the nurses and nurse executive in an organization became deciding factors in which vendor won the deal. The marketplace demand dictated how the clinical solutions were built by the HCIT companies.

Consequently, nurses were put into roles that touched every aspect of a company's operations—from sales support, to content, methodology development, client support, implementation, consulting strategy, and solution development. The numbers of nurses hired by HCIT companies increased dramatically and so did the number of roles and opportunities for leadership responsibility. In this respect, the HCIT industry's demand for nurse informaticians was only slightly ahead of health care organizations. The demand for IT solutions that meet nursing's needs created this explosive growth inside HCIT companies, which, in turn, drove the demand for executive nurse leaders.

Counterbalancing the Chief Medical Officer (CMO) Limitations

Another urgent need was for HCIT companies to interface broadly with client organizations' clinical leaders. The HCIT industry has commonly had a chief medical officer (CMO) role, and all three of the authors' employers have had this role filled for fifteen years or longer. Yet the IT industry had difficulty communicating to the whole clinical team with the CMO as the only clinical leader. Operationally, CMOs often lacked experience with planning strategy and managing daily operations in a health care system, and their lack of business experience detracted from their ability to communicate effectively. In playing key roles in system selection on the health care organization side of the industry prior to their move to HCIT, the authors all dealt with CMOs who viewed the role of the nurse as limited to completing physician-directed tasks. Thus, in interactions with the CNO, COO (chief operating officer), or CEO (chief executive officer), the CMOs' communication gaps could actually harm their companies' prospects in the IT selection process. Another role was needed to bridge the gap.

Creating the IT Corporate CNO Role

Discovering Why the Role was Created

In preparation for this chapter, the authors interviewed the executives in their respective organizations who originally defined the need for the CNO role and participated in our hiring. We asked two basic questions: why did you create this role, and what were you looking for when hiring for the position? In comparing our interview findings, similar trends and strategies emerged.

Cerner Corporation's (Kansas City, Missouri) chairman defined the concept of a CNO in early 1998, understanding that success with nurse stakeholders meant that the company's nursing solutions had to be leading edge and superior to those of all other competitors. Prior experience had taught Cerner that acute care work processes and nursing's work flow were extremely difficult for non-nurses to understand sufficiently to translate into system requirements and design. The initial focus was to hire an experienced IT nurse leader with business and operational background to fill the CNO role. For Weaver, hired in July 1999 as the first CNO in the HCIT industry, the road map adopted for the role was not much different from that of her previous IT roles: defining requirements, managing projects, managing teams, managing alpha implementations, creating budgets, and developing strategic plans. Increasingly, however, the operational aspect lessened as the need to be more market-facing became a pressing priority. Six years after taking the position, Weaver finds that her role is still evolving, with her areas of responsibility and accountability defined at the highest level: success in sales of nursing solutions and adoption in client organizations. The road map for how to get to these end points is left up to Weaver to figure out.

Role ambiguity is a common theme in all three authors' experiences. Eclipsys Corporation (Boca Raton, Florida) selected Cato as their CNO in March 2002. Cato's primary responsibility was to provide the vision and direction for their nursing solutions strategy. Of equal importance, however, was representing Eclipsys' nursing vision to the market, providing a nursing voice, and serving as a thought leader in the industry. Previously, Cato was a CNO/COO in a large community hospital system with extensive hospital operational responsibility, as well as oversight for the implementation of a highly successful nursing and acute care team clinical system. During his three years as CNO at Eclipsys, Cato's experience is that, although he may have been given a basic mandate to "make a difference," defining the role is up to him. Cato's job has two major components: fulfilling a market-facing role and providing oversight for solution development strategies. He defines striking a balance between the two demands as key. Being with clients or at conferences means being away from the home office at which development work is conducted. To juggle both aspects of his role effectively, Cato manages his time to stay available for key decision and solution review meetings.

Latimer joined Siemens Medical Solutions, USA, in June 2004 after being a Siemens customer for ten years. Leveraging her background as a CNO and COO, she proactively worked with Siemens to define her role as having oversight of clinical solutions encompassing the whole care delivery team. The role involves three areas of responsibility: (1) outreach to external organizations, e.g., the Joint Commission on Accreditation of Healthcare Organizations and the American Organization of Nurse Executives to ensure that industry requirements are met, (2) regular communication with customers so that their strategic and tactical priorities are accommodated, and (3) internal advancement of the clinical agenda within Siemens so that management and the development staff are continually aware of the clinical issues. Latimer is therefore not only charged with the oversight of clinical product development but also charged with the culture change required to deliver products that will lead to clinical advancement and health care transformation. In addition to her role in clinical research and development, she manages the Office of Government and Industry Affairs. Latimer sees her first year as one of "shock and awe" with a steep learning curve. During the assimilation process, her most significant challenges were learning the cultural nuances of the corporate executive world and combining the role of business executive with that of clinical thought leader.

Background Traits: Similarities and Differences

Driving the creation of the nurse executive position was the need for nursing systems that nurses would embrace and love. Yet, as important as the systems themselves were, our companies saw the need to mirror client organizations with peer-to-peer clinical and operational counterparts, during both the sales process and the ongoing partnership. Thus, in the search for CNO candidates, the two deficit areas (client peers and nurse-focused clinical systems) dictated the required skill sets.

Among the most notable attributes that our company executives were looking for in a CNO was the ability to be charismatic and visionary as a nursing thought leader; in its simplest form, the deciding question was is this person likable? A winning personality is the first criterion of candidate evaluation. Both in sales and in consulting, success depends initially on being liked and trusted. This characteristic takes precedence over what one knows or what educational background or kind of job title one has. As nurses, we do not often see personableness as our number one success factor, but on the vendor side of the industry it is.

Our interviewers were also looking for the basics: an educational level of at least a master's degree, preferably with fellowships at Wharton, Robert Wood Johnson, or a school of similar caliber. Such high requirements were necessary if the candidate was to demonstrate thought leadership and the ability to be a peer with our clinical leader counterparts in health care organizations. Leadership evaluation was based on previous job titles, professional organization involvement, and offices held, as well as on publications and presentations at national and international conferences.

Just as important as leadership, however, was the ability to be a good team player and to work harmoniously with diverse types of people from different professions and backgrounds. Informatics skills were key in Weaver's evaluation but not for Cato and Latimer. Prior business, budget, and operational experience, however, were carefully evaluated and fully vetted for all of us.

What Does the IT CNO Do?

Advocacy

At its essence, the role of the CNO in an HCIT company is similar to that of the CNO in a health care organization. Each focuses on patient safety and on delivering solutions and strategies that bring value to clinicians, helping them to focus on patient care.[1] Nurses are patient advocates; they "nurse the system" to ensure care is delivered. The public rates nurses as the most trusted professionals and expects that they will act as their advocates. Although nurses work in an industry (HCIT) in which trust is not a paramount attribute, in the CNO role, their responsibility for advocacy is transferred to clients. They exercise this responsibility through close, personal work with clients (the nurse executive team, project team, etc.) and through translating the insider's view for those in their companies. It is much like the nurse's integrator function within the organizational complexities of a hospital,[2] that is, when nurses navigate across organizational divisions to coordinate and ensure safe and appropriate care delivery for their patients.

The Disruptive Innovation

The advocacy activities of nurses from their insiders' view of health care production processes can disrupt the company's operations and engineering segments. Inside an HCIT company, CNOs, as well as the other IT nurse leaders, function as advocates on behalf of clients, bringing this advocacy into product reviews. Formally or informally, CNOs oversee clinical solutions with the authority to validate whether a solution design promotes safe care delivery and work flow efficiencies for the entire care team. When the design is out of compliance with these principles, the CNO's disapproval can often cause a major disruption inside the engineering operations. After the first honeymoon year, the full disruptive impact of the CNO role hits the "nonclinician" business and engineering management segments of the company. Inevitably, the question becomes hard to ignore: Can we sideline this disruptive person? The question affects other nurses in leadership roles in the HCIT company. As nurses are assigned responsibility for leading solution development and having a final say, the disruption ensues in full.

Those of us who have watched the HCIT industry for more than three decades know that the clinicians' exercise of power and control over development has been a tug-of-war at best. Historically, the HCIT industry kept clinicians on the outside looking in, but the need to deliver the type of clinical solutions demanded by the marketplace caused the culture to shift fairly rapidly and extensively. Nurses and physicians alike describe an uneasy truce in the industry, with the clinical advocate tolerated as the "necessary evil." With the advent of the CNO position, nurses could channel their issues, concerns, and recommendations with an organized voice that had broad access to all levels of the company.

Driving the Vision and Strategy

In each of our companies, large numbers of nurses are in varying degrees of leadership positions. They are responsible for developing solutions and for defining the best practices methodology for implementing the solutions to deliver maximum value. Often the CNO's function, in guiding development initiatives, starts with evaluating a current state and critiquing it against marketplace trends to define the vision and strategy for going forward. This sounds simple but it is not. *When a company waits to respond to current market demand, it will be up to five years too late in delivering.* The challenge therefore is to stay current with technological advancements, with changing health policy and economics; with what is being done broadly across the market, both domestic and international; and then finally to project this knowledge into future trends. CNOs must leapfrog over day-to-day marketplace demands and anticipate needs three to five years into the future. They must read extensively and constantly synthesize new knowledge about the design and use of technology in health care delivery. Publishing in peer review journals on a variety of topics is a highly effective way to stay current because of the extensive literature reviews required. Similarly, giving presentations at major conferences and teaching at local universities also support this requirement.

CNOs drive nursing vision by "selling ideas" within their companies and its different teams. Their "likableness" plays just as important a part inside their organizations as it does for success with clients. It has to be this way because CNOs generally do not have the authority to mandate changes. All three authors became CNOs from positions of formal power, with direct budget responsibility, with hiring and firing authority for director levels down, and with a broad span of control. As corporate CNOs, however, because of the intense market-facing nature of the role, they do not carry operational or line responsibilities, which was not only a major shock but also a huge role challenge for all three of them. In the HCIT company, they have little formal power and their effectiveness is built on their ability to build consensus and respect. They have learned to navigate along the top of the executive team, as well as from bottom up. They message, persuade, champion, teach, and bring information to the right people, all in an effort to make something happen or to keep something from happening. *This is power, and it is real.* To achieve this level of influence in the corporate world, nurses have to acquire the communication skills of a diplomat—slow to be offended, always pleasant and poised in the face of adversity, objective and reasoned in the face of emotion, and quick to use humor.

There is an outward facing side of the CNO role: CNOs must sell their vision in the marketplace. They translate how technology can be used to address current challenges in patient safety, efficiencies, and teamwork. They present their interpretations to clients to help them see how to go from their current processes to a future state using the HCIT firm's technology tools. The translation of vision—offering hope for a better future—is at the heart of the selling that nurse executives do. Acquiring and improving the communication skills required to sell effectively to different audiences, cultures, and organizational personalities is a lifelong journey. The journey is humbling when nurse leaders fail miserably, yet energizing when, through their efforts, they connect and know that they have helped an organization move to a better place.

The Unique Challenges of the Corporate CNO Role

There is no mentor, there are no books, and there is no road map for being a successful CNO; for the authors, the learning has been by the seat of their pants! Role ambiguity arises from the uncertainty of knowing what they will be held accountable for and how best to prioritize their focus and time. Inevitably, CNOs undergo a period of trial and error as they learn. Perseverance in the face of initial failure or criticism is an important trait. It is not a question of working hard, but rather a question of working strategically for maximum impact and value. Most CNOs work eighty hours or more a week, but they get no brownie points for that unless they produce results. The authors recognized another common and important requirement: demonstrating the value of the CNO role within the company and to the client. They all had to identify how to do this, so as to clarify the difference they make and the value they contribute. Making a difference and delivering value are not enough; CNOs have to market what they do so that it is recognized. Nurses are not good at "self-advertisement;" they tend to wait to be recognized and find "bragging" offensive. But in the HCIT corporate world, waiting to be recognized can be deadly. Executives are too busy to do the discovery work about other people's work; CNOs have to publicize their own contributions.

Similarly, when identifying the unique aspects of their role in their companies, CNOs have to recognize the financial imperatives, constraints, and language that set HCIT firms apart from health care organizations. Strategies, advocacy, and sign-offs on enhancements or new solutions must be done against the backdrop of the quarterly profit and loss. When making recommendations that might disrupt or somehow affect the bottom line, CNOs must frame them in terms of the appropriate business concepts and use appropriate business language. And importantly, they have to do the financial analysis to be able to include estimates in their recommendations. CNOs must balance their actions, strategies, and recommendations with the interests of stockholders. This means delivering on business imperatives so as to meet targeted metrics, such as earnings per share, as well as quarterly bookings, revenues, and available cash. CNOs have to be skilled in finance. They have to understand the terms, to think strategically, and to translate initiatives into the language of financial concepts and business imperatives. Without these skills, CNOs risk being dismissed from the core business leadership team, and nursing's voice would not be at the table when business decisions are made.[3]

Finally, the biggest challenge all the authors identified is the extensive travel—long sedentary hours in planes and meetings. With well over 80 percent of our time spent away from the home office, the travel requirement entails very real physical and emotional demands, including fatigue and the effect on home life. Just like professional baseball players who continue to play into their forties, surviving this amount of travel means that you must take exceedingly good care of yourself.

Why Be a Corporate CNO?

Embracing Power to Make a Difference

Each of the authors moved into the corporate CNO role with a sense that their previous roles, education, and professional activities gave them the credentials and skills to take on the position. In their view, they had an opportunity to drive strategy and change in a more influential way than they could in a single health care organization. The corporate CNO role puts the player in a position to make a global difference in health care. Accepting the responsibility of such an opportunity also comes from the deep-seated belief that nurses are the best people to define how nursing solutions should be designed. The CNO, as the nurse leader at the executive table, can represent the recommendations and strategies from the nurse teams across the organization, thereby empowering nursing with a voice in the organization. And it is this nursing voice—across all levels, but most importantly at the executive cabinet—that results in nursing and clinical solutions that bring value to all clinicians and patients.[4]

In the face of worldwide nursing shortages, the declining throughput capacity of university nursing schools, the increasing health care demands of aging populations, and ever increasing costs, the health care industry must transform itself to survive. IT is the major enabler of that transformation.

The stakes are high and the quality of patient care is at the very heart of the challenge. Each of the authors accepted the CNO role as an opportunity to influence change and make that happen. Leveraging the opportunity is what keeps us in the CNO role long after the honeymoon period, when many would like to see us out the door.

Going Over to the Dark Side

As the first CNOs in the industry, the authors have experienced reactions from professional colleagues who refer to their career choice as "going over to the dark side." In preparing this chapter, the authors discussed the reaction and felt it important to address. They acknowledge that joining the industry is puzzling to other nurse leaders for at least a couple of reasons. For one, the HCIT industry does not enjoy a high trust ranking among health care providers. Another is the profession's discomfort with the deliberate pursuit of power. Florence Nightingale founded modern nursing based on the core values of altruism and care of the individual patient. Yet, just as dedication and patient advocacy are the sources of nursing's strength and of the public's trust in nurses, they also present the greatest liability for effecting system-level change. As professionals, it is crucial for nurses to add to their skill set a readiness to seek power and to be comfortable with having it.[5] To be active participants in influencing how organizations bring solutions to health care delivery, nurses have to be players at the executive cabinet level—on all sides of our industry.

Without a doubt, when nurse education was placed in the university setting in the late 1960s, the move paved the way for this generation to be the first to acquire broader management and business leadership credentialing. Over the last forty years, academic preparation and good mentoring have allowed nursing leadership to develop skill sets beyond clinical skills. Increasingly, nurses are promoted to assume operational responsibility in the CEO and COO roles. And it is not unusual for nurses to engage with a client organization that has a nurse in the chief information officer (CIO) position or as COO, CEO, or a combination of such roles. If power is the ability to cause something to happen or to keep something from happening, clearly nurses from all corners of the industry are stepping into positions of power. The authors see this opportunity to make the voice of nursing heard inside corporate boardrooms as the opportunity to deliver solutions and implement strategies that will enable transformation in health care.

Why be a corporate CNO? The authors answer by saying, "If we get this right, we get a huge improvement in patient safety. We can make nursing an evidence-driven profession. We can make the workplace an energizing, attractive place for nurses and other clinicians to work. We can help education incorporate technology into its curriculum and keep education aligned with practice. We can support nursing in practice and science, and we can allow nurses to function as professional knowledge workers with high touch enabled by high tech. That is our vision, and it is our invitation to the next generation who will follow in our footsteps."

Paving the Road for the Future

The authors have several recommendations to help nurses in the future step into the corporate CNO role with a full toolbox. First, one of the most important assets is a network. Set out to develop a broad set of relationships among peers and colleagues throughout the industry. Networking skills are critical to a CNO's effectiveness in moving throughout the industry to make things happen. Having an extensive network allows nurses to gain entry for themselves and their company, when otherwise the door might remain closed. Having broad, personal connections enables them to navigate effectively across all sides of the industry. Connectedness can be one of the most important things a nurse brings to a company.

When networking does not come naturally, learn the skill. Become an active participant in professional organizations, work on committees, volunteer for task forces, and/or run for office. Do all this at national and international levels. At meetings, be prepared to exchange business cards. Carefully maintain contacts and use the database for messaging, holiday cards, or other personal greetings, as well as for business. Deliberately set aside time for communication, contact, and face-to-face meetings.

Another important activity consists of writing papers and making conference presentations. When it makes sense, do these activities in collaboration with other colleagues. Especially look for opportunities to collaborate across the boundary lines of industry, health care, and academe. Such collaborations are powerful; you can leverage the strength of each domain to accomplish more than by staying in the same segment of the industry. In the context of professional organizations, committees, or task force work, make yourself known to the professional leaders in the industry.

Use such opportunities not only to interface with the thought leaders in the profession, but also, when possible, to recruit your mentors. Mentors are crucial. Each of the authors' biographies contain the names of wise individuals who guided them through skill deficits, who helped them define their messages, and who guided them toward strategies vital to navigating unfriendly or critical waters. Choose your mentors from within and outside your current organization or professional setting. You cannot have too many mentors, and at no time in your career should you be beyond having one.

The authors hope that this insiders' description of the corporate CNO role sheds light on its broad importance to nursing. To those who will follow in their footsteps, they offer a commitment of mentoring and support.

References

1. Heath J, Johanson W, Blake N. Healthy work environments: a validation of the literature. *JONA*. 2004; 34(11):524-530.
2. McClure M. Magnet hospitals and unique role functions of nurses. Paper presented at: Discussions in the Desert at American Organization of Nurse Executives 2004 Conference; April 2004; Phoenix, AZ. Available at: Margaret.McClure@med.nyu.edu.
3. Matisoff A. Chief nursing officers: a seat at the table. *Health Leaders*. 2004;April:36-40.
4. Johnson T. Executive synergy: the artful balance of vision, strategy, and innovation. *Nurse Leader*. 2004; 2(3):23-25.
5. Weaver CA. Nurses in corporate America: embracing power through influence. *Seminars in Nursing Management*. 2002;3(2):28-32.

CHAPTER 14

Nurses in Project Management Roles

By Judy Murphy, BSN, RN, and Brian Gugerty, DNS, MS, RN

Tree Health Care System (a fictional compilation based on known entities) is an integrated health care delivery network in a U.S. midwestern city with a population of 350,000. Tree is the result of a merger of three hospitals in 1995, one with a modest university teaching service. It has since acquired another small hospital and has built a fifth. There were problems with the merger, but most organizational members now feel, ten years later, that Tree is strong, unified, and fulfilling its mission.

One of Tree's most significant challenges was reconciling disparate hospital and related information systems in an effort to centralize information technology (IT) functions across all the Tree entities. Tree hired Susan Eply as corporate chief information/informatics officer (CIO) in 2000 to lead the system consolidation effort. Susan, with a background of twelve years in nursing followed by ten years in IT, had been a project manager and IT director at another hospital. She had taken two project management (PM) courses at the local university and attended a PM workshop and two PM conferences from 1995 to 1997.

Under Susan's direction, in 2000 and 2001, Tree eliminated 50 percent of the pre-2000 hospital information systems, consolidating them into Acme's Electronic Health Record integrated system. They also adopted three non-Acme products as corporate standards: Alpha Pharmacy Information System, Beta Perioperative Information System, and Gamma Radiology/PACS. In 2002, Tree formed a clinical informatics group with a chief medical informatics officer (CMIO), chief nursing informatics officer (CNIO) and six trained nurse informaticians, two of whom were certified as project management professionals (PMPs). IT Services, led by Susan, the clinical informatics group, and many functional departments, created a clinical transformation plan that yielded significant cost reductions and demonstrable quality improvements. In 2004, computerized provider order entry (CPOE) and electronic medication administration were implemented, and electronic clinical documentation implementation is currently under way. Staff satisfaction with these three highly clinically interactive applications is high.

In this case, a nurse with IT training and experience successfully led a transformation project. In this chapter, we explain why nurses are suitable for such a role. Then, to frame an understanding of this powerful approach, we explore several areas: (1) the effect of PM on success; (2) the roots of PM in nonhealth care industries and the relationship between PM and other management and leadership frameworks; and (3) the opportunities for PM education, training, professional organization membership, and certification. A classic PM model is presented, giving the reader an overall view of a PM life cycle. We then refocus on nursing and explore efforts by nursing professional organizations, nursing educators, and health care informatics professional societies to assure that PM principles are incorporated within the best practice of nursing informatics (NI). Finally, we draw conclusions and make recommendations to adopt more widely the practices and principles of PM into health care to bring projects in on time and within budget, as well as to meet customer expectations.

The Nurse as Project Manager

When adequately trained and experienced in the practices and principles of PM, nurses make good candidates as project leaders and managers for the electronic health record (EHR) and clinical transformation projects that are sweeping health care organizations in many parts of the world today. Nurses take naturally to PM primarily because, as the authors believe, the similarities between the nursing process and the PM life cycle outweigh the differences (Figure 14-1). Others have drawn similar parallels in the two processes.[1] For example, the first phases of the processes, shown in Figure 14–1, demonstrate how they are related. Similar to assessment in the nursing process, the PM phase of initiation is critically important to success. What would happen if a nurse failed to assess a patient's vital signs or pulmonary and cardiac status prior to administering an unusually high dose of a diuretic? Similarly, what would happen if a project manager jumps into developing implementation and training plans before the project team understands the vision of what is to be done and has worked out clear objectives with the project sponsors? Other reasons that nurses easily assimilate and effectively apply PM are their experiences with high levels of responsibility, with management, and with supervision. Finally, as managers of IT projects that have significant clinical components, nurses have a huge advantage over nonclinicians because they are intimately familiar with the health care organizational culture and work flow processes.

On the other hand, nurses have at least one disadvantage—a propensity to be risk averse. By their very nature, complex EHR and clinical transformation projects involve risk taking at many levels, and nurses not trained in project risk management tend either to fail to identify risks or to be paralyzed by them.

Project Management's Impact on Project Success

EHR and clinical transformation projects tend to be large. Some cost millions of dollars or more and last two to four years or longer. With so much money and time at stake, failure is not a desirable option. Yet, as we all know, these projects sometimes fail, run past their due date, or run over budget. The 2001 *Extreme Chaos Report,* the latest IT project management success survey available on the Standish Group's Web site, indicates that there has been considerable improvement since the original 1994 *Chaos Report.*[2] Project success, defined as project completion on time and within budget, was up to 28 percent from 16 percent. Failed projects were down from 33 percent to 23 percent. The percentage of "challenged" projects changed less, down from 56 percent to 48 percent, but the time and cost overruns—which constitute the "challenge" in challenged IT projects—improved dramatically, with time overruns decreasing to 63 percent from 222 percent and cost overruns decreasing to 45 percent from 189 percent. It is reasonable to assume that a 2006 survey would show continued improvement but not as dramatic a difference as that between 1994 and 2001, because many of the easy project performance gains have already been achieved. When we apply these data to challenged new IT projects in health care, just the cost overruns in 2005 would amount to $1.32 billion (based on an $8 billion new health care IT project expenditure rate in the U.S.), even when we assume that only 40 percent of the projects were challenged and the amount of cost challenge was

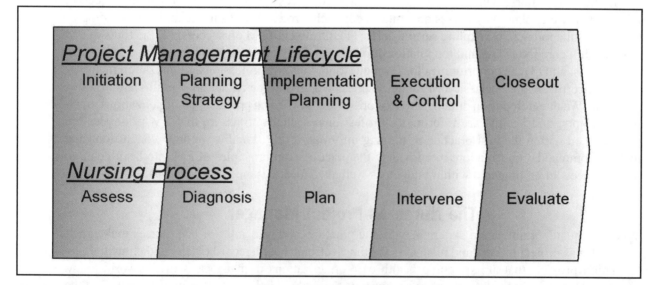

Figure 14-1. *Correlation of the Project Management Life Cycle and the Nursing Process.*

a 33 percent overage. Similar projected losses from failed projects could add up to $1.8 billion in 2006.

There is clearly room for further improvement. The questions are whether these estimates are valid and whether they apply to health care, which is perceived to be farther behind in IT PM practices than other industries. The answer seems to be yes to both questions. Preliminary data analysis of a survey of health care IT project managers comparing their project outcomes to nonhealth care IT project managers indicates two conclusions: "(1) the common perception that health care IT PM practices lag behind other industries is untrue; (2) there is no significant difference in project outcomes between the two groups," according to Richard D. Lang.[3] Although these conclusions are encouraging, advocates for health care IT PM cannot rest on their laurels. As in other industries, there is considerable room for improvement in project management practices that can affect positive health care organizational outcomes.

How can health care leaders and managers foster continued improvements to these powerful PM approaches? Our experience and the literature on critical IT project success factors give us some answers.[4-8]

1. We need to define project success in PM terms. Project success is usually measured by time (deliverables on time), cost (within budget), customer expectations (met), and project objectives (achieved).
2. Upper management support is on the top of many lists of requirements for project success. The support must be sustained and, to some degree, active.
3. Rewards for achieving project success are usually seen as a potent upper management tool.
4. The competence of the project manager, project team members, and their combined technical ability is another critical success factor.
5. Effective communication throughout the project, along with a clear project vision or mission, is seen as imperative.
6. Mutual understanding of the project vision, objectives, and deliverables by the project team, the projects' customers, and the stakeholders is key to success.
7. Adequate resources to carry off the project is another frequently mentioned factor.

The Roots of Project Management

No one has yet discovered a project plan for the pyramids, but many project managers suspect such a plan must have existed. How else could the ancients have organized thousands of manual laborers, hundreds of skilled craftspeople, and dozens of knowledge workers? Possibly, however, they did what manufacturing enterprises, governments, and other large organizations from the industrial revolution through the mid-twentieth century have done to organize their project work—they used many-layered organizational structures and low spans of supervisory control.

The Influence of Scientific Management

The practice and discipline of project management have their roots in scientific management, even though the reasons might not be immediately clear. The focus of scientific management was fundamental work analysis and redesign, as well as structuring organizations to supervise new and more productive work processes. It was based on repetitive tasks and rigid, hierarchical management structures, not on project plans that empowered workers to be creative within the limits of agreed-upon goals. Why, then, are project management's roots in scientific management? The fundamental scientific management principle of breaking a work process into irreducible steps was adopted by project managers to create comprehensive lists of important project activities early in the project planning process. The basic management tenet that "managers must manage," born of the scientific management movement, led to principles and techniques of project execution and control. Additionally, Henry Gantt's simple, elegant, and powerful adaptation of the bar chart, which bears his name, was originally used for set work processes, and was adapted yet again to form the basis of several key project management tools and technical methodologies, notably the Critical Path Method.

Project Management Comes of Age

After World War II, management theories progressed from human relations theory to systems theory to total quality management theory to value chains and chaos theory. These attempts to explain and understand rapidly changing organizations, although not perfect, helped to build management science into a powerful discipline by the end of the twentieth century. Knowledge of and skill in PM are now seen as basic management science competencies across many industries. How did that come about?

The principles and practices of PM were widely adopted by the construction industry, especially on large projects, during the postwar era and continue to be widely used in construction today. During the 1950s and 1960s, the engineering, scientific, and government communities adopted project management techniques. In the 1980s, they were adopted by the IT industry. By 1990, project management was declared a core business competency across all industries.[9]

If, as some contend, PM is a core management competency, where does it fit within management frameworks and approaches? Project management is a management framework, not a leadership framework. Stephen R. Covey describes *leadership* as providing the vision, overall direction, and high-level motivation to an organization. Management's task, according to Covey, is to make the vision a reality.[10] Thus, in most cases, an organization's leadership charters projects consistent with its organizational vision. Management can then use PM techniques to balance project costs, schedules, and quality in order to successfully complete projects that actualize the organizational vision. Within this context, PM is consistent and works well with a variety of effective management frameworks and approaches. Communication, motivation, control, and many other management principles apply to PM as well.

Project Management Education, Training, Membership, and Certification

Education and Training

Project managers learn their trade through a variety of mechanisms within and between industries. They can receive formal education in PM, either as a degree or as a minor concentration of course work within a discipline's program of study. They can receive an undergraduate, master's, or doctoral degree in project management. However, today, a degree in PM is not the usual entry into a project manager position. Most project managers, are exposed to one or two project management courses as part of their professional or discipline's degree, and then go on to receive additional PM training in the form of continuing education, e.g., workshops, seminars, and conferences. Having sufficient time in the role, a project manager may sit for certification in project management, which is offered by the Project Management Institute (PMI).[11,12]

The Project Management Institute (PMI)

PMI is a not-for-profit professional organization dedicated to education, standards setting, and advocacy for its 150,000 members. PMI has published its third *Guide to the Project Management Body of Knowledge, 2004 Edition,* also known as the *PMBOK Guide.*[13] The *PMBOK Guide* is PMI's largest selling publication and has the added distinction of being an American National Standard of the American National Standard Institute. The *PMBOK Guide's* PM knowledge areas are

1. Integration management
2. Scope management
3. Time management
4. Cost management
5. Quality management
6. Human resource management
7. Communications management
8. Risk management
9. Procurement management

PMI also offers certification in several aspects of PM, but by far the most certifications it grants are for PMP. There are more than 75,000 PMPs in more than 120 countries worldwide. Those aspiring to become PMPs must meet education and experience requirements and must agree to adhere to a code of professional conduct. They are then eligible to sit for a rigorous multiple-choice examination. If they pass it, they may use the PMP title.

A Project Management Framework

Although the *PMBOK Guide* is widely used and respected by project managers, instructors, faculty, and students, there are many other quality sources of PM information, some of which give a better overview or starting point for project manager novices and experts alike. The Lewis Method®[13] is one such comprehensive, general project management model (see Figure 14-2). The Lewis Institute is one of several registered education providers for PMI; thus this model includes all the core PM knowledge areas. The Lewis model uses classic project management components, such as work breakdown structure, critical path methodology, and earned-value analysis, while including unique components, e.g., many of the steps in the strategy planning phase.[14]

The Lewis Method® consists of five phases. The project initiation phase is a particularly important part of this model. Lewis reminds us that a successful passage through this phase is needed to prevent a "headless chicken project" (an accepted term in PM parlance). Great project objectives, mutually understood by the project team and select stakeholders, are the milestones for completion of this phase. Project and technical strategies that the organization and project team can use to make the project objectives a reality are the output of the strategy planning phase. The implementation planning phase consists of identifying all the important project activities, estimating their durations, assigning resources to them, and scheduling them all so as to successfully attain the project objectives. In the execution and control phase, the project activities are performed. Management control is exercised during this phase through several mechanisms, one often being earned value analysis, a technique that integrates cost and schedule data. Finally, the closeout phase consists of project closure and a "postmortem." The postmortem serves as a method to identify lessons learned from the just completed project, which can be applied to future projects.

Selecting the Project Manager

Despite the progress in PM frameworks, educational programs, and professional organizations, many managers still make the mistake of considering the planning phase to be the entirety of project management. The project manager role is often assigned to a low-level leader who has demonstrated leadership skills. The individual is provided with PM software and sent off to do the job. In this case, neither the organization nor the new project manager takes advantage of all the powerful principles and tools of a holistic PM approach:

1. Leading a project team in crafting mutually agreed-upon project objectives that align leadership vision and support organizational goals
2. Identifying risks to the project and managing them
3. Breaking a project's tasks down quickly and effectively and managing them at the right level
4. Catching a critical task that is about to derail and keeping it on track
5. Knowing when a change in scope, time, budget, or quality needs to be reported to upper management and when it does not
6. Learning from the current project so that the next one is better

All this goes by the wayside when the project manager is ignorant of the practices and principles of PM

The Project Management Office

The *PMBOK Guide* defines a project management office (PMO) as "an organizational unit to centralize and coordinate the management of projects under its domain."[12] Health care, like other knowledge worker-intensive industries, has begun to use PMOs. Although PMOs are present less than 10 percent of the time in health care, based on anecdotal surveys these authors have conducted

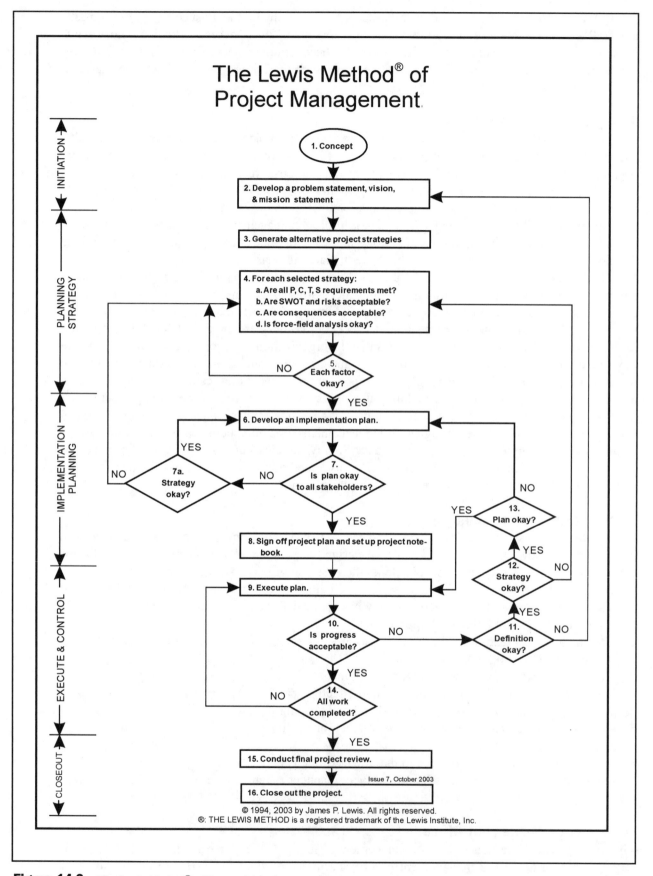

Figure 14-2. *The Lewis Method® of Project Management.*

in health care IT PM workshops in the past two years, this percentage represents an increase from the 1990s.

Some people are opposed to the use of PMOs on the grounds that they merely introduce more hierarchy and bureaucracy. But even those who disfavor them tend to advocate an intra-organizational PM support group. Whether organized as a PMO or as a PM support group, a centralized project function can provide consistent methodologies, training, and support to sustain PM practice and principles in an organization.

IT Versus Non-IT Project Management

It is helpful to consider the differences between management of IT projects and non-IT projects. Schwalbe[15] describes the aspects of IT projects that make them different from non-IT projects. Essentially, IT projects are different because the technology involved and the people involved combine to have an impact on processes, or work flow. Because of the intense competition in all forms of IT hardware, software, and services, new technologies are being developed all the time, and they have a relatively short shelf life. Organizations often desire, or the market demands, that new and sometimes cutting-edge technology be developed and deployed. Therefore, IT projects have an unusually high rate of change, steep learning curves for project team members, and much technological risk.

Then there is the specialization factor. Network engineers, programmers, systems analysts, and many other specialized IT personnel have unique competencies. Often, especially on large IT projects, it takes many different kinds of specialized people, with complementary skills, to make up a project team. Non-IT organizational members may see them as homogeneous, but they and the project manager see themselves as a heterogeneous team. With diversity there can be strength to be sure, but IT diversity definitely demands management care and feeding. Finally, because of the specialized technical requirements of IT projects, there tend to be a large number of contract workers in a typical large IT project.

Project Management in Nursing Informatics Practice

To appreciate the role that PM plays in the practice of nursing informatics (NI) today, it is important to understand the history of NI development as a specialty and the evolution of the NI role in practice. PM, including related implementation responsibilities, was not a major skill set expected of nurses practicing in informatics positions until the last five years. In fact, there is little mention of, much less a focus on, PM or implementation in many of the early NI publications. However, this changed as time passed, and the NI role became more pervasive in the health care industry and as more informatics nurses began working in health care delivery settings.

NI started on the road to becoming a recognized specialty in the 1980s and is one example of a discipline-specific informatics practice within the broader category of health care informatics. It expanded and evolved as health care organizations around the world implemented varied and increasingly complex clinical information systems (CIS). The American Nurses Association (ANA) formally recognized NI as a nursing specialty in 1992. The ANA defines NI as "a specialty that integrates nursing science, computer science, and information science in identifying, collecting, processing, and managing data and information to support nursing practice, administration, education and research; and the expansion of nursing knowledge."[16] There is no specific mention of PM in their definition.

Project Management and the Scope of Practice for Nursing Informatics

The *Scope of Practice for Nursing Informatics,* published by the ANA in 1994, was the first document to address NI. This fifteen-page text elaborates on system design and development, including information gathering, handling, communication, and clinical transformation. There is a reference to project management–like skills in one of the eighteen "Preparation for Practice" competencies: "Ability to coordinate projects of various sizes involving diverse team members and constituencies."[16]

The *Scope and Standards of Nursing Informatics Practice,* published by the ANA in 2001, revised and expanded the scope of NI practice: "… Nursing informatics facilitates the integration of data, information, and knowledge to support patients, nurses, and other providers in their decision making in all roles and settings. This support is accomplished through the use of information structures, information processes, and information technology." The fifty-one-page document adds much detail to the 1994 publication and elaborates on the roles of the informatics nurse specialist, including project manager, which is one of the seven roles described. Additionally, *Standards of Practice* describes implementation of informatics solutions as a competency and Standard IV lists "Demonstrates expertise as a project manager" as a measurement criterion.[17]

Project Management Criteria in the Nursing Informatics Certification

The American Nurses Credentialing Center (ANCC), a subsidiary of the ANA, offers certification in more than forty specialty areas of nursing practice, including one for NI. So far, since NI certification began in 1995, 645 nurses have passed the NI certification examination (as of Q3, 2004). The ANCC description of NI practice indicates, "The work of an informatics nurse can involve any and all aspects of information systems including theory formulation, design, development, marketing, selection, testing, implementation, training, maintenance, evaluation, and enhancement." Examination topics include System Life Cycle; Human Factors; Information Technology; Information Management and Knowledge Generation; Professional Practice, Trends, and Issues; and Models and Theories.[18] Notably, project management is not singled out as a definition or as an examination topic, but some aspects of it are covered in the "Systems Life Cycle and Professional Practice" sections.

Project Management in Nursing Curriculum

Nursing (General) Undergraduate and Graduate Programs. A positive trend in undergraduate nursing education programs, especially bachelor degree programs, in the past fifteen years is the inclusion of management science concepts and principles in professional socialization courses. Such courses provide a good foundation on which to build PM knowledge and understanding. There are now a few programs in health care informatics, at least one of which offers a course in basic PM. PM courses are beginning to be offered in NI graduate specialty programs, and a promising trend is that nursing administration and other non-nursing informatics students are sometimes taking these courses (see below).

Nursing Informatics (Specialty) Graduate Programs. Master's and doctoral NI programs are available at a variety of universities, through both traditional onsite course work and online distance programs. When the first of these programs began in the very late 1980s, only two universities offered NI degrees. Now there are more than eighteen with programs, and still others offer a concentration in NI within a nursing administration graduate program. PM course work is increasingly available in the form of electives in NI graduate programs, although these authors know of only one NI program that *requires* a health care IT PM course.

Recent Surveys

There were 307 CIO respondents to the *15th Annual Healthcare Information and Management Systems Society (HIMSS) Leadership Survey,* conducted by means of a Web-based questionnaire from November 2003 to January 2004.[19] Although there were many interesting findings, the two most germane to this chapter are related to IT priorities and IT staffing needs. Other than security and compliance issues, CIO priorities are focused on implementing IT systems to promote patient safety (52 percent) and on replacing/upgrading inpatient clinical systems (38 percent). In the staffing area, CIOs reported needing staff for clinical transformation (25 percent), clinical champions (24 percent), and clinical informaticians (24 percent). These two findings are related; the CIOs understand that, to implement complex clinical systems like bar-coded medication administration and CPOE, an increasing number of clinical staff have to be involved in the projects. And some of these staffers need to be nursing informaticians skilled in PM.

To gain a better understanding of the background of nurse informaticians, the issues they address on a daily basis, and the tools they turn to for completing their jobs, HIMSS also conducted a Web-based *Nursing Informatics Survey* in October 2003.[20] A total of 537 responses were received, making it the largest ever survey of nurse informaticians. Two-thirds of respondents reported system implementation as a top job responsibility, with system development and coordination/administration of activities rounding out the top three, suggesting that increasing numbers of nurses are playing a critical role in the development and implementation of clinical systems. Two-thirds of respondents worked in hospital or health care system settings, and an additional fourth worked for vendors or consulting firms. This finding reinforces the assertion that a majority of nurse informaticians have job responsibilities and are practicing at settings in which PM is an essential job skill.

Interestingly, more than half of the respondents indicated that their knowledge of informatics came from on-the-job training, and, whereas nearly half of them held a graduate degree, only 10 percent had a formal informatics degree. Only one-quarter of the respondents had ten or more years of informatics experience, and nearly 40 percent had fewer than five years' experience. This emphasizes the need for PM training on the job or through continuing education, in addition to being incorporated into NI formal education programs.

Summary

Today, as so often has been the case in history, health care resources are limited. Yet participants in the health care industry are dramatically changing support systems and designing new processes, with many advances in IT and pressures from patient safety and care management initiatives. There are many, varied, and complex health care IT projects demanding resources. So how does one ensure that health care dollars and clinician time are spent wisely on projects that guarantee patient-driven outcomes? In addition to selecting and funding the projects wisely, the authors believe, good PM also minimizes risk and enhances success. We further contend that clinicians, and particularly nurses, are excellent candidates, once trained in PM techniques, to be good project managers. Executive management should support, and maybe even demand, PM training for the organization's clinical IT project team leaders.

NI has been evolving since its inauguration some twenty-five years ago. More and more, PM skills are being included in training and formal education programs. And increasingly, nursing informaticians are stepping up to the plate and taking on key roles in the planning, selection, implementation, and evaluation of the critical clinical systems needed in health care today. We hope that we have provided a glimpse as to why that is a trend to not only be watched, but also promoted. Good PM skill holds part of the key to consistent success with clinical IT system implementations in health care settings.

References

1. Hunt E, Sproat S, Kitzmiller R. *The Nursing Informatics Implementation Guide.* New York: Springer; 2003:30.

2. Standish Group, The. The extreme chaos report. Available at: http://www.standishgroup.com/sample_research/index.php. Accessed February 27, 2005.

3. Lang RD. IT project management in healthcare: Improving the odds for success. *J Healthcare Information Manage.* 2005;19(1): 2-4.

4. Belassi W, Tukel OI. A new framework for determining critical success/failure factors in projects. *Int J Project Manage. 1996;*14(3): 141-151.

5. Hartman F, Ashrafi R. Project management in the information systems and information technologies industries. *Project Manage J.* 2002;33(3): 5-15.

6. Jiang J, Chen E, Klien G. The importance of building a foundation for user involvement in information system projects. *Project Manage J.* 2002;33(1):20-26.

7. Jiang J, Klien G, Margulis J. Important behavioral skills for IS project managers: the judgments of experienced IS professionals. *Project Manage J.* 1998; 29(1): 39-44.

8. Jiang J, Klien G, Balloun J. Ranking of system implementation success factors. *Project Manage J.* 1996; 27(4): 49-53.

9. Peters T. *Liberation Management.* New York: Knopf; 1992.

10. Covey S. *The 7 Habits of Highly Effective People.* New York: Fireside; 1989.

11. Project Management Institute. Project Management Institute Web page. Available at: http://www.pmi.org/info/default.asp. Retrieved February 22, 2005.

12. Project Management Institute. *A Guide to the Project Management Body of Knowledge.* 3rd ed. Newton Square, PA: Project Management Institute, Inc.; 2004.

13. Lewis JP. The Lewis method® of project management [Lewis Institute Web site]. Available at: http:// www.lewisinstitute.com/pdf/83.pdf. Retrieved February 22, 2005.

14. Lewis JP. *Project Planning, Scheduling, and Control.* 3rd ed. New York: McGraw-Hill; 2001.

15. Schwalbe K. *Information Technology Project Management.* 3rd ed. Boston: Course Technology; 2004.

16. American Nurses Association. *The Scope of Practice for Nursing Informatics.* Washington, DC: American Nurses Publishing; 1994:3,14.

17. American Nurses Association. *Scope and Standards of Nursing Informatics Practice.* Washington, DC: American Nurses Publishing; 2001:vii,18,32,36.

18. American Nurses Credentialing Center. Informatics nurse certification. Available at: http://www.nursing-world.org/ancc/certification/cert/certs/informatics.ht ml. Accessed February 25, 2005.

19. Health Information Management System Society. 15th annual health information management system society (HIMSS) leadership survey. Available at: http://www.himss.org/2004survey/ASP/healthcarecio_ final.asp. Accessed December 15, 2004.

20. Health Information Management Systems Society. HIMSS nursing informatics survey. Available at: http://www.himss.org/content/files/nursing_info_ survey2004.pdf. Accessed December 15, 2004.

Case Study 14A

The Nurse Project Manager as a Critical Success Factor: Australia's CHIME Community Health System

Mary-Jane Fry, BN, RN, and David Willock

Nurses are focused and outcome-driven, and these are the exact qualities needed for managing project initiatives, including information technology (IT). Nurses bring their clinical expertise and knowledge of management and work processes to system implementation project teams. In this case study, we examine the strategy and project team structure adopted by Queensland Health for implementing the Community Health Information Management Enterprise (CHIME) project. We propose that the project's clinical leadership was a critical factor in the successful implementation of CHIME.

Community Health within Queensland, Australia

All Australians are eligible for primary and acute care services delivered by general practitioners and public hospitals. This service is federally funded through Medicare. Public health services in Queensland are provided through a centralized government entity called Queensland Health. Although community health in Australia is federally funded, each state manages its own service delivery. Figure 14A-1 illustrates a map of Australia with Queensland highlighted.

A mix of government and nongovernment organizations, including Christian, provide community health in Queensland. The federally funded Home and Community Care is the major supplier of community services and includes the Australian government's aged care program for frail, aged, and younger people with disabilities, and their careers. Other services include child and youth health, mental health, sexual health, drug and alcohol services, palliative care, domiciliary nursing, and allied health. Queensland Health's management is divided into three geographical areas called *zones* that comprise thirty-eight districts divided as shown in Figure 14A-2. Queensland Health is a large, complex organization, employing more than 65,000 people and covering a land area of 1.73 million km. Queensland's land mass is seven times the size of Great Britain.

The Need for a Standardized Community Health Application

Historically across Australia, including Queensland, the use of information systems in community health had evolved as either service-specific or area-specific applications. In some cases, no system was used at all. By the 1990s, the federal government was looking for standardized reports on services delivered across the states to evaluate the effectiveness of those services. From Queensland's perspective, its highly complex, dispersed, and diverse community health network was becoming difficult to manage without an IT system. Simply put, a standard application used across all of Queensland's community health services would enable collection of basic service data, greater access to patients' clinical data, and development of an important component of the electronic health record (EHR).

A Partnership Approach

In the early 1990s, the state of New South Wales began working on a conceptual model for a community health information system and standardized data dictionary. During the mid-1990s, Queensland, South Australia, and the Australian Capital Territory joined in partnership with New South Wales to underwrite the cost and otherwise support the effort to develop this prototype. This multimillion dollar project ran for seven years; the end product was CHIME.

Queensland's Approach to CHIME Implementation

Once the CHIME system was available, Queensland Health, in contrast to other states in the partnership, wanted to implement quickly and broadly. To recoup its financial investment and address its business challenges, Queensland Health committed to a pilot implementation across a single district's community health services and geographic areas. To guide the pilot implementation, Queensland Health developed several

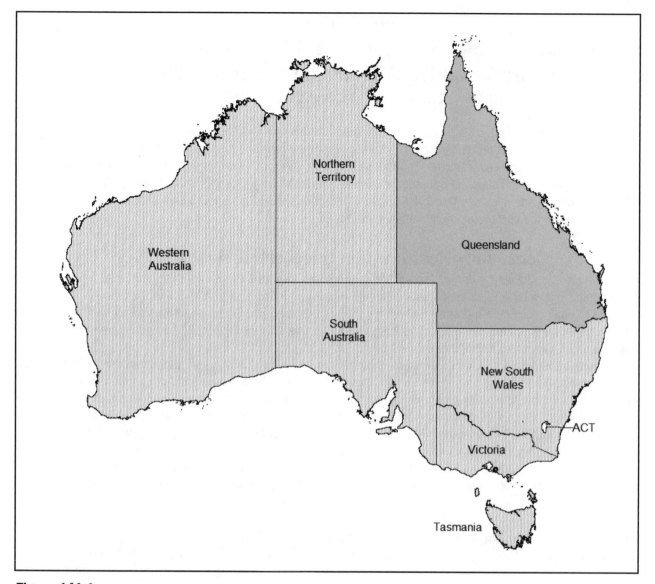

Figure 14A-1. *Queensland is located in the northeast region of Australia.*

principles: (1) there would no dual running of applications, (2) the timeframe to implement the application would be as short as possible, (3) it would test both scalability and all application functionalities, and (4) lessons learned would be incorporated into the development schedule, which would then be quickly rolled out statewide.

At the outset, the CHIME pilot project had to answer many questions and gain statewide acceptance on four levels. At the core user level, it had to be clinically relevant, simple, accessible, and fast. At the zonal and district levels, it had to provide standard and consistent information for activity, outcomes, health delivery planning, and mandatory reporting. At a corporate level, it had to provide a single, affordable solution that could be integrated to other parts of the e-health record. Brisbane South Community Health Services (BSCHS) was selected as the pilot site because of its large size, existing IT infrastructure, and strong executive support for the project. BSCHS offers almost the full spectrum of community services to two Queensland Health districts: Princess Alexandra Hospital District and Queen Elizabeth II Hospital District (Figure 14A-2, Inset B). BSCHS employs more than 400 staff, mainly clinicians and support personnel.

The Project Team and Clinical Leadership

Figure 14A-3 shows the governance structure of the CHIME project team. The project executive sponsor was a highly respected executive with a long tenure in Queensland community health, who came from a nursing

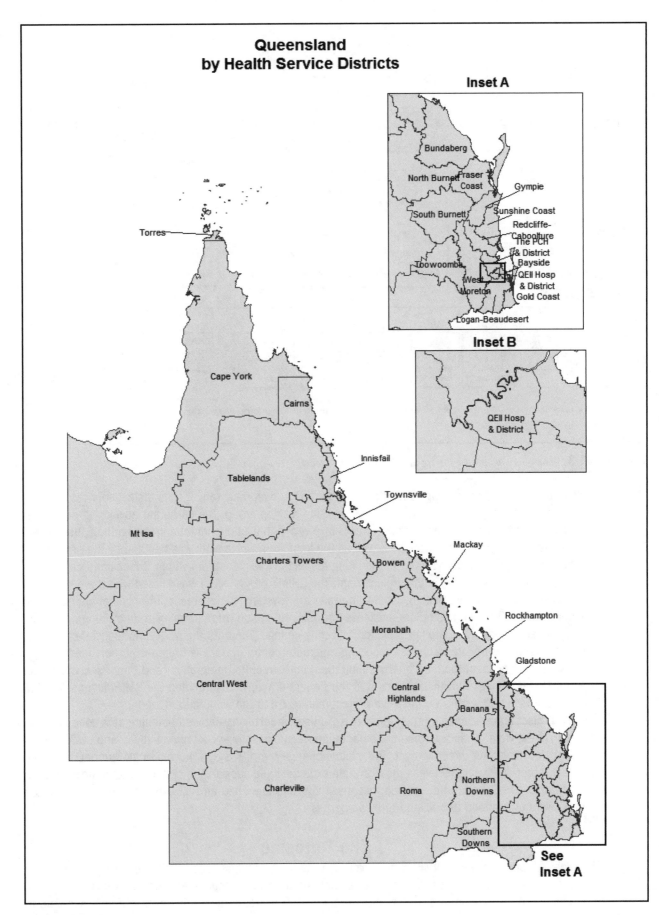

Figure 14A-2. *Queensland Health's thirty-eight districts.*

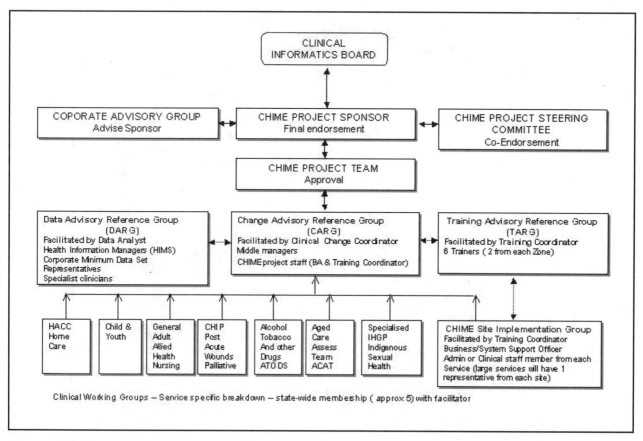

Figure 14A-3. *The governance structure of the CHIME project team.*

background. The project steering committee consisted of core representatives from district services throughout Queensland, and they constituted the key decision-making group. The corporate advisory group represented the heads of all corporate departments involved in the implementation. Recognizing that CHIME would affect the way clinicians worked as well as the manner in which work was handled by the administrative staff, careful attention was given to recruiting respected clinicians from within Queensland community health to lead and participate in the project team. The CHIME project team was formed with three key areas of expertise in mind: clinical change, data analysis, and system management. The clinical change team included within it three other streams—business analysis, education (broader focus than training), and benefits management—as these are key tools for delivering change. The data analysis team focused on consistency and definition of core data sets, reporting, migration, entry of data, and import/export functionality. The system management team covered configuration, infrastructure, integration, and ongoing second-level support. Underpinning all of these teams was the project office, which handled the PM functions. The PM leadership was a partnership between the project manager and the work stream leads.

The project team focused on their areas of expertise, undertaking detailed planning as a cohesive unit. Inevitably there were occasions when the balance between clinically acceptable usability and system management needs were in direct conflict. The clinical change team, led by a nurse, would support the clinicians and other core users; whereas the IT system experts would support the system. The important lesson is not that these conflicts were resolved, but that they were identified and all aspects and impacts of the solution were understood and agreed to by all parties.

The Outcome

The project team delivered CHIME to the seven services in its original scope. It delivered a patient record that not only acted as a registration and referral tool but included clinical notes, images, assessment tools, alerts, and care path templates. Five trainers brought 250 users, stationed in seven different sites, up to speed on the system in five months. Ten thousand client records were manually entered. The project was delivered on time and within budget. In short, the BSCHS was brought up on the CHIME system in five months from initial go-live at the first site.

Strategies and Tactics for Success

The CHIME project governance structure allowed for clinician leadership and focus. The clinical change team had a formal responsibility to function as change agents. The fact that this team was led by a senior nursing clinician was critical to the CHIME implementation success in Queensland. All education, business analysis, and benefits were undertaken within this team. As a consequence the core user was always the focus, and put simply, this is because it was clinically-led. Users openly expressed confidence in the project team, knowing that a clinician was leading the change process. Peer respect is important, particularly for clinical acceptance. Clinicians accept change more readily from a trusted source, given their evidence-based approach to practice. This is an important dynamic when dealing with multidisciplinary teams covering multiple facets of health service delivery within multiple delivery settings. Additional steps to success are outlined below.

Identify Benefits that Are Relevant to All Stakeholders. If they are to deliver true benefits to an organization, clinical system implementations cannot only be systems. They must be about fully considering the way work is done, and then envisioning the way work could be done. Immediate benefits were evident to the core users when one site was implemented, and this proof of concept was helpful in developing statewide plans.

Communicate, Communicate, Communicate. One of the success factors in such a diverse organization as Queensland Health is to communicate, communicate, and then communicate some more. The corporate, and to a certain extent, district engagement was relatively easy compared with a core user community consisting of more than 5,000 users based at 270 sites. The team used many mechanisms to deliver targeted messages and held multiple forums for engagement on a statewide basis. They addressed major concerns, including how the system would affect people's roles, specifically the time spent in front of a computer versus time spent with the client. The team also had to engage an aging workforce with different levels of technical literacy; therefore, careful attention and support was given to this group. Clinicians had concerns about the privacy, security, and confidentiality of patient information given the goal of sharing this within the CHIME system. New policies and procedures had to be developed, communicated, and taught throughout each phase of the project to reach organizational readiness on this important issue. The issues raised were common to all clinical system implementations. The important lesson is to intentionally address each of them throughout the project and, most importantly, as they occur with live use of the system.

Cultivate Strong Executive Sponsorship. The CHIME project was supported by a clinical sponsor who was committed and provided strong leadership. She also provided a considerable amount of intelligence, experience, and context with an extensive background in community health. For the clinical project manager, having access to this executive sponsor to consult, broker, and engage at the most senior level within the organization was crucial to the success of the project. In turn, the project relied on the executive sponsor to articulate the CHIME project benefits to the organization executive leadership as well as staff.

Target Your Training. Training materials need to integrate business rules and local user scenarios to ensure that the training is targeted and relevant to the audience. Much time was spent defining the current processes and how they would change with the new application. This, in turn, helped focus the training on supporting new ways of working.

Provide Visible Support. Post go-live support is key to success, ie, acceptance of the system. From the beginning, we focused on the essential aspect of supporting core users on the ground. Every member of the project team was trained as a super-user and was expected to provide go-live support. Users were supported through the CHIME help desk (technical issues); by the CHIME mobile phone hotline that was used to provide immediate user assistance; by floorwalkers who provided daily on-site support; and with one-to-one training sessions for those needing more in-depth help. Post-go-live support was kept in place for three months at all sites.

Notable Hurdles

The following section attempts to review known hurdles in this process as opposed to new, surprising obstacles.

Do Not Disadvantage the Local Site. The project leveraged heavily off the existing resources within the district to form the project team; although only four team members out of twenty-four were taken from the district, they were key resources within their local environment. Put simply, key local resources are required to ensure project success; therefore, incorporating them within the project team can compromise local readiness. Resources needed from the local site tend to be underestimated, and there is dynamic balancing that must be done to retain sufficient resources to handle workload as well as provide support at go-live.

Gain Early Access to the Product. When we were planning the CHIME implementation, it had yet to be released. We were planning, to a degree, in a vacuum. This had major implications for such key factors as the development and availability of training materials, system management, and business process change. The configuration of an application has an impact on many business processes. The planning process should allow for a reasonably lengthy configuration testing period incorporating user scenarios. It was only after establishing a full understanding of the CHIME system that key business representatives comprehended the impact of their decisions surrounding business processes. It was time-consuming to go back to some areas and adjust these processes, not to mention frustrating for users.

Control Scope and Expectations. The project changed in scope for various reasons, including a rapidly evolving community health environment. A continual change of key stakeholders both within the state and across the partnership led to different expectations that had to be managed. Changes in reporting requirements at the federal level altered the scope of the project on an ongoing basis. With each service, there were differing reporting requirements, some defined by the state, which is considerably easier to manage than national reporting requirements. Changes to scope were expected, and expectation management was a known facet of delivery. The key was to maintain the original project scope, while accommodating new requirements in future plans by documenting agreed-on changes.

Make Learning Easier. It was known that the IT skill base of the new users would be low overall. This included use of intranet, Internet, and e-mail; therefore, a basic training course was provided early and made easily available. We also had the challenge of standardizing language and terminology across the multiple disciplines that cross community health. We empowered the people involved to analyze the problem in the context of patient care quality. This helped them reach consensus and avoid turf wars.

Unanticipated Lessons Learned

The following section describes the lessons that were learned that were not initially anticipated.

What Is the Source of Truth? The application did not have the ability to combine multiple patient master indices; because the pilot site had three patient administration systems (PAS) it therefore had three patient master indices. Furthermore, the quality of data in some systems was known to be poor. This led to the decision to manually enter all "live" patients into CHIME prior to go-live. The magnitude of this effort required an urgent hiring of additional resources to keep the project on schedule. Additionally, the application could not track the hard copy records, which was essential to acceptance of the application, not to mention medico-legally. Some patients had up to four hard copy records over four different sites. The project therefore had to develop a separate Web-based tracking solution. This means that, to find a patient, users often have to search three databases: the legacy application, the CHIME application, and the tracking database.

Understand the Security Model Early On. The CHIME application has the ability to accept scanned records; however, all scanned images were located in an area that was used for storing images required under the Opioid replacement program. Given the serious potential breach in confidentiality, only drug and alcohol clinicians were granted access to this area of the system until the images of Opioid-dependent patients could be moved to a restricted area. This affected other users who relied on the ability to measure improvement via images.

Maintain Dynamic Lists: A Major Difficulty. Access to up-to-date demographic information for external service providers is imperative in community health. External service providers are referred to and contacted by clinicians daily. CHIME has the capacity to store such information; however, the effort required to maintain this database was insurmountable.

Investigate. When determining a perfect fit for a system within business processes, it is essential to know how the business operates. We determined this by interviewing the business representatives themselves. On a number of occasions, we completed this process only to find out down the track that this was not the manner in which business was conducted in that unit at all. The business representatives thought they knew how the business was run; however, what we needed in the end was a set of targeted questions to targeted key representatives to get a true understanding of that area's work.

Summary

Clinicians should lead these change transformation initiatives because they involve "selling ideas" to other clinicians. Whether or not it is warranted, when clinicians know that a peer is leading the process of change, they are reassured. They believe their interests and, more importantly, the interests of their patients are being made a priority. A clinical leader not only understands how fellow clinicians complete their tasks but also has an understanding of their tangential issues. As we have highlighted, the user, particularly the clinician, was foremost in our decision-making process. Clinicians witnessed a united approach to change from the project team; we could promote the vision for the proposed change with a united voice. As a team, we knew and could appreciate why decisions were made, and that allowed us to be united champions. On our project team we had systems and technology experts, project managers, business analysts, change specialists, and clinicians. All contributed their expertise to make for a strong and capable project team. Nurses are a new addition to such teams. Nurses need to participate in both leadership positions and as team members to give the needed clinical focus in the planning and deployment of CIS.

CHAPTER 15

The Case Management Role and Informatics

By Diane L. Huber, PhD, RN, FAAN, CNAA, BC

Case management is a provider intervention, a collaborative process that involves communication, care coordination, resource management, and advocacy. Its aim is cost-effective, coordinated care delivery that enhances clients' knowledge, involvement, empowerment, and adherence to treatment to achieve desired outcomes. Although most case managers are registered nurses, case management is a multi-interdisciplinary field of practice. Since the 1980s, case management has been recognized for its value in achieving quality while containing or stabilizing costs.[1] It has grown and expanded in areas, e.g., hospitals, health systems, and insurance companies. Case management is part of an integrated approach to meeting the health care needs of large populations. It often is targeted to the top 10 percent to 20 percent of a patient population; those who have complex care needs and are most in need of integration of clinical care and financial benefits. Figure 15-1 offers an integrated model of how case management strategies fit within a larger view of comprehensive care for an entire population.

Nurses' Roles in Case Management

All nurses are really managers, to some degree. McClure[2] describes the nature of a nurse's role as having two parts: the caregiver role and the integrator role. The caregiver role is described as what nurses do: the one-on-one direct care of clients. In this capacity, nurses use organization, management skills and knowledge to assess, plan, implement, and evaluate clients' health care needs and subsequently manage clinical services delivery. Within this role, two levels emerge: one-on-one direct care and a more aggregate level of clinical care management, e.g., disease management.[3]

The integrator role is often associated with nursing administration. This is the management of the context of care delivery and the structuring of the care delivery environment so that the safest, highest-quality, lowest-cost care occurs. The integrator role comprises care coordination across the care team and venues of care as well as systems administration levels.[3] An example of care coordination is case management. There is an area of overlap between the caregiver and the integrator roles within the coordination of clinical care.[3] Figure 15-2 displays this conceptualization of the roles of nurses.

As seen in Figure 15-2, the overlap area is the domain of care coordination and management. This describes the reality of nurses' work within a complex, multidisciplinary health care delivery setting. Nurses have their own area of practice and yet operate at the pivotal intersection of coordinating the work of many disciplines. Fragmentation of health care delivery is a patient safety issue; it also is a key area for the work of nurses. Case management is the health care services strategy used to coordinate and manage care. Along with its twin, disease management, case management has become the preferred intervention by payers for managing quality while controlling costs. This has become possible because of the growing use and sophistication of informatics applications in case and disease management.

Definitions and Models

Case management incorporates client-focused strategies designed to coordinate care.[4] It targets the coordination and integration of health services for clients with complex or extraordinarily costly health problems[5] and has a strong interdisciplinary component. The Case Management Society of America (CMSA) is the professional organization representing case managers. CMSA defines case

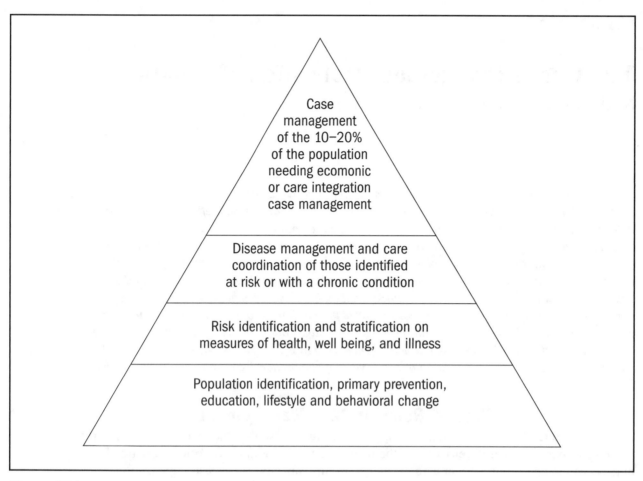

Figure 15-1. *Integrated Model. Source: ® 2005, Coggeshall Press.*

management as "a collaborative process of assessment, planning, facilitation, and advocacy for options and services to meet an individual's health needs through communication and available resources to promote quality cost-effective outcomes."[6]

Case management has also been defined as a system of health assessment, planning, service procurement, service delivery, service coordination, and monitoring through which the multiple service needs of clients are met.[7,8] A more recent definition by the American Nurses Association (ANA) is found in the American Nurses Credentialing Center's (ANCC) Nursing Case Management catalog. Their definition is:

> Nursing case management is a dynamic and systematic collaborative approach to provide and coordinate health care services to a defined population...Nurse case managers actively participate with their clients to identify and facilitate options and services for meeting individuals' health needs, with the goal of decreasing fragmentation and duplication of care, and enhancing quality, cost-effective clinical outcomes.[9]

In general, case management is any method of linking, managing, or organizing services to meet clients' needs, using elements of client assessment, service integration, and follow-up.[10] Thus, case management is the coordination and sequencing of care, aimed at tightening the plan of care and linking direct caregivers and services across facility and service boundaries. The nurse case manager coordinates care across the continuum of settings, sites, and services. Hospital nursing case management (a specific subset of case management) is usually targeted to high-risk populations. Although all clients need some degree of coordinated care, case management functions are most cost effective when used to coordinate health care services for high-risk populations across community, ambulatory, acute, and long-term care settings. The focus is on the individual client.[1]

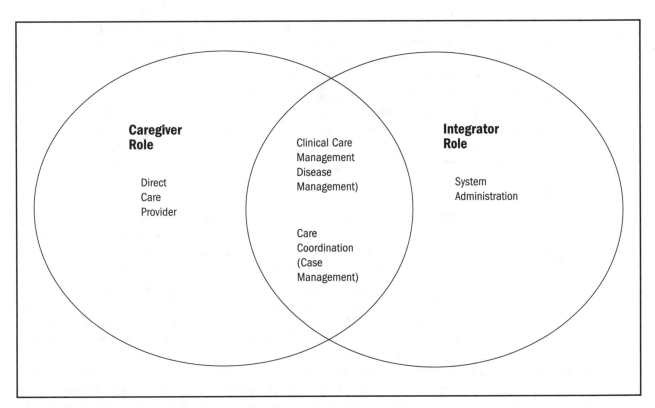

Figure 15-2. *Roles for Nurses. Source: ® 2005, Coggeshall Press*

A term used in conjunction with case management is *disease management.* Case management and disease management have been described as two sides of the same coin.[10] Disease management looks at aggregate client populations, e.g., persons with diabetes. The professional association representing disease management is the Disease Management Association of America (DMAA). Disease management is defined by the DMAA as

> "...a system of coordinated healthcare interventions and communications for populations with conditions in which patient self-care efforts are significant."[1] The DMAA identifies the following disease management components:
> 1. Population identification processes
> 2. Evidence-based practice guidelines
> 3. Collaborative practice models to include physician and support-service providers
> 4. Patient self-management education (may include primary prevention, behavior modification programs, and compliance/surveillance)
> 5. Process and outcomes measurement, evaluation, and management
> 6. Routine reporting/feedback loop (may include communication with patient, physician, health plan, and ancillary providers, and practice profiling)[11]

Because much of case management is directed at chronic care, the Chronic Care Model[12] is most often used as the conceptual framework. This model identifies six essential elements of a health care system that facilitate quality chronic illness care: the community, the health system, self-management support, delivery system design, decision support, and clinical information systems (CIS). Care coordination falls under both the health and CIS as a subconcept; case management falls under delivery system design.

Informatics and Case Management

The success of case management strategies is predicated on the use of targeted informatics strategies. Computerized support for case management begins with having a user-friendly documentation system, ideally as a part of an electronic health record (EHR). Then, informatics applications are needed to support case management processes and functions. Some case managers carry a caseload of fifteen to thirty clients, whereas others manage caseloads of hundreds or thousands. The management of large numbers of cases is feasible only with computerized support, but the complexity of case management as a health care service requires a strong informatics infrastructure in all situations. This can be done even with limited financial resources. Unable to afford expensive software programs specifically designed for case management, Skeels et al[13] customized Microsoft Outlook to fit their case management program. Two specific informatics applications in case management are programs that support predictive modeling and programs that augment demand management.

Predictive Modeling

Both case and disease management rely on the ability to identify members of a population who have a particular condition or who are at risk for adverse clinical or health care financial outcomes. In managed care, it has been found that five percent of health plan members will generate about 50 percent of total health plan expenditures.[14] This high risk group includes a yet again one percent segment that can account for 20 percent to 30 percent of all costs, usually about twenty times or more the average cost in the insured population.[14] In order to best manage this highest-risk one percent, it is necessary to precisely pinpoint specific individuals before high costs or complications occur. An effective identification process for high-risk individuals is needed, and it needs to be supported by software applications. The data are collected using survey instruments, e.g., mailed health questionnaires, more of which are becoming psychometrically tested for reliability and validity (e.g., Brody et al's work),[15] or by mining claims or administrative databases. Commercial applications are available that produce registries of high-risk individuals based on predictive algorithms. These software solutions act to scan the population and identify members in the top risk levels.

Meek and Citrin[16] noted that organizations should look for an application that can provide the following functions: find high-risk individuals before they incur; identify both high-risk individuals and those interested in being helped; manage varied populations; and be able to hold an entire population's health record. *Predictive modeling* is a methodology designed to stratify a population on its risk for an outcome.[16] The objective is to easily and effectively segment the group of high-risk clients. It is especially valuable in finding individuals at high risk for needing acute care hospitalization so that timely interventions might prevent adverse outcomes. The two important uses of predictive modeling are controlling near-term costs and improving how care management resources are allocated.

The three major statistical techniques used to develop predictive models are rules-based, statistical regression, and neural network technology.[16] *Rules-based techniques* identify individuals who meet certain criteria (e.g., diagnosis) or reach cost or utilization of services thresholds. Claims or pharmacy databases are most often used to reveal cost or utilization of services data. In this type of predictive modeling, when an individual gets a preidentified type of prescription, has a preidentified diagnosis, obtains preidentified health care services, meets a predetermined cost threshold, or has some predetermined unique combination of these factors, a high-risk score is triggered, the insurer is alerted, and the individual may be put on a nurse contact list for case or disease management.

Statistical regression models contain a series of predetermined factors that affect care use (may be based on evidence-based protocols) and that are evaluated in order to find high-risk individuals. The ideal computer-generated model would select factors that are most relevant to predicting care use, weight each factor appropriately, and then generate a probability value that indicates which members are more likely to incur high costs or seek higher levels of near-term care.[16] A risk score is thus computed, which identifies individuals for referral to case or disease management.

Neural network technology is similar to regression. It weights predetermined factors related to care and then searches for relationships between what is targeted for prediction and factors that are most predictive. Requiring very large data sets with lots of elements, neural network technology can nevertheless converge prediction outcome with actual occurrence in order to more precisely profile a population.[16]

Predictive modeling is a powerful tool for identifying, reaching, and intervening early on with individuals in high-risk populations. Engaging such individuals early in self-care and initiating health behavioral change sets the stage for improved personal health in individuals and for stabilization or reduction in the cost of care. Informatics applications and statistical analysis methods have contributed to the power of case and disease management interventions.

Demand Management

Case and disease management have developed into various forms depending on the setting and providers involved. In managed care organizations, telephonic and informatics-based initiatives have been used. These go beyond screening and health risk assessment in the attempt to reduce the demand for health care by teaching enrollees to become more skilled users of care. This activity is called *demand management.* It is defined as "the use of self-management and decision support systems to enable, educate, and encourage people to improve their health and make appropriate use of medical care."[17] The widespread access to health information through television, publications, and the Internet has influenced the perceived need for health care. Methods of demand management designed to encourage appropriate health care utilization focus heavily on teaching self-care through guides and manuals, utilizing Web sources for health information, and providing nurse telephone health counseling (telephone triage). The outcome is an informed client who is in a position to be an active participant in their care and to make informed choices about their care alternatives.[17]

The increasing demand for health care challenges the delivery system to better manage demand (and the resultant costs) by investigating how health care demand is initiated and expressed and then to use this knowledge to more effectively manage the whole system.[18] Thus, it is important to know how people navigate through the health care system and how to help them make better decisions about the appropriate use of health care services based on considerations of risk and benefit. Demand may be managed by reducing, substituting, or encouraging the use of care services.

Demand management employs two basic strategies: reducing the need for care by improving health and improving clients' decisions about service use through teaching, counseling, and self-care augmentation.[19] Wellness, health promotion, health advocacy, risk reduction, prevention, and early detection are key demand management initiatives aimed at improving health. To influence clients' decisions, strategies of giving advice and clarifying information are used. Patient education materials and telephone help lines (sometimes referred to as nurse call centers) are used to guide decision making regarding when to see a primary care provider or how to manage a condition at home. The informatics applications are computerized software programs that give the nurses protocols for responding to a wide variety of call-ins. For example, in one comprehensive demand management program, nurses used a Windows-based computer software application to customize their explanations of various care options. Clients were encouraged to make decisions for themselves based on in-depth medical and health care information.[20]

The future promises even more advanced information management technologies to supplement and enhance case and disease management. In one disease management program, new information technology helped to achieve 50 percent to 60 percent reductions in health care costs.[21] Specific examples of emerging information technologies being used in case and disease management are interactive, disease-specific Web sites designed to engage clients in self-care activities; home-based biometric measurement devices, e.g., digital scales or blood pressure monitors; work flow and care coordination software programs that have guideline-initiated alerts; registries generated from predictive modeling; and electronic linkages that connect insurers, providers, and clients to deliver patient education and communication support. These informatics-based strategies can surmount limitations found in traditional care delivery and provide a useful infrastructure to assist nurse case managers in their care interactions with clients and other providers.[21]

Summary

Case management is one area of practice in which nurses are often used as the primary care coordinator. Informatics applications are being developed and refined with greater sophistication for case management practice. As more powerful software programs emerge, case managers will be able to more precisely manage scarce resources in the delivery of cost-effective, high-quality health care. The development and use of such informatics applications is absolutely critical to the ongoing evolution and effectiveness of case management practice.

References

1. Huber DL. *Disease management: a guide for case managers.* St. Louis: Elsevier Saunders; 2005.
2. McClure M. Introduction. In: Goertzen I, ed. *Differentiating nursing practice: into the twenty-first century.* Kansas City, MO: American Academy of Nursing; 1991:1-11.
3. Huber DL. *Nurses' roles: CNL, nursing administration and case management.* Unpublished paper. Iowa City: University of Iowa; 2005.
4. Bower KA. *Case management by nurses.* Kansas City, MO: American Nurses Publishing; 1992.
5. Grimaldi PL. A glossary of managed care terms. *Nurs Manage.* 1997; 27 (suppl): 5-7.
6. Case Management Society of America. *Standards of practice for case management.* Little Rock, AR: Case Management Society of America; 2002.
7. American Nurses' Association. *Nursing case management* (Publication No. NS-32). Kansas City, MO: American Nurses' Association. 1988.
8. Zander K. Case management: a golden opportunity for whom? In: McCloskey J, Grace H, eds. *Current issues in nursing.* 3rd ed. St. Louis: Mosby. 1990: 199-204.
9. American Nurses Credentialing Center. *Nursing case management catalog.* Washington, DC: American Nurses Credentialing Center. Available at: http://nursingworld.org/ancc/certification/cert/certs/specialty.html. Accessed June 11, 2005.
10. Zawadski R, Eng C. Case management in capitated long-term care. In: *Health Care Financing Review,* Annual Supplement. 1988;75-81.
11. Disease Management Association of America. *Definition of disease management.* Washington, DC: Disease Management Association of America. Available at: http://www.dmaa.org/definition.html. Accessed June 11, 2005.
12. Wagner EH. Chronic disease management: what will it take to improve care for chronic illness? *Effective Clin Pract.* 1998;1:2-4.
13. Skeels MF, Wilsker D, Roberts K, Stinson C. Case management communication on a shoestring budget. *The Case Manager.* 2004;15(4):45-49.
14. Glynn K, Patel K. Ensuring quality of highest-risk population care management in a teleworking environment. *The Case Manager.* 2004;15(3):61-64.
15. Brody KK, Maslow K, Perrin NA, et al. Usefulness of a single item in a mail survey to identify persons with possible dementia: a new strategy for finding high-risk elders. *Dis Manage.* 2005;8(2):59-72.
16. Meek J, Citrin RS. Predictive modeling and its application to disease and case management. In: Huber D, ed. *Disease Management: A Guide for Case Managers.* St. Louis: Elsevier Saunders. 2005:21-31.
17. Peterson KW, Kane DP. Beyond disease management: population-based health management. In: Todd WE, Nash D, eds. *Disease Management: A Systems Approach to Improving Patient Outcomes.* Chicago: American Hospital Publishing; 1997:305-342.
18. Pencheon D. Managing demand: matching demand to supply fairly and efficiently. *BMJ.* 1998;316:1665-1667.
19. White B. Demand management: putting patients first. *Family Practice Management.* Available at: http://www.aafp.org/fpm/980900fm/patfirst.html. Accessed June 11, 2005.
20. Gray BB. *Demand management helps patients make choices.* Available at: http://www.nurseweek.com/features/0796/demand.html. Accessed June 11, 2005.
21. Nobel JJ, Norman GK. Emerging information management technologies and the future of disease management. *Dis Manage.* 2003;6(4):219-231.

CHAPTER 16

Every Organization Needs Them: Nurse Informaticians

By Joyce Sensmeier, MS, RN, BC, CPHIMS, FHIMSS

In their primary role as health care providers, registered nurses (the largest group of health care providers in the U.S.[1]) need access to patient information whenever and wherever they are delivering care. Because they understand the potential impact of new systems and technology on their work flow, nurses frequently act as change agents. Health care organizations, vendors, and consulting groups are recognizing the importance of nursing involvement in the design, implementation, and evaluation of information systems. This recognition is driving the demand for nurse informaticians with the knowledge and skills to develop and implement information systems that will enhance nursing work flow, promote patient safety, and elicit clinical outcomes to improve patient care.

The Growing Demand for Nurse Informaticians

The 2000 National Sample Survey of Registered Nurses projects that 8,406 of the 2.7 million registered nurses in the U.S. identify nursing informatics (NI) as their nursing specialty.[1] To achieve a national vision for the majority of Americans to have interoperable electronic health records (EHRs) and personal health records within ten years,[2] it has been suggested that additional physician and nurse informaticians are needed in health care. According to Charles Safran, MD, chair of the American Medical Informatics Association (AMIA) board, "There is a critical need for trained informatics professionals if we seriously hope to implement the president's vision concerning EHRs. I would like to see 6,000 physicians and 6,000 nurses with high-level clinical informatics training—one for every hospital and care setting by 2010." (C. Safran, CSafran@cstlink.com, e-mail, March 1, 2005.) The recently formed Alliance for Nursing Informatics, a collaboration of twenty distinct nursing informatics groups, will provide a vehicle for a single, unified voice for NI, allowing consistent representation and participation in the public health care policy process; information technology (IT) standards development; information systems design, implementation, and evaluation; and shared communication and networking opportunities.[3]

The Increasing Emphasis on Core Clinical Systems

Health care provider and payer organizations in the U.S. spent $36.7 billion on IT in 2003.[4] Increasingly, clinical systems are moving to the head of the class with system implementations. In a recent survey of health care chief information officers (CIOs), bar-coded medication management systems, clinical information systems (CIS), and computerized provider order entry (CPOE) systems were rated among the most important IT applications to implement in the next two years.[5] Respondents in this survey also identified clinical informatics as a key staffing need in their organizations.

Using Technology to Improve Patient Safety

Using information systems to reduce medical errors and promote patient safety is the number one IT priority identified by CIOs today.[6] Reducing medical errors is also identified in this same 2005 survey as the top business issue facing health care. The central role of nurses in patient safety initiatives was validated in a patient safety survey conducted in 2003, which cited nurses more often than any other constituency (95 percent) as participants on patient safety committees.[7]

Mounting evidence shows that clinical information systems have a big impact on reducing medical errors. Approximately fifty-one medication errors were prevented each day after implementation of a bedside bar-coded medication management system at a 623-bed regional tertiary-care medical center.[8] The rate of medication error prevention has since remained consistent at 10 to 11 per 1,000 administrations. The University of Wisconsin Hospital and Clinics performed a direct-observation study of medication errors before and after the implementation of a bar-coded medication management system. The hospital demonstrated that medication administration errors decreased by 87 percent with the use of bar codes.

CPOE is another application that can impact medical errors. After a large tertiary care hospital in the Midwest implemented an integrated CIS that incorporated CPOE, medication error rates were reduced by 35 percent, and transcription errors were eliminated.[9] However, depending on the computer system's design and user competence, automated computer systems for administering medications can contribute to mistakes. A United States Pharmacopeia study of 570 hospitals and other health facilities found 235,159 medication errors in 2003. About 20 percent of those errors involved automated drug administration systems. However, it was determined that the mistakes arising from computerized systems were about half as likely to harm patients.[10]

The role of CPOE in facilitating medication errors was explored in a recent study of house staff interaction with a CPOE system at a tertiary-care teaching hospital. Study results demonstrated that the CPOE system exacerbated or caused twenty-two types of medication error risks, including fragmented medication views, ignored antibiotic renewal notices, and inflexible ordering formats generating wrong orders.[11] However, further analysis of the study questions its validity in terms of its methodology and subsequent outcomes. The study does not compare errors resulting from paper ordering to computerized order entry, and it is based on interviews with ordering physicians and observations of them at work, rather than providing actual measurement of errors or adverse events.

According to PricewaterhouseCoopers,[12] hospitals that invest sufficiently in technology are found to have improved clinical processes, increased revenue, and fewer errors. The Indiana Heart Hospital, which opened in 2002, is the first all-digital heart hospital in the U.S. Metrics compared to previous cardiac facilities in the health system show that in its first year of operation, the Indiana Heart Hospital achieved:

1. An 85 percent reduction in medication errors
2. A 65 percent reduction of inappropriate denials and delays with respective payers
3. Reduction of chart management costs from $15 to $3 per chart
4. A 45 percent reduction in medical transcription and dictation costs

The report says that digital hospitals spend between 3 and 5 percent of their operating budgets on IT, whereas a typical hospital spends only 2.5 percent

Launching the Decade of Health Information Technology

In April 2004, President George W. Bush established the position of national coordinator for health information technology (HIT) and called for the majority of Americans to have an interoperable EHR within ten years. As the appointed national coordinator, David Brailer, MD, PhD, has responsibility for coordinating programs and policies regarding HIT across the federal government. At a summit in July 2004, he launched "the Decade of Health Information Technology" and outlined a plan for accomplishing four major goals. These goals, described in the Framework for Strategic Action[13] as the means for realizing a vision for improved health care, are

- Inform clinical practice
- Interconnect clinicians
- Personalize care
- Improve population health

Informing clinical practice focuses on efforts to bring EHRs directly into clinical practice. As primary caregivers, nurses will benefit from timely, accurate information that is available at the point-of-care. Patients will benefit from a reduction in medical errors and duplicative work, enabling clinicians to focus on improved patient care.

Dr. Brailer recently sought the input of nurses in helping to achieve the goal of EHR adoption. At a meeting with nurse informaticians from a variety of roles and settings, Dr. Brailer expressed concern as to whether enough nurse informaticians are available. Moreover, he confirmed his commitment to utilizing the nurses currently working within federal agencies to implement his agenda. After revealing that his mother has been a nurse for fifty years, he promised a continuing dialogue with nursing and announced that his office would soon be establishing a nurse fellowship program.

The Nurse Informatician's Key Roles in Clinical Systems Success

Nurse informaticians play many key roles in creating an effective health care information technology infrastructure. As project managers, they help develop and implement CIS. They educate others in NI, and they develop research agendas related to evaluating the impact of informatics on quality and nursing care.[14] Some of these experts purchase information systems for hospitals, outpatient settings, and community and home care nursing environments. They also contribute to decision support, outcomes management, advocacy, and policy development. Increasingly nurse informaticians are taking executive-level positions and are being recruited for the position of CIO or chief nursing information officer (CNIO).

Nursing Informatics Survey and Implications

In a recent survey of 537 nurse informaticians, two-thirds of respondents reported that systems implementation is their top job responsibility.[15] In addition, these nurses have implemented about one-quarter of the CPOE systems in the U.S. The results suggest that nurse informaticians play a critical role in the implementation of clinical information and documentation systems. Although two-thirds of respondents work in a hospital or health care system, nearly one-quarter work for a vendor, a supplier, or a consulting firm.

Methodology

To better understand the background of nurse informaticians, the issues they address daily, and the tools they use in their job-related roles, the Healthcare Information and Management Systems Society (HIMSS) conducted a Web-based survey in October 2003. Input to the survey came from a number of NI groups, including the Puget Sound Nursing Informatics Group (PSNIG), Capital Area Roundtable on Informatics in Nursing (CARING), Nursing Information Systems Council of New England (NISCNE), American Nursing Informatics Association (ANIA), Boston Area Nursing Informatics Consortium (BANIC), Delaware Valley Nursing Computer Network (DVNCN), and Midwest Alliance for Nursing Informatics (MANI). Support was also received from the Utah Nursing Informatics Network (UNIN).

Nurse informaticians who were part of these organizations, as well as HIMSS members, were invited to participate in the survey. A total of 537 usable responses were received, making it the largest ever survey of nurse informaticians. A summary of this survey follows.

About the Respondents

A hospital setting is the work environment for more than half of the survey respondents, with another 13 percent working at the corporate level of a health care system. Almost one-quarter (21 percent) are employed by a vendor, supplier, or consulting organization. The remaining 15 percent of respondents work for other facilities, including academic settings, government or military facilities, payer or managed care employers, and ambulatory care locations.

In terms of geographic location, one-quarter of the respondents (26 percent) work in the South and Middle Atlantic (Delaware, Florida, Georgia, Maryland, North Carolina, South Carolina, Virginia, West Virginia, and Washington DC) region. The second and third largest geographic areas represented include the East North Central (Illinois, Indiana, Michigan, Ohio, and Wisconsin) region (18 percent) and the Pacific (Alaska, California, Hawaii, Oregon, and Washington) region (16 percent). Five percent or fewer respondents came from each of the following regions: Mountain (Arizona, Colorado, Idaho, Montana, Nevada, New Mexico, Utah, and Wyoming), New England

(Connecticut, Maine, Massachusetts, New Hampshire, Rhode Island, and Vermont), West South Central (Arkansas, Louisiana, Oklahoma, and Texas), and East South Central (Alabama, Kentucky, Mississippi, and Tennessee).

Survey respondents go by a wide variety of job titles, including application analyst, clinical analyst, clinical applications specialist, consultant, director of nursing informatics, informatics nurse specialist, nursing informatics specialist, project manager, and senior application specialist. No single job title emerged as a standard, illustrating the diversity of roles and related job titles in this emerging field. This variability was confirmed by a recent review of NI–related job titles that identified 30 different titles, with clinical analyst and clinical systems analyst listed in the top ten (S. Newbold, snewbold@umaryland.edu, e-mail, March 15, 2005).

Clinical Background and Education

Nearly half of the nurses in this survey have achieved a postgraduate degree. One-third of the respondents (31 percent) hold a master's degree in nursing, and another 14 percent hold a master's degree with a non-nursing focus, e.g., an MBA. Only 3 percent of respondents have achieved a doctorate degree in nursing, whereas 1 percent has a different kind of doctoral degree.

Prior to beginning an informatics career, half of the respondents indicate they had at least sixteen years of clinical experience. Nearly half of the respondents have a background either in critical care or in medical or surgical nursing. One-quarter of the respondents (25 percent) report critical care nursing—also a high-tech specialty—as their background. Another 22 percent report a background in medical/surgical nursing, and an additional 15 percent report a background working in multiple departments. The nursing backgrounds of other respondents include specialties, e.g., emergency medicine, surgery, and pediatrics. Only 3 percent of nurses report having a background solely in informatics. Previous clinical experience is key to enabling a nurse informatician to understand the potential impact of technology on work flow and to using the technology to transform rather than negatively affect the nurse's work environment.

Informatics Training and Experience

As a result of the recent demand for clinical informaticians, most of those surveyed have been involved with informatics for only a few years (see Figure 16-1). Only one-quarter of the respondents have ten or more years of informatics experience, and nearly 40 percent have fewer than five years. Nearly one-quarter of respondents (23 percent) have only one to two years of experience.

In contrast to medical informaticians, most of the nurse informaticians in this survey do not continue in active clinical practice. Nearly three quarters of the respondents (74 percent) reported that they spend no time performing clinical functions, whereas another 18 percent spend less than 25 percent of their time on clinical responsibilities. Only 8 percent of respondents reported devoting more than 25 percent of their time to clinical activities once they assume an informatics-related role.

More than half of the respondents indicated that their informatics knowledge and skills came from on-the-job training. And although nearly half of the survey respondents hold a postgraduate degree, only 10 percent hold a formal degree in their informatics specialty. Three percent reported that they completed informatics training as a concentration or minor within another degree program.

Nearly half of the survey respondents hold at least one professional certification relevant to their work. Among those who indicated that they are certified, nearly 50 percent have achieved the NI certification offered by the American Nurses Credentialing Center. More than one-third (37 percent) indicated that they are certified in another nursing area, e.g., perioperative nursing (Certified Nurse Operating Room—CNOR) or critical care nursing. Four percent reported that they hold the Certified Professional in Healthcare Information Management Systems (CPHIMS) certification offered through HIMSS.

Workplace Setting

Adding fuel to the continuing debate over the ideal reporting structure, no single reporting department emerges for nurse informaticians in this survey. Approximately 37 percent indicated that they

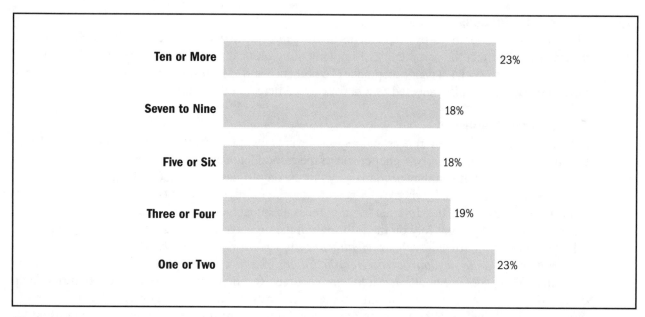

Figure 16-1. *Number of Years as a Nurse Informatician. Source: HIMSS 2004 Nursing Informatics Survey*

report to the information systems department, whereas 26 percent report directly to the nursing department. Respondents also indicate that they report to other areas, including administration, sales and marketing, implementation, or quality improvement.

Job Responsibilities

Most of the surveyed nurses work in an independent role with minimal supervisory requirements. Of those with supervisory responsibilities (fewer than 50 percent of the respondents), 48 percent oversee four or more employees. Only 25 percent indicated that they had managerial responsibility for eight or more individuals.

Systems implementation, defined to include training, supporting, and preparing users, was reported as the top job responsibility by 67 percent. Systems development, which includes the customizing and updating of a vendor system or the creating and updating of an in-house system, was identified by 52 percent of the respondents as a top job responsibility. Thirty-three percent of the respondents identified the last of the top three job roles, acting as a liaison or communicator, which includes working with administration and coordinating activities. Leading quality initiatives (e.g., system evaluation and problem solving, quality improvement, and patient safety) and informatics education (e.g., training, planning, and continuing education) were each identified by approximately 25 percent of the respondents. Less than 10 percent of respondents identified policy development, operations, sales and marketing, and informatics research.

Respondents to this survey were most likely to identify systems development and implementation as critical components of their day-to-day role. The extensive clinical backgrounds of these respondents lend themselves nicely to these tasks, because nurses have an intimate understanding of the environment, work flow, and procedures necessary for a successful implementation.

Respondents were also asked to identify the applications they were involved in developing or implementing. Seventy-four percent indicated they were involved with a clinical documentation system. Another 71 percent reported that they were implementing a CIS. Fifty-two percent were implementing CPOE systems, and 48 percent were implementing an EHR. Fewer than 25 percent of the respondents were involved with the development or implementation of the following systems: barcoded medication management, ICU technology, enterprise master patient index, picture archiving and communications, and utilization review.

Barriers to Success

Three key areas, identified by respondents as the greatest barriers to success in their role as nurse informatician, reflect the complexity of implementing clinical systems: (1) availability of financial resources (18 percent), (2) user acceptance (16 percent), and (3) administrative support (16 percent). Software design was also selected as a barrier by 12 percent of the respondents.

Educational Resources

Attendance at national conferences and regional events most frequently meets the respondents' continuing education needs. Sixty-eight percent of the respondents indicated that their preferred method for getting the information they need to carry out the day-to-day requirements of their positions was from a national conference, whereas 58 percent depend on regional events. Many nurses depend on multiple sources, with the Internet as the most frequent source of information (78 percent). Approximately 60 percent rely on the information they receive from listserves, whereas 52 percent rely on industry journals, such as *Healthcare Informatics, Journal of the American Medical Informatics Association, Journal of Healthcare Information Management,* and others. Slightly more than 33 percent use books as a frequent resource. Respondents were least likely to turn to help desks (17 percent) and survey research (15 percent) for their daily needs. Formal education venues, either in a traditional classroom setting or over the Internet, are sources of continuing education for nearly half of the respondents.

"Nurse informaticians are most likely to be interested in learning more about professional practice trends and issues"; this response was chosen by 59 percent of the respondents. Information on informatics careers (45 percent) and database design and management (43 percent) was also considered important. Systems integration, report writing, and Web technology each received a nearly 40 percent response, confirming the broad scope of the nurse informatician's role.

Professional affiliation is important to more than 90 percent of survey respondents, who indicated they were members of at least one professional association. One-third of respondents belong to only one organization, with another 47 percent belonging to two or three organizations. Of the respondents who indicated they were members of a professional association, nearly 40 percent held a HIMSS membership, 37 percent are members of CARING, and 35 percent belong to the ANIA. More than one-third of respondents also indicated they are members of the Sigma Theta Tau International Honor Society for Nursing, and nearly 20 percent are AMIA members.

Compensation

The average salary earned by respondents is $69,500. Approximately one-third of nurses responding to this survey report an annual salary of less than $60,000; another third earn a salary of between $60,000 and $75,000. Respondents living in the New England and Middle Atlantic regions tend to earn higher salaries. Those living in the West South Central and West North Central regions are more likely to earn salaries of $60,000 or less.

More than half (58 percent) of the respondents who work for vendor organizations earn a salary in excess of $75,000 (see Figure 16-2). Those working in hospital and health system settings tend to earn lower salaries; only 20 percent of those working for a stand-alone hospital and 35 percent of those working for a health system earn $75,000 or more annually.

Not surprisingly, individuals with managerial responsibilities tend to earn higher salaries. Among respondents who manage eight or more individuals, 64 percent earn a salary of $75,000 or more. Conversely, among respondents who manage only one individual, nearly half earn $60,000 or less.

Education, years of experience, and salary are also related. Only 20 percent of individuals with a graduate education earn $60,000 or less annually, compared with 46 percent of individuals who do not hold a graduate-level degree. Among individuals with ten or more years of experience as nurse informaticians, 59 percent earn $75,000 or more. Conversely, only 17 percent earn $60,000 or less.

Clinical Applications, Current and Future

Patient safety is a well-documented priority for health care organizations,[16] and nurses play a vital role in providing safe, high-quality patient care. As reflected in the Nursing Informatics Survey,

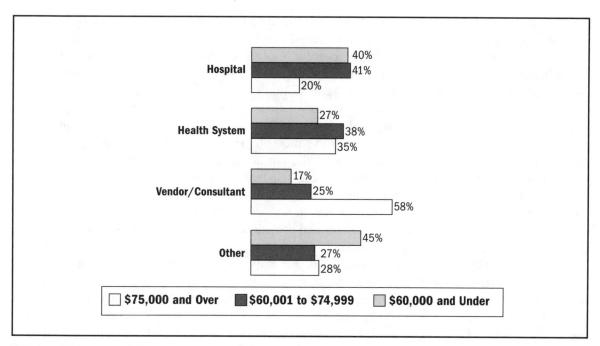

Figure 16-2. *Salary By Type of Organization. Source: HIMSS 2004 Nursing Informatics Survey*

nurses play a critical role in the implementation of safety-oriented systems. Newly emerging technologies, e.g., biometrics, genomic messaging, wearable computers, robotics, and implantable medical devices, e.g., radio frequency identification—will also be a focus for health care organizations within the next several years.[17]

Future Directions and the Role of the Nurse Informatician

Major drivers for the use of technology in the health care industry will likely influence the future role of the nurse informatician. New drug discoveries, applications such as genomics research to practice, and the advancing use of medical devices as special-purpose computers, will enhance the opportunities for applying technology to new and emerging systems. Regulation and compliance activities, including new and ongoing requirements from the Health Insurance Portability and Accountability Act of 1996 (HIPAA), Joint Commission on Accreditation of Healthcare Organizations (JCAHO), and Centers for Medicare & Medicaid Services (CMS) will continue to affect current and future systems, processes, and applications, creating new opportunities for evaluating outcomes.

Flat or declining reimbursement, rising overhead costs, and the drive for pay-for-performance initiatives will add pressure for providers. Physician and nurse recruitment, retention, and productivity issues will continue to stretch needed resources, increasing the demand for traditional "back office" systems, and encourage the evaluation of work flow. Government activities that encourage the industry to achieve the goal of widespread use of EHRs will continue to drive standards-based systems that can support the necessary integration and meet the interoperability requirements. Consumer demand for better information, greater choice, and more control over their health care will influence the usability of systems and provide impetus for the development of personal health records.

Consumer Informatics

Patients are demanding a greater role in their health care decision making. More data are accessible to them on the Internet, and increasingly they are coming to their health care encounters armed with this information—hence the current administration's strong commitment to advancing quality, consumer-driven health care and to encouraging collaboration and productivity in the medical services sector. Consumer empowerment and active interaction between consumers and the Internet have been rapidly increasing since the early 1990s. In research among 2003 adults surveyed by telephone in June and August 2004, Harris Interactive® found that 156 million (74 percent) of adults are now online, up from 69 percent in late 2003, 67 percent in late 2002, 64 percent in late 2001, 63 percent in 2000, and 56 percent in 1999. When Harris Interactive® first began to track Internet use in 1995, only 9 percent of adults reported that they were online.[18]

Collaborative healthware is the application of information and communication technologies designed to enhance decision making and communication among providers, patients, and their families.[19] This software will enable caregivers and patients to act as partners, enhancing their trust and confidence in provider–patient relationships. With their understanding of technology and the application of related software, nurse informaticians can help both caregivers and patients with knowledge transfer and shared decision making. A new nursing role—that of Internet guide—has developed as patients are given prescriptions to find information resources at recommended Web sites.[20]

Patient-centric portals that allow patients and providers to communicate across the Internet are increasing. According to Manhattan Research, about 16 million consumers reported using a hospital Web site in 2005, up by 6 million from 2004.[21] Portals can be used as forums for secure e-mail requests for prescription refills, for test results, or for nonclinical needs, e.g., scheduling appointments and asking questions about billing and referrals. Approximately 35,000 patients use the Beth Israel Deaconess Medical Center portal each month, and on average, a patient sends 1.2 e-mails per month, 90 percent of which are handled by a nurse practitioner or other staff member.[22] Key to portal success is its effective and secure use of e-mail communication, which can improve the delivery of timely, quality health care.

Knowledge-Driven Decision Support

The term clinical decision support provides the capability to recognize knowledge as a critical asset. It broadly refers to providing clinicians or patients with clinical knowledge and patient-related information to enhance patient care.[23] The application of clinical decision support can enable the clinician to improve outcomes in health care organizations. Key to its success is the link with documentation and its relationship to work flow. Opportunities exist for nurse informaticians to advance this technology for applying evidence to practice. Toward that end, nurse informaticians need an international standard for a nursing minimum data set that supports evidence-based practice and outcomes research, along with informatics processes that provide a mechanism by which they can view the effectiveness of evidence-based practice over time.[24]

Electronic Health Records

The president's call for the majority of Americans to have an interoperable EHR within ten years has energized the industry and given impetus for collaboration among stakeholders to embrace IT. The Physicians Electronic Health Record Coalition has been formed to "assist physicians, particularly those in small- and medium-sized ambulatory practices, to acquire and use affordable, standards-based EHRs and other HIT for the purposes of improving quality, enhancing patient safety, and increasing efficiency."[25] The Certification Commission for Health Information Technology[26] was founded to accelerate the adoption of interoperable HIT by creating an efficient, credible, sustainable mechanism for the certification of such products; the goal is certification of ambulatory care EHR products by summer 2005. The commission has formed work groups to address the following four areas:

1. **Functionality**—the features and functions that the EHR product must provide
2. **Security and reliability**—the protection of the privacy of data with sufficient robustness to prevent data loss
3. **Interoperability**—the ability of the EHR product to perform standards-based data exchange with other sources of health care information
4. **Certification process**—determining how vendors will apply for certification, how product compliance will be tested, and how the database of certified products will be maintained and publicized

Nearly two-thirds of the CIO respondents in the HIMSS 2005 Annual Leadership Survey indicate that an EHR is the most important application in the next two years. Although only 18 percent have a fully operational EHR system, 42 percent are currently installing one. As seen in the 2004 HIMSS Nursing Informatics Survey, 48 percent of the nurse respondents are involved with an EHR implementation. And nearly half of adults (45 percent) say that it is very important for patients to be able to track their own personal health information in an electronic record.[27] Outcomes from the implementation of an EHR at the Mayo Clinic[28] resulted in improved accessibility of patients' medical information, documentation quality, patient safety, and patient and staff satisfaction. The system also enabled the reduction of support staff by 25 percent. The acceleration of EHR implementations will increase the demand for nurse informaticians who can provide the expertise needed for evaluating the impact of EHR systems on the delivery of patient care.

Pay-for-Performance

CMS has recently identified the physician practices that will participate in the first public pay-for-performance demonstration. CMS will implement a process intended to lower Medicare costs and improve health care quality by offering to return to physicians a portion of the money that they save the government program.[29] The fundamental concept of pay-for-performance models is to tie payment to how well providers adhere to practice standards.[30] As leaders in the design and implementation of CIS that enhance work flow and capture the necessary data for optimal care delivery and reporting of outcomes, nurse informaticians will play many key roles in these models. The challenge for nurses will be to identify the necessary elements of nursing documentation that can be used for performance measurement and to activate industry-wide collaboration for their use.

References

1. 2000 National Sample Survey of Registered Nurses. Available at: http://bhpr.hrsa.gov/healthworkforce/. Accessed March 26, 2005.

2. Thompson TG, Brailer DJ. *The Decade of Health Information Technology: Delivering Consumer-centric and Information-rich Health Care.* Washington, DC: Department of Health and Human Services; 2004.

3. Alliance for Nursing Informatics. Nursing informatics groups form alliance through HIMSS and AMIA to provide unified structure. Available at: http://www.himss.org/ASP/topics_News_item.asp?cid=57813&tid=30. Accessed March 26, 2005.

4. Frost and Sullivan. How big is the health IT market? *Health Data Management.* 2004;12(10): 28.

5. Healthcare Information and Management Systems Society. 16th annual HIMSS leadership survey, sponsored by Superior Consultant Company. Available at: www.himss.org. Accessed February 28, 2005.

6. *Ibid.*

7. Healthcare Information and Management Systems Society. 2003 HIMSS patient safety survey, sponsored by McKesson Corporation. Available at: http://www.himss.org/content/files/PatientSafetyFinalReport8252003.pdf. Accessed February 28, 2005.

8. Galusha C. The challenges and success of implementing a bedside barcoding system. *HIMSS 2005 Annual Conference Proceedings.* Chicago: HIMSS; 2005.

9. Jacobs B, Price T. Success with CPOE and ICIS. *HIMSS 2005 Annual Conference Proceedings.* Chicago: HIMSS; 2005.

10. United States Pharmacopeia. Computer entry a leading cause of medication errors in U.S. health systems. Available at: http://www.onlinepressroom.net/uspharm/. Accessed Feb. 28, 2005.

11. Koppel R, Metlay JP, Cohen A, et al. Role of computerized physician order entry systems in facilitating medication errors. *JAMA.* 2005:293(10): 1197-1203.

12. PricewaterhouseCoopers. Reactive to adaptive: transforming hospitals with digital technology. Available at: http://www.pwc.com/digitalhealth. Accessed March 19, 2005.

13. Thompson TG, Brailer DJ. *The Decade of Health Information Technology: Delivering Consumer-centric and Information-rich Health Care.* Washington, DC: Department of Health and Human Services; 2004.

14. American Nurses Association. *Scope and Standards of Nursing Informatics Practice.* Washington, DC: American Nurses Publishing; 2001.

15. Healthcare Information Management and Systems Society. 2004 HIMSS nursing informatics survey, sponsored by Omnicell, Inc. Available at: www.himss.org. Accessed March 26, 2005.

16. Healthcare Information Management and Systems Society. Patient safety and nursing: transforming the work environment with technology, sponsored by McKesson. Available at: http://www.himss.org/content/files/Nursing_Informatics_Toolkit/White%20paper/McKesson%20Nursing%20Pt%20Safety%20Paper.pdf. Accessed March 1, 2005.

17. Featherly K. Emerging technologies. *Healthcare Inf.* 2005:22(1), 25-34.

18. Harris Poll. More than one-third of internet users now have broadband. Harris Interactive, The Harris Poll #63, September 8, 2004. Available at: http://www.harrisinteractive.com/harris_poll/index.asp?PID=432. Accessed March 26, 2005.

19. Goldsmith D, Safran C. Collaborative healthware. In: Nelson R, Ball MJ, eds. *Consumer Informatics: Applications and Strategies in Cyber Health Care.* New York: Springer-Verlag; 2004.

20. Ball MJ. Nursing informatics of tomorrow. *Healthcare Inf.* 2005:22(2), 74-78.

21. Beusekom MV. Patient-centric portals. *Healthcare Inf.* 2005:22(2), 58–60.

22. *Ibid.*

23. Osheroff JA, Pifer EA, Sittig DF, Jenders RA, Teich JM. *Clinical Decision Support Implementers' Workbook.* Chicago: HIMSS; 2004.

24. Bakken S, McArthur J. Evidence-based nursing practice: A call to action for nursing informatics. *J Am Med Inf Assoc.* 2001:8(2), 289-290.

25. Physicians' Electronic Health Record Coalition. Available at: http://www.centerforhit.org/x199.xml. Accessed on March 26, 2005.

26. The Certification Commission for Health Information Technology. Available at: http://www.cchit.org/. Accessed on March 26, 2005.

27. Landro L. Electronic medical records pose risks, Americans say. *The Wall Street Journal Online,* February 24, 2005. Available at: http://online.wsj.com/public/us.

28. Moore DN, Ferguson JA. Show me the benefits: implementing an EHR. In: *2005 HIMSS Annual Conference Proceedings.* Chicago: HIMSS; 2005.

29. Glendinning D. Medicare tests pay for performance. *American Medical News.* Available at: http://www.ama-assn.org/amednews/2005/02/21/gvl10221.htm. Accessed on March 26, 2005.

30. Kimmel KC, Sensmeier J, Reeves R. Pay for Performance: An Economic Imperative for Clinical Information Systems. Available at: http://www.himss.org/content/files/PayForPerformance.pdf. Accessed on March 26, 2005.

SECTION III

Nursing Education and Information Technology

SECTION III

Introduction

Connie White Delaney, PhD, RN, FAAN, FACMI

Illustrations of nursing's responsiveness to technological innovation pervade the chapters and education exemplars included in this section. These chapters and case studies build on the changes in nursing's knowledge work, the nature of nursing as a care discipline, and the emergence of new education strategies that depend on informatics competencies. The contributions in this section reflect the permeating extension of information technology (IT) into daily clinical practice, the demand for informatics competencies in existing roles as well as a plethora of new roles that cross all domains of the healthcare industry—from bedside to the corporate boardroom.

Section III's contributors exemplify the reach of transformative educational models with national and global import. Initially, in Chapter 17, Connors describes an innovative strategy for using the electronic paperless clinical mandate to transform the learning methodology of a professional curriculum. Watkinson and colleagues in Case Study 17A from the United Kingdom and Honey in Case Study 17B from New Zealand provide further examples of using technology to teach clinical skills and to support classroom teaching. The case studies from Hovenga (17C) and Delaney and colleagues (17D) illustrate the power of collaboration and partnership. In fact, collaboration is a theme reflected as essential to the success of most innovations presented in all the contributions to this section. In Chapter 18, Paget and colleagues describe an influential partnership which has transformed informatics preparedness throughout Europe. Section III culminates with Ball and McBride's powerful description of the essential integration of informatics competencies in the preparation of all nurses. You are invited to enjoy these chapters and case studies that exemplify the boldness of educators in testing innovations that extend the classroom into the home and out to a global presence.

CHAPTER 17

Transforming the Nursing Curriculum: Going Paperless

By Helen R. Connors, PhD, RN, FAAN

The most important challenge in the education of health professionals is not preparing them to do well on high-stakes tests. Rather, it is fostering twenty-first century knowledge and skills so that they are prepared to provide quality, safe, efficient, and effective health care in a consumer-centric, global, knowledge-based society. Crossing the Quality Chasm, *an Institute of Medicine (IOM) report released in March 2001, calls for a major overhaul of the health care system, including the education of health care professionals. Specifically, the report's chapter "Preparing the Workforce" outlines the enhanced skills required of health professionals to practice in the renewed and evolving health care environment.[1] In 2003, the IOM issued a second report outlining specific core requirements for educating health professionals. The authors of this highly acclaimed report recommend that all clinicians, regardless of their disciplines, possess five core competencies:[2]*

1. *Provide patient-centered care*
2. *Work in interdisciplinary teams*
3. *Employ evidence-based practices*
4. *Apply quality improvement*
5. *Utilize informatics*

Health care informatics is viewed as the enabler that will (1) enhance patient-centered care, (2) address safety issues and continuous quality improvement through evidence-based practices and decision support protocols, and (3) provide a communication infrastructure that sustains interdisciplinary teams and promotes the measurement of outcomes and care processes.

The Old Paradigm

Despite the advances in health care information technologies (HCIT) and the numerous calls for new skills and competencies for health care providers, the fundamental approach to the clinical education of health professional students, for a variety of reasons, has not changed substantially in the last fifty years. One very important contributor to the status quo is the fact that faculty qualifications are the same as they were years ago. Faculty tend to teach in the same mode that they were taught, and most were taught in a teacher-franchised, industrial age, as opposed to a learner-franchised information age. Today's information-age students are calling for learner-driven education environments that provide access to powerful learning tools, to information and knowledge bases, and to scholarly exchange networks for the delivery of learning.[3]

It is highly apparent that, if we are to transform health care systems through the advancement of health information technologies, we need to transform the educational practices to prepare graduates who are more able to become the absolute core of this environment. We can no longer continue to educate in a low-tech paper environment when the clinical setting is "going paperless."

The New Paradigm

Imagine a learning environment in which, instead of knowledge being primarily imparted from the professor to the student, there is a culture of learning in which everyone is valued for his or her contribution and is involved in a shared effort of continually advancing the collective knowledge and skills. Imagine also less reliance on lecture notes, PowerPoint slides, and paper generation and more reliance on emerging technology to produce more efficient and effective learning and knowledge management, as well as increased academic productivity. Just as information technology (IT) has changed how we live and work, it must change how we educate our future health care providers. However, at this point, we are far behind the curve because the technology is either not being used or is being used inappropriately.

The new learning environment for health professional schools is a radical departure from the traditional view of education, which relies heavily on individual knowledge and performance and on the expectation that students acquire knowledge and skill in a linear route through the written and spoken word. The transformation requires a shift in thinking and challenges the primary assumptions of the current curriculum models. Altering such deeply ingrained beliefs, values, assumptions, and cultures and starting the process of transformation that creates next-generation educational practices requires intellectual, emotional, and social support.

Envision that we are going paperless in the academic environment. The knowledge, information, and data needed for enhanced learning and quality patient care will be readily available anytime and from anyplace through an array of technological tools. Virtual health care delivery systems and simulators will be primary learning environments for gaining clinical know-how and developing clinical expertise. The faculty will be facilitators who guide the learning process in this learner-centric environment that promotes a community of scholars.

Driving Forces for Change in Health Professional Education

Through its efforts to address the quality of health care in America, the IOM is building a basis for supporting the needed change in health care delivery systems and the related transformation in health professional education. An essential element of any attempt to change a health care system must be the education of future clinicians who will practice new approaches in new environments.

In 2000, the Institute's Quality of Care Committee issued its first report, *To Err is Human: Building a Safer Health System.*[4] This report startled the country with the assertion that 44,000 to 98,000 Americans die annually as a result of preventable mistakes. Even more startling is the fact that these numbers may be low, because, in many cases, errors are frequently unrecorded. Also, these figures did not include nursing home and ambulatory care deaths. One of the recommendations from this report has direct relevance to educating health professionals: medical schools should consider educating medical students in conjunction with nursing students, so that they learn how to do joint problem solving in the same way that health care institutions are trying to deal with real-world patient safety issues.

The education of all health professionals needs to reflect team functioning and orientation to micro- and macro-systems of care to a far greater extent than it has. The complex problems and questions faced in health care today are too complicated to be confronted by any one discipline. We need to prepare health professional students to be lifetime learners, knowledge workers, and citizens in a rapidly changing, complex, interconnected, and global environment.

Of the many challenges facing health professional education, one of the most difficult to manage is IT's impact on health care. Emerging information technologies are fundamentally changing health care and will change how we educate health professionals. Academic institutions must have strategies for dealing with the impact of these new technologies on teaching, learning, and ultimately on patient care outcomes. The knowledge and skills that health care professionals need to work in today's environment are increasingly interdisciplinary, problem-focused, and process-based, rather than linear, routine, and well-defined.

The message has been clear for some time now: nurses and other health professionals need to have informatics knowledge and skills, and acquiring the knowledge and skills should be part of their education process.[5-8] Others are making similar pleas for the incorporation of "telehealth" competencies into the curriculum as these technologies expand and become an integral part of mainstream health care.[9] Despite these appeals, the evidence shows that schools send nursing graduates off to practice without the knowledge and skill base to function in this IT age.[10] Clearly, there is a gap between competencies taught in the world of education and those required to function efficiently and effectively in emerging health care delivery settings. It is a fact that nurses and other health professionals currently in practice do not have the required skill set to meet the national goal for improved health care through IT.[11,12]

Meanwhile, the need for trained health care informaticians has increased dramatically over the last few years, as health care organizations try to meet the challenges of the Health Insurance Portability and Accountability Act (HIPAA), the Leapfrog Group, the Joint Commission on Accreditation of Healthcare Organizations (JCAHO), the National Health Information Infrastructure (NHII), the Patient Safety initiative, and other regulatory influences. In response to these regulatory challenges, medical and nursing informatics (NI) academic programs are rapidly increasing; however, little research is available to support the assertion that the competencies gained in these specialized programs are being applied to clinical practice. Also, it is highly apparent that many of these informatics skills need to be integrated at all levels of the curriculum and not only offered as a specialty focus in graduate or post baccalaureate certificate programs. Indeed, specialists are needed, but they should not be the only result of our efforts to incorporate informatics skills. As government, regulatory agencies, and purchasers of health care besiege our health care industry to use IT to address challenges of medical error, inefficiencies, labor shortages, and increasing costs, the application of advanced ITs to address these challenges becomes more ubiquitous.

As a follow-up to the IOM reports, in April 2004, President George W. Bush issued the Executive Order "Incentives for the Use of Health Information Technology and Establishing the Position of the National Health Information Technology Coordinator." The goals of this order are to:

1. Provide leadership for the development and nationwide implementation of an interoperable health IT infrastructure to improve the quality and efficiency of health care
2. Ensure that the health records of most Americans are available in electronic format within ten years[13]

On the heels of this order in 2004, then Secretary of Health and Human Services Tommy Thompson appointed David Brailer, MD, PhD, to the role of National Coordinator of Health Information Technology. Dr. Brailer is charged with implementing the strategic plan outlined in Secretary Thompson's report, "The Decade of Health Information Technology."[14]

With these national forces as drivers, nurses need to take action and adopt IT faster than they have in the past or action will be taken for them. Armed with these facts and incentives, leaders in the nursing profession and particularly in the health care IT sector are joining forces to identify solutions to address the challenges and to assist professionals in doing their part in reaching the national goal. The opportunity to transform nursing education through the use of technology has never been more apparent or more unified. The government; regulatory boards; policy makers; health care delivery systems; health care technology vendors; and health professional schools, including nursing, medicine, and allied health, are all united on this front.

It Takes a Village to Transform Health Professional Education

The IT and knowledge management marketplace is designed to assist in the management and processing of data, information, and knowledge to support the practice of health professionals. Health professional programs need to provide the environmental framework and context to develop the unique skill sets required to function in this automated world. Transforming education to meet the demands of the health care system is therefore critical to the future of nursing and other health professions. Models to integrate the necessary competencies into the curriculum need to be developed, implemented, evaluated, disseminated, and replicated.

Knowledge management and the development of knowledge workers require a heavy investment; yet, when properly applied, this investment can leverage the human potential to create unprecedented levels in health professional education and ultimately in health care delivery. As with any significant change in education, the cost to implement technologies effectively is high in terms of human and financial resources. On the other hand, the cost of *not* making the shift is just as high in terms of the quality of the program, faculty, and graduates.

The critical nature of this call to reform over the next ten years has brought together a village of stakeholders to discuss unique partnerships for enhancing health information technologies in the curriculum. It will take all of us working together to change the paradigm. Through collaboration, we can leverage resources to get us closer to the national goal. There are no doubts that it will take a village to make this shift. The following sample project exemplifies a unique innovative partnership for advancing health IT. The development, implementation, and outcomes are described.

An Academic-Business Partnership

In 2000, shortly after the first IOM report on quality and efficiencies in health care, Dean Karen Miller of the University of Kansas School of Nursing and Neal Patterson, CEO of Cerner Corporation, Kansas City, Missouri, U.S., a supplier of health care information systems, embarked on a partnership to advance health care informatics competencies, beginning with the nursing curriculum. The vision from the start was to launch the use of an electronic health record (EHR) system embedded in curriculum to teach content, process and new IT competency skills needed in the marketplace. Named the Simulated E-hEalth Delivery System (SEEDS) project, our plan was to begin with the School of Nursing and then to include additional partnerships with the other health professional schools on the health center campus. This venture marks the first time a live-production, clinical information system designed for care delivery is being used as a simulation in teaching curricula content to nursing students.[15]

The purpose of the academic-business partnership model is to fully integrate applied clinical informatics into an academic setting to bridge the gap between education practices and the competencies required in real-world clinical practice. This was accomplished by establishing the set of clinical solutions that make up Cerner's EHR system as a teaching platform throughout the curriculum, beginning with new undergraduate nursing students. The goal is to familiarize the students with the automated health care environment while keeping the technology transparent to the pedagogy. In this model, the live EHR, adapted for the education environment, permeates the nursing curriculum and follows the educational work flow. The EHR forms are designed to support the level of student learning in class, in the laboratory, and in assigned readings. Also, students are required to submit care plans and other clinical course assignments on the forms. The faculty uses the adapted EHR for teaching in the classroom, clinical seminar groups, and skills laboratory. The adapted system resulted in the development of the Academic Education Solution (AES), a new service offering that is being adopted by other universities today.

Once the automated system was initiated as a teaching platform in the curriculum, faculty quickly appreciated its power and realized they could use it to teach far more than just documentation. They can teach students to use data to make decisions, acquire information at point-of-learning, understand evidence-based practice, use decision-making tools and protocols, acquire patient teaching materials, and work more efficiently.

Initially, students are introduced to the CIS through a virtual health care delivery system using case studies and simulated experiences. Later, students use the same CIS environment to document patient assessments (these are "scrubbed" of all identifying information) and care planning for patients they encounter in various clinical settings as part of their course requirements. This unique partnership enables the academic environment to simulate more closely the reality of practice in an automated health care system, thereby assisting future nurses to develop core IT competencies.

Initiating the Partnership

The integration of the CIS into the curriculum required significant preplanning. In fact, this phase of the project took more than one year, with a large part of the time spent in translating curriculum content. During this phase, both the academic institution and the software supplier needed to assess their environments, examine necessary resources, and make substantial commitments. The technical teams from the University and the software supplier met to discuss, analyze, and implement strategies necessary for the system to run in an academic environment and to support teaching and learning. This innovative partnership—a first of its kind—challenged both organizations. Both participants needed to establish that they had the technical capacity, as well as the staff and faculty, to develop, implement, and manage the project. The University needed to demonstrate that it had the support staff to connect, support, and maintain the software applications through the campus network, desktop PC, and printers. The software supplier needed to be certain that the hardware, client-server platforms, and application software could be installed, built, and maintained through the vendor's remote hosting center. The software supplier also needed to commit resources to assist University personnel to adapt the system to fit the educational processes and work flow. Neither side had experience in using a CIS in this manner and therefore had no previous knowledge of the problems that might arise when a clinical system is adapted for an academic environment; however, both were willing to take the risks.

The school installed the supplier's full data repository, clinician order entry, documentation and clinical decision support tools to run in a live-production environment. The system's hardware and software is run and supported through a remote hosting center. A distinct advantage of a live environment is that the remote hosting center pushes the latest software updates out to the school. This means students are always working with the latest version of the software and are aligned with the current technology in the workplace.[16] In recognition of academic work patterns and the impact of new releases on faculty and students, the updates are taken once a year in early August, between semesters, allowing the faculty time to train and troubleshoot the system before implementing its use with students in the fall semester.

The Project Director as Point Person

Key to the successful implementation of this partnership was the hiring of a project manager to serve as point person with the faculty team. The right person in this position is critical to the success of any project. The academic-business partnership, however, brings together two exceedingly different cultures that need to be bridged to bring about equity and to ensure success. In the case of this project, the manager needed to be a nurse with strong informatics skills who was conversant with both sides of the partnership. That meant someone who was eligible for a faculty position *and* who had the expertise in how clinical information systems work in the real world. We sought an individual who could relate to the faculty and faculty role and who had the ability to communicate and understand the vendor side. In addition, we sought good interpersonal and communication skills, which are essential qualities in helping faculty to envision teaching through a CIS as a teaching platform and in communicating those concepts to the vendor community and others. Lastly, as with any innovation, the work is not easy; so it helps to have a project director who is high on energy and low on stress to handle the unexpected.

The tasks of the project manager are to (1) develop the technical skills to build, troubleshoot, and maintain the AES environment or to oversee these functions; (2) work with faculty to translate and adapt successful teaching strategies into ones that are transformed by the AES; (3) recognize opportunities for research and scholarship enriched by the AES environment; and (4) provide vision for transforming the learning environment to support evidence-based teaching and learning strategies, which help faculty to work more efficiently and effectively. Through meeting with the faculty and learning about the various courses in the curriculum, the project manager can generate ideas for the use of the technology in the academic environment.

The SEEDS Environment

One of the first things the project manager did was to create a simulated health care delivery system so that the students and faculty could play with the EHR in the virtual environment.

This led us to call the pilot project the Simulated E-hEalth Delivery System (SEEDS). The acronym is appropriate for this project because we truly are planting the seeds for developing future health professionals with informatics competencies. In Table 17-1, the objectives for the SEEDS project are listed and compared with the informatics competencies addressed in the literature and the IOM report.

The virtual care delivery system supported by the EHR includes an acute care hospital, as well as outpatient settings, e.g., school-based clinics, public health clinics, ambulatory care clinics, health

Table 17-1. SEEDS Objectives and Related Competencies

SEEDS Objectives	Competencies for Health Care Informatics[2,8]
1. Enhance the development of critical thinking and problem solving	a. Demonstrate thinking in a data-driven way b. Redesign teaching strategies to incorporate explicit views of data, information, and knowledge c. Recognize the use and/or the importance of nursing data for improved practice d. Assist patients to use data to make informed decisions
2. Integrate online patient assessment, problem identification, treatment, and evaluation	a. Reveal the components of the professional standards of practice b. Support the integration of recognized guidelines of quality patient care c. Identify the basic components of CIS d. Recognize that CIS will become more common
3. Demonstrate the impact of structured data and information on patient care	a. Appreciate the requirement for the use of standardized clinical terminology b. Promote the integrity of nursing information within an integrated EHR c. Define the impact of computerized information management on the role of the nurses d. Deliver patient-centric care
4. Provide the information infrastructure for evidence-based clinical practice	a. Understand the use of networks for electronic communications b. Develop competencies in information management c. Develop competencies in knowledge management d. Practice evidence-based nursing e. Discuss principles of privacy and security
5. Promote the dissemination and evaluation of knowledge and research	a. Demonstrate the value of clinicians' involvement in design, selection, implementation, and evaluation of systems b. Identify general applications available to research c. Assess the accuracy of health information on the Internet d. Focus on quality improvement e. Evaluate the applications to support best practices in nursing education

fairs, and home settings. These environments reflect all aspects of the nursing curriculum and are used with virtual patient case studies created by the faculty. In didactic, clinical seminar courses and skills learning laboratories, the cases are presented to students, who process and analyze the clinical data while using the EHR as a framework for documentation and care management. The faculty can review the students' work electronically and quickly see whether or not they are on target. Faculty also have the capability to share all student documentation on a spreadsheet embedded in the system and can point out trends and discrepancies. This provides students with rich, rapid feedback and reinforces learning.

The long-term vision is to have all health professional students interacting in the virtual environment with the same virtual patients, whose cases are adapted to the learning needs of the respective health disciplines (medicine, nursing, occupational therapy, physical therapy, nutrition, etc.). At this level, students can come to understand not only the power of the EHR, but also the multidisciplinary team approach to patient care. Other technologies, such as patient simulators, handheld computer devices, and standardized patients, can be coupled with the virtual training environment to provide safe, active learning situations for students. Use of these technologies increases clinical competencies in a controlled environment and standardizes the learning experiences.

Curriculum Transformation

Once the virtual health delivery system was created to house the EHR in the curriculum, the faculty updated previously used case studies to present virtual patients who capture the data elements, analysis, and decision-making skills required for student learning at the various levels of the curriculum and supported by the EHR. In turn, the EHR was adapted to follow the educational work flow and matched to the competencies of the curriculum. It is essential to structure the learning activities to follow clearly the novice-to-expert pathways. At first, keeping the forms simple, easy to follow, and grouped by learning concepts is important. Later, as students progress in the program

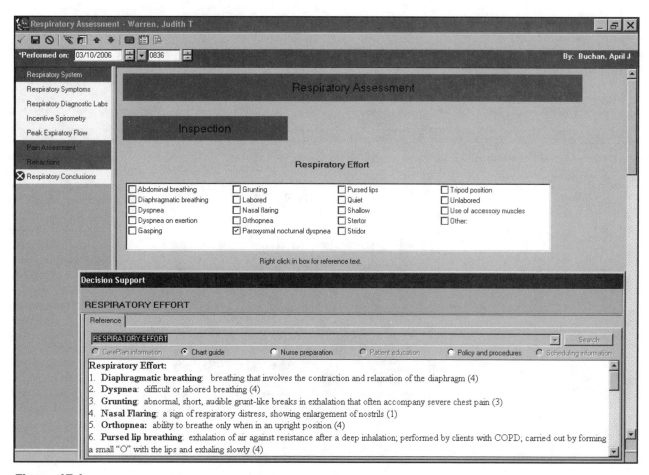

Figure 17-1. *Information at Point of Learning with Reference Text.*

and become more competent, the forms can be adapted to bring them into alignment with the EHR in real-world applications. The novice-to-expert framework supports this learning strategy.

In the first semester of nursing school, the students learn nursing process, clinical documentation, and care planning by means of the electronic system. They also develop critical thinking, decision-making skills, and experience with the concepts of data-driven management plans and evidence-based practice. Students became skilled at acquiring information at point-of-learning with a simple right click. Figure 17-1 demonstrates how medical terminology definitions are embedded in the system and readily available to students when it is important to their learning.

Students became accustomed to using the system to seek out the drug information, guidelines and protocols, and health education information that they would incorporate into their plan of care. Through this method of learning, students begin to organize, process, and manage data and information differently.

As a result of the way the system is organized, students are taught to arrange data and information in clusters, which help them to view these more efficiently and to develop their critical thinking abilities. Now more than ever, students are basing decisions on data, not assumptions. This view of the EHR as a teaching platform in the curriculum provides a visual framework on which to hang the elements of the nursing process, making it easier for students to see how the process works in patient care. Students have commented that visualizing the nursing process through the EHR allows them to have a better understanding of the relationships within the process because it provides them with a "mental picture." It is not hard to believe that a tool that helps them visualize creates increased understanding because this generation of students grew up with computers and video games and are accustomed to "mental pictures." They expect to see this technology in the classroom.

Stimulated by early changes in the learning outcomes, the faculty began to envision that, with the EHR integrated into the curriculum, they could teach more than just process. They began to experiment with teaching content and concepts through the system. For example, the faculty developed a cluster of case studies centered on a fictional three-generation Hispanic family. The family

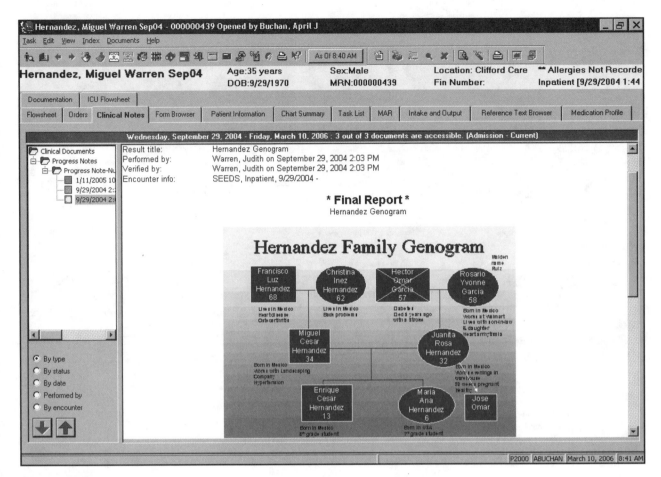

Figure 17-2. *Family Genogram.*

genogram (see Figure 17-2) and the individual family case studies are electronically integrated into the EHR. The individual case studies are developmental and follow the students throughout the curriculum. For example, Maria Ann, the six-year-old daughter of Miguel and Juanita Hernandez, is first introduced to students through the school-based clinic during the Foundations and Health Promotion course in the first semester. Later, Maria Ann is encountered in the acute care setting in the pediatric course with a different set of problems appropriate to the level of learning in that course. Other Hernandez family members are encountered in various courses throughout the curriculum. These virtual patients are used to teach content, develop central competencies important to the curriculum, and demonstrate cultural differences. Now we are exploring opportunities to use these case studies with human patient simulators. Through this virtual family, in addition to developing the knowledge, skills, and competencies related to health and disease-state management, the students develop cultural competencies related to better understanding of the Hispanic culture.

These virtual case simulations, integrated in the EHR, provide very powerful learning tools. More virtual cases, representing a variety of ethnic groups, are under development. The intent is to use these case studies across disciplines and to develop a repository of learning objects in the form of case studies to be used by many.

During the past three years of using the EHR as a teaching platform, faculty members have expressed that they are just beginning to see the tip of the iceberg in terms of how we can enhance learning through this embedded technology. Currently, some faculty members are experimenting with incorporating aspects of the EHR in their nonclinical courses. Faculty who teach undergraduate research are teaching evidence-based practice through student assignments that search for and evaluate research supporting documentation and specific management plans. This evidence-based practice research is then incorporated into the EHR so that it is readily available to students

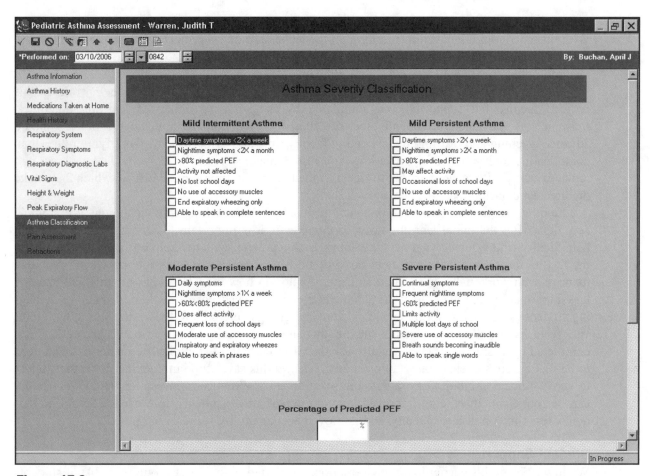

Figure 17-3. *Evidence-Based Protocol.*

(see Figure 17-3). In this manner, students are consistently reminded of the research supporting their practices.

Other faculty members are exploring opportunities to use examples from the EHR to demonstrate legal and ethical practices or to enlighten students regarding the financing of health care. Graduate students are involved in practicum projects within SEEDS, researching guidelines and evidence-based protocols that can be incorporated into the EHR to support student learning. Additionally, PhD students are involved in research and dissertation work that evaluates outcomes of the teaching and learning strategies employed when introducing the technology into the curriculum.

Integrating the EHR system into the curriculum has encouraged optimism for our dream of going paperless in the academic environment. As we move case studies and course work into the electronic format, there is no real need for paper copies. Everything can be done online: students can view cases and prepare care plans, and faculty can grade, monitor students' progress with assignments, and provide feedback.

Faculty Development and Support

As with the integration of any technology in the curriculum, there is a learning curve. The faculty need *time to learn the new skills* required of them and to develop expertise for incorporating the AES into their teaching practices. Release time for the faculty or additional assistance with course load helps them find this time.

Access is another important factor. The faculty need to be able to use the technologies at the office, at home, and away from home. For the SEEDS project, they gained access by loading the Citrix client on their desktop computers in classrooms and laboratories and by working with Cerner to provide an Internet protocol to accommodate anytime, anyplace access. As we supply faculty with handheld apparatuses and require students to have them too, we will achieve more ubiquitous access to and increased familiarity with the EHR system.

Additionally, the faculty appreciates and deserves *recognition and rewards* for their efforts. With this curriculum innovation and through the leadership of the project director, the faculty were able to find a variety of opportunities for scholarship (presentation and publication), resulting in recognition and rewards in terms of merit increases based on scholarly productivity.

Finally, the faculty must be *technically and administratively supported* in their work. In this project, faculty felt supported and stimulated by the students' enhanced learning outcomes. Inasmuch as the faculty frequently feel threatened by technology, strategic technology should advance teaching and learning by leveraging faculty time and resources, by simplifying rather than complicating their job, and by increasing their research and scholarship capacity. The goal is not to replace faculty with technology but to free up valuable faculty time for the areas in which they make the greatest contribution.

Finding the elusive *return on investment* for faculty when teaching with technology is extremely complex. After the initial learning curve is completed, it is important to search for measures that help faculty find value in what they are doing. In this project, with the help of the project manager, the faculty discovered that they could not only push out course work through the system, but also manage such work and manage their students. Exploring how the CIS allows providers to manage tasks, the faculty discovered that the same electronic flow sheet forms could be applied to managing student assignments. With the clinical students groups entered into the system along with their various tasks or course assignments, the faculty can electronically monitor whether the student has completed the assignment. They can also use the CIS to monitor the clinical competencies that need to be met before students enter a clinical area. Clearly this saves time in tracking down the student to verify clinical eligibility or progression. In summary, the return on investment (ROI) for faculty can be found in values, e.g., improved learning outcomes of students, improved feedback to students, less time on task for faculty, and improved accountability for teaching practices.

Student Support

When we began this curriculum transformation, we started with a pilot group ($N = 34$) of students to test the innovation and to learn from the experiment. Students were initiated into the project in small group seminar sessions conducted by the faculty and took to the adapted EHR system with little difficulty. Students today are computer-savvy, and the Windows environment made it easy for them to navigate the system. Because this was a new teaching strategy, we wanted to be sure to maintain open communication with the students, to anticipate their concerns, and to provide them with encouragement and support. We tried to keep the technology transparent to the learning, and certainly we did not want the technology to interfere with the students' achievement in the course.

Initially, the students' biggest criticism was that the faculty was not proficient with the system. This was expected because the faculty was in a learning phase as well. Once the faculty developed skills, the students became more comfortable. Students in this pilot also expressed concern that this technology was not required for the entire class ($N = 120$). They did not like being singled out; however, the pilot was essential to understand and resolve the issues that might be encountered in this innovation. After the first year of the pilot, we rolled out the EHR-integrated curriculum to all beginning nursing students. To maintain the pilot group's interest and buy-in for the project, each student received a certificate as a Clinical Informatics Scholar to include in his or her portfolio. The certificate was signed by the dean of the School of Nursing and the chief executive officer (CEO) of Cerner Corporation.

Once students completed the first semester, which is primarily on campus, they needed anytime, anyplace access to the system because many of the clinical practice sites are at a distance from the campus. Students did not want to return to the campus to complete assignments that required the use of the CIS. At this time, we were able to work with Cerner to provide Internet access for students and faculty. This approach made the use of the CIS more convenient and efficient.

As we gained experience in this virtual learning environment, we found that students need little support. The system is easy to access and navigate. We encountered few technical glitches. The biggest challenge we faced from students is their inability to remember their password to access the system.

What Have We Learned?

By incorporating applied health care informatics into the curriculum as a teaching platform, the University of Kansas School of Nursing is providing its students and graduates with a competitive advantage in the marketplace and a comprehensive understanding of how IT is playing a vital role in improving the *quality* of patient care and reducing medical errors. This integrated system brings data, information, and knowledge to students at the point of learning. It helps them better conceptualize documentation practices and the nursing process by providing a visual frame of reference. Structuring learning concepts and providing information at the point of learning, with reference text to support data-driven care and evidence-based practices, help students to better organize learning and understand conceptual relationships. This approach encourages students to build on prior knowledge and mentally organize their thoughts before new concepts are introduced. The evidence-based practice protocols embedded in the AES assist students to integrate research into practice, a concept that is very difficult to teach in isolation. However, when it is related to the plan of care for virtual or real patients, the research becomes more meaningful and useful to students.

By using the EHR as an underlying framework to organize the curriculum and integrate learning, the faculty began to see that students learn more efficiently and effectively. The data, information, and knowledge are at their fingertips and are consistent with the course objectives and the student's level of learning. The AES-enhanced curriculum provides an information-rich learning environment that, through actively conceptualizing, applying, analyzing, synthesizing, and evaluating information, supports critical thinking behaviors. It also allows students to learn at their own pace because they can access information anytime. This aspect, coupled with the visual learning features of the technology-enhanced curriculum, provides an improved learning environment for English-as-a-second-language students, who frequently need more time and alternative ways of learning the material.

The faculty perceived that students were better able to assimilate more data and information earlier in the curriculum. This was a result of the fact that the CIS, with its various assessment forms and decision-making tools, was triggering requests for more information. Previously the faculty believed that students could only grasp a certain amount of information at any one time. The ability to grasp more information became clear when the case scenarios used in the initial courses did not have sufficient data elements for the students to effectively process information in the EHR. Students challenged the faculty for more information about the cases, and the faculty responded by redesigning the cases to include data and information that normally came later in the course or curriculum. The new teaching platform provides an excellent opportunity to present information when needed and to reinforce learning, especially when students are challenged to learn. The system supports not only good teaching practices, but also the informatics competencies required for nurses[7] and the changes required for health professional education emphasized in the IOM report.[2]

As health care organizations become increasingly more automated, new skills are needed by clinicians to use these new technology tools. There is no doubt that today a gap exists between the skills needed in practice settings and those being taught in academic programs for health care professionals. This gap will only widen if education transformation like the one described in this chapter is not made now. As has been demonstrated, these changes require a unified effort aimed at an efficient and effective transformation of education to enhance a required skill set of critical competencies and to support the use of health care IT in the clinical setting. In addition to changes in knowledge and behaviors, a change in attitudes that support cultural revolutions in health care management and systems is essential to the transformation.

Although leaders in the nursing profession, and especially IT zealots, have been pushing for some time to expand informatics competencies at all levels of the nursing curriculum, the opportunities to embrace this initiative were never more prominent. The window of opportunity for change is now, if we can unite and strategically overcome the challenges. It will, however, take a village to make the transformation happen.

References

1. Committee on Quality Health Care in America, Institute of Medicine. *Crossing the Quality Chasm: A New Health System for the 21st Century.* Washington, DC: National Academy Press; 2001.

2. Institute of Medicine. *Health Professions Education: A Bridge to Quality.* Greiner AC, Knebel E, eds. Washington, DC: National Academy Press; 2003.

3. Dolence MG, Norris DM. *Transforming Higher Education: A Vision for Learning in the 21st Century.* Ann Arbor, MI: Society for College and University Planning; 1995.

4. Committee on Quality Health Care in America, Institute of Medicine. *To Err Is Human: Building a Safer Health System.* Kohm LT, Corrigan JM, Donaldson MS, eds. Washington, DC: National Academy Press; 2000.

5. American Association of Colleges of Nursing. *Essentials of Baccalaureate Education for Professional Nursing Practice.* Washington, DC; American Association of Colleges of Nursing; 1998.

6. Gassert C. The challenge of meeting patients' needs with a national nursing informatics agenda. *J Am Med Inf Assoc.*1998;5:263-268.

7. Bellack JP, O'Neal EH. Recreating nursing practice for a new century: recommendations and implications of the Pew health professions commission's final report. *Nurs Health Care Perspect.* 1998;21:14-21.

8. Staggers N, Gassert CA, Curran C. Informatics competencies for nurses at four levels of practice. *J Nurs Ed.* 2001;40:303-316.

9. Whitten P, Cook D, eds. *Understanding Health Communication Technologies.* San Francisco: Jossey-Bass; 2004.

10. McNeil BJ, Elfrink VL, Bickford CJ, et al. Nursing information technology knowledge, skills and preparation of student nurses, nursing faculty and clinicians: A U.S. survey. *J Nurs Ed.* 2003;42(8):341-349.

11. Pravikoff D, Pierce S, Tanner A. Are nurses ready for evidence-based practice? *Am J Nurs.* 2003;103(5):95-96.

12. Westbrook JI, Gosling AS, Coiera E. Do clinicians use online evidence to support patient care? A study of 55,000 clinicians. *J Am Inf Assoc.* 2004;11:113-120.

13. Incentives for the Use of Health Information Technology and Establishing the Position of the National Health Information Technology Coordinator. Available at: http://www.whitehouse.gov/news/releases/2004/04/20040427-4.html. Accessed December 30, 2004.

14. Thompson TG, Brailer DJ. *The Decade of Health Information Technology: Delivering Consumer-centric and Information-rich Health Care: Framework for Strategic Action.* Washington, DC: Department of Health and Human Services, U.S. Federal Government; 2004.

15. Connors H, Weaver C, Warren J, Miller K. An academic-business partnership for advancing clinical informatics. *Nursing Education Perspectives.* 2002;23:228-233.

16. Warren J, Fletcher K, Connors H, Ground A, Weaver C. SEEDS: from health care information system to innovative educational strategy. In: Whitten P, Cook D, eds. *Understanding Health Communication Technologies.* San Francisco: Jossey-Bass; 2004.

Using Technology to Teach Clinical Skills

Graham Watkinson, EdD, RN, MA, PGCE, MIHPE; Anne Spencer, BA (Hons), RN;
Eloise Monger, BSc (Hons), RGN; Mike Weaver, PhD, PGDipR, PGCTLHE;
and Mary Gobbi, PhD, DipNEd

Using Technology to Teach Clinical Skills

This case study describes a two-year pilot project using virtual case simulation to enable the acquisition of clinical skills at the University of Southampton School of Nursing and Midwifery (SONAM), the second largest such school in the United Kingdom.

The projected shortfall of the required numbers of health professionals, especially in English-speaking nations and particularly among nurses[1] is being addressed in the United Kingdom primarily by means of a significant increase in education and training. The SONAM responded to this imperative by expanding its preregistration education programs by approximately 300 percent over the past six years, with an annual intake of 750 students. Ironically, as student enrollments have increased, our service organizations' ability to absorb students and provide clinical experience has decreased markedly.[2,3]

Clinical Practice Experience in Short Supply

Interestingly, the "supply and demand" gap appears to be a widespread phenomenon, challenging universities in Australia, the U.S., and Canada, as well as in the United Kingdom. Consequently, schools of nursing within universities are rapidly turning to virtual health care delivery laboratories as a way to augment the teaching of clinical skills and to ensure that their graduates are safe to practice and can meet regulatory requirements.[4] In the United Kingdom, these changes have occurred so rapidly, however, that the educational innovations are out of synchronization with regulatory and legal requirements for nursing education. Currently, all student nurses in the United Kingdom and European Union whose nurse registration is covered by the European Commission Directive[5] must undertake a general nursing program of three years or 4,600 hours, of which at least 50 percent must be in defined areas of clinical practice "in direct contact with patients."[6]

The Virtual Interactive Practice (VIP) Laboratories Project is one response to the challenge of enabling nursing students to acquire clinical skills and judgment in the face of ever-declining clinical practice opportunities. Currently, time spent in skills laboratories cannot count toward the required 2,300 hours of practice because it is not considered to be "in direct contact with patients" by the competent authority, the Nursing and Midwifery Council. This issue as to what constitutes "clinical instruction/practice" is subject to current debate as the "realism" of VIP "skills laboratories" increases.[7] The impact of current and predicted educational technologies may require revision or reinterpretation of the European Union Directives themselves.[5]

Synergy Between Practice and Education: Evolution of the VIP Simulation Laboratories

The University of Southampton has developed a strong synergistic partnership with clinical placement providers, particularly Portsmouth Hospitals National Health Service (NHS) Trust. In May 2002, this Trust implemented a fully integrated clinical information system (CIS) within its Department of Critical Care and, in so doing, initiated the Trust's first formal step toward the electronic patient record. This initiative within the department includes direct bedside links to the monitoring systems and ventilators and to other key clinical departments, e.g., pathology and diagnostic imaging. The CIS is utilized by all members of the multidisciplinary team to record patient observations, interventions, and treatments. This is in line with the objectives of the National Programme for Information Technology (www.npfit.nhs.uk), which is currently being implemented within the NHS in England.

From Bedside to Classroom

The wealth of clinical data stored within the CIS provides an excellent data bank from which contextual data can be extrapolated and constructed into patient-focused scenarios. There is also the additional functionality of being able to video stream interventions "live" into the classroom. The media and clinical data can also then be formulated into scenarios and/or used to develop the patient simulation material incorporating a number of SimMan mannequins (http://www.laerdal.com/simman/simman.htm). The incorporation of SimMan mannequins has distinct benefits of assuming physiological characteristics and the additional flexibility to make scenarios exceedingly real. The ability to then synthesize and integrate this into the learning environment is the ethos of VIP and sets it apart from virtual reality and the conventional delivery of nurse education.

Facilities within the VIP Laboratories

Recently, the university has made a significant investment in terms of equipping the SONAM with high-specification clinical skills laboratories with the additional capability of linking directly to practice areas. This enables the students to engage clinicians, specialist practitioners, and other health care professionals at the point-of-care. Two VIP laboratories have been equipped to meet the challenge of providing realistic simulated clinical environments for twenty-first-century practice. The infrastructure of each VIP laboratory replicates the real clinical environment.

Teaching and Learning in Virtual Clinical Areas

Scenario-based simulation is developing as a forceful tool for professional health care skills training,[8] with worldwide adoption. At SONAM, we built a virtual interactive practice environment in which live and recorded data are acquired from a hospital's CIS and fed directly into the skills laboratory. The material for inclusion within the scenarios is acquired from practice areas. (Issues relating to consent, confidentiality, and data security are addressed with all individuals.)

Description of the Virtual Interactive Practice

The integration of digital images (still and video), sounds (breath and heart sounds), and anonymized clinical data enables real patient scenarios to be synthesized. These scenarios are developed to meet specific practice learning outcomes from the various nursing and midwifery curricula and are therefore grounded in sound educational principles, meeting required student assessment of practice competencies. For the purposes of VIP with preregistration students, we have defined *virtual reality* as "a real learning experience from an interaction, which has no steer or effect(s) on patients' or client outcomes, being separated from the event by time and or distance."[9]

The recording of the student–scenario interaction is carried out by a series of overhead pan-tilt-zoom cameras (see Figure 17A-1) and directional microphones, which have been installed at the foot of each bed or cot and above the nurses' station to record key dialogue during the scenarios. Extra lighting was installed to ensure good-quality photography. The audiovisual footage from each bed is then fed back through a matrix to a series of digital video disk (DVD) recorders and may also be directed to plasma screens in the adjacent laboratory and seminar rooms for observers to view the scenario.

Camera operation, recording, and playback are all controlled via a Creston touch screen panel from within the central control room. This has been specifically programmed with the requirements of the VIP project in mind, enabling an operator to oversee, record, and play back all activities within both laboratories (ten beds and two nurse stations). In addition, the operator can control the level of ambient sound, recorded in authentic clinical environments, which is sent to ceiling speakers within each laboratory to provide background clinical noise. By connecting a laptop to the Virtual Graphics Adaptor (VGA) input of the plasma screens, students may also be shown supplementary audiovisual footage, as well as clinical data such as x-ray and MRI images. Currently twelve DVD recorders are housed alongside the audiovisual matrix, Crestron control unit, and audiocassette player in a single fan-cooled rack.

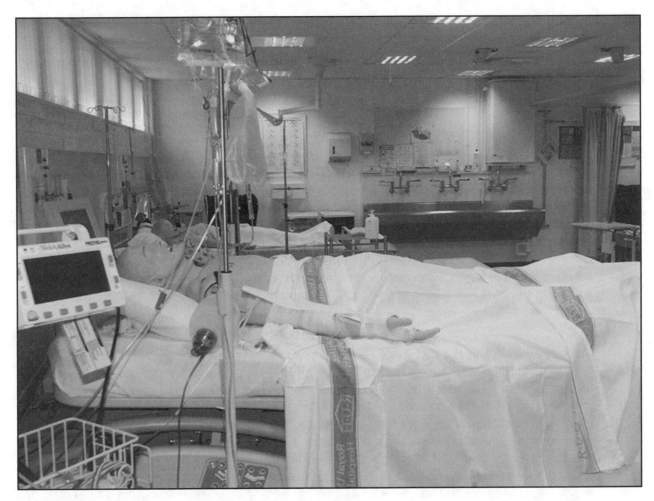

Figure 17A-1. *VIP Laboratory with Ceiling-mounted PTZ Cameras and SimMan. Photo by Dr. Graham Watkinson.*

Student Learning

To enable students to access the clinical data related to the scenarios in progress, each is assigned a laptop that has been configured to access a dedicated media server through a wireless network connection. They may then access a series of interactive Web pages, PowerPoint presentations, computer-aided assessment exercises, and streamed video and audio files to work with and to prepare for their scenario experiences with SimMan. Thus, students' decision-making skills can be formally assessed or compared with those made in practice. The software program, Perception,[10] was used to ascertain the number of attempts taken to complete a scenario and the level of success.

DVD recordings of the students' interaction with SimMan enable the teaching staff to gain insight into their verbalized thoughts and psychomotor skills and to evaluate their performance on an individual or group basis. Being able to see the team working is especially useful when a scenario requires an acute and rapid response, such as to an anaphylactic reaction. Students have also found the immediate facilitated critical appraisal of their performance, both as individuals and as members of a team, to be beneficial. They can, as neophytes, learn safely from their mistakes and feel positive about examples of safe practice. The VIP laboratories are also equipped with a mobile videoconferencing unit that enables students to be connected to and, when appropriate, interact with a live clinical environment or an external expert, anywhere in the world.

The learning environment, student behavior, and reflective practice focusing on clinical reasoning are three key constructs utilized to enhance practice learning within VIP. In addition, VIP allows the students to explore their personal feelings in relation to professional identity, self-esteem, and confidence at the end of each scenario and module.

Tracking Students' Competencies

The student's Assessment of Practice document, which outlines the student's learning objectives for each of the individual clinical placements, is the key tool used to identify and formulate the content for the scenarios. Approximately thirty key objectives on the Assessment of Practice document must be achieved in each clinical placement, and these can be themed into core learning outcomes, e.g., communication and interpersonal skills, ethics and professional development, fundamentals of nursing practice, and management and decision-making skills.

Curriculum Development

Reference groups were established with educationalists and practitioners to ensure that the content of each scenario is evidence-based and credible in relation to the patient experience. The scenarios depict differing elements of the patient journey—for example, clinical emergencies, management issues, and evidence-based research. The deliberate emphasis on research-based practice helps to steer the students to explore differing resource sites on the Internet, e.g., the National Electronic Library for Health (www.nelh.nhs.uk). VIP offers a new pedagogy within nursing and midwifery curricula. To this end, our work was carefully evaluated with summary findings from the first pilot groups.[11]

Evaluation of VIP

Students were surveyed to ascertain their curriculum and pedagogic satisfaction scores, including their skill level competencies (self-evaluated) before and after their VIP experience. The scenarios were scored with respect to realism and comparison with practice-based learning. In addition to observational accounts, there were individual and group video and online assessment data. For all survey responses, students were given a five-point Likert rating scale, from which the scores were elicited, with "five" being the best score. In an attempt to measure the impact of the week on subsequent performance, a postintervention survey was conducted for Cohort 2003, six to eight weeks after they had completed their clinical placement following the VIP week. Follow-up for Cohort 2004 was in progress at the time of writing. In response to their overall degree of satisfaction with the week as a clinical learning experience, 88 percent (2003) or 92 percent (2004) gave a mean score ≥ 4. Individual scenarios received mean score evaluations ranging from 3.65 to 4.4. The scenarios utilizing SimMan scored higher than those without simulation.

It is beyond this case study to report fully on these data, so we offer a "slice" representing the data concerning an individual scenario. This scenario required students to deal with a relative complaint (which excluded simulation) and received a "middle" mean ranking evaluation between 3.8 and 4.16 respectively from the two cohorts. When asked to compare the simulated experience with learning in a real clinical situation, 22 percent (2003) or 50 percent (2004) rated the complaint component "as good as live training," with 77 percent and 50 percent respectively indicating that they learned it "more effectively." In addition, 62.5 percent (2003) or 83 percent (2004) of the students reported that their competence had improved in relation to their ability to "respond appropriately if complaints are made." Further work is needed to establish the appropriateness and impact of these interventions with different students, curricula, cohorts, clinical environments, and topics.

How Can VIP Enhance Clinical Skills Acquisition?

VIP assures all students an equitable experience with the programming and timetabling of scenarios and other interrelated activities—something that cannot always be guaranteed in real practice (see Table 17A-1 for a timetabling example). Students cannot disengage or withdraw as their participation is being monitored and recorded. Thus there is no avoidance, and students are required to encounter elements of practice in which they may have previously assumed a passive role. A typical comment from students was, "It was good to learn in an environment where you can make mistakes and feel more confident to ask questions." (Student 29).

Five groups of students undertook each scenario in a sequenced rotation. Students' qualitative comments revealed their appreciation and experience of the VIP week. The following comments typically demonstrate the realism of the experiences in the VIP laboratories:

Table 17A-1. Timetabling Example for Two of the Five VIP Days

Monday	Tuesday
Welcome to Badger Ward, including staff introductions; followed by health and safety lecture and online pediatric drug calculation quiz	HANDOVER
Tour of VIP laboratories and introduction to SimMan	Skills lab poser—safety assessment of clinical environment
Individual group projects assigned	Fluid management of fifteen-year-old with diabetic ketoacidosis (SimMan) combined and member of staff suffering latex allergic reaction
HANDOVER	Anaphylaxis—nut allergy and how to use an Epipen; ward-based teaching session
Relative complaint (Part 1)—Web-based	
COFFEE BREAK	COFFEE BREAK
Online asthma quiz—Web-based	Virtual tour of pediatric emergency department
Domestic slipping (management scenario)—Web-based	Observe A& E team preparing to receive eleven-year-old involved in road traffic accident
LUNCH	Assume care for eleven-year-old following a road traffic accident in VIP laboratory (SimMan)
Relative complaint (Part 2)—Web-based	
Asthmatic attack—twelve-year-old (SimMan)	Fire safety interactive quiz—Web-based
IT skills workshop	1:1 Review AOP competencies
Review scenarios, debrief, observer group feedback	Review scenarios, debrief, observer group feedback

"Although it was a very stressful week, the content was all relevant and the experience was not unlike it could be in practice. We were definitely pushed to our limits ... It was extremely stressful; emotionally, physically, psychologically and mentally draining (however this is probably a good thing as I've learned a lot about myself)." (Student 6).

However, we noted that the students' professionalism and self-confidence grew the more they were actively participating. It was quickly evident that some students were able to demonstrate leadership, and the VIP scenarios stimulated such behavior.

"I understand better my role in leadership which affects decisions in practice. I now have an awareness of how I react under pressure and how that affected the decisions I made." (Student 11).

Ethical Issues Associated with VIP

VIP demands rigor in relation to the acquisition, use, and storage of patient images and clinical data to protect patient, staff, relative, and student confidentiality. A robust ethical protocol was developed using examples from other sensitive applications, like genetic databases. Within the protocol, a formal consent form was devised by SONAM, and each subject is asked to agree to the use and distribution of their images and/or clinical data.[12] The consent forms are archived so that all linked data can be accessed, and data pertaining to any individual can be collated and withdrawn when requested. Patients and student participants may "opt out" at any stage if they wish.

A different group of data is unidentifiable and can be extracted from clinical information systems. This kind of data has been traditionally used for educational purposes without consent and continues to be a legitimate strategy for the use of such data; however, there are now procedures that should be followed. In the United Kingdom, the NHS Trust Caldicott Guardian[13] must formally agree to the use of all anonymized patient-related data to ensure that the patient's statutory rights under the Data Protection Act (1998)[14] are safeguarded. The data are then stored to a dedicated secure server.

Students' Consent Required

Students undertaking the VIP experience are also formally requested to consent to the use of recording equipment, both video and audio, during the VIP experience and also to the subsequent publication of selected footage. A student who withholds consent is not included in any published footage.

The challenges of the ethical considerations should not be underestimated. The rapidly changing political climate in relation to data demands that the protocol continually evolves to comply with current legislation. The team has taken a cautious approach and, when in any doubt, has limited the scope of VIP in favor of patient protection. Every step in the development of VIP has required ethical scrutiny, and collaboration and discussion with a wide range of experts, both lay and professional, have been the cornerstones of the development and evolution of the protocol.

Lessons Learned

1. Partnership between practice and education was and remains crucial in developing VIP successfully and embedding it into educational programs.
2. Although curricula integration is ideal, this project has been incremental in its implementation.
3. The power of the scenarios (especially when simulation, computer-based interaction, and role-play are blended together) can be very realistic, as depicted in the students' comments.
4. Some students required individual and group support and encouragement, not dissimilar to that associated with real clinical practice, particularly in times of stress when they are either personally or professionally challenged.
5. Ensuring engagement and collaboration from senior nurses at director level within the school or faculty and at the NHS executive level is crucial to drive and finance such a project.

Acknowledgement

We are grateful for the support of Professor Dame Jill Macleod Clark, head of SONAM, and Ursula Ward, chief executive of Portsmouth Hospitals NHS Trust.

References

1. Rothert M, Wehrwein T, Andre J. *Informing the Debate: Health Policy Options for Michigan Policy Makers; Nursing Workforce Requirements for the Needs of Michigan Citizens.* Institute for Public Policy and Social Research and Institute for Health Care Studies; Michigan State University; 2002.
2. Department of Health. *Working Together—Learning Together: A Framework for Lifelong Learning for the NHS.* London: Her Majesty's Stationery Office; 2001.
3. Humphris D, Macleod-Clark J. *Shaping a vision for a "New Generation" workforce. Future Health Worker Project.* University of Southampton; Institute for Public Policy Research; May 2002.
4. United Kingdom Central Council. Fitness for practice and purpose. In: *Report of the UKCC's Post-Commission Development Group.* London: United Kingdom Central Council for Nursing, Midwifery and Health Visiting; 2001.
5. United Kingdom Central Council. Registrar's letter 15/2000 European Commission directive 77/453/EEC. Available at: http://www.nmc-uk.org/nmc/main/employers/RL1500.pdf. Accessed August 11, 2005.
6. Nursing and Midwifery Council. Standards of proficiency for pre-registration. Booklet standards 0204. London: Nursing and Midwifery Council; 2004.
7. Nursing and Midwifery Council. Skill labs for students. 11 June 2004. Available at: http://www.nmc-uk.org/nmc/main/news/Skill_labs_for_students. Accessed November 7, 2004.
8. Sheba Medical Centre at Tel Hasomer Israel. Available at: www.http://eng.sheba.co.il. Accessed January 28, 2005.
9. Watkinson GE. From virtual to virtual reality—bringing clinical practice to the student. Conference presentation at: University of Southampton School of Nursing and Midwifery; July 4, 2002; Southampton.
10. Perception Software. Available at: http://www.pearsonncs.com/perception/. Accessed February 15, 2005.
11. Gobbi M, Monger E, Watkinson GE, et al. Virtual Interactive Practice™: a strategy to enhance learning and competence in health care students. In: Fieschi M, et al. eds. *MEDINFO 2004 Proceedings.* Amsterdam: IOS Press; 2004:874-878.
12. Willison DJ, Keshavjee K, Nair K, Goldsmith C, Holbrook A. Patients' consent preferences for research uses of information in electronic medical records: Interview and survey data. *BMJ.* 2003;326:373-376.
13. Roch-Berry C. What is a Caldicott guardian? *Postgrad Med J.* 2003;79:516-518.
14. Data Protection Act 1998. Available at: http://www.hmso.gov.uk/acts/acts1998/19980029.htm#aofs. Accessed January 24, 2005.

Bringing Technology into the Classroom

Michelle Honey, MPhil (Nursing), RGON, FCNA

This case study presents an account of nurse teachers' experiences with introducing e-learning into a university-based school of nursing in New Zealand. Data were collected as part of a doctoral study on the principles and practices of flexible learning and on their impact on learning, using a case study method. This account focuses on the nurse teachers' stories and discusses the accomplishments, issues, examples of hurdles, and lessons learned.

Background

Established in 1999, the School of Nursing at the University of Auckland offers both undergraduate and postgraduate nursing education. The school has developed a range of programs to meet the needs of contemporary nursing practice. The courses within these programs have been offered in increasingly flexible formats to better meet the needs of students and also the strategic goals of the University. Undergraduate nursing study prepares students for beginning practice as registered nurses. Postgraduate studies are designed for registered nurses seeking to advance their professional knowledge and skills. The University postgraduate nursing students work in diverse areas of clinical practice, as well as in different physical locations. These nurses are predominantly mature female students with an average age of 37 years.[1] Most are employed for more than thirty hours per week[2] and combine employment and study with other commitments.

Recognizing the important role of technology in education and professional practice, the University of Auckland has encouraged increased flexibility in teaching and learning, as stated in its Mission, Goals, and Strategies, "to become rapidly responsive to changing information systems and capture the benefits of technology for its staff and students."[3] To support e-learning, the University developed its own in-house Web-based learning management system (LMS). The LMS was designed to support student learning within the University and from a distance. The benefits of using the LMS include online course material and details accessible from any computer twenty-four hours a day, enhanced communication through announcements and discussion groups, and student course marks provided by the system.

A strategic plan for e-learning within the School of Nursing, which aligned with the university's goals, supported the progressive increase in e-learning by all courses. The e-learning plan, approved by the school in 2001, consisted of five stages, with clearly outlined criteria for each stage alongside the advantages for teachers and students. Crucially, e-learning was not seen as an all-or-nothing option, but rather as a continuum; on-campus courses can be electronically supported while delivered on-campus, partially electronic, or fully electronic.

Undergraduate courses are predominantly on-campus and supported by e-learning. With undergraduate nursing including both hands-on practical skill and theoretical components, both of which need to be developed in the novice, there is no plan to replace face-to-face teaching. Examples of supported e-learning for undergraduate students include online resources, course information, multichoice questions, assignment of marks, and class announcements. Postgraduate courses are either supported or, more commonly, are partial or full e-learning courses. To enable nurses at a distance to complete a program of study, selected core postgraduate courses are offered, fully utilizing e-learning, rather than just offering a few random courses. Although the flexibility of e-learning makes access to study easier for nurses working shifts and at a distance, the nurses and their teachers were not necessarily familiar with e-learning.

Accomplishments

The significant increase of e-learning within the School of Nursing by 2004 is a major accomplishment. E-learning, supported by the LMS, is now evident in most courses. The undergraduate program has become well established and easily fills its annual intake of eighty-five students. The numbers of postgraduate courses and students have increased more than threefold.

Having readily accepted a supported e-learning approach, undergraduate students now expect and request it. Of particular note for undergraduate students has been the success of the online multichoice questions related to and supporting their inquiry-based learning case studies.[4] The students' early acceptance of e-learning in the undergraduate program, along with the demonstrated proficiency and increased confidence of undergraduate nurse teachers, had a "flow-through" effect on the postgraduate teachers.

Although most postgraduate courses use e-learning, the developmental approaches have varied. Some teachers favored altering their existing courses to an e-learning format, whereas others preferred developing a new course directly for the e-learning mode. Another approach that proved successful was a pharmacology course that was offered both in on-campus and in e-learning modes—giving students the option of enrolling in either. Both modes were equally popular with students and, once established, demonstrated equivalence in the quality of learning.[5] Within courses, a number of e-teaching strategies have been tried; most of them have focused on interaction either between students or between students and teacher. Examples of successes include online discussions that have created a sense of a learning community among nurses, small groups established and supported through the LMS for group project work, the timely feedback given to students related to assessed work, and the ongoing communication with students during the semester.

The nurse teachers' increased competence in e-learning has been dramatic, including, for some, improved computer skills. However, underlying the technical skills has been a sharper focus on teaching. The awareness of alternative approaches to teaching has been heightened and so has interest in the art of teaching. Teaching has become more student-focused. The School of Nursing needed to celebrate these e-learning successes and so held a showcase in late 2004. The showcase was a half-day seminar at which teachers in the school shared their experiences. Nurse teachers were asked to address three questions: (1) What motivated you to get started online? (2) What are some of the significant issues or experiences you found? (3) What new learning that occurred for you do you want to pass on to others? Although there was much to celebrate, areas needing improvement and issues were identified.

Issues

Introducing e-learning into the School of Nursing raised a number of issues, most of which were resolved to some degree along the way. However, four issues worthy of particular mention are student computer proficiency, health informatics, teaching practice, and teacher workload.

Student Computer Proficiency

Computer skills are essential for e-learning, given its reliance on the use of information and communication technology (ICT). A survey of 450 undergraduate medicine, pharmacy, and nursing students' technology skills in 2001 found that 88 percent of students used e-mail and 72 percent accessed the World Wide Web at least weekly.[6] A survey of all postgraduate nurses enrolled at the School of Nursing in 2002 found that 94 percent had access to their own personal computer, 87 percent had home access to the Internet, most (60 percent) rated their proficiency as "adequate," and more than 80 percent rated themselves as either "adequate" or "good."[2]

Establishing the level of computer access and the proficiency of postgraduate and undergraduate students was an important basis for planning the introduction of e-learning. This information assisted in identifying that not all students have convenient access to technology for study purposes, nor are they at the same level in terms of their using technology, highlighting the importance of providing self-directed "upskilling" or skill development opportunities. Of the many technological e-learning options, teachers must be cognizant not only of the viable ones (in terms of student access and proficiency), but also of the need to clearly explain the requisite computer skills in course descriptions.

Health Informatics

The School of Nursing had to consider the place of informatics in undergraduate and postgraduate education for nurses. In the undergraduate curriculum, health informatics has been integrated as a thread that runs through the three years of the bachelor of nursing program. The curriculum model is three-dimensional, linking theory and clinical practice. Content threads run through each semester, and health informatics is one of the curricula threads that permeate each semester and level of the program. With informatics integrated in this way, it is expected that all graduates will be equipped with fundamental skills in information literacy. Alongside the planned curricula learning, students also undertake placements in clinical settings and are exposed to health informatics in practice; clinical experience consolidates and further develops informatics skills. The concern is that, when health informatics is integrated within the curriculum, it may seem less significant. This may downplay the importance of health informatics as a speciality in its own right. Additionally, as informatics touches on so many other aspects of the curriculum, it may be so hidden as not to exist.[7]

Postgraduate health informatics courses are offered by a department other than the School of Nursing. This has been the result of a pragmatic development within the University, related to the early support of health informatics coming from another department, and also recognizing that health informatics is beyond the purview of nurses alone. In their current position, the health informatics courses attract a range of health and allied professionals, and the interests of nurses are still served.

Teaching Practice

Issues pertaining to teaching practice included the visibility of teaching practice, teaching preferences, intellectual property, and copyright questions.

In e-learning, more of the teacher's work or practice is *visible* to others, and this can concern teachers. In a face-to-face class, no record of lectures and discussions is kept, except for perhaps handouts or student notes. In a closed learning management system, although only enrolled students can access the course, learning resources might be visible to individuals other than the course students, such as to administrators and to other teachers. Some e-learning materials are prepared and available in written format, often as "published" Web pages. Learning material can be read and scrutinized again and again. Even a discussion, such as an asynchronous online discussion, is visible beyond the moment. Students can read, consider material in depth, and then challenge the teacher in ways not possible in a face-to-face class. Teaching practice, once captured electronically, is often saved and archived, subjecting it to scrutiny and challenge not just from students but from peers too. Teachers may feel vulnerable with the visibility of their practice.

Interviews with nurse teachers revealed that their own experiences as students affected their *preferences* in teaching. The underlying teaching mode that many nurse teachers preferred was face-to-face, because that was what they knew best. Starting with such a preference, however, might limit a teacher's ideas for e-learning developments in his or her courses. It was notable that teachers' previous experiences as students, or the lack of experience in teaching, and more specifically, in e-learning, limited their consideration of options for e-learning. The effect of other nurse teachers' experiences and successes with e-learning were significant in expanding entrenched ideas of teaching.

The University has a clear position on ownership of *intellectual property* related to teaching material, and it is recognized that resources that teachers develop while employed by the University belong to the University. Although it has been common practice for teachers to share resources within the School of Nursing, they have expressed concern about resources being made available more widely. Although there are silos of resources, e.g., medical images, that nurse teachers would like to access, the collegial sharing of learning resources does not extend as readily to other departments. Attempts to create an in-house database of potential electronic resources and learning objects have been unsuccessful, because of a lack of understanding of what e-resources might be able to accomplish, how the resources would be used, and where and how they might be used with limited control.

Nurse teachers have a new awareness of *copyright issues*. With the common use of presentation tools, e.g., PowerPoint, teachers often look for graphics to enliven a topic. With the Internet so easily accessible, they can locate and copy resources from the Web, possibly without considering the copyright implications. The University has taken steps to ensure that all academics are aware of the need to work within licensing agreements and copyright laws, including how those apply to electronic sources. The pressure for teachers is between using learning material that already exists and working within the constraints of copyright law.

Teacher Workload

Nurse teachers, working in a university-based school of nursing, must always balance the demands of teaching, practice, and research. To date, there has been little recognition that introducing innovative approaches to teaching takes time and that a steep learning curve is associated with new technology. Teachers identified that the start-up preparation for e-learning courses took longer than for face-to-face classes, although, once established, the courses took slightly less preparation time. One reason for the initial extra time is the need to prepare the entire course before it is offered. One experienced teacher reported that adapting an existing course for e-learning mode took four months of intensive work, despite already having determined the course aims, learning outcomes, assessments, and much of the learning material.[5] Furthermore, the first-time preparation took teachers longer because they had to develop expertise with both a different mode of teaching and the technology.

Workload is an issue that has contributed to slowing the introduction of e-learning. Yet developments in the School of Nursing have occurred because teachers showed interest and personal commitment to improving quality education. The achievements described have been made not because of extra time allocations or reductions in workload, but because of a genuine interest in the educational needs of the students. In other words, E-learning developments have occurred in addition to, not instead of, other work.

Hurdles

The hurdles in this project were related to technical issues, resources for students, and teacher support.

Technical Issues

Students around the country experienced technical problems. Access to broadband is limited in New Zealand, although it is becoming increasingly available and more realistically priced. Modem speed is generally 56 kilobits per second, and at that speed, access and download time for learning resources can be frustrating and slow. These problems were compounded by different levels of service by Internet service providers (ISPs) around the country, with some areas being better served than others. For example, in one course, when pop-ups were automatically disabled by ISPs, a glossary page failed to display. Other ISPs disconnected the user when they determined the connection was idle. Furthermore, students reported that the LMS disconnected them after it was idle for twenty minutes, but for some students, it could take that much time to thoughtfully compose a reply to an online discussion.

By sharing their experiences, some students helped reduce the isolation others felt. Students also shared their strategies for managing issues, e.g., finding the best ISP in a region, composing a discussion reply offline and then posting it when connected to the LMS, and logging on to the LMS at off-peak times when accessing was faster. For nurse teachers, these technical problems highlighted that, although more technologically advanced options might be available, a priority was to ensure that e-learning was consistently and reliably accessible to the students.

Resources for Students

Resources are needed to support students' e-learning. Preliminary familiarization with the LMS, initially provided as part of a general orientation to the University, forms a sound basis for successful e-learning. Before their course begins, postgraduate nursing students are posted information that includes a pamphlet about getting started on the LMS. Courses that use partial e-learning have included a hands-on session with the LMS as early as possible in the semester. For full e-learning courses, some teachers ask students to introduce themselves on the LMS with a preparatory discussion; this is designed as much to ensure they can access and use the system as to get to know each other. The University has a central Help Call Center, which responds to phone and e-mail, and help desks are also situated in the library. Despite these resources, students often still seek help from the nurse teachers who are identified as their course coordinators. Teachers recognize that the first weeks of the semester, until students became familiar and confident with the LMS, are the busiest and most stressful. Providing practical help, as well as emotional support, for anxious students is an effort for nurse teachers.

Teacher Support

The hurdles related to technical issues and student resources led to another hurdle: supporting the teachers. A variety of tactics arose within the School and the University to meet this need. In the School of Nursing, a nurse teacher with an interest in e-learning was given the responsibility of facilitating and coordinating efforts. The teacher, who became the champion of e-learning, began using e-learning in her teaching and developed some skill with the LMS. As she shared her experience with other teachers beginning to use the LMS, and having a slow start, e-learning rapidly expanded. With more experience in e-learning than others, the e-learning champion was able to offer practical education in the LMS and support for its use. The support was available when it was needed; because the faculty offices were all in close proximity, assistance was always close at hand. Peer sharing among nurse teachers disseminated ideas for e-learning and supporting students.

The library proved to be a vital support for nurse teachers, especially important was the subject librarian. The library has implemented a range of services to help develop information literacy skills in undergraduate and postgraduate students, including tutorials supported in face-to-face, online, and workbook modes. The subject librarian supports nursing students and teachers to ensure that course-specific electronic resources are easily accessible.

As the e-learning effort progressed, staff development in using the LMS was provided on-site, rather than centrally within the University, which made attendance more convenient for nurse teachers. They preferred short, specific courses so that they could learn about specific areas of interest and have the opportunity to use the information before attending the next session. Phone and e-mail help was also extended and is now more readily available than when the School first introduced e-learning. The establishment of a unit to provide technical assistance in developing e-resources at the departmental level and a central Flexible Learning Unit to provide direction and leadership within the University have further supported the development of e-learning.

Lessons Learned

The School of Nursing has learned three key lessons while introducing e-learning. First is the importance of a shared goal, which was articulated through an e-learning strategy. To be effective, the e-learning strategy is best aligned with organizational goals and vision. Although the strategy guided the direction of e-learning development, it was not so prescriptive that individual teachers' creative energy was stifled. Instead it supported a collaborative effort because of a shared goal and a focus on quality learning. The use of increased e-learning and technology became the means to achieve quality learning, not an end in itself. The second key lesson is to know your student population. Rather than guessing what students can do or want to do, it is essential to base plans on a full assessment of the prospective students, including their technology skills and ability to access technology for study. The final lesson is to have an e-learning champion. The School's champion, the nominated facilitator, understood the curriculum and programs, the nurse teachers, and the student body. As the champion, she could combine her contextual knowledge with e-learning strategies that supported curriculum and instructional design, led development, and provided valuable support to others.

References

1. Division of Nursing. *Graduate Student Profile July 1999-July 2001*. Auckland: The University of Auckland; 2001.

2. Honey M. Flexible learning for postgraduate nurses: a basis for planning. *Nurse Ed Today*. 2004;24(4):319-325.

3. University of Auckland. Mission, goals and strategies. Available at: http://www.auckland.ac.nz/cir_visitors/index.cfm?action=display_page&page_title=goals2# Teaching and Learning. Accessed on April 3, 2002.

4. Honey M, Marshall D. The impact of on-line multi-choice questions on undergraduate student nurses' learning. In: Crisp G, Thiele D, Scholten I, Barker S, Baron J, eds. *Interact, Integrate, Impact, Proceedings of the 20th Annual Conference of the Australasian Society for Computers in Learning in Tertiary Education (ASCILITE)*, December 7-10, 2003. Adelaide, Australia: ASCILITE; 2003: 236-243.

5. Lim AG, Honey M. On-line pharmacology course for postgraduate nurses: impact on quality of learning. In: Crisp G, Thiele D, Scholten I, Barker S, Baron J, eds. *Interact, Integrate, Impact, Proceedings of the 20th Annual Conference of the Australasian Society for Computers in Learning in Tertiary Education (ASCILITE)*, December 7-10, 2003. Adelaide, Australia: ASCILITE; 2003:304-313.

6. Lamdin R, Wickham H. *Faculty of Medical and Health Sciences Information Technology Student Survey*. Auckland: The University of Auckland; 2001.

7. Honey M, Baker H. Integrated undergraduate curriculum for health informatics. Paper presented at: HINZ 2004 Third National Health Informatics Conference: Towards a Healthy Nation, July 27. Wellington, New Zealand: HINZ; 2004.

Industry-Government-Academic Partnership: The Australian Story

Evelyn JS Hovenga, PhD, RN, FACHI, FCHSE, FRCNA, MACS
and Derek Louey-Gung, B App Sc

A Nationwide Curriculum Transformation Initiative

The Australian Health Information Council has made building the health workforce capacity in health informatics (HI) a priority.[1] An HI workforce capacity, Think Tank, undertaken in 2003 by the Australian Department of Health and Ageing, identified a dearth of HI expertise among health professionals as a significant impediment to providing better health care outcomes, safety, quality, and cost efficiencies. The need to apply information technology (IT) in care delivery is urgent. Studies on medical error in Australia and the United States have indicated that fragmented, disorganized, and inaccessible clinical information adversely affects the quality of health care and compromises patient safety.[1] The resulting action plan led to the creation of a national statement with thirteen recommendations in late 2004 and in early 2005, which was endorsed by the Australian Health Ministers' Advisory Council (AHMAC). This case study is about implementing the following recommedation, which is one of the thirteen recommendations included with the action plan:

> A consortium is established to make available the tools and to manage the necessary infrastructure needed to enable all Australian universities to access and make use of a simulated and fully integrated health information system to support all health professional and HI education.[2]

The case study reports on the collaborative partnership that enabled this initiative and the planning process undertaken toward implementation of this recommendation. The proposed curriculum transformation project is novel and ambitious in a number of respects. It is a first in health care as a partnership among multiple industry partners, the federal government, and academia. It is also nationwide in scope. There is no other national initiative to bring IT into the classrooms of all health professional schools.

Proposed Project and Approach

Our goal is to integrate an enterprise-wide, electronic health record (EHR) system into the teaching curricula for nurses, physicians, pharmacists, and allied health schools, as well as for health informaticians and computer science specialists. Central Queensland University (CQU) will serve as the initial alpha partner for "Australianising the existing U.S. pre-built database" and establishing proof of concept. Rollout to all other Australian universities will follow the pilot in an implementation phase. The industry partner, Cerner Corporation, is supplying the software as well as its system implementation expertise. Because of the complexity of managing a fully loaded EHR system with clinical decision support and evidence-based knowledge content, the system will be remotely managed. Our overall objective is to improve the preparation of health professional, IT, information system, and computer science students by providing them with the skills and knowledge required in the health industry's work environment.

Why Put IT in the Core Curriculum?

Having a simulated health enterprise system is seen by university-based health academics as key to facilitating the understanding of the use of ITs to support health care delivery. Students undertaking any degree program in the health professions are already exposed to experiential simulated learning strategies in the classroom and skill-based laboratories. Simulation is incomplete, however, when students do not have access to the information systems actually in use in their future work environments. Such exposure is essential for students to obtain practice competencies and to develop or improve their evidence-based clinical decision-making abilities. The latter is an essential foundation for providing safe health care and good patient outcomes.

Graduates need to hit the ground running once employed in the health workforce. Access to current software enables students to learn from hypothetical case studies, taking advantage of a knowledge base that, for example, issues alerts based on best practice protocols. This kind of access enables them to learn critical thinking skills faster, working through all aspects of patient management, care documentation, and system management in a nonthreatening learning environment. These benefits have been demonstrated by the outcomes resulting from using an academic education solution as a tool for teaching health professionals. Specifically, the University of Kansas School of Nursing, Kansas City, initiated a project known as the Simulated E-hEalth Delivery System[3-5] and the U.S. College of St. Scholastica[6] created the Advancing Technology and Healthcare Education Now at St. Scholastica project. The latter project was supported by a $1.8 million federal U.S. Department of Education five-year project grant (2002–2007) to create clinical information software and to incorporate the use of the technology into its nursing, physical therapy, occupational physiology, and health information management curricula.[7,8] Advancing Technology and Healthcare Education Now at St. Scholastica is based on the Simulated E-hEalth Delivery System.

The exposure of future IT and information systems (IS) professionals to the unique technical issues encountered in the health industry sharpens their problem-solving skills. CIS are more complex to develop, implement, and maintain than such systems in other industries. As a consequence, graduates who have been exposed to this type of simulated system are better able to solve technical problems in any industry. Learning effectiveness is improved through the use of simulation models.[9]

The health care environment is changing at an ever-increasing pace as a result of the proliferation of new and emerging technologies. Embracing advances in technology enables us to deliver health care in new and innovative ways. Australian governments have invested heavily in the establishment of a health information management infrastructure to support general practice, in the undertaking of a national EHR initiative, in the creation of a broadband national infrastructure, in the implementation of a clinical system in many health care provider organizations, and other enterprise projects. These investments have made it imperative to ensure that the health workforce is able to make the best possible use of these technologies to improve patient safety and health outcomes, resulting in optimal returns on government's investments.

The IT Skill Base in the Current Health Industry's Workforce

The task force on HI capacity building recommended a scoping exercise to determine the current IT and management skill base of the Australian health workforce. CQU's Health Informatics Research Group undertook a national survey of a random sample of health professionals to communicate their perceptions of needed skills and knowledge. Their responses fall within a five-point scale from novice to expert across sixty-nine topics and five skill categories derived from the International Medical Informatics Association's recommendations on education in health and medical informatics. Of the 461 questionnaires that were returned and analyzed, 95 percent of respondents indicated that their primary role in HI was to use IT to support health care delivery. Of this group 50 percent indicated that they were either novice or advanced beginner users. Only 15 percent saw themselves as proficient or expert.

In another Internet survey conducted by CQU in late 2004, nurse subscribers to a national nursing informatics (NI) mailing list were asked to complete an informatics skills questionnaire. Altogether, eighty-two nurses completed the questionnaire. Eighty percent of the nurse respondents were female, compared with 92 percent nationally. A total of 71 percent described their primary role in HI as "I use information technology in health care." Asked for their degree of competency in this role, 11 percent answered "novice," 17 percent "advanced beginner," 35 percent "competent," and 33 percent "proficient." Only 4 percent considered themselves expert in their primary HI role. Because the survey was of nurses who had previously expressed an interest in NI by subscribing to the mailing list, these results reflect the best possible nursing workforce HI capacity. As a summary question, the nurses were asked to assess the overall degree of competency required for each of five categories of HI fields. All were assessed as requiring basic competency but preferring proficiency.[10]

Nurses form a highly significant part of the health care workforce. A very large percentage of acute hospital[11,12] budgets (varying from 40 percent to 70 percent for different kinds of hospitals) are consumed by nursing services. Yet it is becoming more and more difficult to meet nursing workforce demands. In as much as nurses increasingly use IT, and some also deploy, research, or develop health care IT, they need to be adequately educated for their roles in HI. Meeting those educational goals is the purpose of this project.

Project Context, Goals, and Expected Outcomes

A system improvement objective announced by the Australian Health Ministers is to "identify alternative approaches to existing health workforce education and training, through exploring innovative and/or fast-track approaches to qualifications."[13] The 2004 National Statement regarding health workforce HI capacity building was founded on the vision for the Australian health workforce presented in Table 17C-1. This project provides one approach toward accomplishing that objective and is expected to significantly contribute to the realization of the vision.

The personal health record and EHR in the Australian academic sector have to be incorporated into clinical as well as IT and IS curricula. Yet there are many challenges. For the industry software supplier, the challenges are primarily focused on the economic and technology delivery models, which are inextricably entwined. The economic model must be affordable for the payers, yet viable for the industry software supplier and other partnering service providers.

There has been very strong interest in this project from other universities and the health industry sector. This emerging, jointly funded collaborative partnership among government, an industry software supplier, and academia aims to realize benefits for all concerned. Most importantly, it is anticipated that Australian health care consumers and providers of health care services will benefit as a result of implementing this project nationally. Our criteria for success are:

1. Better prepared university graduates entering the health workforce, able to work effectively with health informatics technologies, including EHRs
2. Academic curricula that use the simulated system as a primary teaching resource
3. Academic staff and student satisfaction with the new education delivery methodology
4. An educational solution that attracts the interest and involvement of other tertiary education institutions

Collaborative Partners

The emerging partnership of government(s), an industry software supplier, and CQU is yet to be formalized, although all parties have undertaken considerable work at the time of writing. CQU has been selected by the industry software supplier as the pilot site to support the content development and implementation strategy for nursing education and HI. Both CQU and the selected industry software supplier have established project teams consisting of individuals with proven track records of achievement in government, academia, nursing, and industry, both in Australia and abroad. Within CQU, the team consists of staff from the Division of Information Technology and a substantial number of academic staff from different schools and locations. Both are currently engaged in identifying required resource estimates based on a project plan that has identified specific roles and responsibilities. The full project-planning phase should be completed by September 2005.

Table 17C-1. Vision for the Australian Health Workforce

An Australian health workforce that has the information management (IM) and information and communications technology (ICT) knowledge and skills to:

- Use IM & ICT to improve clinical care and health outcomes

- Manage health information better

- Improve workplace practices

- Undertake and participate in decision making regarding the application and use of information technologies

- Achieve efficiency gains that result in more effective allocation of resources so that the benefits of IM & ICT in health are distributed to all participants in the health sector

Source: Australian Health Information Council (AHIC) 2004 Health Workforce Health Informatics Capacity Building National Statement. Unpublished working document.

Enabling Infrastructures for National Scope

In a full production offering, the technology needs to use economies of scale to reduce costs. The academic education solution will run on a single, large hardware platform. Each university, college, or educational site will connect to the system through the Internet. A remotely hosted data center facility, with Internet connectivity to all users, is the ideal model for Australia, given its size and geography. While in the start-up and pilot phases a few users will require a lot of technology; long-term sustainability will come from running ten or more universities on the system.

Another important asset that Australia has is its national research and education network (AARNet). AARNet is managed by a not-for-profit company, in which thirty-seven Australian universities and the Commonwealth Scientific and Industrial Research Organisation (CSIRO) hold shares. AARNet3 delivers ten to forty gigabits per second over its own optical fiber network. Dual circuits and duplicated points of presence (PoPs) provide superior reliability. The very high-bandwidth, leading-edge, and cost-competitive Internet services are delivered to tertiary education and research sector communities in metropolitan and regional centers. The educational and research network infrastructure is comparable to the most advanced available worldwide and has an end user client base of more than one million member staff and students. AARNet is available to all Australian universities at a minimum electronic communication cost, thus providing an unprecedented opportunity for this type of national initiative.

References

1. Australian Government Accountability Office, Reports and Testimony, August 13, 2004. Available at: http://www.gao.gov/docsearch/abstract.php?rptno=GAO-04-991R. Accessed February 2005.

2. Australian Health Information Council (AHIC). Health workforce health informatics capacity building national statement. Unpublished working document; 2004:7.

3. Connors HR, Weaver C, Warren J, Miller KL. An academic-business partnership for advancing clinical informatics. *Nurs Ed Perspect.* 2002;23(5):228-233.

4. Kansas University Medical Center (KUMC). 2003 Center for Healthcare Informatics announced Nov 18. *KUMC Campus News.* Available at: http://www.kumc.edu/news/publish/article_375.shtml. Accessed October 2004.

5. CERNER. October 11, 2004, media release. Available at: http://www.cerner.com/aboutcerner/pressrelease.asp?id=3001. Accessed October 2004.

6. Frauenheim E. Training tuneup. *NurseWeek*com.* February 21, 2003. Available at: http://www.nurseweek.com/news/features/03-02/schooltech.asp. Accessed October 4, 2004.

7. Advancing Technology and Healthcare Education Now at St. Scholastica—ATHENS project. Available at: https://www.css.edu/programs/athens/. Accessed September 2004.

8. Phal D, Laitenberger O, Ruhe G, Dorsch J, Krivobokova T. Evaluating the learning effectiveness of using simulations in software project management education: results from a twice replicated experiment. *Information and Software Technol.* 2004:46(2):127.

9. Garde S, Harrison D, Hovenga E. Skill needs for nurses in their role as health informatics professionals: a survey in the context of global health informatics education. *Int J Med Inf.* In press.

10. Sermeus W, Goossens L, Vanhaecht K. WISECARE: an overview. In: Sermeus W, Kearney N, Kinnunen J, Goossens L, Miller M. *Wisecare—Workflow Information Systems for European Nursing Care.* Amsterdam: IOS Press; 2000:3-22.

11. Australian Institute of Health and Welfare (AIHW) Australian Hospital Statistics 2002-03. 2004. Available at: http://www.aihw.gov.au/publications/index.cfm/title/10015.

12. Australian Health Ministers' Conference (AHMC) Joint Communique. July 29, 2004. Health ministers agree to national health workforce action plan. Available at: http://www.health.gov.au/internet/wcms/publishing.nsf/Content/health-mediarel-yr2004-jointcom-jc005.htm. Accessed February 2005.

13. AARNet. AARNet 2003 Annual Report. Available at: http://www.aarnet.edu.au/publications/aarnet_annual_report_2003.pdf. Accessed February 2005.

Case Study 17D

Leveraging through Cooperation:
CIC—*Committee on Inter-Institutional Cooperation*

Connie White Delaney, PhD, RN, FAAN, FACMI; Patricia Flatley Brennan, PhD, RN, FAAN, FACMI; Anna M. McDaniel, DNS, RN, FAAN; Josette F. Jones, PhD, RN; Gail M. Keenan, PhD, RN; and Yvonne M. Abdoo, PhD, RN

Nursing has made systematic investments in information technologies to improve the delivery and management of clinical care, to build and disseminate new knowledge through nursing research, and to deliver educational programs that reflect state-of-the-science teaching and learning strategies for an information-intensive discipline. The investments in informatics, traditionally linked to Florence Nightingale, have particularly been made from the early 1970s to present day and have encompassed, for example, vocabulary and essential data set standards, criteria for nursing information systems, "telenursing," and new methods of knowledge discovery. They have included defining a specialty in nursing informatics (NI), setting an NI research agenda, and inspiring interdisciplinary collaborations. Moreover, significant work has occurred in integrating informatics competencies across undergraduate and graduate nursing curricula, as well as in establishing master's and doctoral programs focused on the NI specialty.[1]

Most recently, nursing's commitment to the essential contribution of informatics to every aspect of the profession is clearly evident. For example, the American Association of Colleges of Nursing (AACN)[2] has included informatics competencies as essential curricular content for their Clinical Nurse Leader program and discussed including the competencies in the doctorate of nursing practice initiative. In another effort, the Technology Informatics Guiding Educational Reform initiative focuses on informatics reform across all nursing curricula and competencies for all levels of clinical practice. The work of Connors[3] is one example demonstrating the fundamental transformation of nursing education into a knowledge-driven informatics framework.

Although all of these responses are essential, the most crucial issue remains open: the dearth of informatics scholars (i.e., doctorally prepared academicians and researchers) needed to support the professional initiatives. The Alliance for Nursing Informatics, supported by the American Medical Informatics Association and the Healthcare Information and Management Systems Society, represents more than 3,000 informatics nurses and brings together more than twenty distinct NI groups in the U.S. that function separately at local, regional, national, and international levels. Despite their efforts to rally NI expertise in the U.S., such initiatives still do not address the breadth and depth of the need for experts and scholars in NI.

Therefore, the purpose of this case study is to describe an innovative solution to this professional crisis. The case study briefly describes the context of the dilemma from societal and informatics education perspectives, presents a consortium solution for preparing informatics scholars, and concludes with the future directions of and opportunities for the consortium.

Context of the NI Scholar Crisis

The U.S.' existing approach to training NI scholars is costly and suboptimal, and it has a very low output of research-productive scholars. For more than fifteen years, nurses who sought research training in NI had only two options: (1) an apprenticeship model of training with one of the few NI scholars at a PhD-granting institution or (2) training in a medical informatics PhD program. At best, the apprenticeship model produces two or three graduates a year nationally. Meanwhile, most of the leading medical informatics training programs exist in schools of medicine in universities that lack doctoral programs in nursing (such as Harvard, Stanford, and Rice).[4] Columbia University stands as a notable exception with a strong doctoral program in nursing whose instructors enjoy a close affiliation with a research-intensive medical informatics faculty. However, even Columbia has a very small cadre of research-productive NI scholars, and their areas of expertise do not cover all of the important components of the NI domain.

One of the challenges faced in creating NI doctoral and postdoctoral programs arises from the small numbers of research-productive nurse informaticians. Schools of nursing are fortunate to count even one NI researcher among their ranks, and many leading schools of nursing lack even a single faculty member with expertise in NI. Establishing a sustainable research program and the concomitant training environment with only a single peer in a school of nursing is daunting, even for an outstanding scholar.

There is a critical need for NI researchers who can envision, devise, implement, and evaluate IT that facilitate patient outcomes. Systematic investment by the National Institute of Nursing Research (NINR) in NI research and research training is essential to fulfill nursing's participation in the initiatives under the National Institutes of Health Roadmap. Specifically, nurses trained in NI research must have the capacity "... to find effective approaches to achieving and sustaining good health and to improve clinical settings in which care is provided."[5]

NI training is essentially interdisciplinary. Scholars need to develop skills in collaboration and integration, incorporating multiple strategies to ask and answer complex questions. There is a need both for basic NI research and for integration of NI strategies into research programs that address all the research themes advanced by NINR. Although NI research contributes to all five of the current research themes, scholars in this area are most likely to contribute to "Harnessing Advanced Technologies to Serve Human Needs."

The current nursing shortage will not be solved by labor force development alone; rather, its safe resolution awaits a rebalancing of the human and technological resources deployed to support patient care. Only through NI research can knowledge management strategies be developed that capitalize on emerging informatics developments while preserving the professional dimensions of nursing and nursing science. Situating NI training in strong PhD programs in nursing ensures the development of NI scholars socialized in the discipline.

A Consortium Solution for Preparing NI Scholars

The national NI community enjoys a long history of peer support and collaboration across institutions. This "invisible college" provides the impetus to develop a novel, cross-institutional training program, possibly linking NI scholars from several research schools in a combined effort that would support research training. The collaborative initiative described below capitalizes on the intellectual strengths and research talents of faculty from several universities. This united approach affords emerging scholars the benefits of a rich, diverse cadre of faculty, with access to the range of research environments needed to ensure comprehensive training in NI inquiry.

To respond to the challenges of increasing the number and competence of doctorally-trained NI scholars, the authors capitalized on established relationships among NI scholars across several universities ($N = 4$ initially and now 6), all member institutions of the Committee on Institutional Cooperation (CIC).[6] The universities are The University of Iowa, University of Wisconsin–Madison, Indiana University, University of Michigan, University of Minnesota, and University of Illinois–Chicago.

The CIC has a forty-four-year history of effective voluntary interinstitutional cooperation. The CIC programs clearly demonstrate a mechanism that enables a set of institutions to accomplish collectively far more than they could achieve individually. The programs do not replace or supplant any individual campus-based efforts, but rather augment them while focusing attention on the issues and adding coherence and continuity to activities that might otherwise seem uncoordinated or unrelated. Mechanisms for course enrollment, credit transfer, and tuition payments among the CIC universities have been established and facilitate collaboration among all six sites. Technology support for education and research initiatives is coordinated through the CIC.

The Nursing & Health Informatics Consortium was created within the CIC. In November 1997, at the AMIA meeting in Orlando, Florida, Dr. Connie Delaney (Iowa) convened nurse informaticians to discuss establishing a national informatics educators' collaborative. The discussion built on the early offerings of summer institutes in informatics for faculty organized and taught by Drs. Diane Billings (Indiana), Patricia Brennan (Wisconsin), and Delaney, under the auspices of the Midwest Alliance in Nursing in 1996–1997. The discussions continued a year later in Chicago, with the AMIA Spring Congress focused on informatics education. The group enlisted the support of Deans Melanie Dreher and Angela McBride to guide the notion of national collaboration in informatics among the members of the AACN in the fall of 1998. Simultaneously Dr. Brennan initiated a student exchange under the auspices of the CIC. As each organization increased faculty capacity in informatics, the stage was set in 2001 for Drs. Delaney, Brennan, and Dean McDaniel to hold an organizational meeting to establish a formal nursing and health informatics consortium among the University of Iowa, University Wisconsin–Madison, and Indiana University. The University of Michigan was added a year later, and subsequently, the universities of Minnesota and of Illinois. The vision of the consortium is:

> Grounded in 21st century values of collaboration, creativity, partnering, and community, this consortium of informatics leaders and world-class research institutions is committed to enriching the health of individuals, families, and communities through the design, deployment and evaluation of advanced information technologies. The consortium welcomes the unbounded synergy and convergence among academic, clinical practice, research, products and services of business, and the consumer—all as co-producers of health.[7]

This collaboration (1) situates the research training in well-respected doctoral programs in nursing, (2) offers multiple opportunities for on-site and technology-supported courses and colloquia, (3) provides research practica and supervision by a team of faculty with overlapping programs of research that span the domain of NI, and (4) grants access to the rich interdisciplinary environments in place at each university.

The highly committed core faculty, endorsed and supported by the deans of the initial four schools of nursing (Deans Dreher, May, McBride, and Hinshaw) and respective university administrations, has produced two three-semester-hour innovative doctoral seminars delivered by means of video-over-IP (Internet2), collaborative publications, and a monthly journal club. Moreover, they overcame the logistical barriers of aligning training programs across institutions including securing adjunct faculty appointments in each other's schools. The authors have worked with registrars and academic deans to ensure the integrity of each institution's degree-granting processes while benefiting from teaching and research opportunities.

The integrating conceptual framework for the programming builds on the conceptual model of informatics described by the ANA[8]: the management and processing of data, information, and knowledge. The specific integrating dimensions are knowledge representation, knowledge integration, and knowledge discovery.

1. Knowledge *representation* involves creating and defining formal structures, e.g., languages, vocabularies, terminology models, decision models, and information models that express concepts and processes important to the discipline.
2. Knowledge *integration* involves the processes required to bring knowledge representation tools into practice. It includes the design of computer systems, the strategies to implement them in the practice environment, and the methodologies to support the creation of research repositories used to support knowledge discovery.
3. Knowledge *discovery* addresses the generation of findings about informatics tools and their appropriate use in nursing practice and research. An example is the data mining of large databases derived from clinical nursing practice to determine the link between nursing interventions and patient outcomes and the impact of a Web-based home coaching service on outcomes of patients with chronic disease.

The boundaries among these three subdomains of NI are permeable, and much inquiry occurs at their intersection. Patient outcomes result at the core overlap of the three subdomains.

NI contributes to patient outcomes in both direct and indirect ways. *Direct* contribution of NI to patient outcomes can be seen in the work of our core faculty, McDaniel and Brennan. The research of these investigators employs NI innovations (such as reaching home care patients through computer programs and information networks) to facilitate patient well-being and functional outcomes. The *indirect* contributions occur in several ways, including the early knowledge discovery research of Delaney, which identifies patterns among patient problems, nursing interventions, and related outcomes.[9,10] Gail Keenan's work strives to indirectly improve patient outcomes through better communication and documentation of common nursing diagnoses, interventions, and outcome indicators across various patient care settings.[11] Josette Jones's work is focused on improving nursing practice through efficient access to literature.[12] Yvonne Abdoo's work, synergistic with Keenan's, focuses on knowledge integration. It includes clinician acceptance and data use for multiple purposes, interface, feasible hardware and software solutions; database design; and refining interface languages to ensure utility in nursing practice.[13] Thus, our team of recognized NI researchers pos-

Student Benefits:
- Legitimate entry to experts
- Access to larger set of expertise
- Access to diverse student body
- Peer support

Faculty Benefits:
- Colleagueship
- Development of mentorship and peer consultation

Organizational Benefits:
- More robust curricular offerings
- Ability of each school to admit students that it could not otherwise admit because it did not have the courses available
- Better recruitment (that is, familiarity of faculty with one another, ability to share students)
- Prestige and recognition by other nursing schools, CIC programs, and home institutions
- Increased chance that local faculty will be more productive through the support provided by faculty in other schools
- Ability of faculty with different research programs to participate with informatics faculty
- Enhanced credibility of the research program because of the informatics faculty
- The stimulation of the creative process
- Opportunity to act as a model for other collaborations

Figure 17D-1. *Benefits to Consortia Participants.*

sesses the necessary breadth of knowledge to develop nurse researchers who can devise, implement, and evaluate knowledge management strategies to enhance patient outcomes.

Many of the initiatives undertaken by NI researchers complement and extend those addressed by colleagues in HI. For example, Delaney's work in minimum data sets complements Bakken's[14] work in terminology modeling, which in turn complements that of physicians. Brennan's home care computer interventions address problems similar to those addressed in the Comprehensive Health Enhancement and Social Support project.[15] The unique and important aspects added to the field of HI by nurse investigators include attention to the domains of patient experiences that fall within the purview of nursing (human responses to disease and diagnosis) and the expansion in vocabulary and other representation tools by the systematic application of nursing knowledge and perspectives. Because of the increased knowledge base needed to ensure the development and evaluation of robust innovations, it is necessary to offer ample opportunities and resources to enhance the disciplinary study of NI under the interdisciplinary umbrella.

The consortium has been functioning since 2004, and outcomes measures have been established. Figure 17D-1 outlines the benefits to students, faculty, and consortia partners. Moreover, outcomes included collaborative publications and presentations.[16-21] Faculty mentoring contributed to applications for academic and other types of awards.

Future Directions

Clearly, this innovative model for preparing a cadre of NI scholars is effective. The effectiveness is predicated on the existence of cooperative tuition and credit transfer agreements. Most importantly, the model demands a collaborative, rather than competitive, value system. Clearly, the ingredients for the success of such programs include executive leadership and support, faculty commitment, excellent and supportive student services, a high-quality technology infrastructure for course management and synchronous delivery, financial resources, and effective communication, as outlined by Abel.[22] Future priorities include extending the programming throughout the CIC institutions, expanding to include non-CIC institutions, and establishing collaborative research projects. This innovation is the living experience of Marshall McLuhan's assertion, "We have extended our nervous system itself in a global embrace, abolishing both space and time as far as our planet is concerned."[23]

References

1. American Medical Informatics Association. Available at: www.amia.org. Accessed October 11, 2005.
2. American Association of Colleges of Nursing. Available at: www.aacn.nche.edu. Accessed October 11, 2005.
3. Connors H, Transforming the nursing curriculum: going paperless. In: Weaver C, Delaney CW, Weber P, Carr R, eds. *Nursing and Informatics for the 21st Century: An International Look at Practice, Trends, and the Future.* Chicago: Health Information Management Systems Society; in press.
4. National Library of Medicine. Available at: http://www.nlm.nih.gov/ep/GrantTrainInstitute.html. Accessed October 11, 2005.
5. National Institute of Nursing Research (NINR). NINR Mission Statement. Available at: http://ninr.nih.gov/ninr/. Accessed September 1, 2005.
6. Committee on Institutional Cooperation. Available at: www.cic.uiuc.edu. Accessed October 11, 2005.
7. I^4 CIC Nursing & Health Informatics Consortium, Announcement Brochure, November 2001.
8. American Nurses Association. Scope of practice for nursing informatics. *American Nurses Association Publications.* 1994 NP-90:1-15.
9. Delaney C, Clarke M, Ruiz M, Srinivasan P. Knowledge discovery in databases: data mining NMDS. In: Saba V, Carr R, and Rocha P, eds. *Nursing Informatics 2000: One Step Beyond: The Evolution of Technology and Nursing.* 2000: 61-65.
10. Delaney C, Reed D, Clarke M. Describing patient problems and nursing treatment patterns using nursing minimum data sets (NMDS & NMMDS) and UHDDS repositories. In: Overhage JM, ed. *AMIA 2000 Converging Information, Technology, & Health Care.* 2000: 176-179.
11. Keenan G, Stocker J, et al. The HANDS project: studying and refining the automated collection of a cross setting clinical data set. *Computers, Informatics, Nursing.* 2002; 20: 89-100.
12. Poynton MR, Örlygsdóttir B, Jones J, Delaney C. Data preparation for knowledge discovery: a comparison of clinical and research databases. Paper presented at: 28th Annual Research Conference of the Midwest Nursing Research Society; March 2004; St. Louis.
13. Abdoo, YM. Designing a patient care medication and recording system to improve patient care using bar coding. *Computers in Nursing.* 1992; 10: 116-120.
14. Bakken S, Warren J, Lange L, Button P. A review of major nursing vocabularies and the extent to which they have the characteristics required for implementation in computer-based systems. *J Am Med Inform Assoc.* 1998: 321-328.
15. Gustafson DH, Hawkins R, Boberg E, et al. Impact of a patient-centered, computer-based health information/support system. *Am J Prev Med.* January 1999;16(1):1-9.
16. Delaney C, Brennan PF, McDaniel AM, Keenan G, Cullen P. Research in nursing informatics: naming, claiming, and changing health outcomes. Paper presented at: 8th International Nursing Informatics (NI) Conference; June 2003; Rio de Janeiro, Brazil.
17. Volrathongchai K, Delaney C, Phuphaibul R. The development of NMDSs in Thailand. *J Adv Nurs.* 2003;43(6):1-7.
18. Clarke MF, Falan S, McDaniel AM, Keenan GM. Diagnostic reasoning and the use of nursing standardized languages. Paper presented at: 28th Annual Research Conference of the Midwest Nursing Research Society; March 2004; St. Louis.
19. Ford Y, Rukanudding RJ, Thoroddsen A, Jones J, Delaney C. An examination of the proposed international nursing minimum dataset. Paper presented at: 28th Annual Research Conference of the Midwest Nursing Research Society; March 2004; St. Louis.
20. Hardardottir GA, Hsieh Y, Brennan PF. Do nursing vocabularies capture the meaning of terms used by patients in email messages to nurses? Paper presented at: 28th Annual Research Conference of the Midwest Nursing Research Society; March 2004; St. Louis.
21. Weaver C, Delaney CW, Weber P, Carr R, eds. *Nursing and Informatics for the 21st Century: An International Look at Practice, Trends, and the Future.* Chicago: Health Information and Management Systems Society; in press.
22. Abel R. Implementing best practices in online learning. *Educause Quarterly.* 2005; 75-80.
23. McLuhan, M. *Understanding Media.* Cambridge, MA: MIT Press; 1994.

CHAPTER 18

European Collaboration for Teaching Nursing Informatics

By Anthony Michael Paget, MSc, RMN, RGN; Franca Mongiardi, MSc, RGN;
Mary Chambers, PhD; and Hans Springer, BSc, RN

The life and success of the European Summer School of Nursing Informatics (ESSONI) mirrors the development of nursing informatics (NI) across Europe and beyond. When the ESSONI was established in the early 1990s, NI was at an embryonic stage of development around the world. Over the years, it has grown into a major discipline, with nurses playing key roles in decision making about procurements; leading local, national, and international research and practice initiatives; and contributing to and promoting developments in education, e.g., masters degrees in health informatics. The nursing community now has the confidence to contribute to multiprofessional education and research in informatics.

As a result of these activities, there is a well-established body of NI literature. Nurses also contribute to a range of health and medical informatics research and literature. Although these activities cannot be attributed solely to the ESSONI, it is reasonable to suggest that it did play a part in raising not only the profile of NI internationally, but also in enabling the personal and professional development of a number of key nurse informaticians.

Beginnings of the ESSONI

In 1989, a number of senior nurses from across Europe were invited to a conference in the Netherlands (Utrecht) to explore the possibility of developing a European-wide master's level program in a number of areas of nursing. Attending the conference were representatives from many nursing disciplines, such as, mental health, oncology, geriatrics, as well as those interested in NI.

Although the initial intention of the event was to develop a master's level program in NI, discussions held during the three days of the conference led to a decision that the timing of such an initiative was not right. This conclusion was based on the collective view that the basic level of knowledge, skills, and understanding of NI and information technology (IT) within nursing was limited and insufficient to develop or sustain such a high-level course.

In the 1980s, NI was not a well-understood concept, and consequently, was not a part of the day-to-day language of nursing in the United Kingdom (UK) or Europe. Use of the term *NI* was more prevalent in the U.S. and the Netherlands. There were some exceptions, as illustrated by the works of Aarts,[1] Hoy,[2] Coates and Chambers,[3] and others. The language used by some of these authors was reflective of the state of the discipline at that time. Much of what was written, certainly in the U.K., centered on the curriculum in higher education and/or computer-assisted care planning. A survey of universities across the U.K. demonstrated that the inclusion of IT in the nursing curriculum was largely determined by the interests of the academics associated with the programs.[4]

Having decided that a master's level program was not appropriate for European nurses at that point, the challenge was to find a strategy that would enable nurses at different levels to access an NI course, one that would increase overall NI capacity and capability. It was decided that a six-day summer school would be the best initial approach.

A working group representing different institutions of higher education was established to plan for the first summer school. Each of the four countries of the U.K. was involved, as well as the Netherlands, Ireland, and Finland.

The aim of the summer school was to forward NI as a research, education, and practice-based discipline. The following objectives were set into place to achieve that goal:
1. Raise the profile of informatics and promote the interchange of knowledge and skills in all areas of nursing.
2. Prepare educators to introduce informatics into all nursing curricula.
3. Facilitate discussion groups and workshop/study days led by NI specialists to further integrate and disseminate informatics and to encourage nurses to recognize the relevance of informatics and incorporate it into their daily practice.
4. Utilize informatics to further the scientific, theoretical basis of nursing as a professional discipline.
5. Encourage enthusiasm and instill commitment to innovative practice.
6. Facilitate structured development and evaluation of all aspects of NI, and promote participants using informatics as a way to identify and clarify expert practice

Another goal was to provide a hands-on informatics experience for students and faculty. To make that possible, the program would cater to groups of no more than forty students. The culture and philosophy of the program would be one of hard work with maximum challenge and expert support. Small groups of students would participate in practical activities to gain confidence in the use of technology and in the language, skills, and application of informatics to nursing.

A proposal was submitted to the European Commission for funding under the European Community Action Scheme for the Mobility of University Students. The application was successful, and the school received financial support for faculty and student exchange. ESSONI continued to receive annual financial assistance until 1996, when that particular Europeon Commission funding program ended.

An executive committee of volunteers organized the school. Several of those who attended the Utrecht conference were early volunteers, e.g., Mary Chambers, Paul Wainwright, Jos Aarts, and Nikki Eaton. Later committee members included Derek Hoy, Paul Epping, Ulrich Schrader, Diane Skiba, Hans Springer, Franca Mongiardi, and Anthony Paget. The school continued as a not-for-profit organization with no additional financial support after 1996.

Development and Function of the Track System
ESSONI consisted of core topics, or "tracks," with four typically offered at a time. The track approach allowed each student to focus on a specific topic. This gave students time to thoroughly explore the subject and improve their understanding. It also made for active engagement in the group work, thus giving students in-depth knowledge about the track subject.

Each track would focus on major aspects of NI such as:
1. **Education**—curriculum design, development, and teaching of NI
2. **Clinical Applications**—using informatics to support the delivery of care
3. **Management**—management of quality
4. **Formal Nursing Knowledge**—expert systems, structuring, and classification of nursing diagnoses, interventions, and outcomes

The summer school also provided opportunities to use computers, including the Internet, and access international resources.

A typical ESSONI program would proceed as follows:
Day 1 - Plenary lectures by tutors, start of track working groups
Day 2 - Plenary papers, continuation of track work
Day 3 - Track working groups, presentations by exhibitors, and a break for local site visits
Day 4 - Plenary papers, continuing track group work
Day 5 - Plenary papers, continuing track group work
Day 6 - Plenary papers, finalize track group work, and presentations of the track work results

For each track, an expert was invited to guide the learning process. Each year, different experts were invited for each track. This allowed the summer school to retain its fresh, innovative nature. Each student would choose one track to focus on for the entire six-day period. This allowed for active engagement in the group work, providing students with in-depth knowledge of their chosen track subject.

Several changes occurred during the years the summer school ran. Initially, students (see Figure 18-1) and tutors in the education track used the most technology. More recently, all the tracks used technology. Students began bringing their own laptop computers and used such applications as Microsoft PowerPoint, as well as the Internet. Students also increasingly wanted to gain practical experience using applications that would support their practice. This often included software for flowcharting, project management, spreadsheets, and databases.

The summer school also changed when students and teachers began "cross-referencing" each other on specific subject areas. This took the form of discussions during group work sessions. For example:

- One year, students in the Formalizing Nursing Knowledge track, who were studying Nursing Language, teamed up for discussion with those in the Information Resources for Patients track. The purpose of the discussion was to explore how, potentially, patients and service users could use nursing taxonomies to access online health-related information.
- In another case, students in the Clinical Applications track, who were studying the implementation of clinical information systems (CIS), teamed up for discussion with students in the Formalizing Nursing Knowledge track. This discussion explored the importance of communica-

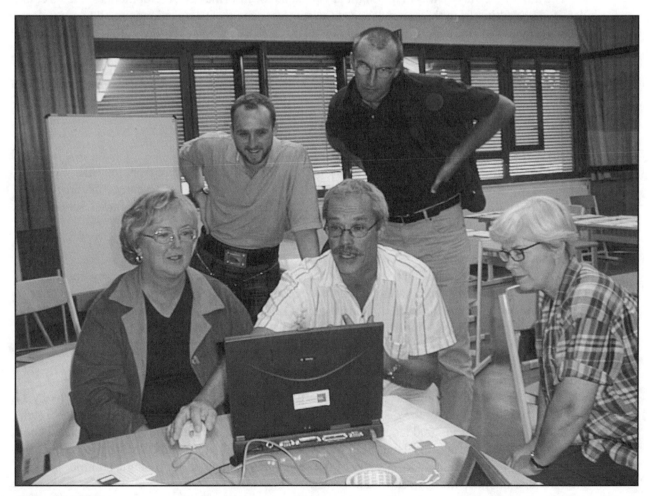

Figure 18-1. *Students from the Clinical Applications track are hard at work, supervised by their tutor. From left: Donna Singleton (Canada), Graeme Elrick (Scotland), Lars T. Rundgren (Sweden), Peter Fehrenbach (Germany), and their tutor Rita Zielstorff (United States).*

tion between system designers and developers and those implementing the system who often in the real world come from two different teams.

The summer school attracted students from many different countries in Europe and beyond. This gave the students, tutors, and organizers opportunities to hear and learn about other health care systems. Although there were many differences, there were also many similarities such as:

- Challenges of computerizing the health care record with all its complexities
- Challenge of achieving consensus—often an enormous undertaking—on a multidisciplinary electronic care record. It would seem that the reluctance of some health professionals to be part of a multidisciplinary record is not confined to any one country.
- Communication between different organizations and professionals involved in delivering care to patients. The patient tended to be in the middle of a complicated arrangement and remained the key information holder for his or her care.

ESSONI—The Students' Perceptions

The organizing committee of the summer school carried out an evaluation after each event, a positive task that helped shape future summer sessions. What such an activity failed to capture was an overview of the school from the students' perspectives, including the potential sequelae of students' attending one or more summer schools. The committee hypothesized that the school was making an important contribution to the development of NI; an online semistructured student survey later tested this theory.

The aim of the survey was to highlight any personal or informatics developments students could identify as resulting from their attendance at the summer school. The questionnaire allowed students to answer in their own words. Thematic content analysis was used to study the replies, and the results are collated here for the first time.

The questionnaire, posted on the ESSONI Web site shortly before the Glasgow ESSONI in 2000, remained available to students for more than one year. E-mail lists were used to encourage all former students to also complete the survey. Twenty-two completed forms were collected. Details about the survey questions follow.

Country of Origin

Respondents were from a wide range of countries. Eleven respondents were from the U.K., two from Denmark, two from the U.S., and one each from Holland, Canada, Japan, Germany, Finland, Austria, and Switzerland. This type of representation is reasonably typical of each summer school. The majority of students over the years came from the U.K.

Professional Background

As may be anticipated, ESSONI mainly attracted nurses. The majority of survey respondents described themselves as nurses, although there were also two information managers, one lecturer in biology, a researcher, and a medical informatician. Of the nurses, several were working in the field of informatics in some way, but the majority (fourteen) were in nurse education. Again, this seems quite representative of ESSONI—nurse educators often were over-represented.

Summer School(s) Attended

The timing of our presenting the questionnaire meant that recent attendees were more likely to respond, and indeed, most of the respondents had attended either the school in Austria in 1999 (ten) or the Glasgow school in 2000 (fourteen). Several respondents had attended more than one school, including those in Northern Ireland, Belgium, Wales, and the Netherlands. The figures reflect the attendance patterns of the school—many of the respondents attended for a single summer session, but a number attended almost year-round.

Track Undertaken

Many respondents listed a range of tracks taken at a number of different schools. This data is not particularly meaningful, except to observe that no single track or topic seems to be over-represented.

"What did ESSONI Contribute to Personal Development?"

This question received a range of positive views. The two most prominent themes were "opportunity to network" (nine) and "broadened knowledge" (ten). These themes were supplemented with views about the "new insights from a global view" (six) and how the school provided "new enthusiasm/inspiration" (six). More specific outcomes related to "new educational perspectives" arising from the school, e.g., new material for lectures, Web-based learning initiatives, and insight into effective group work (six). Two respondents mentioned increased confidence in IT matters and informatics.

"Did ESSONI Attendance Result in New Developments at Work?"

Many would use this as the measure of success for any educational episode, particularly when scarce resources are spent on attending. Most of the respondents were able to cite new developments in a range of activities, with only five offering a "none" or "not yet" response. The over-representation of teachers is evident here as eighteen pointed to new educational developments. These developments include the "introduction of new teaching technologies" (eight), e.g., Web-based learning materials, and "curriculum developments" (ten), e.g., new lectures, modules, and courses. Others mentioned how the school helped "reinforce existing developments" (three), e.g., a new electronic patient record. One respondent spoke of "cascading information to colleagues," another of new "research ideas," and one unspecified new development. In terms of the committee's hypothesis, the results represent a positive and practical impact of the summer school, particularly in the area of informatics education.

"Did ESSONI Help in Any Other Contribution to Nursing Informatics?"

This question captured developments not identified by the earlier questions and provided a checklist for respondents to indicate general areas as shown below.
- Develop an educational module (five)
- Conducting research (three)
- Systems development (two)
- Write an article (five)
- Write/contribute to a book (one)

Respondents were asked to add other contributions not covered by the above; three respondents added "conference papers." These responses again point to a significant contribution to the discipline of NI by students who identify this work as being a direct result of attending ESSONI.

Other Comments

Most of the respondents offered further comments. The range of responses was wide and highly positive. The most frequently occurring theme was that of "opportunity to network" (nine), which was also a factor identified under "personal development." This aspect received very positive comment. An associated theme was how students highly valued gaining the "international perspective" (three), i.e., finding they were not alone in their successes and frustrations. Other students referred to the "positive learning environment" fostered by ESSONI (four), the "specific learning" that occurred (three), a "valuable experience" (three), and, last but not least "an enjoyable experience" (four).

Survey Summary

The responses supported the organizing committee's initial hypothesis: Although the sample was limited and self-selected, it does seem to be representative of the attendance at ESSONI through its history. The fact that many of the identified developments were educational or academic in nature seems to reflect the attendance pattern at many ESSONIs. Nurse educators were over-represented, but they, in turn, were empowered to prepare the next generation of nurses with IT competencies as well as those specializing in NI. ESSONI's largest impact may well be in supporting these educators to be able to further disseminate informatics knowledge via curricula and other educational developments.

A strong feature of ESSONI was the opportunity to network. The week-long informal atmosphere—working alongside colleagues and tutors, eating, drinking, and socializing with them—meant that enduring bonds were made. Many people who met at ESSONI are still in touch with each other, and this is sure to have fostered developments and collaborations that would not have otherwise occurred.

Challenges and Triumphs

As for any such event, there were inherent complications in preparing the necessary infrastructure of the summer schools. Some of these were particular to ESSONI. For example, from its inception, ESSONI was intended to be affordable and accessible to all. To that end, associated costs needed careful management. This often presented a problem, particularly related to finding suitable living accommodations. When the summer school was in the U.K., student accommodations were less of a problem, because suitable facilities are readily available at U.K. universities in August.

In choosing suitable venues, the factor of student accommodations was often a barrier to those wanting to offer their institution as a host. In continental Europe, such accommodation was not as readily available as in the U.K., and the cost of hotels was often prohibitive.

The executive committee, which was responsible for organizing the summer school, attempted to draw up a checklist of the requirements for a potential venue. This included availability of affordable accommodations and catering facilities near the classrooms and computer laboratories. Other challenges included finding a venue with ready transportation access—a local international airport, for example. In addition, the school and its students became ever "hungrier" for more technology. Thus, for the more recent summer schools, a new challenge emerged—to find venues with sufficient IT infrastructure and Internet access.

The exacting nature of these requirements meant that it became increasingly difficult to find suitable venues—particularly outside the U.K. It was always the intention of ESSONI to roam to a different European venue each year, but against increasing technology needs and cost constraints, this goal became difficult. Often very enthusiastic offers from particular venues fell through as problems arose in meeting the school's needs. This occasionally delayed the whole organizing process.

There were many triumphs though, even in adversity. At the 1999 school at Horn, near Vienna in Austria, there were major problems in finding accommodations. One hotelier lost our booking just weeks before the event. Computing facilities were limited, and all funneled through a single Internet access point. However, this turned out to be one of our most successful summer schools.

ESSONI 2001–2003

The last ESSONI was in 2001 in Swansea. Subsequent attempts to run ESSONI in 2002 and 2003 were unsuccessful, because they did not attract enough students to meet the minimum number to make them viable. The reasons for the drop in student attendance were never clear. It may have been that health care organizations did not have sufficient funds for staff to attend such courses. Another view was that the school had achieved its initial aims and that a range of alternative courses had become available, with informatics appearing in more health care curricula, or that the prospects of international air travel became less attractive to potential students.

However, this does not mean that there is a loss of interest in NI or in health informatics. For example, in the Netherlands, every hospital is considering development or is busy with the development of an EHR system. In England, the National Health Service modernization program and the National Health Service (this program is now called NHS Connecting for Health) Program for Information Technology are making NI and health informatics more and more important in health care delivery. The interest in NI is still there. Increasingly, NI is incorporated in basic nurse training and in stand-alone courses, and is available via the Internet.

There is still an interest in summer schools that present informatics. It is clear that ESSONI fulfilled an important role in bringing together interested professionals and world-renowned experts in an effective learning environment. The authors are investigating the viability of a new health informatics summer school drawing on the most successful elements of ESSONI.

References

1. Aarts JEC. 1989: A curriculum in nursing informatics. In: Salamon R, Protti J, Moehr, eds. *Proceedings of the International Symposium of Medical Informatics and Education*. Vancouver, British Columbia: University of Victoria.

2. Hoy D. 1989: *Computer Assisted Nursing Care Planning Systems in the United Kingdom*. Nursing Division Scottish Home and Health Department: Edinburgh, Scotland.

3. Coates VE, Chambers M. Teaching micro-computing to student nurses: an evaluation. *J Adv Nurs.* 1989;14:152-157.

4. Chambers M, Coates VE. Computer training in nurse education: a bird's eye view across the UK. *J Adv Nurs.* 1990;15:16-21.

Chapter 19

Informatics Competencies in Every Nursing

By Marion J. Ball, EdD; and Angela Barron McBride, PhD, RN, FAAN

To hear those in the industry tell it, academic informatics programs have done little to further the development and adoption of information technology (IT) in commercially viable health care applications. A few years ago, in preparing to present on this topic at the Annual Symposium of the American Medical Informatics Association, one of us (Marion Ball) undertook an informal survey at various organizations, hospitals, and academic institutions involved in the development and application of health care IT. She asked them to tell her honestly what they saw academia generating in this field and what they perceived when they interviewed candidates graduating from academic programs. Representatives from the several vendor companies surveyed were hiring the "best and the brightest" candidates. Yet, almost unanimously, they reported finding a pronounced disconnect between academic programs in health care informatics and the real world of health care information technology (HCIT). Although the candidates came from what are considered excellent programs, many were not even familiar with the names of the major companies or organizations in the field. This was a telling story, since these are the very companies with which the candidates would want to interview. The representatives also reported that the candidates they interviewed displayed a basic lack of knowledge about the industry and minimal understanding of how to move theory into practice, that is, how to apply concepts to real-life situations.

Other comments gathered in this informal survey reflected the perception that academics focus on "cool stuff," designed to solve problems in buckshot mode, geared only to challenges in academic medical centers, and having little or no applicability to industry practice. Vendor representatives felt that academics are enamored with the sophistication of the code they write and show disdain for the work developed in mainstream industry. There is little acknowledgment in academia that, when proprietary code runs only at academic institutions, it is not helpful to industry. Overall, industry representatives think that very little of what comes out of academia has sustainable commercial success.

Why Is the Alignment of Theory with Practice so Important?

Health care is at an unprecedented crossroad. Traditionally, the industry has been slow to adopt technologies to enhance the delivery of patient care. Yet today, as David Brailer, National Coordinator for Health Information Technology, noted at the 2005 Annual Healthcare Information and Management Systems Society (HIMSS) Conference & Exhibition, health care has the opportunity to take another path—to transform itself. As each sector of the industry turns in this new direction, academia too must do its part. Just as the industry must grapple with such issues as interoperability, unique patient identifiers and standards, academia must resolve the issue of relevance and ensure that the theoretical foundations they champion have sound practical application. Academia has an unprecedented opportunity to bring the power of enabling technologies to the patient in profoundly significant ways.[1]

What Can Academia Do? Ask the Right Questions.

As Max Planck said when he received the Nobel Prize for physics, "In the correct formulation of the question lies the key to the answer." Academia can begin by asking and addressing the right questions.

One major question: What do companies want to see coming out of the academic informatics arena in the areas of research prototypes, safety research, and decision support content, among other areas? This question is important because it not only enables academics to create prototypes that are useful to industry but also encourages an appropriate mindset in academia. In addition to producing graduates better prepared to deal with the real world, academia would be better equipping candidates to understand the role of informatics research and other advanced knowledge activities in the strategic business of the companies for which they work.

There is another important question: What kinds of skills should academic programs place at the fingertips of the next generation? Nursing informaticians have raised this question and have answered it in key publications.[2-4] As we see it, there must be a concerted effort to focus teaching and technology development on real-world applications.[5] Academia can play an essential role in helping health care provider organizations figure out the best way to transfer and apply what is developed in academic health centers to their environments. For instance, there is a tremendous need to develop code that increases interoperability among products developed by diverse vendors. There is also a real need to help students develop skills for the real world, such as how to develop a project plan, how to engage users in decision making, how to perform process analysis and tie it to functionality, and more. In short, the major areas that will help bridge the chasm between academia and real life include

1. Focusing on the real-world application of technology, not just theory
2. Helping health care providers figure out how to apply technology outside academic medical centers, such as small practice settings, nursing homes, home health care, and so on
3. Developing code to enhance interoperability among multiple vendors
4. Targeting skills needed in real life, such as:
   - How to conduct an organizational readiness assessment
   - How to engage users in decision making
   - How to analyze processes and tie them to functionality
5. Stressing communication skills, the ability to negotiate, managerial know-how, financial savvy, and so on, including the ability to frame issues so IT experts understand the problem(s) to be solved

A New Curriculum for Nurses

Efforts to bridge the gap speak to the need to educate and train nurses and the rest of the health care team differently than in the past. Most of the technology-enabled changes emerging in the health care environment are positive and have the potential to enhance the changing role of nursing.[6,7] All the signs indicate that these changes will gain momentum as technology proliferates. It is therefore time for academia to address how to prepare current and future nurses for the world of tomorrow. Academia needs to play a major role in training nurses differently, preparing them to work in environments that are increasingly interdisciplinary and technology-enabled. Changes must be made in the nursing curriculum to address the evolving interdisciplinary nature of health care, as well as to integrate computing and informatics skills and knowledge at all levels of training, from undergraduate to graduate to continuing education.[8] In sum, academia needs to do a better job of preparing nurses to navigate real work in the new digital era.[9]

In designing a new curriculum, it is useful to identify the skills students need in the real world and should have at the end of their training. Our preliminary assessment indicates that nurses should be able to:

1. Analyze the various types of information (e.g., patient-specific, evidence-based) that a clinician needs to render "timely" and "appropriate" health care and the current trends in providing such information
2. Demonstrate knowledge of how IT has changed and will continue to change patients' involvement in their own health care
3. Demonstrate knowledge of the major functions that a comprehensive computer-based patient record must perform
4. Analyze the attributes of clinical work flow problems that make them especially amenable to informatics solutions, as well as the strategies that informatics solutions might employ to solve those problems

5. Analyze the major barriers to advancing the state of clinical information technology (organizational, financial, technical, political, policy, etc.)
6. Demonstrate knowledge of several general-purpose ITs that are especially well-suited to solving particular problems in health care
7. Analyze the steps that the government has taken to protect the security and privacy of health information and the effect this has had on day-to-day activities
8. Evaluate the extent to which health care information is currently shared across disparate institutions and environments, and discuss the major potential benefits, drawbacks, and barriers to increased connectivity and cultural changes
9. Analyze the factors motivating the current widespread interest in clinical IT and informatics
10. Apply skills learned in IT to specific areas of nursing practice, e.g., pediatrics, geriatrics, the operating room, psychiatry, gerontology, etc
11. Communicate, teach, and interrelate well with people, whether at the personal or organizational level

Nurses have the tremendous opportunity to become agents of change in the health care transformation now under way.[10] Nurses are already taking on new roles as primary care providers, as "Internet guides" for patients who are given Web site "information prescriptions," as managers of environmental safety, and so on. For their work in these areas to be truly effective and recognized, the right educational foundation needs to be in place from the beginning of their training. Academia can be a critical catalyst for change in this respect by staying focused on the requirements of the real world.

This is a tall order, but one that nursing leaders are addressing through a collaborative effort known as TIGER (Technology Informatics Guiding Educational Reform). The seeds for this initiative were planted at the National Health Information Infrastructure (NHII) meeting held in Washington, DC, in July 2004. The conversations there ultimately expanded to include a group of more than twenty-five nurses from academia and industry, who then participated in a seminal meeting at the Johns Hopkins University School of Nursing in January 2005.* The January meeting established a consensus and put an action plan in place. The TIGER initiative is now planning, organizing, and facilitating a summit of nursing leadership on the issue of informatics education and practice reform for nursing students and practicing nurses.

The intent is to ensure that nurses become involved at every level of the "Informatics Revolution." The vision defined in January 2005 at Hopkins calls for nurses who can use informatics tools, principles, theories, and practices to make health care safer, more effective, more efficient, more patient-centered, more timely, and more equitable—in short, to realize the national goals for health care set by the IOM and David Brailer.* To this end, the summit will bring together nursing leadership from the Alliance for Nursing Informatics and the umbrella Nursing Organization Association for nursing specialty groups. The summit will charge them with developing plans, specific guidelines, and agendas to interweave enabling technologies transparently into—and across—nursing practice and education. This is a critical step toward making IT the stethoscope for the twenty-first century, enabling evidence-based care, and transforming nursing and ultimately health care. Nursing education and nursing practice will be at the heart of this transformation, bridging the chasm between industry and academia to improve health care for all.

---

* TIGER Team membership includes Patricia Abbott (Johns Hopkins), Marion Ball (Hopkins, IBM, and Healthlink), Emily Barey (Epic Systems), Jim Cato (Eclipsys), Helen Connors (University of Kansas), Connie Delaney (University of Minnesota), Linda Dietrich (Healthlink), Judith Douglas (Hopkins), Donna DuLong (Thomson MICROMEDEX), Holly Farish-Hunt (Healthlink), Veronica Feeg (George Mason University), Carole Gassert (University of Utah), Brian Gugerty (University of Maryland), Matt Hagg (Hopkins), Lynda Joseph (Unisys), Maria Koszalka (Hopkins Bayview Medical Center), Gail Latimer (Siemens), Angela McBride (Indiana University), Teresa McCasky (McKesson), Anthony Norcio (University of Maryland), Carolyn Padovano (MITRE), Virginia Saba (Georgetown University), Joyce Sensmeier (HIMSS), Patrick Shannon (U.S. Army), Diane Skiba (University of Colorado), Sheryl Taylor (QuadraMed), Michelle Troseth (CPM Resource Center), Mary Walker (MITRE), Charlotte Weaver (Cerner), Bonnie Wesorick (CPM Resource Center), and Rita Zielstorff (HealthVision).

References

1. McBride AB. Nursing and the informatics revolution. *Nurs Outlook.* 2005;53:183-191.

2. Staggers N, Gassert CA, Curran C. A Delphi study to determine informatics competencies for nurses at four levels of practice. *Nurs Res.* 2002;51(6):383-390.

3. Saba VK, Skiba DJ, Bickford C. Competencies and credentialing: nursing informatics. *Stud Health Technol Inf.* 2004;109:75-89.

4. Skiba DJ. Informatics competencies. *Nurs Ed Perspect.* 2004;25(6):312.

5. Ball MJ, Garets DE, Handler TJ. Leveraging information technology towards enhancing patient care and a culture of safety in the US. *Methods Inf Med.* 2003;42(5):503-508.

6. Feeg VD. Campaign for nursing curriculum reform in information technology: Got IT? Part I: IT and Health Care. *Dean's Notes.* 2004;26(2).

7. Feeg VD. Campaign for nursing curriculum reform in information technology: Got IT? Part II: IT and the U.S. government. *Dean's Notes.* 2005;26(3).

8. Billings DM, Skiba DJ, Connors HR. Best practices in Web-based courses: generational differences across undergraduate and graduate nursing students. *J Prof Nurs.* 2005;21(2):126-133.

9. Ball MJ, Weaver C, Abbott PA. Enabling technologies promise to revitalize the role of nursing in an era of patient safety. *Int J Med Inf.* 2003; 69(1):29-38.

10. Ball MJ. Nursing informatics of tomorrow. One of nurses' new roles will be agents of change in the health care revolution. *Health Inf.* 2005;22(2): 74,76,78.

Innovation Applied Through Informatics

Section IV

Introduction

Patrick Weber, MA, RN

Information technology (IT) has permeated health care to the extent that it is being used to apply management rigor to the business side of care delivery, to support transformational quality improvement initiatives, to achieve common codified data sets as an enabler for analyzing nursing care, and for rapid translation of new knowledge into clinical practice. Section IV presents innovative and leading edge work in the areas of research, clinical practice, quality improvement, and fiscal and operations management.

From an international perspective, Sermeus and colleagues in Chapter 20 demonstrate the importance of collecting good nursing data for optimum DRG (Diagnostic Related Groups) categorization and reimbursement. For instance, the authors show that complementing the DRG data with nursing data can improve the prediction of total charges by 80 percent. As the use of DRGs is an important management and financing tool in most nations' health systems, it is basic to nursing's future that its data be included and more visible in these systems. Inclusion of nursing data is also the goal of the International Nursing Minimum Data Set (iNMDS), an international project described in the Chapter 24 by Goossen et al. The iNMDS chapter is an overview of the nursing minimum data set developed to serve as an international standard by the broad team credited as authors. Goossen and fellow authors deliver this important milestone in nursing research and include recommendations for the future that speak to the inclusion of nursing data for clinical, managerial, and research purposes, and most importantly to drive health policy.

Clancy and Carley's report on organization analysis in Chapter 21 presents a methodology for dealing with organizational complexity. "To err is human," starts this chapter, and it could be added that without an ability to perform organization analysis, the risk becomes one of being doomed to repeat errors. Case Study 21A from the Royal Melbourne Hospital reflects an Asian adage: "Little wealth managed thriftily is better than a big treasure misused." Rathgeber describes how he applied IT and quantitative trending and analysis to create a powerful nursing management decision support and management tool that allowed major change in the nursing organization. The Northwestern Hospital case study in 21B is an industry example of the journey to quality that happens when an organization designates quality as its core strategic mission and business imperative.

The chapters on evidence-based practice (EBP) represent a major new frontier in health care and applied informatics. EBP as a concept and approach to care delivery is not new, having been first envisioned by Cochrane in the 1970s.[1] The innovation in its use today is its application to nursing knowledge and its use of IT as a medium for increasing the speed with which new knowledge is brought forth into clinical practice. Titler's Chapter 22 charts a methodology for translating nursing research into evidence-based protocols that can be used in clinical practice and demonstrates the potential impact that evidence-based nursing has on quality. Lang and colleagues (Chapter 23) describe a collaborative partnership between a health care system, university, and business working together to embed EBP knowledge into a clinical information system. While these EBP chapters report on current, on-going work, Betts and Wright's case study (22A) on Florence Nightingale reminds us that Nightingale pioneered the use of outcome data and statistics to determine best practices and demonstrates that she well deserves the title of "first health informatician."

Reference

1. Cochrane AL. 1972. *Effectiveness and Efficiency. Random Reflections on Health Services.* London: Nuffield Provincial Hospitals Trust, 1972.

CHAPTER 20

The DRG Imperative:
Overview and Nursing Impact

By Walter Sermeus, PhD, RN; Patrick Weber, MA, RN; Stephen Chu, BAppSc (AdvNursing, Biomed), PhD, FACS; Wolfram Fischer, MSc, lic.oec.HSG; and Dirk Hunstein, Dipl.-Pflegewirt

Diagnosis-related groups (DRGs) make up a patient classification system that relates the type of patients a hospital treats to the costs the hospital incurs for the treatments.[1] It is a method for grouping patients from a case mix point of view. For a clinician, case mix refers to the condition of the patient being treated and the treatments associated with the care. For an administrator, it refers to the demand for the resources—the personnel, equipment, and materials—that patients place on the organization while it provides their care.

Patients can therefore be categorized into a manageable number of groups called DRGs, on the basis of their economic and clinical homogeneity. *Clinical homogeneity* estimates are based on similarity in medical diagnosis, surgery, complications, birth weight, and, in most DRG systems, age. *Economic homogeneity* is measured first by the classification criterion of the length of stay and later by the complete cost of hospitalization. DRG systems and concurrent medico-economic patient classification systems (e.g., disease staging or patient management categories) were developed in the U.S. in the 1970s.[2-4]

How DRGs Are Put Together

Each patient case is assigned to a single DRG. This is done automatically by a computer program called a *grouper,* based on a set of hospital discharge data commonly known as the *minimum data set.* The minimum data set contains routinely collected data about the patient, e.g., medical diagnoses, birth weight for newborns, age, length of stay and the treatments given, including operating room procedures, certain medical procedures, and other data.

The medical diagnosis that best describes the patient's problem during the hospital encounter is known as the *principal diagnosis.* Within DRG systems, the principal diagnoses, as coded by the International Classification of Diseases, are grouped into twenty-three mutually exclusive groups called the *major diagnostic categories* (MDC). Table 20-1 shows six of the twenty-three MDCs.

Once a DRG is determined in relation to the principal diagnosis, it is "streamed" into surgical or medical groups depending on the procedure (which usually requires the use of the operating room) that was performed on the patient during the inpatient period. Patients who had more than one procedure performed are assigned to the procedure categories with the highest intensity of resource consumption.

The classification system also takes into consideration variables such as "greater than or equal to age severity" and/or "complications and comorbidities." *Substantial complications and comorbidities* are defined as conditions that would likely increase the length of stay by at least one day for 75 percent of the patients. The presence or absence of these variables results in a case being assigned to a different DRG. For example, pediatric patients (age seventeen years or less) and older patients (age seventy years and more) are assigned to separate DRGs. Figure 20-1 illustrates how the surgical group for MDC 11 (diseases and disorders of the kidney and urinary tract) is assigned to different DRGs based on the U.S. Health Care Financing Administration DRGs.

Table 20-1. MDCs defined for ICD-9-CM

MDC	MDC Description
1	Diseases and disorders of the nervous system
2	Diseases and disorders of the eye
3	Diseases and disorders of the ear, nose and throat
4	Diseases and disorders of the respiratory system
...	...
11	Diseases and disorders of the kidney and urinary tract
.....	.....
23	Factors influencing health status and other contacts with health services

Source: Adapted from Lichtig LK, 1986.[5]

The DRG system also accounts for patients whose treatment does not conform to the average and whose length of stay is less or more than the average. Each DRG is said to have a set of *trim points,* which separate a typical from an atypical patient based on the length of stay. Figure 20-2 illustrates the trim points for AP DRG 373 (Cost Weight Swiss v4.1f). Patients whose lengths of stay lie outside the low trim point and the high trim point are categorized as *outliers.* Those within the two points are *inliers.*

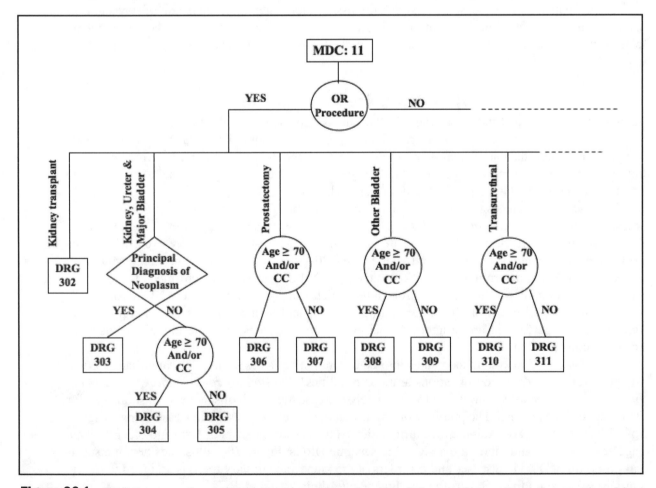

Figure 20-1. *DRG Generation from MDC 11 (Diseases and Disorders of the Kidney and Urinary Tract). Source: Adapted from Lichtig LK, 1986.[5]*

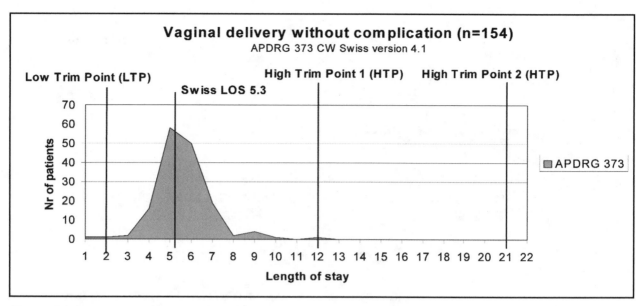

Figure 20-2. *Trim Points for AP DRG 373.*

A Family of DRGs

A wide range of DRG systems are in use, as shown by Fischer (see Figure 20-3).[6,7] The HCFA uses mainstream DRGs (HCFA-DRGs) for hospital payment for Medicare beneficiaries. The All Patient DRGs (AP-DRGs) represent an expansion of the HCFA-DRGs to be more representative of non-Medicare populations; they incorporate the severity of illness and risk of mortality subclasses into the DRGs. Several countries have adapted DRG systems from the U.S. system; examples are the Australian National DRGs (AN-DRGs) and the Australian Refined DRGs (AR-DRGs), the Scandinavian countries (NordDRGs, DkDRGs), Germany (G-DRGs), and France (GHM). Other countries have developed their own DRG-like systems, such as the U.K. (HRG), the Netherlands (DBC), and Austria (LDF), among others.[8] In the original experimental version of 1977 (see Figure 20-3), the Yale DRG system included 383 groups.[9] In the most recent versions of some DRG systems, the number of groups has been increased to more than 1,000.

The original objective of a DRG system was to act as an instrument for the review of hospital resources utilization. This objective was changed later: DRGs became a system for prospective payment, while the HCFA-DRG and AP-DRG systems retained the focus on the original objective.

As the health care industry evolved, the demand increased for a patient classification system that can be used for applications beyond resource use, cost, and payment. Examples of these new objectives are the comparison of hospitals across a wide range of resource and outcome measures, the evaluation of differences in inpatient mortality rates, the implementation and support of clinical pathways, the identification of continuous quality improvement projects, the basis of internal management and planning systems, and other such purposes.[1]

How DRG Is Linked to Nursing

Right from the start, there has been interest in linking DRG systems and nursing. Nursing is resource-intensive, and the obvious question is how well DRGs can capture nursing care information.

In most of the literature, researchers have shown that DRGs are not very homogeneous in respect to nursing.[10-18] DRGs explain only 20 percent to 40 percent of the variability of nursing costs.[19-22] The reported coefficients of variation for nursing cost per DRG vary from 0.22 to 2.56.[11,23-25] Some DRGs are more nursing-intensive than others. The ratio of nursing costs to total costs varies per DRG from 6 percent to 25 percent.[26-31] The most common criticism of DRGs in nursing literature is that they determine the hospital product predominantly by medical condition and medical services consumption. Nursing is thus reduced to a cost factor reflected in intensity of

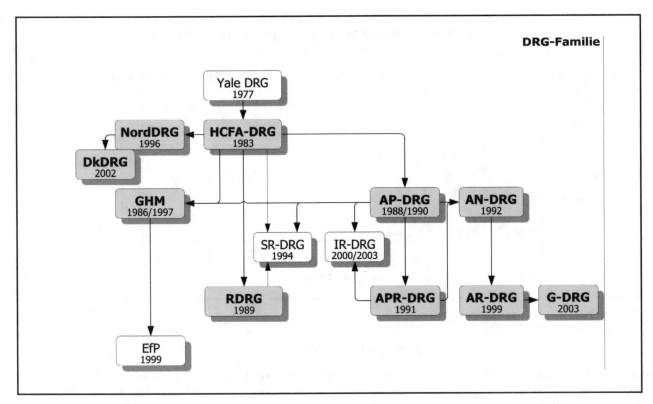

Figure 20-3. *The Yale DRG system.*

nursing care and a measure of how many nurses and minutes of care that are needed. Welton and Halloran[15] show that complementing DRG data with nursing data can improve the prediction by about 80 percent for total hospital days, total intensive care unit (ICU) days, and total charges.

Fischer[32] describes different methods with which DRG systems and nursing care could be linked in determining the actual costs (see Figure 20-4). Fischer sees three approaches to the question of linking nursing data to DRG-groupings:

1. *Make no modification.* The DRG classification remains unchanged and is built solely on medical data (such as medical diagnoses and interventions) and on some patient data (such as age and the like). No nursing perspective is involved in describing the patient product.

2. *Keep the basic structure of DRGs intact except to include the nursing perspective.* Describe complications and comorbidities not only from the medical but also from the nursing perspective, like nursing-related ICD codes or preferably nursing diagnoses and interventions. In the last case, the minimum data set feeding the grouper software would have to be expanded to include nursing-related information.

3. *Develop complementary nursing cost groups.* An example of an independent classification of nursing-related groups[33] is the set of relative intensity measures (RIMs) developed by Caterinicchio and associates.[34-36] In the RIM classification, various DRGs with a similar nursing related groups profile were grouped.

   In describing actual costs, various methods can be used:

- The most common method is using the length of stay as a proxy for nursing costs; variability in nursing costs is expressed as variability in length of stay.
- The use of cost weight per DRG recognizes that nursing care differs among DRGs. This leads to relative nursing cost weights per DRG, which are calculated by linking nursing workload systems to DRGs.
- The variability of nursing costs within DRGs can be described by measuring the variability of nursing care during the stay.
- Other methods include calculating nursing weights separately from the weights of other types of hospital costs or defining trim points based on nursing data (e.g., trim points related to nursing hours).

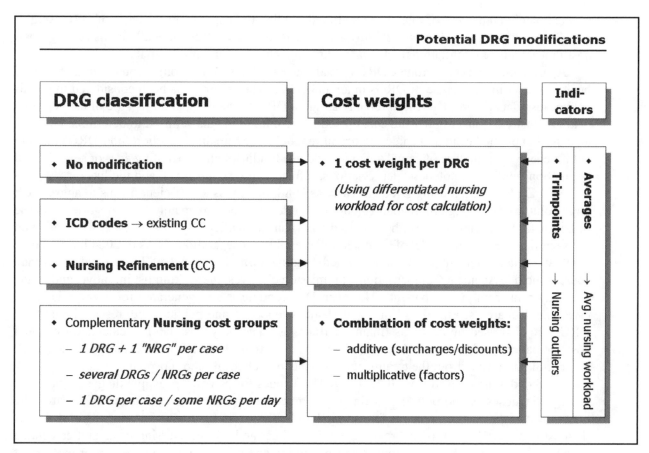

Figure 20-4. *Determining costs by linking DRG systems with nursing care.*

In the first method, no nursing data are required. In the second, DRGs have to be calibrated for nursing from time to time. For the third and fourth methods, continuous nursing data collection is required.

Examples in Linking DRGs and Nursing

Many countries have some experience in linking DRGs and nursing data, using one or more of the preceding methods. Five such initiatives (examples from Australia, New Zealand, Belgium, Germany, and Switzerland) are described and analyzed below. Inasmuch as DRGs are implemented in many Western countries, other nursing systems may also exist.

Australia and New Zealand

Australia introduced DRGs in the early 1990s as a sweeping change to its health care funding model, with the state of Victoria leading the nation in DRG development, implementation, and refinement. The initial effort was an adaptation of the HCFA-DRG system version 12, which had 492 categories. By the end of the 1990s, the Australian DRG system had gone through five iterations of refinements, from AN-DRG-v2 (Australian National DRG version 1) with 527 categories to AR-DRG v5.1 (Australian Revised DRG version 5.1) with 665 categories.

The classification system is generally updated every two or three years. A revision does not necessarily entail adding more classification codes. As each version is reviewed, new codes are added, but existing codes can also be split, deleted, or refined to comply with changes in medicine and technologies.

In Australia, AR-DRG v5.1 is used as the national standard in describing admitted episodes of care under the national health information agreement. Although the DRG weighting for allocating hospital care funding varies from state to state, it represents a significant proportion in hospital funding allocation and cash flow. In the 2004–2005 financial year, the state of Victoria allocated approximately 60 percent of total acute admitted funding to hospitals on the basis of DRG weighting. These weights, called *weighted inlier equivalent separations,* are annually adjusted to general cost movements (e.g., inflations), clinical technology changes, and productivity trends.[37]

Apart from acute care settings, DRGs are also used in "hospital at home" and community-based health care settings. The use of DRGs in an ambulatory care setting has been considered impractical because data are insufficient to reliably assign a DRG to the case, and this type of care episode is not as easily defined as an acute care episode. The minimum data set used to determine DRGs is also used in public health and epidemiological research. The remaining portion (non-DRG) funding is influenced by a mixture of actual activities and needs adjustments, including age- or sex-adjusted population funding, remoteness, depreciations, infrastructure acquisitions, and the like.

New Zealand began using DRGs as early as 1988, merely as an efficient means to aggregate a large volume of data (e.g., more than 20,000 ICD codes) into approximately 500 categories. The use of DRGs for the payment of health services did not start until after July 1995. New Zealand adopted the Victoria (Australian) model of weighted inlier equivalent separations.[38] As of 2004 hospital care in New Zealand went to a population-based funding formula instead of DRGs. Other revenue sources include Accident Compensation Commission electives, the waiting list initiative, and insurance payment from private patients. However, DRG coding is still generated for every episode of care. The data are used for the Ministry of Health's reporting and public health research purposes. DRGs are also used by hospitals (mainly tertiary or quaternary hospitals) to calculate treatment costs on patients referred by other hospitals. Some quaternary hospitals can generate as much as 50 percent of its revenue from the treatment of patients on behalf of other hospitals.

DRG codes are derived from ICD-9 or ICD-10 codes for patients' principle diagnoses and secondary diagnoses (comorbidity) and for major procedures performed during inpatient care. The breakdown of the cost components for sample DRGs is given in Figure 20-5.[39] Nursing cost, one of the cost components, is further broken down into direct and indirect nursing costs and calculated based on the number of nursing hours (determined by time-motion studies) required for the care of the patients in each DRG category. In some Australian hospitals, multidisciplinary clinical pathways have been developed for high-cost, high-frequency DRGs. The clinical pathways map the care provided by all disciplines (including nursing) for these DRGs, from admission to discharge, as a mechanism to ensure that the care is evidence-based and high-quality.

Belgium

Belgium has a long tradition of collecting health care data. The collection of hospital discharge data (Belgian Hospital Discharge Dataset, or HDDS) has been compulsory since 1990 for all inpatients in acute hospitals. The data are extracted from the patient's medical record upon discharge. The HDDS includes data on:

- Hospital identification
- Patient demographics
- Hospital stay (date and type of admission, date of discharge, referral data, admitting department, discharge disposition)
- Clinical data (primary and secondary diagnoses in ICD-9-CM [clinical modification], diagnostic and therapeutic procedures in ICD-9-CM and Belgian nomenclature)

Belgium is one of the few countries that complement its hospital discharge data set with a nationwide uniform nursing minimum data set (NMDS) for a balanced sample of inpatient days. The NMDS contains twenty-three nursing interventions, patient demographics, nine activities of daily living, the number of nursing hours per day of hospital stay, and the qualifications of nurses caring for the patient. The NMDS data make it possible to examine the relationship between nursing care interventions and nurse staffing from 1987 onward.[40] The mandatory collection resulted in an extensive database of more than fifteen million selected inpatient days for some six million selected patients in all nursing units (2,500) from all Belgian hospitals.

The data from the HDDS are used as input for the DRG system. AP-DRGs were used from 1994 until 2001. Since 2001, APR-DRGs are used. For each DRG, severity of illness, and age group, an average length of stay is calculated and used as the basis for financing hospitals.

NATIONAL HOSPITAL COST DATA COLLECTION
FINAL COST WEIGHTS FOR AR-DRG 4.1, Round 4 (1999-00)
AIHW Peer Group A1

V4.1 Public Sector

DRG	DRG Description	Cost Weight	Number of Seps	Number of Days	ALOS (Days)	Average Cost per DRG ($)			Ward Medical		Ward Nursing		Non Clinical Salaries	Pathology		DRG
						Total	Direct	Ohead	Direct	Ohead	Direct	Ohead		Direct	Ohead	
901Z	Ext O.R. Pr Unrel To Pdx	3.32	2,643	28,246	10.69	9,233	6,769	2,464	759	182	1,814	336	342	402	63	901Z
902Z	Non-Ext O.R. Pr Unrel To Pdx	2.26	468	4,217	9.01	6,306	4,407	1,899	562	119	1,391	236	280	267	39	902Z
903Z	Prostatic O.R. Pr Unrel To Pdx	5.13	24	608	25.33	14,296	9,860	4,436	1,101	98	3,570	288	1,057	722	151	903Z
960Z	Ungroupable	2.17	342	3,546	10.37	6,051	4,867	1,184	437	55	1,974	77	99	80	20	960Z
961Z	Unacceptable Principal Dx	0.51	206	332	1.61	1,422	899	523	97	7	194	12	76	46	14	961Z
962Z	Unacceptable Obstetric Dx Comb	0.70	5	15	3.00	1,942	1,406	536	234	56	720	208	28	94	25	962Z
963Z	Neonatal Dx Not Consnt Age/Wgt	7.47	62	1,220	19.68	20,798	14,639	6,159	640	34	1,490	155	551	151	36	963Z
A01Z	Liver Transplant	34.43	53	1,670	31.51	95,895	78,245	17,650	11,455	3,524	14,511	1,931	1,207	4,570	481	A01Z
A02Z	Multiple Organs Transplant	*****	*****	*****	*****	*****	*****	*****	*****	*****	*****	*****	*****	*****	*****	A02Z
A03Z	Lung Transplant	25.57	46	843	18.33	71,226	62,516	8,710	6,808	780	3,238	332	1,573	3,647	208	A03Z
A04Z	Bone Marrow Transplant	11.01	490	11,013	22.48	30,661	25,334	5,327	3,515	845	3,974	1,014	716	1,839	249	A04Z
A05Z	Heart Transplant	19.06	35	630	18.00	53,071	45,482	7,589	4,087	936	2,098	480	916	2,747	260	A05Z
A06Z	Tracheostomy Any Age Any Cond	20.50	3,703	112,348	30.34	57,084	43,671	13,413	2,597	467	4,487	740	847	2,211	380	A06Z
A40Z	Ecmo - Cardiac Surgery	12.57	6	91	15.17	34,996	28,187	6,809	1,789	115	1,557	129	418	1,979	9	A40Z
A41Z	Intubation Age<16	4.23	118	659	5.58	11,791	8,749	3,042	320	17	1,627	73	112	326	73	A41Z
B01Z	Ventricular Shunt Revision	2.90	79	629	7.96	8,065	5,579	2,485	551	142	1,603	335	169	226	33	B01Z
B02A	Craniotomy + Ccc	8.80	864	18,087	20.93	24,513	18,701	5,812	1,580	276	4,142	721	813	912	186	B02A
B02B	Craniotomy + Smcc	4.81	989	11,596	11.72	13,408	10,227	3,181	972	173	2,420	406	423	465	79	B02B
B02C	Craniotomy - Cc	3.80	1,433	12,054	8.41	10,595	8,093	2,502	758	128	1,620	278	283	343	57	B02C
B03A	Spinal Procedures + Cscc	5.51	85	1,204	14.16	15,349	11,679	3,670	1,762	350	3,260	525	510	505	117	B03A
B03B	Spinal Procedures - Cscc	2.45	350	1,735	4.96	6,820	5,283	1,538	585	83	1,078	185	175	83	14	B03B
B04A	Extracranial Vascular Pr +Cscc	3.39	423	3,635	8.59	9,453	6,962	2,491	652	116	1,395	219	359	333	36	B04A
B04B	Extracranial Vascular Pr -Cscc	1.96	918	3,704	4.03	5,456	4,062	1,394	393	84	657	138	148	133	19	B04B
B05Z	Carpal Tunnel Release	0.42	2,920	3,257	1.12	1,160	835	325	90	19	94	23	40	11	3	B05Z
B06A	Cbl Psy,Mus Dysy,Npthy Pr+Cscc	4.06	107	1,801	16.83	11,299	8,214	3,084	1,184	272	2,873	382	706	434	52	B06A
B06B	Cbl Psy,Mus Dysy,Npthy Pr-Cscc	0.85	916	1,864	2.03	2,373	1,739	634	207	47	317	70	87	45	9	B06B
B07A	Prphl & Cranl Nerv & Oth Pr+Cc	3.12	209	1,958	9.37	8,682	6,451	2,230	888	218	1,568	295	273	203	38	B07A
B07B	Prphl & Cranl Nerv & Oth Pr-Cc	1.02	1,381	2,577	1.87	2,853	2,120	733	225	45	293	63	69	28	6	B07B
B40Z	Plasmapheresis + Neurolgcl Dis	1.68	176	929	5.28	4,692	3,542	1,150	307	59	768	110	188	181	23	B40Z
B41Z	Prtngd Mntrng For Cmplx Eplpsy	1.51	162	1,075	6.64	4,199	2,837	1,361	689	244	1,080	280	191	78	9	B41Z
B60A	N-Acute Para/Quad+/-Or Pr+Ccc	6.77	590	16,388	27.78	18,859	13,539	5,320	1,593	580	5,944	1,671	990	513	107	B60A
B60B	N-Acute Para/Quad+/-Or Pr-Ccc	1.88	1,782	11,781	6.61	5,224	3,795	1,429	434	128	1,404	283	302	124	29	B60B

Date Printed: 04/03/2002

* NB: These data should be reviewed in conjunction with section 'Notes to Cost Weights and Tables'

Page 24

Figure 20-5. *Breakdown of cost components for sample DRGs.*

Although medical doctors are still paid on a fee-for-service basis, there is a trend to use DRGs as the basis for a global budget per patient group, including medical fees, medical imaging, physiotherapy, pharmacy, and other services. DRGs have been used for funding the clinical budget of hospitals since 1994. The clinical budget takes up about 55 percent of the operating budget of an average hospital and covers the wages of nurses, medical products for the hospital wards, operating theater, day clinics, emergency departments, intensive care units, and other line items. About two-thirds of the budget is fixed based on minimum standards for the number of nurses per bed. The other third is calculated based on differences in the level of activity and nursing workload.

DRGs are used to determine the number of inpatient days for which the hospital will be funded. The Belgium NMDS is used to partially calculate the variable budget for each hospital. Fixed and variable budget calculations make up the hospital budget per day. The budget per day, multiplied by the number of inpatient days as calculated using DRGs, gives the total hospital budget.[41]

Since 2000, Belgium has been updating its NMDS. One of the aims is to link DRGs and nursing more closely. Because the national length of stay (LOS) per DRG dominates the financing system, most hospitals tend to monitor and shorten the LOS to below the national average. The tendency leads to a vicious cycle: All hospitals try to get their local average LOS below the national average, by which the national average is lowered, driving hospitals to increase their efforts to decrease LOS even further. Because the DRG system and nursing data are not directly linked, the impact of the reduction of LOS on the nursing activity is not seen. It has been shown, by using the NMDS, that the reduction of LOS leads to an increase in patient acuity and thereby an escalation in nursing activity. A central element in future updates will be the integration of NMDS in the hospital discharge data set, which is to be implemented in 2007.[42]

The updated NMDS is expected to lead to new applications in Belgian health care management and policy. A first application is the nursing intensity profile (NIP) per DRG. The NIP describes the nursing intensity per day of stay. An example is given in Figure 20-6, in which the NIP is given for APR-DRG 166.[43]

On the vertical axis, a nursing intensity score (based on NMDS) is given, in which 1 equals independent care. A higher score represents a higher nursing intensity. Average and confidence intervals of the nursing intensity score per day of stay are given.

For surgical conditions, the NIP is low at admission, at its highest point the day after surgery, but decreasing as of the next postoperative day. The NIP is an improvement of the relative nursing cost weights per DRG, used since 1997, which did not take into account the variability in nursing intensity during the stay. The NIP per DRG requires, however, a continuous monitoring of nursing care within and among DRGs.

A second application will be the use of nursing data in appropriate evaluation protocols (AEP).[44,45] These protocols are used around the world to evaluate the appropriateness of hospital admissions and stays. Most protocols are based on the patient's condition and on medical and nursing services. The AEP protocols are mainly evaluated through patient record audits. Part of the Belgium NMDS update efforts will include the evaluation of how the hospital discharge data set complements the NDMS and how it can be used retrospectively to evaluate the AEP.[45] From the study, it became obvious that nursing care is the best predictor of LOS in the hospital, with more than 80 percent of hospital stay explained by it.

Germany

The German Health Reform "(Gesundheitsreform 2000)" introduced a German diagnosis-related group (G-DRG) system in the hospital sector in 2003. This reform will change the current hospital financing system based on the Australian DRG system.[7,47]

The cost of nursing in the G-DRG system is calculated on the basis of PPR (Pflege Personal Regelung—nursing team regulation) intervention data. The system PPR was developed in the early 1990s to calculate the human resource requirements in hospitals. Based on a selection of nursing interventions (e.g., washing the whole body—wholly compensatory), the system PPR allocates

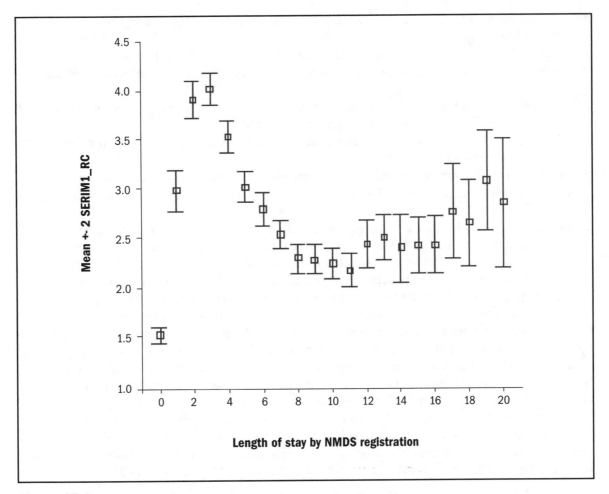

Figure 20-6. *Nursing Intensity Profile: nursing intensity per day of stay.*

patients to one of the nine workload groups for adult patients or one of the twenty-seven groups for children.[46] Every PPR group is associated with a normative time value. For adults, the times range between 52 and 215 minutes per day.

Although the PPR was used from 1993 to 1996, it was abandoned mainly because it was calculating more nurses than could actually be funded. More fundamentally, the system lacks any scientific rationale for validating the results. Nevertheless, some hospitals—among them those that took part in the first G-DRG-calculation—still use PPR for internal management. The use of intervention data to calculate nurses' workload as well as costs needs to be discussed critically. There is evidence that time allocation depends not only on the specific care activities (e.g., washing the whole body—wholly compensatory), but also on the patient's condition (i.e., care dependency or nursing diagnosis).[48]

Because of the lack of agreement on standardized nursing diagnoses and interventions coding, there has been great interest in defining nursing-relevant ICD-10-codes. Hospitals in Germany build their own ICD-10 nursing code lists, containing between 10 and 630 nursing-relevant codes. The underlying assumption is that in some cases, the nurses' workload can be deduced directly from the medical diagnosis and that there is an invariable relationship between medical diagnosis and nursing workload. The DRG-Working-Group University of Witten/Herdecke,[10] however, showed that there is a high variability in nursing interventions for patients with the same medical diagnosis. In particular cases, the relationship between nursing time and the DRG cost weight was even inverse.

Based on the findings that medicine and nursing are complementary and that monoprofessional classification systems like ICD-10 seem to be unsatisfactory for mapping the diversity of multi-professional tasks, the Deutscher Pflegerat (German Nurses Council), assisted by scientists and other experts, recommended that the Institut für das Entgeltsystem im Krankenhaus (INEK), the national institute for the German DRG system, revise the G-DRG. Among other suggestions were the following:

1. Multi-problem patients who require additional effort based on different nursing problems that can be interdependent (e.g., dementia or impaired mobility) should be refunded at a per-diem flat rate.
2. Additional interventions or procedures that may appear besides the main problem but not at all times (e.g., terminal care) should be refunded separately.
3. Alternative or complementary procedures (e.g., palliative care or giving birth in water) should be financed through separate DRGs.
4. In addition to the number of DRG cases, variances of LOS, nursing workload, nursing time, causes for interventions, and the like should be analyzed and published to refine and develop the G-DRG system.
5. Besides established outliers (e.g., extended LOS), an extended nursing workload has to be funded (i.e., nursing outliers). For this purpose data on nursing diagnoses are indispensable.
6. Differentiated sets of cost weights should be used for pediatric or geriatric patients.
7. As in the case of long-term patients, certain medical or nursing data should generate additional refunds (e.g., nursing care outliers or additional nursing interventions).

An essential point in the recommendations is to include not just nursing interventions in the G-DRG system,[49,50] but also data about patients' conditions and abilities. In line with this recommendation, a project was started to develop a standardized assessment tool for signs and symptoms related to basic nursing care needs in an inpatient setting. This research is conducted by Dr. Horst Schmidt Klinik in Wiesbaden and the University of Witten/Herdecke[51] and is promoted by the German Nursing Council. The assessment instrument ePA© (ergebnisorientiertes PflegeAssessment—outcome-oriented nursing care assessment) is based on a standardized collection of data assessing patients' abilities, their impairments (e.g., alimentation—inability to hold cutlery independently and/or inability to bring it to the mouth), and physical conditions (e.g., current nutrition status). The ePA© is still in development and will be published in mid 2006.

Switzerland

In the mid-1980s, Switzerland investigated the introduction of a DRG system for hospital financing. The University Institute for Social and Preventive Medicine, together with the county of Vaud, conducted a study on the possibility of using DRG and case mix for describing the patient at the hospital. The goal was to determine, in the Swiss context, whether a generalized use of a DRG system could improve management of the hospitals. The study started in 1984 and finished with a publication in 1989.[52]

Nurses were not involved in the study. The Swiss Nursing Informatics (SNI) group, established in 1990, followed what the DRG group was doing and made contact with nurses in other countries in Europe, especially those in Belgium. The need for having nursing data together with the medical data for describing the care-related activities in hospitals is evident. The central question of how to describe the nursing activity was addressed at an international symposium organized in Lausanne in 1990 (Systems to Evaluate the Nursing Workload at Hospitals).[53] The conference, at which systems from Canada, the U.S., and Switzerland were presented, was fruitful. Hospitals from the French-speaking part of Switzerland adopted a Canadian tool, PRN (Projet de Recherche en Nursing— Research Project for Nursing), to measure the care needed per shift. In the German part, hospitals in St-Gallen and in Zürich worked first alone, then together to create a well-designed and appropriate tool for evaluating nursing activities: LEP (Leistungerfassung in der Pflege—Nursing Activities Measurement).[54,55] In 1991 in Leuven, the first European NMDS conference was organized, at which a participating member of the SNI group proposed to start a study for evaluating the usefulness of the Belgium Nursing Minimum Data Set (B-NMDS) system. The B-NMDS was at this time the first data collection made at a national level and offered a good scientific background.

A pilot study began in Switzerland, with three hospitals participating for one year and two of them continuing for another year. This study showed that the B-NMDS could be used in Switzerland without major adaptations.[56] Based on this result, several actions were conducted to promote the use of the B-NMDS.[57] Unfortunately there was no support for the development of such a data collection for nursing and the B-NMDS project was set aside.

The university hospitals of Lausanne and Geneva continue using the PRN system, and the German-speaking Swiss continue developing LEP. In the last ten years, use of the LEP grew among the German-speaking Swiss and passed through the language barrier to the French-speaking sections. It is now becoming the de facto system in Switzerland. Germany and Austria are also starting to use the LEP.

Since 1998, the development of the Swiss NMDS (CH-NMDS) started with the support of the government. CH-NMDS will not replace any hospital system already in use. It was designed with the ambition of collecting data from the different sources (hospitals, home care units, elderly homes, and the like) and to map the data into the CH-NMDS classification. A link to the DRG system is a long-term goal and one of CH-NMDS's objectives.

In 1998, a group of insurers, politicians, and hospital representatives began to test the AP-DRG system. Several Swiss counties are using the AP-DRG (All Patient) system to prepare financials for acute-care hospitals. This AP-DRG group is very active, and nearly every year the Swiss cost weights are revised. Thanks to the AP-DRG work, a new four-year (2004–2007) project, called SwissDRG, has been set up. In the SwissDRG group, nurses are invited to participate. The goals of the SwissDRG group are to select a DRG grouper program and to propose a prospective payment system to finance acute care hospitals. The Swiss Federal Statistical Office (SFSO), responsible for medical statistics, is strongly involved in this process.

Some LEP users are working to link LEP results with AP-DRG.[55] The results are shown in minutes of care per shift and per patient and can be used at the hospital level as well as at the national level.[54] A study of the homogeneity of nursing workload, measured by LEP within AP-DRGs, showed that 27 percent of the 30,000 cases of a university hospital, for which the data were available, are in DRGs with a very high variability with regard to LOS (coefficient of variation > 1). In comparison, 40 percent of the cases are in DRGs with a very high variability with regard to nursing workload (measured by LEP hours). The percentages are higher in medical DRGs than in surgical DRGs. The study concluded that research into the reasons for the variability of nursing workload must be intensified. It has to be determined whether refinement can be done more (or less) accurately by using nursing criteria in addition to or instead of using medical secondary diagnoses.

How Nursing Should Participate in the DRG Imperative

Today the DRG system has become an increasingly important tool in the management of health care. It is also the common language of managers and perhaps of clinicians to discuss patient care, resource utilization, and funding. Although nurses are recognized as key partners in the care of a patient, when defining the patient care product in DRGs, they are, unfortunately, practically invisible. One possible explanation is that the DRG system is relatively complex and adding nursing would make it even more complex.

Excluding nursing might reduce the complexity of the classification and costing formulas for DRGs, but simplified rules lead to simplified solutions, not necessarily working and robust ones. As the important role of nursing is increasingly recognized in the health care industry, economists acknowledge that refining DRGs makes no sense when nursing is still only crudely measured. Further, it is extremely important to realize that, when dealing with resource management, either within or outside the DRG system, decreasing patient LOS always has an impact on nursing care intensity and hence nursing staffing.

What elements should we take into account for the DRG debate?

1. First, we have to recognize and accept that the nursing and medical professions are different and complementary. Medical and nursing diagnoses reflect completely different concepts. The medical diagnosis focuses on disease (organic systems, diseases, and body functions). The nurses' focus is more the "ill-being" (i.e., the consequences of the diseases).[58-62] The medical and nursing interventions and goals are different as well. Given the complementary characteristics of

both professions, all efforts to deduce the nurses' activity and workload from medical activity are usually unsuccessful.[63] We have to accept the facts and argue that there is a high variability in nursing care for patients who share the same medical diagnosis.

2. Most of the links between DRGs and nursing data done up to now are based on nursing interventions and time measurement. This approach seriously limits our ability to get a good picture of the complexity of nursing. Nursing is more than time-consuming activities or interventions, and a nurse is more than a cost. Nursing has important and positive impacts on the health status of patients. More effort should be made to incorporate nursing diagnoses.

3. More and more, health care has involved multidisciplinary teamwork, which should be reflected in the information collected about patient care. Complementing medical and nursing data could help to improve DRG classifications as instruments to evaluate and improve the work of the multidisciplinary team in the hospital. The classifications would constitute an improved instrument for communication between doctors and nursing professionals. Research in investigating interdisciplinary classification systems such as the International Classification of Functioning, Disability and Health (ICF)[64] should be recommended.

The Use of ICT to Link DRGs and Nursing: The Challenges to Nurses

Undoubtedly there exists a strong need for information systems capable of collecting clinical data. The use of DRG systems for reimbursement stimulates the development of clinical systems. Thus the pressure to get reliable computerized data is increasing, and obviously the systematic collection of nursing data is a key element. In the late 1980s, Sovie[58] proposed making the NMDS a part of the data requirements for DRG systems. She wrote, "If hospitals are to continue to provide quality care to all patients, regardless of payment source, there must be provision for differential payments based on nursing acuity and severity of illness." In many countries,[65] NMDSs are in use or under development to provide nursing data in a systematic and representative way. A special effort should be made to develop an international NMDS usable for comparing the role of nursing beyond the boundaries of individual health care systems.

The NMDS available today are still limited. In use instead are many nursing workload instruments, which measure nursing workload in terms of points or instrument-specific minutes. In some countries, e.g., Switzerland or Germany, these instruments are used to calculate DRG cost weights, notwithstanding the fact that they often are not scientifically evaluated. Moreover, except the more widely accepted workload instruments, e.g., LEP or PRN, there are almost as many workload systems as there are hospitals, leading almost inevitably to hospital-specific cost weight systems. Because many of the workload systems are commercialized and lack transparency on how cost weights are validated and updated, it is very difficult to use the data generated from these instruments for cross-hospital or cross-country benchmarking. A serious deficit is the absence of causality relationship or linkage between the time consumed in nursing interventions and the patient's problems (e.g., the nursing diagnosis); the workload measurement in normative minutes can therefore at best represent only a small fraction of the real nursing time required.[48] As an aggravating factor, when they are used without taking into account the *causation* of the time-consuming intervention (e.g., the nursing diagnosis), the normative minutes at best can be only a small indicator of the real time. There is an overall need to do more validation work on these instruments.

There is definitely a strong need for developing and implementing standard nursing terminologies that parallel their medical counterparts. Standardized nursing terminologies could then feed the appropriate hospital and clinical information systems (CIS) for nursing resource utilization and outcomes measurement. The challenge is at nursing's doorstep. Electronic health records (EHRs), which are ready or nearly ready to be adopted, should provide highly flexible nursing care planning, documentation, and decision support functionality. Without standardized data about nursing diagnoses, nursing interventions, and outcomes, however, nursing will remain invisible and not measurable. A good example of standardization is the International Classification of Nursing Practice (ICNPv1©), which should provide a common language for describing nursing practice to improve communication among nurses, as well as between nurses and others. Linking with DRGs, ICNP makes it possible for information systems to project trends in patient needs, provision of nursing treatments, resource utilization, and outcomes of nursing care.

When the contribution of nurses can be accurately quantified, nursing will become more visible. Nurse executives, equipped with better information and knowledge, can then engage more assertively and actively in hospital and health care decision making. One of the positive outcomes of the Belgian NMDS is that, because of its direct impact on the hospital budget, nurse executives are invited to play a part in financial decision making. To fulfill this role adequately, nurse executives should be trained to read, effectively analyze, and utilize the complex information that comes before them. In addition, there is a strong need for developing tools, such as costing tools, staff allocation tools, and benchmarking tools, to support the nurse executives when they are at the decision makers' table.

Given the distinct nature of nursing, it might be useful to build some form of nursing-related groups (NRG) as a complementary classification system to DRGs. This could be much more efficient than the endless trials to create so-called "refined" DRGs, all of which consider only medical diagnoses and procedures. Besides nurse-specific classification tools, research in nurse assessment tools is necessary.

Obviously DRGs are playing an important role in the management of health care. The important question is not *whether* nurses should get involved in this matter, but rather *how* nurses should be involved. The five types of initiatives described in this chapter can lead the way to meet this important challenge.

References

1. Averill R, Goldfield N, Steinbeck B, et al. *Development of the All Patient Refined DRGs (APR-DRGs)*. 3M HIS 1997. Available at: http://www.3m.com/us/healthcare/his/pdf/reports/aprdev899.pdf Accessed on August 25, 2005.

2. Fetter RB, Shin Y, Freeman JL, Averill RF, Thompson JD. Case mix definition by diagnosis-related groups. *Med Care.* 1980;18(2):1-53.

3. Gonella JS, Hornbrook MC, Louis DZ. Staging of disease, a case-mix measurement. *JAMA* 1984; 251(5):637-644.

4. Calore KA, Iezzoni L. Disease staging and PMCs: can they improve DRGs? *Med Care.* 1987;25(8):724-737.

5. Lichtig LK. *Hospital Information Systems for Case Mix Management.* New York: John Wiley & Sons; 1986:110.

6. Fischer W. *Patientenklassifikationssysteme zur Bildung von Behandlungsfallgruppen im stationären Bereich. Prinzipien und Beispiele.* Bern and Wolfertswil: Zentrum für Informatik und wirtschaftliche Medizin; 1997. ISBN 3-9521232-2-6

7. Fischer W. Die DRG-Grossfamilie 2003. Available at: http://www.fischer-zim.ch/streiflicht/DRG-Familie-9512.htm. Accessed August 25, 2005.

8. Canadian Institute for Health Information (CIHI). *Acute Care Grouping Methodologies: from Diagnosis-Related Groups to Case Mix Groups Redevelopment.* In: The Redevelopment of the Acute Care Inpatient Grouping Methodology Using ICD-10-CA/CCI Classification Systems. February 2004. Available at: http://secure.cihi.ca/cihiweb/en/downloads/Acute_Care_Grouping_Methodologies2004_e.pdf. Accessed August 25, 2005.

9. Hornbrook MC. Hospital Case Mix: Its Definition, Measurement and Use: Part II, Review of Alternative Measures. *Med Care Rev.* 1982;39:73-123.

10. DRG-Working-Group University of Witten/Herdecke, Germany, Institute of Nursing Science; 2004.

11. Mowry MN, Korpman RA. Do DRG reimbursement rates reflect nursing costs? *Journal of Nurs Adm* 1985;15(7,8):29-35.

12. Halloran EJ, Kiley M, Nosek L. Nursing complexity, the DRG and length of stay. In: Hurley M, ed. *Classification of Nursing Diagnoses: Proceedings of the Sixth National Conference.* St. Louis: Mosby Co.; 1986.

13. Saba VK. The classification of home health care nursing: diagnoses and interventions. *Caring Magazine.* 1992;11(3):50-57.

14. Rockwood K, Stolee P, Fox RA. Use of goal attainment scaling in measuring clinically important change in the frail elderly. *J Clin Epidemiol.* 1993: 46(10);1113-1118.

15. Welton JM, Halloran EJ. A comparison of nursing and medical diagnoses in predicting hospital outcomes. In: Lorenzi N, ed. *Proceedings of the American Medical Informatics Association 1999 Annual Symposium.* Washington, DC: American Medical Informatics Association; 1999:171-175.

16. Mølgard E. *Calculation of Nursing Costs in Relation to the DRG-System.* Viborg: Viborg-Amt; 2000.

17. Baumberger D. *Pflegediagnosen als Indikator der Streuung des Pflegeaufwands in DRGs* [master's thesis]. Universität Maastricht, NL: Maastricht, Aarau; 2001.

18. Fischer W. *Diagnosis Related Groups (DRGs) und Pflege. Grundlagen, Codierungssysteme, Integrationsmöglichkeiten.* Bern: Huber; 2002.

19. Harrell JS. Predicting nursing care costs with a patient classification system. In: Shaffer FA, ed. *Patients & Purse Strings: Patient Classification and Cost Management.* New York: National League for Nursing; 1986:149-164.

20. Atwood JR, Hinshaw AS, Chance HC. Relationships among nursing care requirements, nursing resources, and charges. In: Shaffer FA, ed. *Patients & Purse Strings: Patient Classification and Cost Management.* New York: National League for Nursing; 1986:99-120.

21. Green J, McClure M, Wintfeld N, Birdsall C, Rieder KA. Severity of illness and nursing intensity: going beyond DRGs. In: Scherubel JC, Shaffer FA, eds. *Patients and Purse Strings II.* New York: National League for Nursing; 1988:207-230.

22. Halloran EJ. Nursing workload, medical diagnosis related groups, and nursing diagnoses. *Res Nurs Health.* 1985;8(4):421-433.

23. McKibben RC, Brimmer PF, Galiher JM, Hartley S, Clinton J. Nursing costs and DRG payments. *Am J Nurs.* 1985;85(12);1353-1356.

24. Sovie M, Tarcinale M, Vanputte A, Stunden A. Amalgam of nursing acuity, DRGs and costs. *Nurs Manage.* 1985:16(3);22-42.

25. Wolf GA, Lesic LK. Determining the cost of nursing care within DRGs. In: Shaffer FA, eds. *Patients & Purse Strings: Patient Classification and Cost Management.* New York: National League for Nursing; 1986:165-180.

26. Bargagliotti LA, Smith H. Patterns of nursing costs with capitated reimbursements. *Nurs Econ.* 1985; 3(5):270-275.

27. Dahlen AL, Gregor JR. Nursing costs by DRG with an all-RN staff. In: Shaffer FA, ed. *Costing Out Nursing: Pricing Our Product.* New York: National League for Nursing; 1985:123-134.

28. Fosbinder D. Nursing costs/DRG: a patient classification system and comparative study. *J Nurs Adm.* 1986;16(11):18-23.

29. Reschak GLC, Biordi D, Holm K, Santucci N. Accounting for nursing costs by DRG. *J Nurs Adm.* 1985:15(9):15-20.

30. Riley W, Schaefers V. Costing nursing services. *Nurs Manage.* 1983;14(12):40-43.

31. Trace LD. The total cost of nursing care for patients with acquired immune deficiency syndrome. In: Scherubel JC, Shaffer FA, eds. *Patients and Purse Strings II.* New York: National League for Nursing; 1988:231-248.

32. Fischer W. *Die Bedeutung von Pflegediagnosen in Gesundheitsökonomie und Gesundheitstatistik.* Available at:. http://www.fischer-zim.ch/. Accessed August 25, 2005.

33. Sermeus W. Nursing related groups: a research study. In: Daly N, Hannah K, eds. *Proceedings of Nursing and Computers, Third International Symposium on Nursing Use of Computers and Information Science,* Dublin. St. Louis: Mosby; 1988:177-183.

34. Caterinicchio RP. A debate: RIMs and the cost of nursing care. *Nurs Manage.* 1983;14(5):36-41.

35. Caterinicchio RP. Relative intensity measures: pricing of inpatient nursing services under diagnosis-related group prospective hospital payment. *Health Care Financing Rev.* 1984;6(1):61-70.

36. Caterinicchio RP, Davies RH. Developing a client-focused allocation statistic of inpatient nursing resource use: an alternative to the patient day. *Soc Sci Med.* 1983;17(5):259-272.

37. Victorian Government Health Information. Victorian Cost Weights. Available at: www.health.vic.gov.au/pfg2004/. Accessed August 25, 2005.

38. New Zealand Health Information Service. Technical documentation. Available at: http://www.nzhis.govt.nz/documentation/wies/index.html. Accessed August 25, 2005.

39. Australian Government Department of Health and Aging. *NHCDC Round 4 Report;* 2001.

40. Sermeus W, Delesie L. The registration of a nursing minimum dataset in Belgium: six years of experience. In: Grobe S, Pluyter-Wenting ESP. *Nursing Informatics: An International Overview for Nursing in a Technological Era, Proceedings of the Fifth IMIA International Conference on Nursing Use of Computers and Information Science, San Antonio, Texas, USA, June 17-22, 1994.* Washington, DC: American Medical Informatics Association; 144-149.

41. Sermeus W. *De Belgische ziekenhuisfinanciering ontcijferd.* ACCO: Leuven, Belgium; 2003.

42. Sermeus W, et al. A nation-wide project for the revision of the Belgian nursing minimum dataset: from concept to implementation. In: Roger France FH, De Clercq E, De Moor G, van der Lei J, eds. *Health Continuum and Data Exchange in Belgium and in the Netherlands, Proceedings of MIC2004 & 5th Belgian e-Health Conference.* Amsterdam: IOS Press; 2004: 21-26.

43. Sermeus W. The Belgian nursing minimum dataset, version 2: linking B-NMDS and DRGs. Lecture presented at: The 20th PCS/E (Patient Classification Systems/Europe) Working Conference; October 17–30, 2004; Budapest, Hungary.

44. Panis L, Verheggen F, Pop P. To stay or not to stay: the assessment of appropriate hospital stay, a Dutch report. *Int J Qual Health Care.* 2001;13(4):55-67.

45. Gillet P, Gillain D, Fontaine P, Jacques J. Verantwoord opnamebeleid in de ziekenhuissector, eindrapport fase II. CHU Liège; 2004. Available at http://www.dim-chu.ulg.ac.be/AEP/AEPfr/contexteAEP.htm. Accessed August 25, 2005.

46. Schöning B, Luithlen E, Scheinert H. *Pflege-Personalregelung. Kommentar mit Anwendungsbeispielen für die Praxis.* Dresden, Stuttgart: Kohlhammer; 1993.

47. The German G-DRG. Available at: www.g-drg.de. Accessed August 25, 2005.

48. Bartholomeyczik S, Hunstein D. Time distribution of selected care activities in home care in Germany. *J Clin Nurs.* 2004;13(1):97-104.

49. Hunstein D. Pflege abbilden im G-DRG-System. *Pflege & Manage.* 2003;61(6);21-24.

50. Deutsches Institut für angewandte Pflegeforschung DIP (Hrsg.). *Pflegerelevante Fallgruppen (PRG)— Eine empirische Grundlegung.* Hannover: Schlütersche; 2004.

51. Hunstein D, Dintelmann Y, Sippel B. Developing a screening instrument used as a standardized assessment for signs and symptoms related to basic nursing care needs in an inpatient setting. In: Oud N, ed. *ACENDIO—Proceedings of the 5th European Conference of the Association of Common European Nursing Diagnoses, Interventions and Outcomes in Bled, Slovenia 2005.* Bern: Verlag Hans Huber; 2005, 396-402.

52. Paccaud F, Schenker L. DRG (diagnosis related groups) perspective d'utilisation. Lyon: Edition Alexandre Lacassagne; 1989.

53. Symposium sur les systèmes d'évaluation de la charge de travail dans les secteurs de soins. Quels enjeux? Quels instruments? Croix-Rouge Suisse Ecole supérieure d'enseignement infirmier; 1990.

54. Weber P, Bamert U, Steuer B, Spahni S. Easy tool to collect Swiss nursing workload classification LEP. In: Marin H, Marques P, Hovenga E, Goossen W, eds. *Proceedings of 8th International Congress in Nursing Informatics,* E-papers Serviços Editoriais Ltda: Rio de Janeiro; 2003.

55. Fischer W. Homogeneity of nursing workload measured by LEP within AP-DRGs. In: *Proceedings of the 17th PCS/E International Working Conference.* 2001:154-161. Available at http://www.fischer-zim.ch/paper-en/index.htm. Accessed August 25, 2005.

56. Weber P. Etude pilote dans 3 hôpitaux suisses: evaluation de l'activité des soins infirmiers avec un instrument belge. In: *La pensée médico-economique dans le système de santé: Méthodes et outils informatiques á disposition des médecins, des soignant et des gestionnaires.* Morges: VIII Journées annuelles. La Société Suisse d'Informatique Médicale (SSIM); 1993: 18-19.

57. Weber P. Etude pilote mise en place et évaluation du résumé infirmier minimum (RIM) expérience sur une année. Proceedings of the 5th *Journées Francophones d'Informatique Médicale.* La Société Suisse d'Informatique Médicale (SSIM): Genève; 1994: 163-173.

58. Sovie MD. Establishing the nursing minimum data set as part of the data requirements for DRGs. In: Werley H, Lang N. *Identification of the Nursing Minimum Data Set.* New York: Springer; 1988.

59. Frutiger P, Fessler J-M. *La Gestion Hospitalière Médicalisée.* Paris: EME Editions Sociales Françaises (ESF) ESF éditeur; 1991.

60. Krohwinkel, ed. *Der Pflegeprozess am Beispiel des Apoplexiekranken—Eine Studie zur Erfassung und Entwicklung ganzheitlich-rehabilitierender Prozesspflege.* Baden-Baden: Nomos; 1993.

61. Roper N, Logan WW, Tierney AJ. *Die Elemente der Krankenpflege. Ein Pflegemodell, das auf einem Lebensmodell beruht.* Basel u.a.: RECOM; 1993.

62. Orem D. *Nursing: Concepts of Practice.* St. Louis: Mosby Co.; 1985.

63. Fischer W. Transcodierungsversuch von NANDA-Pflegediagnosen nach ICD-10. *Swiss Medl Info.* 2003;50:17-20.

64. World Health Organization. International Classification of Functioning, Disability and Health (ICF). Geneva: World Health Organization; 2001.

65. Goossen WTF, Epping PJMM, van den Heuvel WJA, et al. Development of the nursing minimum data set for the Netherlands (NMDSN): identification of categories and items. *J Adv Nurs.* 1999;31(3):536-547.

CHAPTER 21

Organizational Analysis: Workflows, Outcomes, and Patient Safety

By Thomas R. Clancy, PhD Candidate, RN, and Kathleen M. Carley, PhD

In 2000, the Institute of Medicine (IOM) released To Err Is Human: Building a Safer Health System[1] *and recommended that hospitals automate their drug use system as one tactic to reduce medication errors. As a result, many hospitals implemented computerized order entry, bar coding, and medication management systems. However, the number of reported fatalities in hospitals as a result of medication errors jumped from three to twenty errors between 2000 and 2002.[2] Although the sudden increase in fatalities may be the result of better reporting, computer-generated medication errors also showed a sudden increase.*

Foreseeing the consequences of new technology can be difficult. For example, laparoscopic surgery was introduced in the 1980s as a major technological breakthrough and heralded a new era of safer and less painful surgical procedures. The popularity of the procedure grew so rapidly that a 1991 study estimated that 400,000 of the 600,000 gall bladder removals that year were conducted by laparoscopy. However, retrospective study now suggests that complications from laparoscopic gall bladder removal may occur ten times more often than they do from traditional methods.[3]

The introduction of e-mail in the 1990s signaled a revolution in communication and promised a transition from paper to a digital medium. The vision of a paperless office appeared on the verge of becoming a reality. However, recent studies show that e-mail use actually increases paper consumption by approximately 40 percent in organizations such as hospitals.[4]

Hailed as a "manifesto for business revolution," Michael Hammer and James Champy's *Reengineering the Corporation*[5] topped the *New York Times* best seller list for business books in 1993. Over the next five years, hospitals religiously applied Hammer and Champy's principles to their own processes in an attempt to streamline systems and to lower costs. However, between 1995 and 2002, there was a 175 percent increase in registered nurse union petitions, in part a result of the reengineering efforts of the 1990s.[6]

The list goes on and on. Clearly these examples typify the difficulty in predicting the effects of new technology and practices in organizations such as hospitals. This is because such organizations are *complex adaptive systems,* which are characterized by "nonlinear interactive components, emergent phenomena, continuous and discontinuous change, and unpredictable outcomes."[7] Complex systems occur everywhere, in such phenomena as weather patterns,[8-11] cell formation,[12,13] animal schooling or flocking behavior,[14] economic markets,[15] and human social networks.[16,17]

In complex systems, the use of traditional planning tools often results in inaccurate predictions.[18] As noted, the consequences of such forecasts can be serious and harmful. A seemingly small error can propagate across multiple interdependent processes and cascade into serious patient harm. Examples in health care include medication errors, wrong side surgery, patient falls, missed treatments, and similar mishaps. Preventing patient harm in hospitals begins with an in-depth knowledge of clinical processes and how information flows through them. By understanding the sequence of tasks that make up processes, nurse administrators can discover system delays, redundant steps, and gaps, all of which can increase complexity and lead to unsafe practices. Work-flow analysis is problematic, however, because it is difficult to isolate cause-and-effect and the dominant feedback mechanisms hidden within the rich network of interacting constituents (physicians, nurses, support staff, equipment, policies, and procedures) that make up health care systems.

Given the complexity of health care today, nurse administrators need a better set of tools and methods to analyze work flow and to assist in decision making. Fortunately, the convergence of knowledge from such diverse fields as sociology, computer science, information theory, physics, biology, economics, operations research, organization theory, and nursing informatics (NI) is beginning to make such instruments available. Examples include electronic flowcharts, data and text mining, social network analysis, and computational modeling and simulation.

This chapter defines the basic concepts underlying complex adaptive systems and then introduces new computational tools to analyze them. A case history regarding the care of heart failure patients provides examples of how the various computer applications can assist nurse administrators in analyzing process work flow.

The Rise of Organizational Complexity

Two forms of organizational complexity are prevalent in hospitals today: combinatorial and dynamic.[19] *Combinatorial complexity* results from the multitude of potential states surrounding a patient's hospital stay. For example, there are more than 400 diagnosis-related groups (DRGs), 1400 prescription medications, and thousands of diagnostic tests and treatments. Add to this the numerous health care disciplines, hundreds of staff roles, and multiple policies and procedures. Collectively, the elements and factors that formulate the processes and systems of a hospital create a vast range of potential states. Attempting to accurately predict which combination of states (complications, response to treatment, mortality, length of stay, and so on) will emerge during a patient's hospital stay is all but impossible.

Dynamic complexity occurs when cause and effect are separated by time and space. Because of the rich social network of physicians, nurses, and support staff working in an environment of tightly coupled processes, hidden feedback loops may delay stimulus and response. Information trapped in negative feedback loops may reappear later as seemingly unrelated events. Conversely, self-reinforcing feedback loops may amplify small events and lead to cascading system behavior. Pinpointing the origin of a problem then can be extremely difficult in such a complex system.

The exponential growth in information in recent years is the driving force behind increased combinatorial and dynamic complexity in hospitals. The "building out" of the information infrastructure has contributed literally to an information explosion.[20] As technological innovation (the Internet, broadband transmission, wireless communication, digital storage, and so forth) has lowered the transactional costs of information processing, a self-reinforcing feedback loop of improved access and diffusion has increased the discovery of new knowledge. For example, more unique information has been created in 2001 and 2002 than is accessible from all of previous human history.[20]

In hospitals, the discovery of new knowledge has increased combinatorial complexity by adding new diagnostic tests, treatment options, procedures, and medications. Dynamic complexity has increased as a result of a growing interdependence between multiple departments to coordinate processes in a precise manner. For example, computerized provider order entry (CPOE) systems manage the flow of information for prescribing, dispensing, administering, and documenting medication use across multiple departments. Because of the tightly coupled interdependencies among these subprocesses, a breakdown in one area can create a chain reaction of errors throughout the entire system. The combined effect of combinatorial and dynamic complexity has created a tangled web of reinforcing and correcting feedback loops that produce nonlinear cause-and-effect relationships. The telltale signs of nonlinearity are unanticipated and often undesirable system behaviors.[19]

Predicting System Behavior in Complex Systems

The difficulty in predicting the effects of change in a complex system has been extensively reviewed in the literature.[18,19,21-24] The human capacity to disentangle the hidden patterns embedded within complex systems is limited. Studies have shown that the human brain can retain only seven to nine discrete pieces of information simultaneously in short-term memory.[25] To cope with environmental complexities, individuals develop heuristics, or "mental models," to recognize and react to perceived patterns of behavior.[19,26]

Mental models act as constructs to manage information processing in highly complex situations. Built on feedback from previous experiences, cultural norms, education, and other factors, mental models allow us to efficiently process information by categorizing events and experiences through "rules of thumb." Two managers experiencing the same event may perceive it differently because of their personal mental models.

There are two fundamental problems with applying mental models to the inflow of information in complex systems. First, the human capacity to interpret accurately the structure and dynamics of complex systems from the information at hand is frequently overestimated.[19] Because of limitations on attention, memory, and time, most individuals are unable to correctly infer the dynamics of all but the simplest causal maps. Second, studies have shown[19] that the filtering of information through individual mental models leads to significant misperceptions of system feedback. Dynamic and combinatorial complexity result in limited information, confounding variables, and ambiguity. The filtering of this information through personal mental models leads to erroneous inferences about system dynamics, judgment errors, bias, and impediments to learning. As a result, the nurse administrator, as a key constituent in the system's reinforcing and self-correcting feedback loops, is often caught in a cycle of responding to one crisis after another.

Traditional Work-flow Analysis in Complex Systems

Many nurse administrators utilize a work-flow analysis approach to clarify and understand processes embedded in a complex system. Work-flow analysis typically involves meeting with content experts to map out a process in standard flowcharting symbols. The objective is to isolate the sequence of steps and subprocesses that constitute a system and thus to understand and predict how changes might affect that system. A good example is to flowchart the surgical process whereby a patient flows through preadmission, admission, surgery, recovery, and discharge. Work-flow analysis is not restricted to the flow of patients. The flow of information can also be mapped among patients, providers, and the medical record.

Work-flow analysis has served nurse administrators well by identifying delays, redundant steps, and nonvalue activities within processes. Performance measures (e.g., turnaround time, process steps, costs per unit of service, and so on) also can be trended on control charts for continuous quality improvement programs. There are many standard and advanced flowchart software programs available on the market. In fact, many standard word processing and slide presentation programs contain extensive flowchart symbols.

The analysis of process workflow through standard flowcharts is most applicable at the local or microsystem, level. At this level, the boundaries of the process are clearly defined, the process steps are limited, and the number of interacting constituents is small. For example, the preoperative, perioperative, and postoperative processes in uncomplicated outpatient cataract surgery are highly predictable. The boundaries of the process are limited to the clinic waiting and changing areas, the operating room, and the postoperative recovery bays. Nearly every cataract surgery patient flows through the same sequence of steps, and the number of physicians and nurses supporting the process is limited. Performance variables, such as waiting times, procedure times, and cost of procedure typically show a bell curve, or normal distribution, when graphed against frequencies.

As processes expand beyond the boundaries of a nursing unit, the ability of standard flowcharts to accurately represent them begins to diminish because complex systems form a "fuzzy," quasitiered structure of interleaved macro-, meso-, and microsystem levels.[23] At the microsystem level, processes are fairly predictable because there are relatively few interdependencies among constituents and entities. However, as processes cut across multiple departments and performance is analyzed at meso- and macrosystem levels, a separate and distinct interaction occurs. For example, the distribution of harmful and nonharmful medication errors is one measure of a nursing unit's medication use process. However, the hospital-wide distribution of such errors is not simply a re-creation of a single unit's distribution. Rather, each nursing unit has its unique interdependent relationships with physicians, coworkers, and supporting departments in the medication use process.

The interactive effect of multiple processes converging at the hospital-wide level emerges as more than just the sum of individual departmental behaviors.

Work-flow analysis, conducted through interviews and standard flowcharts, fails to capture the dynamic nature and interactive effects of interdependent processes in a complex system. Flowcharts provide a static map or snapshot of a process but are only the first step in understanding it.

A System Dynamics Approach to Work-flow Analysis

Processes that extend beyond the microsystem level require a different approach to traditional work-flow analysis. One field that nurse administrators should consider careerwise is system dynamics. "System dynamics is grounded in the theory of non-linear dynamics and feedback control developed in mathematics, physics and engineering."[19] Work-flow analysis using a system dynamics approach identifies and models the essence of complex system behavior and then formulates hypotheses through data mining, social network analysis, computational modeling, and simulation. System dynamics enhances traditional flowcharts by capturing the effects of dominant feedback loops and then analyzing these effects over time. Table 21-1 presents an example of a system dynamics approach to work-flow analysis.

Work flow problems must be approached from an interdisciplinary team perspective that relies on the expertise of individual members. A system dynamics approach to work-flow analysis therefore requires nurse administrators to bring a new expertise to the table: the ability to determine which experts are needed to solve the problem. No one individual has all the knowledge required to analyze a complex system, and the specialty experts include nurse informaticians, industrial engineers, computer programmers, statisticians, simulationists, social network analysts, data mining experts, and even anthropologists. The key role of the nurse administrator is to identify the combination of skills required to solve a problem, build the team of experts, and then keep the project on track and on time. This approach is demonstrated by the following case, based on an actual process improvement project conducted at a midsized community hospital.

Case History: Improving Care of Heart Failure Patients Using a System Dynamics Approach

In 2002, members of the administrative staff at a 234-bed U.S. midwestern community hospital noted that performance indicators for DRG 127, heart failure and shock (HF), were not meeting national benchmarks for quality and cost. Comparison data on risk-adjusted mortality and compli-

Table 21-1. System Dynamics, Computational Modeling, and Simulation

Step	Process
1	Clearly identify the process problem (for example, high length of stay or frequent errors).
2	Specifically describe the desired outcome (reduce length of stay by one day, reduce error rate by a certain percentage).
3	Data mine electronic data sets to search for hidden patterns, feedback loops, and cause and effect relationships that may add to or validate key elements in the process.
4	Meet with content experts (nurses, physicians, unit clerks, support staff) and build consensus around the current processes to be evaluated.
5	Collectively identify the sequence of steps in the process using standard flow-charting methods. Include dominant reinforcing and balancing feedback loops.
6	Utilize social network analysis tools to build social networks from information collected during interviews with content experts.
7	Collectively build with content experts a computational model of the key processes using modeling and simulation software.
8	Revise the computational model in a stepwise fashion, with content experts to verify and validate that the model accurately represents the process.
9	Run virtual experiments in the computational model to test hypothesis and achieve the desired process outputs.
10	Select process improvement projects to implement in the real world.

ance, with accepted clinical guidelines, indicated significant opportunities for improvement. To meet the quality indicators for HF patients, the administrative team took a system dynamics approach to performance improvement. Rather than carving out work flow processes for just HF patients, the team decided to view them as one constituent in the complex systems of the entire hospital. As a result, the administrative team first embarked on a project to map all the hospital's main clinical and nonclinical processes using standard flowcharts. Once the main processes had been mapped, a project team focused on performance improvement for HF patients. The vice president of nursing was charged with developing a team of experts to complete the project in twelve months. The name given the project was FLOW (Fresh Look at Operational Workflow). Given the enormous scale of the project, the nurse executive decided to temporarily assign 100 percent of one manager's time to the project.

Clarifying and documenting the clinical and nonclinical processes of the hospital into flowcharts required hundreds of interviews of staff in multiple areas of the hospital. To assist with this stage of the project, the nurse executive elicited the help of graduate students in the hospital and health administration program offered by the local university's college of public health. Over the course of one semester, the students interviewed staff throughout the hospital as part of a course project. Information gathered from the interviews was used to build flowcharts for each department's main processes. The students developed more than 250 flowcharts.

Once the hospital-wide flowcharts were completed, the nurse executive reviewed the mix of skills required to analyze the HF process and selected team members. The membership consisted of domain experts (nurses, physicians, pharmacists, and staff with advanced education and extensive experience in HF), a nurse informatician, a statistician with data mining experience, a specialist in computational modeling and simulation, and a social network analyst. When in-hospital expertise was unavailable (e.g., NI, industrial engineering), the nurse executive contacted various departments at the university for assistance.

Clarifying Objectives and Understanding the Process

In their initial meetings, the HF team clarified objectives for the project and mapped out a timeline for its completion. The specific project outcomes included reducing mortality by 2 percent, the length of stay by one day, and costs by $1,000 per admission. In addition, the team was tasked with ensuring that various external requirements, such as the Joint Commission on Accreditation of Healthcare Organizations' Core Measurements for HF, were being met.

The team focused on first developing an in-depth knowledge of the many clinical and administrative processes in the continuum of care for HF patients. Using flowcharts previously developed during the FLOW project, the team's domain experts pieced together the many direct and indirect processes that surrounded the HF patient. These process maps included admission through the emergency care unit, care and treatment on various nursing units, the medication use process, the revenue cycle processes, supply chain management, discharge and disease management outside the hospital, and so forth. The end result was an electronic flow map for the typical HF patient with many interconnecting subprocesses. The subprocesses were later found to be extremely important because they often represented the hidden paths that created feedback loops and dynamic complexity.

Data Mining Applications

To validate the initial flow maps and to search for hidden patterns, electronic data stored in the hospital's repositories were mined using an open source software package. Data mining software allows users to sift through large electronic data sets to discover new information and to validate assumptions regarding a process. The ability of data mining to sort through massive amounts of complex data relies on sophisticated algorithms built into the software.[27] Five common techniques are used in data mining: neural networks, decision trees, K-nearest neighbor, naïve Bayesian, and cluster analysis. A data mining application may apply one or more techniques or operations to distinguish patterns or trends in a complex data set. These operations are categorized as classification and prediction, clustering, associational analysis, or forecasting.

Data mining is rapidly becoming a key component in the analysis of workflow in complex organizations such as hospitals. In the hands of domain experts, data mining results can uncover relationships that are hidden in the combinatorial and dynamic complexity of multiple processes. These relationships can then be added to the flow maps originally developed by the domain experts. In the HF project, a number of hidden relationships were discovered using classification and prediction techniques.

Classification is the process of subdividing a data set with regard to specific outcomes. In the case of the HF project, a specific outcome of interest was a length of stay greater than the geometric mean of five days used for DRG reimbursement calculations. A data set, composed of (1) cases with a primary diagnosis of HF in the last five fiscal years and (2) a comprehensive list of predictor or independent variables, was extracted from the hospital's decision support data repository. The variables included the patient's attending and consulting physicians, total hospital costs, comorbidities, readmissions, the nursing unit, codes for diagnostic procedures, medications, laboratory test results, specialists, and others. The selection of variables for inclusion in the data set was based on interviews with the domain experts and information gathered in a literature search on the subject.

The data mining application used a decision tree technique that successively split the variables into groups defined by the values in the independent variables. The aim was to produce a set of rules or a model that could predict the conditions under which an HF patient would stay in the hospital for more than five days (the dependent variable). The use of data mining to analyze workflow in the HF project proved useful from a number of standpoints. For example, 62 percent of HF patients with a stay greater than five days were admitted through the emergency department in acute failure, had new onset atrial fibrillation, were over the age of seventy-five years, had one prior admission for heart failure within the last year, had two or more comorbidities, and lived in a rural area.

Data mining also assisted the team to understand physician practice patterns. For example, the consensus among domain experts was that HF patients were admitted to either the hospital's medical/surgical floor or the cardiac step-down floor. However, they disagreed on the logic for placing patients on different floors. By choosing nursing units as the dependent variable, the team analyst searched for patterns in the data that might explain the reasons. Data mining classification techniques revealed that patients admitted to the step-down floor either were established patients of a cardiologist or had rhythm problems (frequently atrial fibrillation). Patients admitted to the medical/surgical floor were established patients of an internist or family practice physician and had multiple comorbidities. Patients who presented to the emergency care unit without an established physician were always assigned to a solo practice intensivist who admitted patients to the medical/surgical floor.

Text Mining (Natural Language Processing)

To investigate conditions that may have exacerbated an acute episode of heart failure at home, the team used a text mining application to search documents in the target population's transcribed history and physicals. *Text mining,* a form of data mining, allows users to identify critical data contained in large data sets of electronically stored unstructured text.[27] By indexing keywords, text mining applications can search electronic documents to identify specific details or elements that can be used to show connections or relationships. For example, by searching history and physicals for keywords such as swelling, edema, fatigue, shortness of breath, chest pain, decreased appetite, and so forth, team members were able to verify the most common symptoms leading up to an acute episode at home.

Although the symptoms associated with an acute episode of heart failure are well-established in the literature,[28] text mining provided population-specific information to the team. For example, an HF patient's blood pressure on admission to the Emergency Care Unit (ECU) is a strong predictor of in-hospital mortality.[29] However, the only document in which initial blood pressure was stored electronically was in transcribed ECU reports. Without text mining, team members would have had to manually extract handwritten blood pressures from hundreds of individual charts.

The most frequent symptoms identified in the keyword search were fatigue, edema, and shortness of breath. Team members added this information to the data set to begin building a profile of the typical patient readmitted for HF. By building a profile, team members identified patients at high risk for readmission and targeted them for case management outside the hospital.

Social Network Analysis

The care and treatment of congestive heart failure is a complex process that requires the coordination of many physicians, nurses, and support staff across multiple departments. The fragmentation of care in HF patients is a serious problem that can lead to medication errors, extended length of stay, miscommunication, and other safety issues. Content specialists on the HF team felt there was significant variation in treatment patterns because so many different physicians were involved in the process. For instance, in a six-month period, eighty-eight physicians were involved in various aspects of care for 114 patients admitted with a diagnosis of HF.

To clarify practice patterns, team members decided to study the flow of physician referrals using social network analysis software. *Social network analysis* is a set of methods and analytical concepts that focuses on the structure and pattern of relations in a social network.[30] It is beneficial in workflow analysis because it can uncover explanatory factors or variables, such as communication gaps, that influence individual and group behavior. To prepare for social network analysis, a data set composed of all physicians associated with the treatment of HF patients in the prior year was extracted from the hospital's electronic data repository. The physician status in the data set was identified as "admitting," "attending," or "consulting," depending on the degree of involvement with the patient. The status *attending* indicated the physician in charge of the patient, whereas *admitting* indicated the physician on-call who admitted the patient. The status *consultant* indicated referral to either a cardiologist or internist who frequently became the attending physician.

The preprocessing of data required that analysts develop a matrix that identified relationships, or *ties,* among all physicians in the data set. A tie was represented in the matrix by either a 1 (relationship) or a 0 (no relationship). The data were put through an electronic spreadsheet into the application that transformed the matrix into a visual network of nodes (physicians) and connecting lines (relationships) (Figure 21-1). As suspected, the referral network appeared as a tangled, dense web of interconnecting nodes.

Social network analysis software allows users to uncover patterns that may be hidden in large data sets.[30] For example, although eighty-eight physicians were identified in the HF target population, seven appeared to act as referral "hubs." In social network analysis, a *hub* is an individual with many more links (ties) to other members of the network than is typical in the community. Hubs are important in terms of information diffusion and new product acceptance because they often have their finger on the pulse of consensus in the community. They may also be in a position to influence diffusion and acceptance of a new product. In the HF target population, analysts used the software to distill the referral network down to seven "clusters," with either a cardiologist or an internist as

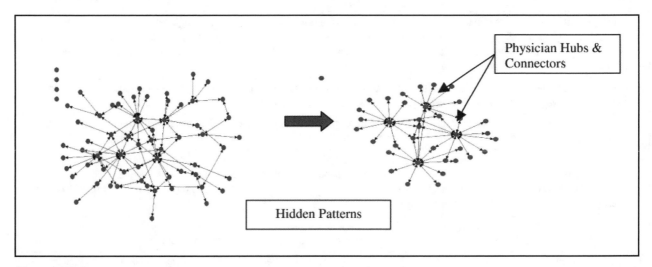

Figure 21-1. *Physician Social Network.*

the HF treatment, seven played a dominant role in influencing practice patterns. Given the social network structure, HF team members realized that, to achieve project objectives, the physician hubs had to play a central role in building consensus on any change initiatives.

Two of the hub physicians (a cardiologist and an internist) not only had multiple links within their own clusters, but were also linked with many other clusters. These individuals served as "bridges" or "connectors" linking the clusters. They were vital to future change initiatives because they acted as an informal channel for the diffusion of information to other physicians. Without help from them, recommendations made by the HF team could get "locked out" of some clusters. Lockout can occur when key information regarding a change initiative never leaves a network cluster, in this case if bridge physicians are excluded from participation in a change initiative.

Because hospitals are complex systems, the social network is only one of the many networks that constrain and enable behavior including the creation, propagation, and discovery of errors. Other networks of relevance connect people, units, knowledge, and tasks; for example, other networks include the knowledge network (who knows what) and the assignment network (who is doing what). The networks evolve over time with the transfer of personnel, the adoption of new technologies, the initiation of on-the-job training, and so on. We can achieve better error reduction management by applying network analysis procedures to such rich relational data, a technique referred to as dynamic network analysis.

Computational Modeling and Simulation

The key objective in the HF project was to improve the overall process of care for HF patients. Successfully achieving the objective meant meeting national benchmarks for quality and cost. Analysis of the process through flowcharting, data mining, text mining, social network analysis, and interviews with content experts yielded the information shown in Table 21-2.

The data supported the notion that HF patients were caught in a complicated spiral of presenting to the ECU in acute failure, an in-patient stay of approximately six days, discharge to home, and the gradual onset of symptoms, ending with an acute exacerbation of heart failure and readmission to the hospital. Team members agreed that one way to meet project objectives was to break the cycle of frequent readmissions to the hospital. The underlying solution was the implementation of a comprehensive HF disease management (DM) program emphasizing ongoing postdischarge care as well as acute inpatient treatment.

Table 21-2. Summary of Findings

• Most HF patients presented to the hospital through the ECU in acute heart failure after a precipitating event. These events often included missing medications, eating a meal high in salt, or suffering from complications of an unrelated illness (flu, diabetes, pneumonia, and so forth).
• The majority of patients recognized the symptoms of cascading failure (swelling, fatigue, shortness of breath) in advance but did not contact their physician until they were in acute failure. Frequently patients stated that they began experiencing symptoms on the weekend but did not want to bother their physician until Monday. A number of patients stated that they were unsure of which physician to contact (their family practice physician, cardiologist, or internist).
• The readmission rate of the HF population was significantly higher than that of other patients in the same age group. Patients over the age of seventy-five who lived in a rural area tended to have a higher readmission rate than the remainder of the population.
• Readmissions tended to have a much longer in-patient length of stay than new onset heart failure patients. These patients frequently stayed longer than the DRG 127 mean of five days, which resulted in overall hospital costs exceeding reimbursement.
• Although many physicians were involved in the treatment of HF patients, five cardiologists and two internists acted as consultants in the majority of cases. Which nursing unit a patient was treated on depended on which physician a patient was referred to. And which physician an HF patient was referred to (cardiologist or internist) depended on whether or not he or she was an established patient with an existing physician or a patient without a primary physician.
• Patients who were treated aggressively upon admission (diuretics administered quickly, frequent regular follow-up to monitor and adjust fluid status, management of atrial fibrillation, and so on) tended to have a length of stay of four days or less.
• There did not appear to be a significant difference in length of stay between patients treated by cardiologists and those treated by internists or by nursing units. However, there was a difference between the physician clusters identified by the social network analysis.

Although there is extensive literature on the merits of DM programs,[31] predicting their costs and benefits is problematic. For example, multiple variables affect the admission and readmission rate of HF patients, including the presence of comorbidities, physician practice patterns, population demographics and insurance plans, as well as complication and mortality rates. Operational variables include defining clinician roles and responsibilities, physician acceptance, program costs, and access to information across the continuum. Combining all these variables to accurately predict the outcome of a DM program on readmission rates, quality, and cost can be challenging.

Predicting the outcome of a new program, e.g., DM, in complex adaptive systems is improved through the use of *computational modeling and simulation.* Although a variety of software applications are available, most packages use algorithms that represent various theories and that produce output simulating dynamic behavior comparable to similar elements in real-world systems.[32,33] Modeling benefits the study of complexity by translating process steps into the language of mathematics and linking theory with data. Simulation is particularly well-suited for modeling complex systems because (1) unanticipated emergent properties may be discovered, (2) studies can be run over many (simulated) years, (3) simulation can be much less expensive than real-world studies, and (4) simulation allows nurse administrators to "test drive," or experiment with, change without costly penalties.

Three common simulation techniques used in the study of complex systems are agent-based modeling, discrete event simulation,[34] and system dynamics.[19] In *agent-based modeling,* a collection of autonomous agents with encoded decision-making abilities is programmed into a virtual system. Guided by a set of rules, the agents respond to parameter inputs in much the same way that real-world networks respond. *Discrete event simulation* utilizes mathematical formulas (differential equations) to model a system as it evolves over time by a representation in which variables change instantaneously at separate points in time.[35,36] Discrete event simulation is most valuable in simulating process flow and design optimization in such areas as operating and emergency department staffing and scheduling.

A *system dynamics approach* to modeling focuses on the information-feedback characteristics of a process or activity. Model processes are represented as *stocks* (knowledge, people, supplies) and continuous *flows* (the information moving between them[19]). Computational models are built on a number of interacting feedback loops that amplify, depress, or balance system behavior. System dynamics utilizes differential equations to represent the nonlinear behavior characteristics of complex adaptive systems.

The team built the HF model using a combination of system dynamics and discrete event modeling techniques in a stepwise fashion with help from an analyst in the hospital's fiscal management department and from the college of industrial engineering at a local university. The output from the model (effects on mortality, readmission rate, length of stay, and cost by a DM program) was used as the basis for considering such a program.

The model output showed a significant increase in costs to implement the program in year one, with little effect on readmission rates, length of stay, and mortality. However, starting in year two, as the program began to take effect, there was a gradual decline in the number of patients most frequently readmitted. This in turn reduced the proportion of HF patients who historically had the longest stays. The result was a lowered readmission rate and lowered lengths of stay. Mortality rate was modeled as declining in a manner similar to other DM programs, but only after readmission rates and length of stay declined. The model's output also showed a significant drop in overall hospital costs associated with HF patients over a five-year period. Without the use of computational modeling and simulation, the positive effect of the program modeled over time would have been missed.

Discussion

This case study provides an illustration of the applied theory underlying complex system behavior in social organizations such as hospitals. Traditional methods of work-flow analysis fail to account adequately for combinatorial and dynamic complexity and, as a result, are poor predictors of future system behavior. As processes cut across multiple hospital departments in a tightly coupled manner, cause and effect become separated in time and space. Unanticipated and often undesirable system behavior emerges from the dense web of interactions and can lead to medical errors, increased cost, and patient harm.

Analyzing work flow in hospitals today means confronting organizational complexity. The vast amounts of data available to managers must be reduced so as to allow them to analyze the essence of a problem. Knowledge discovery through data and text mining, social network analysis, computational modeling, and simulation assist nurse administrators to understand the patterns and interaction effects hidden in complex systems. Armed with this knowledge, nurse administers can steer health care systems toward a safer and more productive environment.

References

1. Institute of Medicine. *To Err Is Human: Building a Safer Health System.* Washington, DC: National Academy Press; 2000.
2. Hicks RW, Cousins DD, Williams RL. *Summary of Information Submitted to MEDMARX in the Year 2002. The Quest for Quality.* Rockville, MD: USP Center for the Advancement of Patient Safety; 2003.
3. Tenner E. *Why Things Bite Back.* New York: Vintage Books; 1996.
4. Sellen AJ, Harper RHR. *The Myth of the Paperless Office.* Cambridge, MA: MIT Press; 2003.
5. Hammer M, Champy J. *Reengineering the Corporation.* New York: Harper Collins Publishers; 1993.
6. Van Drake S. Nurses treat staffing issue with union. *South Florida Business Journal.* Available at: www.bizjournals.com/southflorida/stories/2003/09/22/story3/html. Retrieved February 1, 2005.
7. Zimmerman B, Lindberg C, Plsek P. *Edgeware.* Irving, TX: VHA Inc.; 1998:263.
8. Lorenz E. Deterministic, nonperiodic flow. *J Atmospheric Sciences.* 1963;20:130-141.
9. Lorenz E. The mechanics of vacillation. *J Atmospheric Sciences.* 1963;20:448-464.
10. Lorenz E. The problems of deducing the climate from the governing equations. *Tellus.* 1964;16:1-11.
11. Lorenz E. *On the Prevalence of Aperiodicity in Simple Systems in Global Analysis.* New York: Springer-Verlag; 1979.
12. Kauffman S. *Origins of Order: Self-Organization and Selection in Evolution.* Oxford, UK: Oxford University Press; 1992.
13. Kauffman S. *At Home in the Universe.* Oxford, UK: Oxford University Press; 1995.
14. Camazine S, Deneubourg J, Franks N, et al. *Self-Organization in Biological Systems.* Princeton, NJ: Princeton University Press; 2001.
15. Arthur BW. Positive feedbacks in the economy. *Sci Am.* February 1990:92-99.
16. Carley K, Prietula M. *Computational Organizational Theory.* Hillsdale, NJ: Lawrence Erbaum Assoc.; 1994.
17. Johnson S. *Emergence, the Connected Lives of Ants.* New York: Simon & Schuster; 2001.
18. Perrow C. *Normal Accidents.* New York: Basic Books; 1984.
19. Sterman JD. *Business Dynamics: Systems Thinking and Modeling for a Complex World.* Boston: McGraw-Hill Publishers; 2000.
20. Harris J. Blindsided, how to spot the next breakthrough that will change your business forever. In: *Audio-Tech Business Book Summaries.* Vol 11. Willowbrook, IL: Audio-Tech; 2002:5-6.
21. Clancy TR. Navigating in a complex nursing world. *J Nurs Adm.* 2004;34(6):274-282.
22. Clancy TR. Medication error prevention: progress on initiatives. *JONA's Health care Law, Ethics, and Regulation.* 2004:6(1):3-14.
23. Auyang SY. Foundations of complex-system theories. In: *Economics, Evolutionary Biology, and Statistical Physics.* Cambridge, UK: Cambridge University Press; 1998.
24. Waldrop M. *Complexity, the Emerging Science.* New York: Simon & Schuster; 1992.
25. Bourtchouladze R. *Memories Are Made of This.* New York: Columbia University Press; 2002.
26. Senge P. *The Fifth Discipline: The Art of and Practice of the Learning Organization.* New York: Doubleday Publishers; 1990.
27. Berry MJA, Linoff GS. *Data Mining Techniques.* 2nd ed. Indianapolis, IN: Wiley Publishing, Inc.; 2004.
28. Hunt SA, Baker DW, Chin MH, et al. ACC/AHA guidelines for the evaluation and management of chronic heart failure in the adult. [The American College of Cardiology Web site.] Available at: http//www.acc.org/clinicalguidelines/failure/hf_index.htm. Retrieved on February 10, 2005.
29. Acute Decompensated Heart Failure National Registry (Adhere). Available at: www.adhereregistery.com. Accessed February 15, 2005.
30. Wasserman S, Faust K. *Social Network Analysis: Methods and Applications.* Cambridge, UK: Cambridge University Press; 1994.
31. Grady GL, Dracup K, Kennedy G, et al. Team management of patients with heart failure. *Circulation.* 2000;102:2443-2456.
32. Weiss G. *Multi-Agent Systems: A Modern Approach to Distributed Artificial Intelligence.* Cambridge, MA: MIT Press; 1999.
33. Ilgen D, Huli C, eds. *Computational Modeling of Behavior in Organizations.* Washington, DC: American Psychological Association; 2000.

34. Bonabeau E. Agent-based modeling: methods and techniques for simulating human systems. Presented at: Arthur M. Sackler Colloquium of the National Academy of Sciences, Adaptive Agents, Intelligence, and Emergent Human Organization: Capturing Complexity Through Agent-Based Modeling, held at the Arnold and Mabel Beckman Center of the National Academies of Science and Engineering; October 4-6, 2001. Irvine, CA; 2002.

35. Cassandras C. *Discrete Event Systems.* Boston: Aksen Associates; 1993.

36. Van Merode G, Groothuis S, Goldschmidt H. Workflow management: changing your organization through simulation. *Accred Qual Assur* 1999;4:438-444.

Case Study 21A

Rebuilding the Nursing Workforce at Royal Melbourne Hospital

Danny Rathgeber, MBA, Graduate Dipl Management, Graduate Dipl Critical Care, Certificate Coronary Care, Certificate Cardiothoracic

In August 2002, the Royal Melbourne Hospital (RMH) was investigated by the health services commissioner for Victoria in response to circumstances surrounding the deaths of two patients and allegations of unprofessional conduct that had occurred earlier that year. Just prior to this event, I had been recruited to create a new nursing leadership team at RMH and to rebuild its nursing workforce.

This chapter describes how RMH's nursing leadership team achieved a transformation in nursing over a two-year period. During that time, the organization evolved from one characterized by major staffing shortfalls, high nursing agency costs and staff turnover rates, poor nursing morale, and a reputation as least preferred employer to being among the most sought after graduate nursing placements in Australia.

Background

RMH is a part of Melbourne Health, a major public health provider in Victoria that employs more than 3,000 nursing staff across its services, which comprise North Western Mental Health, North Western Dialysis Service, and Victorian Infectious Disease Reference Laboratory, in addition to RMH. With an operating budget in excess of $550 million, RMH manages 1,050 beds in acute, subacute, and community settings. It serves a population of nearly one million people living in Melbourne's northern and western metropolitan region. It also provides a wide range of specialty services to all Victorians. RMH has been a leading hospital for more than 150 years and enjoys a national and international reputation for quality patient care, research, and education in both the medical and the nursing professions.

Between 1992 and 2002, RMH experienced a series of health care reforms at the government level, including changes in funding models and organizational restructuring, all of which heavily affected hospital-based management practices. The RMH nursing workforce had six successive executive directors of nursing in seven years (1996–2002), and this leadership instability was accompanied by staff shortfalls exceeding 300 effective full-time (EFT) nursing positions. The constant change in leadership resulted in lack of a shared vision, a loss of direction, and a focus on costs rather than on care. A disconnect developed between those providing professional nursing care and those who were charged with managing nursing services. Nursing staff who had initially been attracted to practice at the hospital did not stay. Confrontation was the norm, wards became insular, and nurses lost their voice.

Just as members of the new nursing management team were settling into their roles, the health services commissioner for Victoria released to hospitals and to the public at large an extensive report detailing the findings of its 2002 investigation. "The Royal Melbourne Hospital Inquiry" stated that nursing standards had suffered as a result of large staff shortfalls, significant reliance on casual staff, lack of clinical support, and limited professional development opportunities. The report also documented RMH's lack of clearly defined nursing standards, which limited the ability to monitor and evaluate patient outcomes. Also during 2002, the Office of the Victorian Auditor General identified inefficiencies in workforce planning and data collection throughout the province's public health system.

The Problem

In 2002, RMH was suffering from the classic dilemma in workforce management: rich in data, poor in information. As in many other hospitals in the Australian public health system, the nursing service at Melbourne Health was strategically blind and logistically compromised. The new nursing leadership team believed that in order to make good decisions related to staffing requirements, accurate, real-time, meaningful data must be available.

Nursing leadership sought to identify the following variables:

- How many nursing staff were needed?

- How many nurses staff the hospital on a daily basis?
- What were their sick leave trends?
- How often were casual staff used?
- What were the nursing shortfalls, both current and projected?

Because these variables were unknown, it was not possible to accurately identify staffing demands and trends in a timely manner beyond immediate day-to-day requirements. The organization was buried in piles of paperwork, with little useful data available to nursing decision makers. Similar to other Australian health care services, Melbourne Health's chosen data collection methodology consisted of nonlinked Microsoft Excel spreadsheets in which the data were entered some time after the event. This data collection system led to multiple entries of the same data, often by different individuals who lacked a common understanding of the meaning of specific data elements; for example, there were two definitions for "short-term sick leave." The result was that critical staffing decisions were being made on the basis of inaccurate or redundant data. The financial arm of the organization was disconnected from the operational wing. And the operational wing could not articulate staffing needs or clinical pressures to the management group.

The Solution

Solving the problems confronted by RMH started with the development of a nursing information system that reflected the needs of the organization. The nursing leadership team recognized that the current RMH nursing information system could be converted from a closed system that was being fed inaccurate, redundant data into an open system that would support the right person entering the right information at the right time throughout the organization.

As executive director of nursing services, I served as the primary designer, programmer, and developer of the new information system. Early in my management career, I discovered the limitations of nursing management systems. While a nurse unit manager at a rural hospital, I began developing the system to serve as a tool for tracking the activities of nursing staff in the intensive care unit. This system was then expanded to meet the demands of several wards, and later it was used as the primary nursing staff management tool for a moderately sized rural general hospital. As the system was developed, defects were removed and modifications were made to meet the challenges of increased workforce size and complexity.

At RMH, we developed the system to the point where it could be networked across a large metropolitan health care organization and integrated with key services, e.g., the finance department. The availability of this powerful nursing information management system provided the basis for immediate application, while we developed the remaining features. Fortunately, because we had used the standard Microsoft Office suite that was already loaded on every manager's desktop, no new software was required to implement this application.

The nursing leadership team was under enormous pressure to restore the effective professional operation of the RMH nursing workforce, so the nursing leadership team decided to implement the first of four software applications, the Nursing Workforce Management Database. Nurse unit managers welcomed the new system because it proved to be a direct aid in managing their wards and departments. To facilitate compliance with the data set, each ward received staff replacement for sick or annual leave, roster vacancy, or patient acuity, based on whether its data entry into the system was complete. This strategy proved effective, and we quickly obtained 100 percent compliance in system use by unit managers. The database is linked directly to the hospital's staffing allocation service, which is responsible for providing casual staff replacement for all wards and departments.

No Data, No Replacement

The workforce management tools were a perfect fit for tracking the activity of all nursing staff across RMH, but the success of the software application was directly proportional to uptake by nurse unit managers. No sophisticated implementation strategy was developed; rather, the change process was aided by a series of educational forums for key stakeholders. These forums were designed to acquaint them with current workforce issues and the solutions that would be provided by the workforce management tools.

Within two weeks, the workforce management database software was rolled out across the entire organization. The assumption was made that the change management process would be trouble-free if the product actually improved staff management at the ward level, as well as the functions of budgeting, staff recruitment and replacement, leave management, and casual workforce monitoring. The system was designed from the bottom up; therefore, there were obvious advantages to nurse unit managers, and prompt feedback was received.

The Nursing Workforce Management Tool-Kit

The Nursing Workforce Management Tool-Kit has four interrelated multi-user databases: the EFT Profiler, the Nursing Workforce Management Database, the Nursing Allocations Package, and the Nursing Yearly Planner.

EFT Profiler

The EFT Profiler is a software program that consists of tables, queries, forms, reports, and macros. The application is a budgeting tool, driven by a series of uniquely developed algorithms and formulae for estimating staffing requirements for a given ward, department, or cost center. In determining the ward's EFTs, the program considers such variables as direct and indirect nursing hours, nursing ratios (number of nurses for each patient, as mandated by industry agreement), ratio of full-time to part-time employees, accrued day-off entitlements, amount of potential sick leave, study leave entitlements, shift lengths, ward configuration, hours of operation, and patient demand.

Nursing Workforce Management Database

The Nursing Workforce Management Database contains vital information entered by the nurse in charge of the shift in each ward or department. Roster schedules, staff levels, sick leave, workloads, and staffing requirements can be easily entered into the database. The database uses a three-step process that collects, collates, and facilitates data into meaningful workforce information.

Data that are identified include roster numbers of permanent staff; staff vacancy levels; sick leave and staff overtime hours; nursing agency and bank hours and shifts, and the cost of usage for each; number of staff required to safely staff a shift for each ward; and number of staff actually on the ward for each shift. All of these data are available to line managers in real time, and the database seamlessly links to the Nursing Allocations Package.

Nursing Allocations Package

The Nursing Allocations Package is a software program that manages the casual workforce from a central location. Casual staff profiles and preferred work requests are stored in the program to allow auto-generated allocation of staff to wards or departments. In the simplest terms, this program matches work demands with the most appropriate qualified member of the casual workforce. And when staff vacancies persist, it facilitates the employment of nursing agency staff. The costing module built into the system allows real-time calculation of salary expenditures and is used to pay and audit all casual staff employed at RMH.

Nursing Yearly Planner

The Nursing Yearly Planner is a Microsoft Access program installed on the hospital's Intranet to provide managers with a means for proactive human resource management. The aim is to minimize inconsistencies with regard to leave management, study day approval, and staff recruitment and to delineate EFT position requirements and skill mix.

Each cost center manager collects and collates the following: staff member assignments, employment status (full-time, part-time, or limited tenure), contracted hours, job classification, staff member activity, duration of employment, and entrance and exit interviews.

Results

Using data from the Nursing Workforce Management System, we developed basic, sound recruitment and retention strategies. These strategies included designing a career pathway, conducting entrance and exit interviews, capturing related data in the system, and establishing continuing education programs in response to knowledge or skill deficits. By creating an interface between the workforce management tools

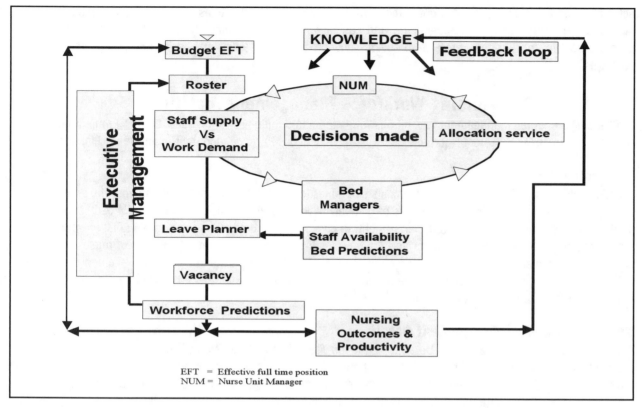

Figure 21A-1. *Melbourne Health Nursing Workforce System Model.*

and the financial system, we were able to obtain evidence we could use to gain executive and board-level support for key initiatives. We trained middle managers in system use and in developing financial and budgeting skills. We also actively mentored them in their continuous data monitoring and analysis skills.

As a result of these strategies, unit managers and directors across all units were actively using the new system within a twelve-month-period. A major achievement was the improved management of casual staff by the Allocations Department. By setting up a central command and control system, we were able to rigorously monitor the deployment of these staff, allowing us to cut inappropriate use and costs by more than 32 percent, thereby safeguarding this important resource pool that comprises 10 percent of our nursing workforce.

Other key achievements included:
- Decreased nurse shortfalls from more than 300 to 50 EFT positions
- Increased graduate nurse recruitment per year from thirty staff in 2002 to 110 in 2003 through 2005
- Reduced nursing agency-related expenditures from $1.5 to $0.2 million a month
- Development of a nursing education center, with an increase in support staff from fifteen to thirty-three employees

Accurate forecasting for resource and budgeting needs was another major achievement. The nursing leadership team can now reliably forecast how many nurses will be required across the system, determining when and where they should be deployed, costs, and number of beds needed for a given budget year.

The results achieved and the quality of data generated by the Nursing Workforce Management System have acquired such credibility with the executive team that nursing's budget and resource staffing requests are now endorsed with little challenge. The leadership team now understands the nature and operation of its workforce. This understanding is encapsulated within the Melbourne Health Nursing Workforce System Model (see Figure 21A-1).

Conclusion

The databases described above form the hub of RMH's innovative Nursing Workforce Management System, which allows ward-level data entry, centralized data collation, and informed decision making. Innovation requires people, technology, and process improvements. The Nursing Workforce Management System incorporates these elements successfully and has had many positive benefits for the organization.

Lessons learned from this initiative include the following:

- Frontline staff are the right people to enter data.
- Data should be entered only once and at the right time.
- Adoption of the system requires buy-in from all stakeholders to be successful.
- The budget process must interface with the financial system.
- System and process redesign are more likely to be successful when a bottom-up approach is used.
- IT staff should not be relied on to design and develop software solutions, because the bulk of their time is spent in defining the problems.

RMH's knowledge-based Nursing Workforce Management System provides accurate, real-time data to the nursing leadership team, enabling it to make informed operational decisions and to validate the effectiveness of its strategies. The system is unique and supports the nursing leadership team's vision of "taking nursing into the future."

Reports

The database is accompanied by preformatted reports that nurse unit managers, finance managers, directors of nursing, and executive staff can access. The following figures, Figures 21A-2, 21A-3, and 21A-4 are examples of the auto-generated reporting function.

References

1. Health Services Commissioner. *Royal Melbourne Hospital Inquiry Report.* Melbourne: Department of Human Services; August 2002.

2. Auditor General of Victoria. *Nursing Workforce Planning.* Melbourne: Office of the Auditor General; May 2002.

3. Cornell P. *Accessing and Analyzing Data with Microsoft Excel 2003.* Redmond, WA: Microsoft Press; 2003.

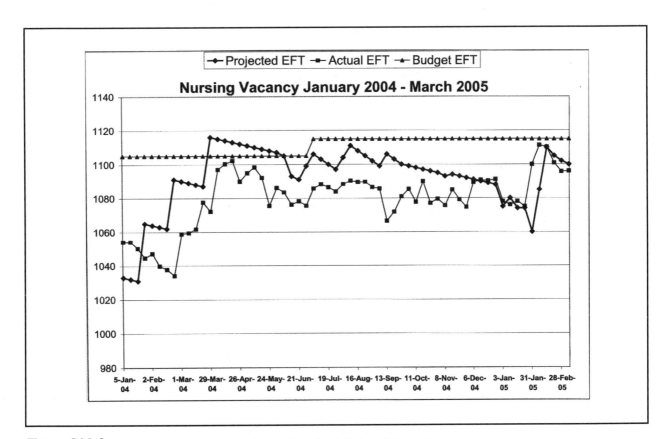

Figure 21A-2. *Effective Full-time EFT Budget vs. Actual and Projected Expenditures.*

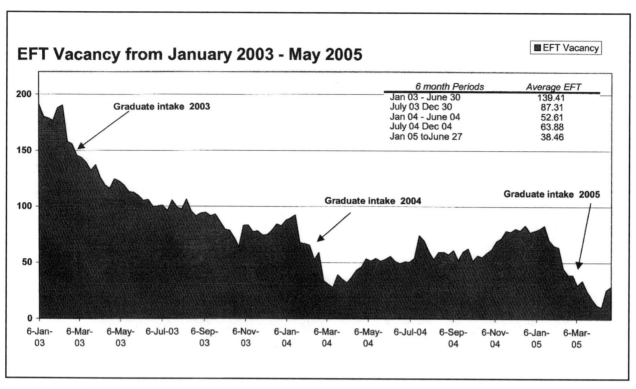

Figure 21A-3. *Nursing Effective Full Time Positions at RMH (City Campus).*

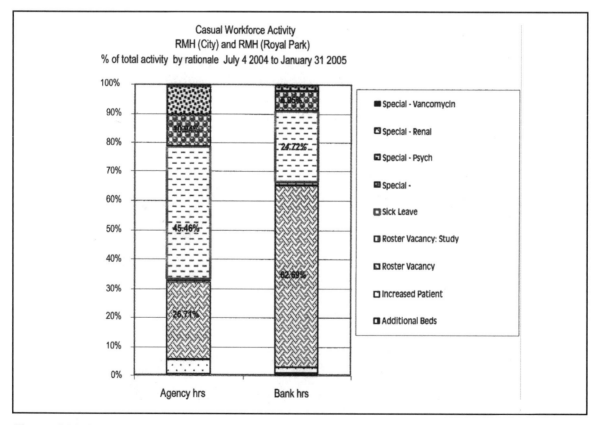

Figure 21A-4. *Activity by Rationale.*

Case Study 21B

Pursuing Quality: Opportunity and Change for Nursing

Julie Creamer, MS, RN

The U.S. National Quality Agenda

The national quality and patient safety agenda has challenged hospitals and other providers to seek new answers to a complex set of problems.[1] The solution set includes improved measurement, robust process improvement, and system redesign. However, to significantly improve outcomes in these areas, information technology (IT) must be made a critical element of system infrastructure. The successful implementation and effective use of this technology is becoming a core competency for the health care workforce, including physicians, nurses, other clinicians, and support staff, as well as health care executives. The following case history illustrates how an academic medical center embraced the call for action to improve health care quality and patient safety in the U.S., using clinical IT as a key enabler.

Northwestern Memorial Hospital Case History

Background, Mission, and Strategy

Northwestern Memorial Hospital (NMH), located in downtown Chicago, is a 750-bed academic medical center with more than 1,300 physicians representing almost every specialty and 6,000 additional employees. Guided by its "Patients First" mission and a culture of ongoing improvement, Northwestern Memorial constantly strives to deliver the safest, most effective, and most advanced care to its patients. As one of America's top teaching hospitals, Northwestern Memorial is bonded in an essential academic and service relationship with Northwestern University's Feinberg School of Medicine.

In 1999, Northwestern Memorial created a new strategic plan to address challenges, e.g., forecasted workforce shortages, decreased reimbursements, and increased operational and capital requirements. The new strategic plan focused on three fundamental principles: (1) every patient deserves the best possible care and service, (2) employees and staff are the organization's single most important asset, and (3) strong financial performance is essential to meeting its responsibilities to the community. Correspondingly, the current strategic plan for the organization includes three overarching goals:
1. To provide the *best patient experience* from the patient's perspective
2. To recruit, develop, and retain the *best people,* who share the organization's values and achieve results
3. To develop the resources to achieve the organization's mission and vision through *exceptional financial performance*

To actualize this plan, a set of objectives was outlined for each goal. Early on, the hospital's leadership recognized that achieving the goals would require a secure, reliable, and scalable IT infrastructure. This case describes how Northwestern Memorial is using technology to advance the best patient experience from the patient's perspective and to achieve marked improvements in nursing care. Figure 21B-1 illustrates how the organizational objectives are aligned with Northwestern Memorial's strategic plan for achieving *best patient experience.*

Infrastructure to Support the Strategic Plan

To meet the plan objectives, three key constructs of hospital infrastructure were designed and implemented:
1. Advanced capabilities in process improvement, measurement, monitoring, and change acceleration.
2. A centralized staff training engine through the creation of an in-house academy.
3. Customized information systems that support clinical care practices.

Incentives were developed to align staff across all levels of the organization to adopt and own the new innovations and process changes. Because funding for these infrastructure strategies competes directly with other budget demands, careful attention was given to framing these initiatives in a business case structure with clearly defined, sustainable, and measurable goals.

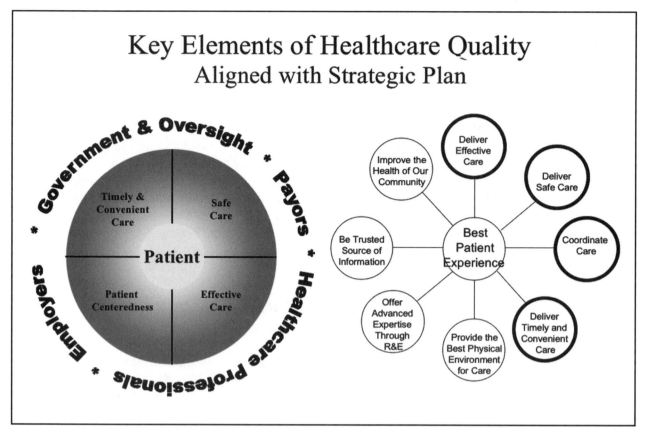

Figure 21B-1. *Aligning organizational objectives with Northwestern Memorial's strategic plan.*

The Significant Role of Clinical IT

To maximize the value of designing and implementing a powerful CIS, the organization recognized the need to clarify exactly how the system would support the achievement of the strategic plan. Thus, as strategic plan deliverables were identified each year, the function, capabilities, and needs of the information system implementation plan were linked so as to accelerate achievement of the outcomes. Figure 21B-2 illustrates the connection between the strategic plan and the applications within the information system.

The alignment with strategy helped guide the overall timeline for the implementation of major system components. Other considerations for the timeline included (1) the maturity of the software, (2) the risk of disrupting clinical work flow, (3) the dependency of one application on the information generated from another system component, and (4) the timing of other key activities within the organization. Figure 21B-3 illustrates the long-range IT plan for the implementation of key components of the CIS.

Hardwiring Quality and Patient Safety into the Clinical Information System

To redesign health care at Northwestern Memorial and to advance the best patient experience goal, an important set of guiding principles was adopted to support decision making and the prioritization of initiatives. These principles, adapted from a variety of leading patient safety sources, include:

1. Providing access to all pertinent information
2. Reducing reliance on memory
3. Developing fail safes and forcing functions
4. Standardizing and simplifying processes
5. Eliminating precursors to error
6. Making the safest thing the easiest thing to do

The CIS has been critical to hardwiring these principles into clinical operations and the daily practices of health care providers. For example, the CIS provides anytime, anywhere access to legible patient infor-

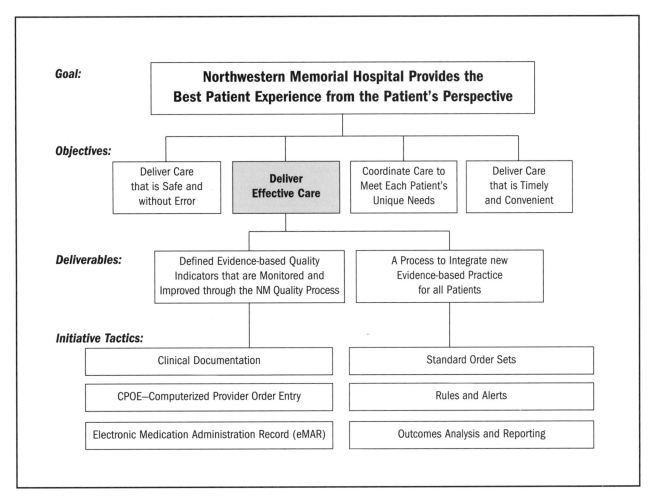

Figure 21B-2. *Connection between Northwestern Memorial's stratgeic plan and applications within the information system.*

mation, from any computer networked to the hospital system or through a secure Web-based connection. Information entered at the time of care delivery is immediately and broadly available, current, and secure. Additionally, the EHR allows the application of evidence-based care guidelines through the utilization of standard order sets. Within the functionality of the CPOE application, standardized order sets are developed and accessible to clinicians based on the patient's diagnosis or episodic needs. Care can be individualized as needed, and variance from the guidelines tracked and measured. Such monitoring supports the ongoing dialogue essential not only to allow modifications to the order sets based on evolving evidence, but also to measure the impact of variation on the overall course of treatment.

Another important component of the CIS is the rules and alerts function, which enables automated "intelligence" in the context of the clinicians' natural work flow. As caregivers use the system to do their work, they are presented with clinical decision support in the form of pertinent patient and reference data. The rules and alerts can be linked to different components of the information system, e.g., results viewing, nursing documentation, and CPOE. For example, when an order is placed into the system, the rules engine checks for relevant information, e.g., laboratory results and patient weight, and presents an alert automatically, when necessary, thereby enabling the physician or pharmacist to act on safe practice information relevant to treatment choices and dosing decisions.

The rules and alerts function can also be linked to other system components such as nursing documentation. As nurses become more comfortable with the system, they identify opportunities to leverage its powerful capabilities to solve problems and improve patient care. Two recent examples at Northwestern Memorial demonstrate the creativity of the nurses in system design to maximize the quality of care and patient safety.

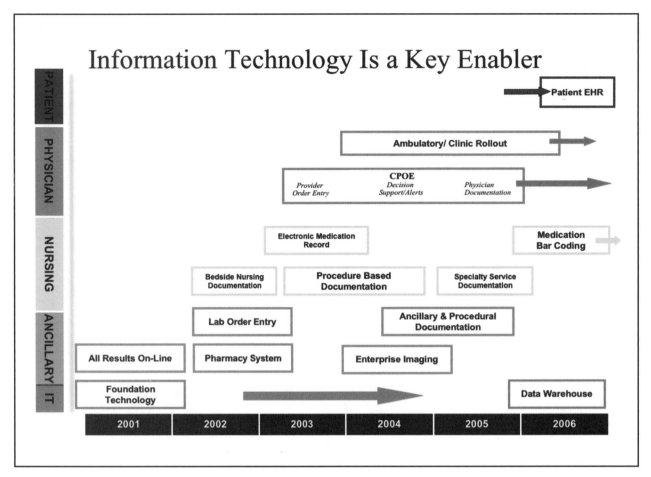

Figure 21B-3. *Long range IT plan for implementing key components of the clinical information system.*

Nursing Example I: Improving Pain Management

Effective pain management is a fundamental component of providing the best patient experience. Pain assessment and treatment are also required under the standards of the Joint Commission on Accreditation of Healthcare Organizations.[2] Patients must receive appropriate initial assessment of their pain, appropriate intervention for pain, and then timely reassessment of the success of the interventions. Yet, when using manual patient record and documentation systems, the consistent recording of all assessments and interventions, as well as easy access to real-time information, proved challenging. This changed with the implementation of electronic nursing documentation and the electronic medication administration record, which actualized the patient safety guiding principles. The system design features real-time access to information with a standardized process, reduced reliance on memory, and automated forcing functions to make the safest thing the easy thing to do.

For example, documentation of pain assessment is integrated with mandatory clinical and vital sign documentation. The task list is updated with a reminder to the nurse to complete and document the initial pain assessment as part of routine care processes. The reminder stays on the electronic task list until the pain assessment is documented. Then, if a moderate to severe pain score requires intervention (defined as a score of four or greater on a zero-to-ten scale), the nurse is prompted to complete and document a comprehensive pain assessment and appropriate pain intervention. Completion of the documentation triggers a reminder on the nurse's task list for a patient reassessment and documentation one hour later. This set of rules and alerts was instrumental in improving the timely documentation of patient pain assessments from 67 percent to 98 percent and the timely reassessment following intervention from 50 percent to 96 percent within two calendar quarters. As noted in Figure 21B-4, these improvements were seen as soon as the system designs were implemented, and they have been sustained.

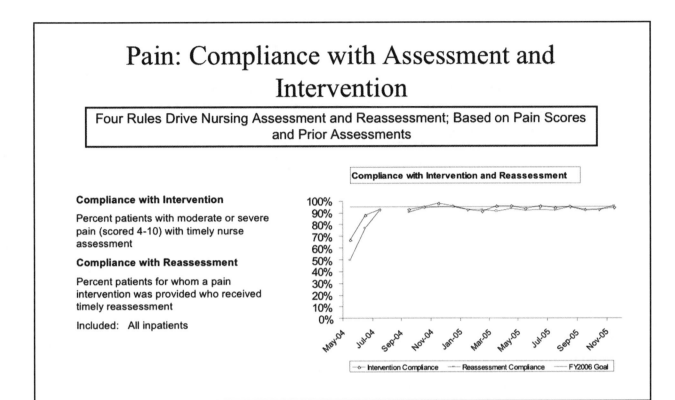

Figure 21B-4. *Rate of improvements following implementation of pain assessment documentation.*

Nursing Example II: Improved Care for Pneumonia Patients

Another example of system-based care improvements based on the patient safety guiding principles is the compliance measure on smoking cessation counseling for pneumonia patients. Research shows that patients who receive even brief smoking cessation advice from their health care providers are more likely to quit than those who receive none.[3] Thus, such evidence-based intervention is important to Northwestern Memorial's best patient experience objective to deliver effective care based on clinical evidence. As illustrated in Figure 21B-5, with the introduction of nursing documentation (May 2003), the provision and documentation of smoking cessation counseling improved from 30 percent to 90 percent. With the implementation of mandatory rules for documentation of smoking history in May 2004, full (100 percent) compliance with this standard has been achieved and sustained. Furthermore, in addition to the improved access to smoking cessation education during hospitalization, an automatic consultation request is sent to the Northwestern Memorial Wellness Institute so that follow-up with a professional smoking cessation counselor is offered to patients after discharge.

Summary

As this case history demonstrates, many of the challenges of implementing an EHR in an acute care hospital setting can be successfully navigated with effective leadership and strategic planning. Rather than trying to achieve an EHR as a goal unto itself, Northwestern Memorial has accelerated the progress and achievement of its strategic goals by leveraging the powerful tools found in an integrated CIS. Involvement of staff throughout the organization in the design, implementation, and evaluation of the system led to a high level of acceptance and the ability to optimize the system to improve the quality and safety of patient care.

Pneumonia: Compliance with Documentation of Smoking Cessation Counseling

Clinical Documentation Implemented in May 2003 which improved performance. Process Variability Addressed by Mandating Nursing Documentation Field in May 2004

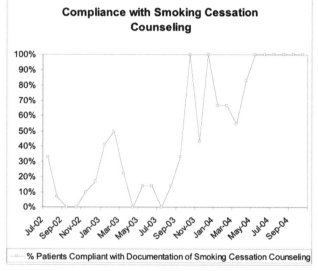

Included Populations: Discharges with principal Diagnosis of Pneumonia AND a history of smoking cigarettes anytime during the year prior to hospital arrival

Excluded Populations:

• Patients < 18 years of age
• Patients transferred to another acute care hospital, expired, left AMA, discharged to hospice
• No working diagnosis of pneumonia at the time of admission, patients who receive comfort measures only

Figure 21B-5. *Improvements in provision and documentation of smoking cessation counseling after introducing nursing documentation.*

References

1. Institute of Medicine. *Crossing the Quality Chasm: A New Health System for the 21st Century.* Washington, DC: National Academies Press; 2001.

2. Joint Commission on Accreditation of Healthcare Organizations (JCAHO). *Comprehensive Accreditation Manual for Hospitals.* Oakbrook Terrace, IL: JCAHO, 2005. Standards RI.2.160–Right to pain management, PC.6.10–Patient education, PC.8.10–Pain assessment and treatment, PC.13.40–Sedation and anesthesia, PI.1.10–Performance improvement data collection.

3. Fiore MC, Bailey WC, Cohen SJ, et. al. *Treating Tobacco Use and Dependence. Quick Reference Guide for Clinicians.* Rockville, MD: U.S. Department of Health and Human Services, Public Health Service; October 2000. Available at: www.surgeongeneral.gov/tobacco/ tobaqrg.pdf. Accessed September 7, 2005.

CHAPTER 22

Evidence-Based Practice

By Marita G. Titler, PhD, RN, FAAN

The stark reality [is] that we invest billions in research to find appropriate treatments, we spend more than $1 trillion on health care annually, we have extraordinary capacity to deliver the best care in the world, but we repeatedly fail to translate that knowledge and capacity into clinical practice.[1]

Introduction

In the U.S., the failure to rescue, decubitus ulcers, and postoperative sepsis accounted for 60 percent of all patient safety incidents among Medicare patients hospitalized from 2000 through 2002. Decubitus ulcers accounted for $2.57 billion in excess inpatient costs to Medicare over three years (2000–2002), and postop pulmonary embolism or DVT accounted for $1.4 billion in excess inpatient costs to Medicare over three years (2000–2002).[2]

Given the annual expenditure on health care in the U.S., why do such costs persist? Research is only the first step to improving practice.[3,4] To bridge the gap between the discovery of knowledge and its use in practice, concentrated efforts must focus on methods to speed the translation of research findings into practice.[4-10] The development and dissemination of evidence-based practice guidelines are essential steps, but alone they do little to promote knowledge uptake by direct care providers.[6,8,9] Promoting the use of evidence in practice is an active process that is facilitated, in part, by a number of strategies: modeling and imitation of others who have successfully adopted the innovation, an organizational culture that values and supports use of evidence, the localization of the evidence for use in a specific health care setting, incorporating evidence-based information into clinical information systems (CIS), and use in electronic decision support tools.[4,11-15]

The *translation of research into practice* (TRIP) is a multifaceted, systemic process of promoting the adoption of evidence-based practices (EBPs) in the delivery of health care services, and it goes beyond the dissemination of evidence-based guidelines.[4,9,11,12,16] Promoting knowledge uptake and changing practitioner behavior require active interchange with those in direct care. Although the science of translation is young, the effectiveness of interventions for promoting the adoption of EBPs is being studied, and federal funding is supporting research in this area.[9,17,18] Additionally, today more evidence is available to guide the selection of strategies for translating research into practice than was available five years ago.[4,9,19-24]

This chapter presents an overview of EBP and the steps of the EBP process and describes the use of CIS in supporting the implementation of EBPs.

Overview of EBP and the Steps of the EBP Process

Evidence-based practice (EBP) has been defined by some experts as the synthesis and use of scientific findings only from randomized clinical trials,[25-29] while others define it more broadly to include the use of empirical evidence from other scientific methods (e.g., descriptive studies) and information from case reports and expert opinion.[30,31] Sackett et al[31] define evidence-based practice as "the integration of best research evidence with clinical expertise and patient values." The application of research findings in practice may not only improve quality care but may also create new and exciting questions for future research.

Multifaceted, active dissemination strategies are needed to promote the use of research evidence in clinical and administrative health care decision making. The strategies need to address *both* the individual practitioner and the organizational perspective. When nurses decide individually on which evidence to use in practice, considerable variability in practice patterns occurs and can result in adverse patient outcomes. For example, an individual EBP perspective would leave the decision about the use of evidence-based endotracheal suctioning techniques to each nurse. Some nurses might be familiar with the research findings for endotracheal suctioning, while others might not. Such a situation is likely to result in different and conflicting practices compounded by the fact that nurses change shifts every eight to twelve hours. From an organizational perspective, written policies and procedures are based on research, the evidence-based information is integrated into the CIS, and the adoption of practices by nurses is systematically promoted in the organization.

Models of Evidence-Based Practice

Multiple models of EBP and translation science are available.[4,12,24,32,33-42] Common elements of these models are syntheses of evidence, implementation, evaluation of the impact on patient care, and consideration of the context or setting in which the evidence is implemented (reviewing these models in more detail is beyond the scope of this chapter). To implement evidence in practice, a conceptual model is required to organize the strategies used and to elucidate the extraneous variables (e.g., behaviors and facilitators) that may influence the adoption of EBPs (e.g., organizational size, characteristics of users). The conceptual models used in the TRIP I and TRIP II studies, funded by the Agency for Healthcare Research and Quality (AHRQ), were adult learning, health education, social influence, marketing, organizational, and behavior theories.[9]

The Iowa Model of Evidence-Based Practice

The Iowa Model of Evidence-Based Practice to Promote Quality Care is an example of an EBP *practice* model (see Figure 22-1[24]). This model has been widely disseminated and adopted in academic and clinical settings.[24,43] It is an organizational, collaborative model that incorporates the conduct of research, the use of research evidence, and other types of evidence.[24]

The authors of the Iowa Model define EBP as the conscientious and judicious use of current best evidence to guide health care decisions.[44] The levels of evidence range from randomized clinical trials to case reports and expert opinion. In this model, knowledge- and problem-focused "triggers" lead staff members to question current nursing practice and to ask whether patient care can be improved through the use of research findings. If through literature review and the critique of studies, it is found that there are not a sufficient number of scientifically sound studies to use as a basis for practice, consideration is given to conducting a study. Nurses in practice collaborate with scientists in nursing and other disciplines to conduct clinical research that addresses practice problems encountered in the care of patients. The findings from such studies are then combined with findings from existing scientific knowledge to develop and implement the practices. If there is insufficient research to guide practice and conducting a study is not feasible, other types of evidence (e.g., case reports, expert opinion, scientific principles, theory) are used and/or combined with available research evidence to guide practice. Priority is given to projects in which a high proportion of practice is guided by research evidence. Practice guidelines usually reflect research and nonresearch evidence and therefore are called EBP guidelines.

Based on the relevant evidence, practices are recommended and compared with current practice, and a decision is made about the necessity for the practice change. When a change is warranted, it is implemented. Aligning the clinical documentation system components with the evidence-based components is essential for implementation. The practice is first implemented with a small group of patients, and an evaluation is carried out. The EBP is then refined based on evaluation data, and the change is implemented with additional patient populations for whom it is appropriate. The patient, the family, the staff, and fiscal outcomes are monitored.

Throughout the process, organizational and administrative support is important for success in using evidence in care delivery.

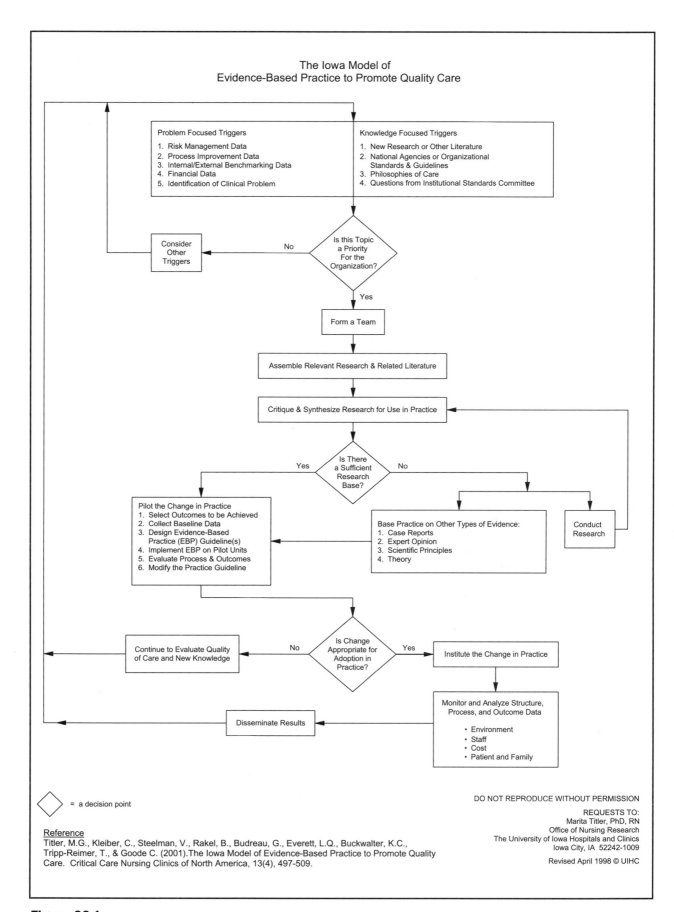

Figure 22-1. *Example of an Evidence-based Practice Model.*

Steps of Evidence-Based Practice

The Iowa Model of Evidence-Based Practice to Promote Quality Care[24,43] (see Figure 22-1), in conjunction with Rogers' Diffusion of Innovation Model[4,45,46] provides the guiding steps in actualizing EBP. A team approach is most helpful in fostering a specific EBP, with one person in the group providing the project leadership. The steps of EBP are outlined in Table 22-1, and the reader is referred to other sources for a more detailed description.[24,43] Table 22-2 illustrates using PICO—Patient/Population/Problem, Intervention/Treatment, Comparision Intervention, and Outcome(s)—to formulate the EBP question.

Table 22-1. Steps of Evidence-Based Practice

Step	Comment
Select a topic (e.g., pressure ulcer prevention).	Consider problem-focused and/or knowledge-focused triggers. Involve staff in topic selection.
Consider the priority of the topic for the organization.	Aligning the topic with organizational priorities assists in garnering administrative support and resources.
Form a team.	Consider stakeholders and disciplines affected by potential changes in practice related to the topic. An important task for the team is to formulate the evidence-based practice question (see Table 2).
Retrieve the evidence from the literature.	Include meta-analyses, research, synthesis reports, integrated literature reviews, and EBP guidelines.
Critique and grade the evidence.	Select a critique and grading system for research using a common form. Select a critique method and form for guidance (http://www.agreecollaboration.org/). Synthesize the reports and conduct an integrative review (http://www.sign.ac.uk/).
Synthesize the evidence and set forth practice recommendations.	Select evidence sources for inclusion in the synthesis based on specific criteria (e.g., age, patient population, quality and type of evidence source). Clearly indicate the type and strength of evidence for each practice recommendation.
Describe whether evidence findings are appropriate for use in practice.	Criteria to consider include: • Consistency of evidence from several sources • Characteristics of research samples similar to those of patient populations for whom they will be used • Risk/benefit ratio • Feasibility for practice • Cost-effectiveness
Write an evidence-based practice standard specific to the organization (e.g., localize the evidence).	Use a consistent format to reflect the type of evidence. Evidence sources should be reflected in the written standard. Provide key stakeholders with an opportunity to revise the written EBP standard.
Implement the EBP change in a pilot unit or area, and evaluate the process and outcome.	Multifaceted methods are needed to implement and sustain EBPs. Delete reference. Evaluate adherence to EBP and patient outcomes.
Revise or modify the EBP standard and/or implementation strategies based on the pilot and decide whether the EBP will be adopted by other units or in other areas.	Piloting an EB practice change is recommended to determine its effectiveness and feasibility in a clinical setting and to modify implementation strategies. Based on the pilot, determine the appropriateness of implementation in other clinical areas and develop an implementation plan for them.
Implement the EB practice changes in other areas as appropriate.	Strategies for implementation are available from Titler.[43]
Evaluate EBP changes.	Process and outcome indicators are selected and used as part of the quality improvement process.
Provide evaluative data to users.	Feed back data to users on an ongoing basis to illustrate the impact on quality of the care.
Continue to monitor new evidence and modify the EBP standard accordingly.	

Table 22-2. Using PICO to Formulate the EBP Question

	P **Patient/Population/ Problem**	**I** **Intervention/ Treatment**	**C** **Comparison Intervention**	**O** **Outcome(s)**
Tips for building the question	How would we describe a group of patients similar to ours?	Which main intervention are we considering?	What is the main alternative to compare with the intervention?	What can we hope to accomplish?
Example 1	Pain management for elders admitted to a hospital with a hip fracture	Pain assessment – pain tool Patient controlled analgesia	Standard of care Nurse administered analgesic	Regular (e.g., q 4 hrs.) pain assessment Less pain intensity Earlier mobility Decreased length of stay (LOS)
Example 2	Pain assessment of cognitively impaired elders	Pain assessment tool designed for assessing pain in cognitively impaired elders in long-term care setting	Not assess pain Yes/no question	Regular pain assessment with treatment of pain; fewer residents in pain

Source: Redrawn from University of Illinois at Chicago, PICO Model for Clinical Questions—http://www.uic.edu/depts/lib/lhsp/resources/pico.shtml.

The Role of Clinical Information Systems in the Implementation of EBPs

The emerging health information technology (HIT) revolution makes it possible to push the evidence to the point of care and to determine where practice and evidence diverge.[47] Rogers' seminal work on the diffusion of innovations[11] is an extremely useful framework for selecting strategies that promote the adoption of EBPs. According to this model, the adoption of innovations such as EBPs is influenced by the nature of the innovation (e.g., the type and strength of evidence, the clinical topic) and by the manner in which it is communicated (disseminated) to members (nurses) of a social system (an organization, the nursing profession).[4,45] CISs play an important role in actualizing strategies for each of these areas,[48] but the selection of health care information technology (HCIT) functions must be considered within a framework of EBP adoption to effectively use HCIT as a tool in fostering EBPs in clinical care delivery.

Nature of the EBP

The nature of the EBP topic influences adoption. For example, credible evidence (strength of practice recommendations) promotes knowledge uptake. EBPs developed from high-quality synthesis reports, guidelines, and research are more likely to be adopted than those with lower levels of evidence, but the strength of the evidence alone does not guarantee adoption.[49] The complexity of the evidence-based practice topic influences the length of time for implementation and overall adoption.[43,50,51] For example, the EBP for acute pain management is more complex than that for influenza immunization or breast cancer screening, and thus it will require more effort and take longer to implement. The potential advantage of the EBP to improve effectiveness, as perceived by clinicians, fosters evidence uptake; relative advantage alone, however, does not guarantee adoption.[52] If the implementation process encourages adaptation or the reinvention of guidelines by practitioners for use in their local agency, adherence to the EBP is increased.[4,43,52] Studies suggest that clinical systems, computerized decision support, and prompts that support practice (e.g., decision-making algorithms, equianalgesic chart) have a positive effect on aligning practices with the evidence base.[9,43,53-57] To move evidence from the "book to the bedside," information from EBPs must (1) have perceived benefits for patients, nurses, physicians, and administrators; (2) be "reinvented" and integrated into daily patient care processes; (3) impart evidence in a readily available format; and (4) make EBPs observable for practitioners.[11,12,47]

CISs should deploy the evidence base to the point of care and incorporate computer decision support system (CDSS) software to integrate evidence for use in clinical decision making about individual patients.[47,48] Evidence is infrequently available in a form that can be acted on at the time the clinical decision is made. In clinical encounters, there are few clear pathways from the evidence available through peer-reviewed synthesis reports to the point of decision making. Clinicians searching for the evidence all too often find that existing knowledge is not accessible in real time and may not necessarily map to the issue at hand.[47] Thus, CIS functionality must allow clinicians to see and learn the credibility of the evidence relevant to the clinical topic. An example is assessing pain in individuals with dementia. A CDSS that alerts users to assess acute pain every four hours should be linked to a detailed evidence source that explicates the evidence for this practice and that allows the user to pull up the evidence source as needed. As clinicians and others use computer-interpretable guidelines, it is essential that the evidence source, as well as the level and strength of evidence, be transparent.

CDSSs must meet three key criteria to be useful: (1) they must be based on the correct type of evidence for the decision; (2) they must take into account variations in patients and incorporate individual patient profiles and data; and (3) they must offer tailored advice that informs decision making.[49] Functions of CDSS for clinical decision making include:

1. **Alerting** (e.g., the values are out of range) and reminding (e.g., the patient is due for an influenza vaccine)
2. **Critiquing** (e.g., the dose is too high)
3. **Interpreting** (e.g., analyzing EKG rhythms)
4. **Diagnosing** (e.g, what are the possible differential diagnoses—heart failure, hypovolemeia, sepsis—for hemodynamic data, along with other clinical patient data?)
5. **Predicting** (e.g., what is the risk for pressure ulcer development from the Braden scale?)
6. **Assisting** (e.g., orders, such as antibiotics for individual patients, are tailored according to evidence-based parameters)
7. **Suggesting** (e.g, what actions can be taken to adjust mechanical ventilator settings to achieve better oxygenation?)[48]

Having clinicians notice and tend to computer-generated alerts, reminders, and critique messages involves complex system and screen design factors. Design factors (e.g., the user interface, the nature of the message, screen designs, and the context of care) are key to the safe and effective use of CDSS by clinicians.[58] Getting the attention of the person who can take action is one of the most difficult aspects of making these systems effective.[48] Thus, embedding the evidence base into the CIS is helpful but does not guarantee the use of the EBPs. Although HCIT and CDSSs can provide evidence at the point of care and assist with the application of the evidence in practice, additional strategies are necessary for knowledge uptake and use. These strategies are described in the following sections.

Methods of Communication

How the EBP standard is communicated to those delivering care affects the adoption of the practice.[45,59,60,61] The education of staff, the use of opinion leaders, change champions, core groups, and consultation by experts (e.g., advanced practice nurses) in the content area are essential components of the implementation process. *Continuing education* alone does little to change practice behavior.[28, 54,62,63,64] Interactive and didactic education, used in combination with other practice-reinforcing strategies, has more positive effects than education alone.[54,65-68] The staff must know the scientific basis for the changes in practice and the improvements in quality of care anticipated by the change. Disseminating this information to staff needs to be done creatively, using various educational strategies, including computer-assisted instruction and competency testing. Although it is unrealistic for all staff to participate in the critique of the evidence, they should know the myths and realities of the practice. The education of staff must also include ensuring that they are competent in the skills necessary to carry out the new practice. For example, when a pain assessment tool is being implemented to assess pain in cognitively impaired elderly individuals, caregivers must have the knowledge and skill to use the tool in their practice setting.

Several studies have demonstrated that *opinion leaders* (OLs) are effective in promoting the adoption of EBPs.[50,54,66,69-71] OLs are from the local peer group, viewed as respected sources of influence, considered by associates as technically competent, and trusted to judge the fit between the EBP and the local situation.[54,69,72,73] OLs use the EBP, influence peers, and alter group norms.[11,74] The key characteristic of an OL is that he or she is trusted to evaluate new information in the context of group norms. To do this, an OL must be considered by associates as technically competent and a full and dedicated member of the local group.[1,54,69] Social interactions such as hall-way chats, one-on-one discussions, and addressing questions are important but often overlooked components of translation.[11,12] Thus, having local OLs (early adopters) discuss the EBPs (e.g., four-hour pain assessments and use of pain assessment reminders in the CIS) with members of their peer group is necessary to translate research into practice. When the EBP change being implemented is interdisciplinary (e.g., pain management), it is best to select an opinion leader for each discipline (nursing, medicine, pharmacy).[75]

Change champions are necessary for implementing EBP changes in practice.[11,51,76-78] They are practitioners within the local group who are expert clinicians, passionate about the clinical topic, committed to improving the quality of care, and able to work positively with other health profession-als.[11,76,78-80] They circulate information, encourage peers to align their practice with the best evidence, arrange demonstrations, and orient staff to the EBP.[51,77] Change champions believe in an idea, do not take no for an answer, are undaunted by insults and rebuffs, and above all persist.[72] For potential evidence-based changes in practice to be enacted at the point of care, one or two change champions must be identified for each patient care unit or service for which the change is being made.[81]

Outreach and consultation by an expert promote positive changes in the practice behaviors of nurses and physicians.[82,83] *Outreach (academic detailing)* is accomplished by an expert who meets one on one with practitioners in their setting to provide not only information about the EBP, but also feedback on provider performance.[54,82-85] This strategy alone or in combination with others results in positive changes in health care practices.[82,83,85-88] Advanced practice nurses (APNs) can provide one-on-one consultation to staff regarding the use of the EBP with specific patients, assist staff in troubleshooting issues in the application of the practice, and provide feedback on provider perform-ance regarding the use of the EBPs. Studies have demonstrated that the use of APNs as facilitators of change promotes adherence to the EBP.[81,82,89]

Users of the Innovation/EBP

Members of a social system influence how quickly and widely EBPs are adopted.[11] Performance gap assessment (PGA), audit and feedback, and trying the EBP are strategies that have been tested.[11,24,90-96] PGA and audit and feedback have consistently shown a positive effect on changing the practice behavior of providers.[85,92,95,97,98]

BPP (baseline practice performance) informs members, at the *beginning* of change, about a practice performance and opportunities for improvement. Specific practice indicators selected for performance gap assessment are related to the EBPs that are the focus of change, such as every four-hour pain assessment for acute pain management.

The strategy of *audit and feedback* is the ongoing audit of performance indicators (e.g., every four-hour pain assessment) throughout the implementation process and the discussion of the find-ings with practitioners *during* the practice change.[51,99] This strategy helps staff know and see how their efforts to improve care and patient outcomes are progressing throughout the implementation process. Audit and feedback should be done at regular intervals throughout the implementation process (e.g., every four to six weeks).[95,99] Performance gap assessment and audit and feedback data can be provided in run charts, statistical process control charts, or bar graphs.[100]

When planning CISs, developers and users should consider architecture and functionality that can aggregate and report real-time indicators for core clinical care processes and outcomes, includ-ing symptom management, function, and self-care management. The system should be flexible enough to allow the modification of indicators to aggregate specified clinical indicator data for performance gap assessment prior to implementation, the audit and feedback of data during implementation, and the evaluation of improvements in care quality following implementation. This type of functionality automates data collection and analyses of clinical care to illustrate where and why practice diverges from the evidence base. A well-designed health information infrastructure reduces the burden of quality assessment, enables timely feedback of performance, and provides the necessary electronic data repositories to conduct large-scale outcomes effectiveness research.[47,101] Using real-time detailed clinical data from large patient cohorts can expedite enrollment in prospective studies, as well as data collection and management.[63]

Characteristics of users (such as educational preparation, practice specialty, and views on innovativeness) influence the adoption of an innovation.[11,64,77,102,103] Users of an innovation usually try it for a period before adopting it in their practice.[11,104] When *trying an EBP* (piloting the change) is incorporated as part of the implementation process, users have an opportunity to use it for a period, provide feedback to those in charge of implementation, and modify the practice when necessary. Piloting the EBP as part of implementation has a positive influence on its adoption.[11,24,77,91] The CIS and its user interface should facilitate this trial rather than hinder the adoption of the EBP. Thus the CDSS functions and those explicating the evidence base also need to be tried in practice to make it easy to do the right thing.

Social System

The social system (context) has a high degree of influence on the adoption of an innovation.[11,14,24,105-110] Chief nurse executives and their leadership staff set the stage and culture for EBP in their settings.[12,41,43,111-118] How they do this varies, but the essential components include expressed verbal and written support, along with the provision of the necessary resources, materials, and time to fulfill assigned responsibilities.[43,111,119] Additional organizational variables that influence adoption include (1) access to inventors and researchers, (2) the authority to change practice; and (3) support from and collaboration with peers, other disciplines, and administrators to align practice with EBPs.[43,71,112,120,121]

Organizational and unit practice standards, as well as documentation systems, must support the use of the EBPs.[51,119] The role of the nurse manager is critical in making EBP changes a reality for staff at the bedside. Nurse managers must expect that staff will participate in the change to EBP, model it in their practice, and provide written and verbal support for it. When selecting a potential topic, the nurse manager has to value the idea and support the potential changes.

As part of the work of implementing the change, the social system—unit, service line, and/or clinic—must ensure that the policies, procedures, standards, clinical pathways, and documentation systems support the use of the EBPs. Documentation forms or CISs might need revision to support changes in practice; documentation systems that fail to readily support the new practice thwart change. For example, if staff members are expected to reassess and document pain intensity within thirty minutes following the administration of an analgesic agent, then documentation forms and CISs must reflect this practice standard. The role of upper- and middle-level leadership is to ensure that organizational documents and systems are flexible and supportive of the EBPs. In summary, making an EB change in practice involves a series of steps and a process that is often nonlinear. Implementing the change takes several weeks to months, depending on its nature. Those leading the project must be aware of change as a process, and they must continue to encourage and teach peers about the change. The new practice must be continually reinforced and sustained, or the change will be intermittent and soon fade, allowing more traditional methods of care to return.

Evaluation of EB (Evidence Based) Changes in Practice

Evaluation provides an opportunity to analyze data on the use of a new EBP and then to modify the practice as necessary. The EB change has to be evaluated, both in the pilot area and later in the additional patient care areas. The importance of the evaluation cannot be overemphasized; it provides information for performance gap assessment, for audit and feedback, and for determining whether the EBP should be retained, modified, or eliminated. Well-designed CIS can reduce the burden of data collection and provide a rich data source for evaluation and timely feedback on performance. A desired outcome achieved in a relatively controlled environment, when a researcher is implementing a study protocol for a homogeneous group of patients (conduct of research), might not be the same when the practice is implemented in the natural clinical setting, by several caregivers, to a more heterogeneous patient population.

Evaluation should include both process and outcome measures.[39,43,122] The *process* component focuses on how the EBP change is being implemented. Are the staff using the practice in care delivery, and are they implementing the practice as noted in the organization's EBP standard? Process data can be collected from staff and/or patient self-reports, from electronic medical records or other electronic data sources, or from the observation of clinical practice.

Outcome data are an equally important part of evaluation to assess whether the expected patient, staff, and/or fiscal outcomes are achieved. Therefore, the baseline data must be used for a pre- and postcomparison.[24] The outcome variables measured should be those that are projected to change as a result of the new practice.[39,40] For example, research demonstrates that less restricted family visiting practices in critical care units result in improved satisfaction with care. Thus patient and family member satisfaction should be an outcome measure that is evaluated as part of changing visiting practices in adult critical care units. Outcome measures should be measured before the change is implemented, after implementation, and every six to twelve months thereafter. Findings must be provided to clinicians to reinforce the impact of the change in practice and to ensure that the findings are incorporated into quality improvement programs.

The evaluation process includes planned feedback to staff who are making the change. The feedback includes verbal and/or written appreciation for the work and a visual demonstration of progress in implementation and improvement in patient outcomes. HCIT developers should consider data aggregation and feedback as essential components in a well-designed CIS. The key to effective evaluation is to ensure that the EB change in practice is warranted (i.e., it will improve quality of care) and that the intervention does not bring harm to patients.[122] For example, when instituting a change in practice for assessing the return of bowel motility following abdominal surgery in adults, it was important to inform staff that using markers other than bowel sound assessment for the return of bowel motility did not result in increased paralytic *ileus* or bowel obstruction.[123]

The HCIT and EBP Interface: Challenges for the Future

Most hospitals lack an information infrastructure to use evidence at the point of care or to measure performance easily. The recently announced decade of HIT, however, offers unparalleled opportunities to develop and implement strategies that bring evidence-based information to the point of care.[47] Yet developing and implementing HCIT that supports EBP faces several challenges, including:

1. Making the evidence base for the practice transparent to the user
2. Keeping the evidence-based information current
3. Forging collaborative relationships between the public and private sectors to understand which HCIT functions promote the adoption of EBPs
4. Developing interoperable electronic health records that can be used across systems, sites, and levels of care delivery

Clinical decision support for EBP must be implemented in a way that balances the transparency of the data source and the strength of evidence with legitimate private sector incentives to deploy workable electronic solutions for clinicians and consumers. Implementing EBPs requires more than bringing evidence to the point of care through HCIT technology. Advances in HCIT must be linked with the redesign of care processes, the development of ways to deliver the right information at the right time to the right patient, and constructing infrastructures to ensure that the evidence underlying CDSS remains current. Knowledge databases that house EB information should be maintained in computer-interpretable formats to facilitate effective care in practices that adopt EHR.[124,125] Will computer-interpretable guidelines require governance and oversight to ensure the application of the most recent evidence? Although experts suggest that the customization of evidence should be left to individual organizations and clinicians, at what point might this practice increase variations in care rather than decrease them? The flexibility and integrity of HCIT tools are essential for evidence to be delivered at the point of care.

The Veterans Health Administration, the largest health system in the U.S., has transformed care delivery through performance measurement, timely data feedback, and information systems that increasingly support clinicians, managers, and patients in achieving EBP. Because these improvements involved several interventions (e.g., HCIT, performance measurement, patient-centric focus) that were initiated as strategic initiatives rather than as an experimental design, it is difficult to understand the unique contributions of each intervention such as new HCIT.[126] It is reasonable, however, to conclude that some aspects of the EHR—such as critical alerts, reminders, and CPOE—have contributed to these improvements. Clinical performance in selected areas at the VA improved more rapidly and substantially than in other health care settings, and the measured performance improved more substantially than unmeasured performance even within the VA.[126] The EHR and HCIT were integral components of these transformations.

Capitalizing on HCIT to promote the use of evidence at the point of care is not about limiting options or replacing clinical judgment; it is about assisting clinicians in choosing options that are most likely to improve health outcomes while containing costs.[47] Shojania and Grimshaw[57] warn, however, that many strategies are being suggested as the magic cure for delivery of evidence-based care with minimal empirical evidence and that "the wonder pill most frequently encountered currently is in fact the 'wonder clinical information system' despite the often glaring discrepancy between the promise of systems in showrooms and the way they perform in the real world."[57] HCIT alone does not guarantee the adoption of EBPs, but it can be a tool that drives EB information to the point of care for use. The interface between the user and HCIT is an important component of the agenda, and so is integration with additional strategies that promote EBPs, such as the context of care, the communication mechanisms, the perceived importance of the clinical topic, and the users of the EBP information.

Future Directions

For organizations to take advantage of EBP projects from various sites throughout the country, a national center for EBP and translation science is needed. Such a center would encompass an electronic data repository of EBPs that includes:
1. The relevant policy and procedure or practice standard with links to evidence references
2. The population to which it applies
3. The quality improvement indicators (data definitions) and data collection forms used in evaluation
4. A list of references
5. The suggested strategies for implementation
6. The type of institutions where the EBP has been implemented
7. Contact people at each agency
8. The EBP topic content expert

This information should be available online through electronic communications, e.g., a dedicated list serve, the Virtual Hospital System, or some other form of electronic media. The center could facilitate networking among health care professionals working on similar EB topics and provide helpful consultants and educational materials.[127] It could also serve as an electronic data repository for interventions and strategies that have been tested to translate research into practice and provide a "tool kit" of interventions for use by all types of health care agencies.[128-130] For example, the tool kit on the use of opinion leaders to translate research into practice might include a definition of opinion leader, the characteristics of an opinion leader, how to select an opinion leader, the function of the opinion leader, in what types of settings and projects opinion leaders have been used effectively, and methods to evaluate the effect of using opinion leaders in promoting the adoption of certain EBPs. Lastly, such a center would also conduct translational research and provide consultation regarding research methods and design for translation science.[51]

Acknowledgement

The author would like to acknowledge Kim Jordan for her superb assistance in preparing the manuscript for publication.

References

1. Institute of Medicine. *Priority Areas for National Action: Transforming Health Care Quality.* Washington, DC: National Academy Press; 2003.

2. Health Grades Inc. *Health Grades Quality Study: Patient Safety in American Hospitals.* Golden, CO: Health Grades, Inc.; 2004.

3. Goode C, Bulechek GM. Research utilization: an organizational process that enhances quality of care. *J Nurs Care* Quality. 1992; (special report):27-35.

4. Titler MG, Everett LQ. Translating research into practice: considerations for critical care investigators. *Crit Care Nurs Clin North Am.* 2001a;13(4):587-604.

5. Feldman PH, Kane RL. Strengthening research to improve the practice and management of long-term care. *Milbank Q.* 2003;81(2):179-220.

6. Lavis JN, Robertson D, Woodside JM, et al. for the Knowledge Transfer Study Group. How can research organizations more effectively transfer research knowledge to decision makers? *Milbank Q.* 2003; 81(2):221-248.

7. Dopson S, Locock L, Chambers D, Gabbay J. Implementation of evidence-based medicine: evaluation of the Promoting Action on Clinical Effectiveness programme. *J Health Serv Res Policy.* 2001;6(1):23-31.

8. Dopson S, FitzGerald L, Ferlie E, Gabbay J, Locock L. No magic targets! Changing clinical practice to become more evidence based. *Health Care Manage Rev.* 2002;27(3):35-47.

9. Farquhar CM, Stryer D, Slutsky J. Translating research into practice: the future ahead. *Int J Qual Health Care.* 2002;14(3):233-249.

10. Jennings BM, Loan LA. Misconceptions among nurses about evidence-based practice. *J Nurs Scholarship.* 2001;33(2):121-127.

11. Rogers EM. *Diffusion of Innovations.* 5th ed. New York: The Free Press; 2003.

12. Berwick DM. Disseminating innovations in health care. *JAMA.* 2003;289(15):1969-1975.

13. Gillbody S, Whitty P, Grimshaw J, Thomas R. Educational and organizational interventions to improve the management of depression in primary care (a systematic review). *JAMA.* 2003;289 (23):3145-3151.

14. Institute of Medicine. *Crossing the Quality Chasm: A New Health System for the 21st Century.* Washington, DC: National Academy Press; 2001.

15. Institute of Medicine. *Patient Safety: Achieving a New Standard for Care.* Washington, DC: The National Academies Press; 2004.

16. Silagy CA. Evidence-based health care 10 years on: is the National Institute of Clinical Studies the answer? *Med J Australia.* 2001;175(3):124-125.

17. Demakis JG, McQueen L, Kizer KW, Feussner JR. Quality Enhancement Research Initiative (QUERI): a collaboration between research and clinical practice. *Med Care.* 2000;38(6,suppl I):I17-25.

18. Agency for Healthcare Research and Quality. Available at: http://www.ahrq.gov. Retrieved August 1, 2003.

19. Doebbeling BN, Vaughn TE, Woolson RF, et al. Benchmarking Veterans Affairs Medical Centers in the delivery of preventive health services: comparison of methods. *Med Care.* 2002;40(6):540-554.

20. Dykes PC. Practice guidelines and measurement: state-of-the-science. *Nurs Outlook.* 2003;51:65-69.

21. Eisenberg JM, Kamerow DB. The Agency for Healthcare Research and Quality and the U.S. Preventive Services Task Force: public support for translating evidence into prevention practice and policy. *Am J Prev Med.* 2001;20(3S):1-2.

22. Katz DA, Muehlenbruch DR, Brown RB, Fiore MC, Baker TB. Effectiveness of a clinic-based strategy for implementing the AHRQ Smoking Cessation Guideline in primary care. *Prevent Med.* 2002;35:293-302.

23. Vaughn TE, McCoy KD, Bootsmiller BJ, et al. Organizational predictors of adherence to ambulatory care screening guidelines. *Med Care.* 2002;40 (12):1172-1185.

24. Titler MG, Kleiber C, Steelman VJ, et al. The Iowa Model of Evidence-Based Practice to Promote Quality Care. *Critical Care Nursing Clinics of North America.* 2001;13(4):497-509.

25. Dickersin K, Manheimer E. The Cochrane Collaboration: evaluation of health care and services using systematic reviews of the results of randomized controlled trials. *Clin Obstet Gynecol.* 1998; 41(2):315-331.

26. Estabrooks CA. Will evidence-based nursing practice make practice perfect? *Canadian J Nurs Res.* 1998; 30(1):15-36.

27. Estabrooks CA. Thoughts on evidence-based nursing and its science: a Canadian perspective. *Worldviews on Evidence-Based Nursing.* 2004;1(2):88-91.

28. Geyman JP. Evidence-based medicine in primary care: an overview. *J Am Board Fam Pract.* 1998; 11(1):46-56.

29. Mion LC. Evidence-based health care practice. *J Gerontological Nurs.* 1998;24(12):5-6.

30. Cook D. Evidence-based critical care medicine: a potential tool for change. *New Horizons.* 1998; 6(1):20-25.

31. Sackett DL, Straus SE, Richardson WS, Rosenberg W, Haynes RB. *Evidence-Based Medicine: How to Practice and Teach EBM.* London: Churchill Livingstones; 2000.

32. Rycroft-Malone J, Kitson A, Harvey G, et al. Ingredients for change: revisiting a conceptual framework. *Quality and Safety in Health Care.* 2002; 11:174-180.

33. Barnsteiner JH, Ford N, Howe C. Research utilization in a metropolitan children's hospital. *Nurs Clin North Am.* 1995:30(3):447-455.

34. Dufault MA. A program of research evaluating the effects of collaborative research utilization model. *Online J Knowledge Synthesis Nurs.* 2001;8(3):7.

35. Dufault MA. Testing a collaborative research utilization model to translate best practices in pain management. *Worldviews on Evidence-Based Nursing.* 2004; 1:S1,S26-S32.

36. Goode CJ, Piedalue F. Evidence-based clinical practice. *JONA.* 1999;29(6):15-21.

37. Logan J, Harrison MB, Graham ID, Dunn K, Bissonnette J. Evidence-based pressure-ulcer practice: the Ottawa Model of Research Use. *Canadian J Nurs Res.* 1999;31(1):37-52.

38. Olade RA. Evidence-based practice and research utilization activities among rural nurses. *J Nurs Scholarship.* 2004;36(3):220-225.

39. Rosswurm MA, Larrabee JH. A model for change to evidence-based practice. Image: *J Nurs Scholarship.* 1999;31(4):317-322.

40. Soukup SM. The center for advanced nursing practice evidence-based practice model. *Nurs Clin North Am.* 2000;35(2):301-309.

41. Stetler CB. Role of the organization in translating research into evidence-based practice. *Outcomes Manage.* 2003;7(3):97-105.

42. Wagner EH, Austin BT, Davis C, et al. Improving chronic illness care: translating evidence into action. *Health Affairs (Millwood).* 2001;20:64-78.

43. Titler MG. Developing an evidence-based practice. In: LoBiondo-Wood G, Haber J, eds. *Nursing Research.* 5th ed. St. Louis: Mosby-Year Book, Inc. In press.

44. Sackett D, Rosenberg W, Gray J, Haynes R, Richardson W. Evidence based medicine: what it is and what it isn't. *BMJ.* 1996;312:71-72.

45. Rogers EM. *Diffusion of Innovations.* New York: The Free Press; 1995.

46. Rogers EM. Innovation in organizations. In: Rogers EM, ed. *Diffusion of Innovations.* 5th ed. New York: Free Press; 2003.

47. Clancy CM, Cronin K. Evidence-based decision making: global evidence, local decisions. *Health Affairs.* 2005;24(1):151-162.

48. Thompson CJ, Dowding D, Guyatt G. Computer decision support systems. In: DiCenso A, Guyatt G, Ciliska D, eds. *Evidence-Based Nursing: A Guide to Clinical Practice.* St. Louis: Mosby, Inc.; 2005.

49. Grimshaw JM, Thomas RE, MacLennan G, et al. Effectiveness and efficiency of guide dissemination and implementation strategies. *Health Technol Assess.* 2004;8(6):i-xi,1-72.

50. Berner ES, Baker CS, Funkhouser E, et al. Do local opinion leaders augment hospital quality improvement efforts? A randomized trial to promote adherence to unstable angina guideline. *Med Care.* 2003;41(3);420-431.

51. Titler MG. Methods in translation science. *Worldviews on Evidence-Based Nursing.* 2004;1: 38-48.

52. Greenhalgh T, Robert G, MacFarlane F, Bate P, Kyriakidou O. Diffusion of innovations in service organizations: systematic review and recommendations. *Milbank Q.* 2004;82(4):581-629.

53. Cook DJ, Greengold NL, Ellrodt AG, Weingarten SR. The relation between systematic reviews and practice guidelines. *Ann Intern Med.* 1997;127(3):210-216.

54. Oxman AD, Thomson MA, Davis DA, Haynes RB. No magic bullets: a systematic review of 102 trials of interventions to improve professional practice. *Can Med Assoc J.* 1995;153(10):1423-1431.

55. Hunt DL, Haynes RB, Hanna SE, Smith K. Effects of computer-based clinical decision support systems on physician performance and patient outcomes: a systematic review. *JAMA.* 1998:280(15):1339-1346.

56. Schmidt KL, Alpen MA, Rakel BA. Implementation of the Agency for Health Care Policy and Research Pain Guidelines. *AACN Clinical Issues.* 1996; 7(3):425-435.

57. Shojania KG, Grimshaw JM. Evidence-based quality improvement: the state of the science. *Health Affairs.* 2005:24(1):138-150.

58. Fung CH, Woods JN, Asch SM, Glassman P, Doebbeling BN. Variation in implementation and use of computerized clinical reminders in an integrated health care system. *American Journal of Managed Care.* 2004;10(Part 2):878-885.

59. Carroll DL, Greenwood R, Lynch KE, et al. Barriers and facilitators to the utilization of nursing research. *Clin Nurse Specialist.* 1997;11(5):207-212.

60. Funk SG, Tornquist EM, Champagne MT. Barriers and facilitators of research utilization: an integrative review. In: Titler M, Goode C, eds. *The Nursing Clinics of North America.* Vol 30. Philadelphia: W.B. Saunders Company; 1995:395-408.

61. Wells N, Baggs JG. A survey of practicing nurses' research interests and activities. *Clinical Nurse Specialist.* 1994;8:145-151.

62. Dalton JA, Blau W, Carlson J, et al. Changing the relationship among nurses' knowledge, self-reported behavior, and documented behavior in pain management: does education make a difference? *J Pain Symptom Manage.* 1996;12(5):308-319.

63. Mazmanian PE, Daffron SR, Johnson RE, Davis DA, Kantrowitz MP. Information about barriers to planned change: a randomized controlled trial involving continuing medical education lectures and commitment to change. *Academic Med.* 1998;73(8):882-886.

64. Retchin SM. The modification of physician practice patterns. *Clin Performance Quality Health Care.* 1997:5:202-207.

65. Anderson JF, McEwan KL, Hrudey WP. Effectiveness of notification and group education in modifying prescribing of regulated analgesics. *Can Med Assoc J.* 1996;154(1):31-39.

66. Bero LA, Grilli R, Grimshaw JM, et al. Closing the gap between research and practice: an overview of systematic reviews of interventions to promote the implementation of research findings. *BMJ.* 1998; 317:465-468.

67. Elliott TE, Murray DM, Oken MM, et al. Improving cancer pain management in communities: main results from a randomized controlled trial. *J Pain Symptom Manage.* 1997;13(4):191-203.

68. Bookbinder M, Coyle N, Kiss M, et al. Implementing national standards for cancer pain management: program model and evaluation. *J Pain Symptom Manage.* 1996;12(6);334-347.

69. Soumerai SB, McLaughlin TJ, Gurwitz JH, et al. Effect of local medical opinion leaders on quality of care for acute myocardial infarction: a randomized controlled trial. *JAMA.* 1998;279(17):1358-1363.

70. Locock L, Dopson S, Chambers D, Gabbay J. Understanding the role of opinion leaders in improving clinical effectiveness. *Soc Sci Med. 20*01;53:745-757.

71. Thomson O'Brien MA, Oxman AD, Haynes RB, et al. Local opinion leaders: effects on professional practice and health care outcomes (Cochrane Review). *The Cochrane Library.* 2002;2.

72. Greer AL. The state of the art versus the state of the science. *Intl J Technol Assess Health Care.* 1988;4:5-26.

73. Goodpastor WA, Montoya ID. Motivating physician behavior change: social influence versus financial contingencies. *Int J Health Care Quality Assurance.* 1996;9(6):4-9.

74. Collins BA, Hawks JW, Davis RL. From theory to practice: identifying authentic opinion leaders to improve care. *Managed Care.* July 2000:56-62.

75. Backer TE. Research utilization and managing innovation in rehabilitation organizations. *J Rehabil.* 1987;54:18-22.

76. Backer TE. Integrating behavioral and systems strategies to change clinical practice. *Joint Commission J Quality Improvement.* 1995;21(7):351-353.

77. Shively M, Riegel B, Waterhouse D, et al. Testing a community level research utilization intervention. *Appl Nurs Res.* 1997;10(3):121-127.

78. Titler MG, Mentes JC. Research utilization in gerontological nursing practice. *Journal of Gerontological Nurs.* 1996;25(6):6-9.

79. Titler MG. Use of research in practice. In: LoBiondo-Wood G, Haber J, eds. *Nursing Research.* 4th ed. St. Louis: Mosby-Year Book, Inc.; 1998.

80. Harvey G, Loftus-Hills A, Rycroft-Malone J, et al. Getting evidence into practice: the role and function of facilitation. *J Adv Nurs.* 2002;37(6):577-588.

81. Titler M. *TRIP intervention saves healthcare dollars and improves quality of care (abstract/poster).* Paper presented at: Translating Research into Practice: What's Working? What's Missing? What's Next? Sponsored by the Agency for Healthcare Research and Quality; July 22-24, 2003; Washington, DC.

82. Hendryx MS, Fieselmann JF, Bock MJ, et al. Outreach education to improve quality of rural ICU care. results of a randomized trial. *Am J Respir Crit Care Med.* 1998;158(2):418-423.

83. Thomson O'Brien MA, Oxman AD, Davis DA, et al. Educational outreach visits: effects on professional practice and health care outcomes. *The Cochrane Library.* 2003;2.

84. Hulscher ME, van Drenth BB, van der Wouden JC, et al. Changing preventive practice: a controlled trial on the effects of outreach visits to organise prevention of cardiovascular disease. *Quality Health Care.* 1997;6(1):19-24.

85. Thomson O'Brien MA, Oxman AD, Davis DA, et al. Audit and feedback versus alternative strategies: effects on professional practice and health care outcomes. *The Cochrane Library.* 2003;2.

86. Pippalla RS, Riley DA, Chinburapa V. Influencing the prescribing behavior of physicians: a meta evaluation. *J Clin PharmTher.* 1995;20:189-198.

87. Jiang HJ, Fieselmann JF, Hendryx MS, Bock MJ. Assessing the impact of patient characteristics and process performance on rural intensive care unit hospital mortality rates. *Crit Care Med.* 1997;25(5):773-778.

88. White CL. Changing pain management practice and impacting on patient outcomes. *Clin Nurse Specialist.* 1999;13(4):166-172.

89. Bauchner H, Simpson L. Specific issues related to developing, disseminating, and implementing pediatric practice guidelines for physicians, patients, families, and other stakeholders. *Health Services Res.* 1998;33(4):1161-1177.

90. Titler MG, Kleiber C, Steelman V, et al. Infusing research into practice to promote quality care. *Nurs Res.* 1994;43(5):307-313.

91. Titler MG, Moss L, Greiner J, et al. Research utilization in critical care: an exemplar. *AACN Clinical Issues.* 1994;5(2):124-132.

92. Eisenberg JM. Other approaches to changing physicians' practice. *Doctors' Decisions and the Cost of Medical Care: The Reasons for Doctors' Practice Patterns and Ways to Change Them.* Ann Arbor, MI: Health Administration Press Perspectives; 1986:125-142.

93. Schroeder SA. Strategies for reducing medical costs by changing physicians' behavior: efficacy and impact on quality of care. *Int J Technol Assess Health Care.* 1987;3:39-50.

94. Berwick DM, Coltin KL. Feedback reduces test use in a health maintenance organization. *JAMA.* 1986;255:1450-1454.

95. Eagle KA, Mulley AG, Skates SJ, et al. Length of stay in the intensive care units: effects of practice guidelines and feedback. *JAMA.* 1990;264:992-997.

96. Winickoff RN, Coltin KL, Morgan MM, Buxbaum RC, Barnett GO. Improving physician performance through peer comparison feedback. *Med Care.* 1984;22:527-534.

97. Fiore MC, Bailey WC, Cohen SJ, et al. *Smoking Cessation: Information for Specialists.* Rockville, MD: U.S. Department of Health and Human Services, Public Health Service, Agency for Health Care Policy and Research and Centers for Disease Control and Prevention; April 1996. AHCPR Pub. No 96-0694.

98. McCartney P, Macdowall W, Thorogood M. Feedback to general practitioners increased prescribing of aspiring to patients with ischaemic heart disease. *BMJ.* 1997;315:35-36.

99. Jamtvedt G, Young JM, Kristoffersen DT, Thomson O'Brien MA, Oxman AD. Audit and feedback: effects on professional practice and health care outcomes (Cochrane Review). *The Cochrane Library.* 2001;1.

100. Carey RA. *Improving Healthcare with Control Charts: Basic and Advanced SPC Methods and Case Studies.* Milwaukee, WI: American Society for Quality; 2002.

101. Titler MG, Dochterman J, Reed D. *Guideline for Conducting Effectiveness Research in Nursing and Other Healthcare Services.* Iowa City, IA: University of Iowa College of Nursing, Center for Nursing Classification & Clinical Effectiveness; 2004.

102. Rutledge DN, Greene P, Mooney K, Nail LM, Ropka M. Use of research-based practices by oncology staff nurses. *Oncol Nurs Forum.* 1996;23(8):1235-1244.

103. Salem-Schatz SR, Gottlieb LK, Karp MA, Feingold L. Attitudes about clinical practice guidelines in a mixed model HMO: the influence of physician and organizational characteristics. *HMO Pract.* 1997; 11(3):111-117.

104. Meyer AD, Goes JB. Organizational assimilation of innovations: a multilevel contextual analysis. *Acad Manage J.* 1988;31:897-923.

105. Morin KH, Bucher L, Plowfield L, at al. Using research to establish protocols for practice: a statewide study of acute care agencies. *Clin Nurse Specialist.* 1999;13(2):77-84.

106. Thompson CJ. The meaning of research utilization: a preliminary typology. *Crit Care Nurs Clin North Am.* 2001;13(4):475-485.

107. Foxcroft DR, Cole N, Fulbrook P, Johnston L, Stevens K. Organisational infrastructures to promote evidence based nursing practice (Protocol for a Cochrane Review). *The Cochrane Library.* 2002;2.

108. Ciliska D, Hayward S, Dobbins M, Brunton G, Underwood J. Transferring public-health nursing research to health-system planning: assessing the relevance and accessibility of systematic reviews. *Can J Nurs Res.* 1999;31(1):23-36.

109. Fraser I. Organizational research with impact: working backwards. *Worldviews on Evidence-Based Nurs.* 2004a;1(S1):S52-S59.

110. Fraser I. (2004b). Translation research: where do we go from here? *Worldviews on Evidence-Based Nurs.* 2004b;1(S1):S78-S83.

111. Omery A, Williams RP. An appraisal of research utilization across the United States. *Nurs Adm.* 1999;29(12):50-56.

112. Shortell SM, O'Brien JL, Carmen JM, et al. Assessing the impact of continuous quality improvement/total quality management: concept versus implementation. *Health Services Res.* 1995;30:377-401.

113. Carr CA, Schott A. Differences in evidence-based care in midwifery practice and education. *J Nurs Scholarship.* 2002;34(2):153-158.

114. Antrobus S, Kitson A. Nursing leadership: influencing and shaping health policy and nursing practice. *J Adv Nurs.* 1999;29(3):746-753.

115. Baggs JG, Mick DJ. Collaboration: a tool addressing ethical issues for elderly patients near the end of life in intensive care units. *J Gerontological Nurs.* 2000;26(9):41-47.

116. Nagy S, Lumby J, McKinley S, Macfarlane C. Nurses' beliefs about the conditions that hinder or support evidence-based nursing. *Int J Nurs Pract.* 2001;7(5):314-321.

117. Retsas A. Barriers to using research evidence in nursing practice. *J Adv Nurs.* 2000;31(3):599-606.

118. Titler MG, Mentes JC, Rakel BA, Abbott L, Baumler S. From book to bedside: putting evidence to use in the care of the elderly. *J Quality Imp.* 1999; 25(10):545-556.

119. Rutledge DN, Donaldson NE. Building organizational capacity to engage in research utilization. *JONA.* 1995;25(10):12-16.

120. Tranmer JE, Coulson K, Holtom D, Lively T, Maloney R. The emergence of a culture that promotes evidence based clinical decision making within an acute care setting. *Can J Nurs Admin.* 1998;11(2): 36-58.

121. Walshe K, Rundall TG. Evidence-based management: from theory to practice in health care. *Milbank Q.* 2001;79(3);429-457.

122. Lepper HS, Titler MG. Program evaluation. In: Mateo MA, Kirchhoff KT, eds. *Using and Conducting Nursing Research in the Clinical Setting.* 2nd ed. Philadelphia: W.B. Saunders Company; 1999:90-104.

123. Madsen D, Sebolt T, Cullen L, et al. Why listen to bowel sounds? Report of an evidence-based practice project. *Am J Nurs.* In review.

124. Sim I, Gorman P, Greenes RA, et al. Clinical decision support systems for the practice of evidence-based medicine. *JAMIA.* 2003;8(6);527-534.

125. Casalino L, Gillies RR, Shortell SM, et al. External incentives information technology, and organized processes to improve health care quality for patients with chronic diseases. *JAMIA.* 2003;289(4):434-441.

126. Perlin JB, Kolodner RM, Roswell RH. The Veterans Health Administration: quality value, accountability and information as transforming strategies for patient-centered care. *Am J Managed Care.* 2004; 10(part 2):828-836.

127. Titler MG. Research utilization: necessity or luxury? In: McCloskey JC, Grace H, eds. *Current Issues in Nursing.* 5th ed. St. Louis: Mosby; 1997.

128. Registered Nurses Association of Ontario. Implementation of clinical practice guidelines. Available at: http://www.rnao.org/bestpractices/completed_guidelines/BPG_Guide_C1_Toolkit.asp. Accessed November 30, 2004.

129. QUERI. Available at: http://www.hsrd.research.va.gov/queri/implementation/section_2/default.cfm. Accessed November 30, 2004.

130. Titler MG. *Toolkit for Promoting Evidence-Based Practice.* Iowa City, IA: Department of Nursing Services and Patient Care, University of Iowa Hospitals and Clinics; 2002.

Case Study 22A

Lessons on Evidence-based Practice from Florence Nightingale

Helen J. Betts, EdD, RN, and Graham Wright, DN, RN, RMN, RNT, RNCT, MBCS, CITP

Florence Nightingale was born in Florence, Italy, on May 12, 1820, the second daughter of William and Frances Nightingale. The family had two grand homes, one in Derbyshire and the other in Hampshire, England. However, they had a fairly nomadic lifestyle, moving between homes, going to London for the "season," and taking extensive tours of Europe. The sisters were educated at home, initially by a governess but later by their father.[1,2] Their education went beyond that expected of young Victorian ladies, and both girls were accomplished in many areas, including Latin, Greek, history, and mathematics. Nightingale was tutored in mathematics by James Sylvester, the celebrated mathematician who developed the theory of invariants with Arthur Cayley.[3] Statistics became a tool that Nightingale used to support her case in many of the reports she wrote on her return from the Crimean War. Indeed, some primarily regard Miss Nightingale as a great statistician, rather than as the founder of modern nursing.[4,5]

From Student to Superintendent in One Easy Step

Nightingale recorded in an autobiographical fragment written in 1867[1,2] that she was called to "God's service" on February 7, 1837, aged sixteen years, at Embley, her Hampshire home. It was not until 1845, however, that she asked her family to allow her to go to Salisbury Infirmary for three months of nursing experience. An argument ensued and her request was denied. In July 1850, on the way home from a second foreign tour, Nightingale reached Kaiserswerth, in Germany, an institution that included a hospital for training volunteer nurses as deaconesses. She studied there for two weeks with the pastor and his wife and returned home fired with enthusiasm and determined to dedicate her life to service of the sick.

In July 1851, Nightingale returned to Kaiserswerth for three more months.[1,2] She wrote long, descriptive letters home, telling her family of the work in which she was involved and of the religious instruction that she was receiving. The Institution was a place of training through example and education, and the pastor frequently discussed with the deaconesses any difficulties they were having and ways to overcome them. Educational topics included the education of the young, the ministration of the sick, the art of district nursing, and the work of rescue and reformation. Miss Nightingale was not enamored by the nurse training at Kaiserswerth, however, and would later deny having received her nurse training there. The standards she would set for the Nightingale School at St. Thomas' Hospital nine years later in 1860 would far exceed the standards she considered to be so poor at Kaiserswerth.[1,2]

In April 1853, Miss Nightingale applied for the post of superintendent at the Institution for the Care of Sick Gentlewomen in Distressed Circumstances. The Institute had found itself in difficulties and was looking for someone to supervise a reorganization and a move of premises to Harley Street, London. In this position, she received no salary and had to pay for the services of a matron from the £500 annual allowance that her father gave her. In return, she had complete control of the management of the Institution and its finances.[1,2]

The Crimean War

After a year or so at the Institution on Harley Street, Nightingale became restless and was planning a move to King's College Hospital in London and becoming superintendent of nurses. However, in 1854, the British went to war in the Crimea, and, worthy of note, for the first time in history a war correspondent, William Howard Russell, sent news of the terrible scenes of the war, which were extensively reported in the *Times*.[1] Eight days later, Nightingale and her nurses set sail for Constantinople in response to the overwhelming public concern for the horrors of modern warfare.

Nightingale was based at the Scutari Barrack Hospital on the Turkish coast, across the Black Sea from the Crimea. Her role was as "Superintendent of the Female Nursing Establishment of the English General Military Hospitals in Turkey,"[1] with no jurisdiction whatsoever in the Crimea. She became the chief organizer and administrator of the hospital. It was a struggle at first, both against the unsanitary conditions of the hospital and the medical doctors who resented the intrusion of women. Nightingale herself did little actual nursing in Scutari; she was too busy administrating the affairs of the hospital.

The Nightingale Fund was launched in 1855 while Miss Nightingale was involved in the Crimean War effort. The fund's objective was to collect donations from a nation that was grateful for the work accomplished by Nightingale and her nurses. The original intention was to present Nightingale with a memento, but a large sum of money had been collected, so it was decided to use the money "to establish a permanent institution for the training, sustenance, and protection of nurses,"[6] enabling Nightingale to continue her work for others, "as a sort of English Kaiserswerth."[1] The idea was put to her, but she was focused on her own battles with disease and death, jealousies and intrigues in the Crimea. She did finally agree to the plan, although she did not know when she would be able to carry it out.

Nightingale returned to England in August 1856, at age thirty-six. Unknown to all was the fact that her contribution to the improvement of living conditions was only just beginning. She was praised for the contribution her nurses had made during the war and for having raised the status of women by opening a new profession to them. During the time Nightingale worked in Scutari, Queen Victoria sent her a brooch "as a mark of the high approbation of your Sovereign."[1] Upon returning to England in September 1856, Nightingale was presented to Queen Victoria and Prince Albert at Balmoral Castle. During the five years immediately after the war, other priorities, e.g., the reform of the army medical services and the collection of medical statistics, had overtaken her consuming desire to nurse.[2,7] She became heavily involved in matters relating to the health of the army. During this time, the Nightingale Fund was invested, waiting for her to decide how to use the money.

Nightingale was very affected by her experiences in Scutari. Realizing that the great majority of soldiers need not have died,[1] she set about analyzing the war's death rate and causes of death. She devised a statistical diagram originally composed of colored wedges, the "polar area diagram" (see Figure 22A–1), in which the statistic being represented is proportional to the area of a wedge in a circular diagram.[8] The outer areas were in blue, the central darker areas in black, and the central lighter areas in red. The chart categorized the rates and causes of death during the war years, demonstrating that most of the British soldiers had died of sickness (outer wedges) rather than from wounds (pale, central wedges) or other causes (dark, central wedges). The chart also demonstrated that the death rate was higher in the first year of the war, before hygiene in the camps and hospitals was improved, following the arrival of the sanitary commissioners in March 1855.[10] The diagram was appended to various reports, in addition to being privately printed and distributed.

Using statistical techniques, Nightingale and William Farr, MD demonstrated that unsanitary conditions, particularly overcrowding, in the hospitals caused the majority of soldiers' deaths. In Nightingale's hospital at Scutari, 5,000 men had died in the winter of 1854–1855; in fact, her hospital had the highest death rate among all the war hospitals. In today's era of "evidence-based practice," it is interesting to read in a letter Nightingale wrote to Sidney Herbert after the war that he must have documented evidence to support the statements the doctors were making to the Royal Commission, an organization that he chaired.[10] Nightingale wrote her own confidential report, *Notes Affecting the Health, Efficiency, and Hospital Administration of the British Army* (1858), which she sent as her own evidence to the Royal Commission. Although her report was never published, she sent privately published copies to various influential people the following year.

Florence Nightingale is credited with developing the idea that social occurrences could be measured and mathematically analyzed. Her statistical work earned great respect, which culminated in her being recognized in elections in 1858 as a Fellow of the Royal Statistical Society and in 1874 as an honorary member of the American Statistical Association.

Post-Crimea Writings

Nightingale's work as a statistician was evident in 1859 when she wrote about infant and child mortality in *Notes on Nursing,* which is probably the best known of her writings. Nightingale wrote, "The causes of the enormous child mortality are perfectly well known; they are chiefly want of cleanliness, want of ventilation, want of white washing; in one word, defective household hygiene."[11] Child and infant mortality statistics

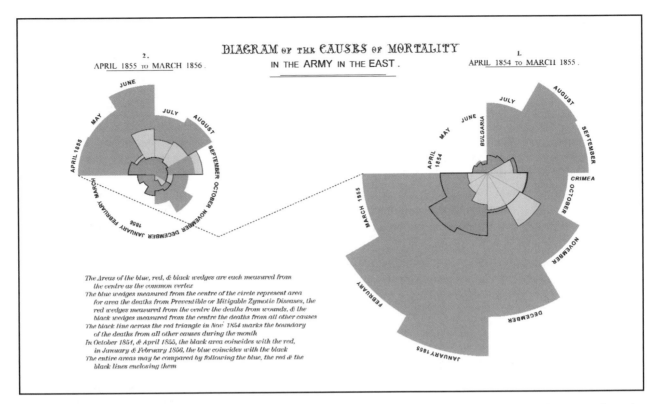

Figure 22A-1. *Causes of Mortality in the Army in the East, April 1854 to March 1855. Source: http://www.florence-nightingale-avenging-angel.co.uk/Coxcomb.htm.*

have been collected in England and Wales since 1837 and were first available as data in 1840[12] (see Table 22A–1). Hence the statistics that Nightingale quoted in 1859 are likely to be fairly accurate for the period. Table 22A-2 contrasts the 2002 mortality rates for children in England and Wales with those published by Nightingale in 1859 as shown in Table 22A-1. While "defective household hygiene"[11] accounted for the higher death rates in 1859, in 2002 the main causes of deaths for children between one and fifteen years were injury, poisoning, and cancer, e.g., leukemia.[13] Nightingale wrote a paper on the subject of hospital

Table 22A-1. Mortality of Children in England in 1859

Age Group	Mortality
0–1 year	142.8 per 1,000 live births (1 in 7)
Under 5 years in London	40,000 per 100,000 children (2 in 5)
Under 5 years in other cities	50,000 per 100,000 children (1 in 2)
Source: Nightingale, F., 1859[11]	

Table 22A-2. Mortality of Children in England and Wales in 2002

Age Group	Mortality
0–1 year	5.2 per 1,000 live births (3,127 deaths)
1–4 years	23 per 100,000
5–9 years	11 per 100,000
Source: Office for National Statistics, 2003[12,13]	

statistics for the International Statistical Congress in London in July 1860. In it, she observed that there was no standardized plan for keeping hospital statistics and proposed a plan that had been tested in some hospitals. The principal objective was to obtain a uniform record of facts from which to calculate statistical results, e.g., the average duration in days and in parts of a day for each disease classified by age and sex, or the mortality rate resulting from each disease classified by sex and age. Nightingale's paper was discussed by the Congress and additions were even suggested. Controversy arose, however, regarding the practicality of collecting the data. A few London hospitals did implement Nightingale's forms, agreeing to start a patient registration system and to publish statistics annually. The plan was later abandoned; however, because of the difficulties and costs involved. Undaunted, Nightingale created forms for collecting data on surgical patients in 1863. The Royal College of Surgeons reviewed the statistical forms but responded negatively.[14]

The collection and analysis of health care data is a significant contribution to nursing administration and management. Nightingale's contribution to the collection and analysis of health care data is consistent with Goossen's definition of nursing informatics, which states that the collection of hospital statistics is a "multidisciplinary scientific endeavour of analyzing, formalizing, and modelling how nurses collect and manage data, process data into information and knowledge, make knowledge-based decisions and inferences for patient care, and use this empirical and experiential knowledge to broaden the scope and enhance the quality of their professional practice."[15] Nightingale had suggested how all health professionals, not just nurses, should collect and analyze data for enhanced patient care.

Toward that end, Nightingale went on to gather vast amounts of English and European statistics on maternal mortality in the nineteenth century for *Notes on Lying-in Institutions,* written in 1871.[16] It was a meticulous investigation of all the statistics she could accumulate on maternal mortality. She argued for an improved system of statistics and noted how they demonstrated a proportion of preventable mortality.[17] It makes for interesting yet sobering reading as the specifics emerge from the pages as to how many women died in childbirth. The detail and dedication with which she researched the issues reveals a passion for statistics and an understanding of the issues involved in maternal mortality.[16] *Notes on Lying-in Institutions* began with a short preface on the rise in the rate of maternal deaths and the subsequent closing of the Kings College Hospital Midwifery School. Nightingale had opened the school in January 1862 to train midwifery nurses to work in poor rural areas, using some of the money from the Nightingale Fund. The school closed five years later in December 1867, because nine women had died that year out of 125 deliveries in her hospital.

Nightingale noted that puerperal fever was the primary cause of death in all maternal deliveries across Europe. Dr. Le Fort, a Frenchman, who had written about the maternal mortality rates in various institutions across Europe, was heavily quoted by Nightingale. While also acknowledging the possibility of inaccuracy in Dr. Le Fort's data, she wrote, "For every two women who would die if delivered at home, fifteen must die if delivered in lying-in hospitals."[16]

It was not until 1843–1844 in the seventh annual report of the Registrar General that deaths in childbirth were even included in the published lists of causes of death.[18] Maternal death in the United Kingdom is now investigated in detail and reported every three years in the expectation that the lessons learned will help avoid women's deaths in the future; the first report of a national inquiry into maternal deaths in England and Wales was published in 1915 by the Local Government Board.[19] The first triannial report for England was published in 1952.[20]

Nightingale's interest in building and designing hospitals convinced her that wards used as training environments should be purpose-built and made as safe for lying-in women as for women who delivered in home settings. Nightingale concluded *Notes on Lying-in Institutions*[16] with her own design for a lying-in institution and training school. The detail was indicative of the amount of research she had undertaken and demonstrated her in-depth knowledge of the subject, as well as her objective of improving the care of mothers and babies through analysis of evidence and recommendations for future care.

Conclusion

Florence Nightingale wrote about nursing, hygiene, sanitation, hospital buildings, training schools, management and administration, and related subjects. In all her writings, she was a meticulous researcher. Her use of evidence to improve the care of patients can be summarized in a passage that she wrote in 1867:

A good nursing staff will perform their duties, more or less satisfactorily, under every disadvantage. But while doing so, their head will always try to improve their surroundings in such a way as to liberate them from subsidiary work and to enable them to devote their time more exclusively to the care of the sick. This is, after all, the real purpose of them being there at all, not to act as lifts, water carriers, beasts of burden or steam engines—articles whose labour can be had at vastly less cost than that of educated human beings.[17]

It is suggested that nurses need liberating from other non-nursing, subsidiary work "to enable them to devote their time more exclusively to the care of the sick."[17] However, this list should not include making "knowledge-based decisions and inferences for patient care, and [using] this empirical and experiential knowledge in order to broaden the scope and enhance the quality of [their] professional practice."[15] EBP is a fundamental component of a twenty-first-century nurse's duty in the care of the sick.

References

1. Cook E. *The Life of Florence Nightingale.* Vol. I. London: Macmillan & Co., Ltd.; 1913.
2. Woodham-Smith C. *Florence Nightingale.* London: Constable; 1950.
3. O'Connor JJ, Robertson EF. *Florence Nightingale.* Available at: http://www-groups.dcs.st-and.ac.uk/~history/Mathematicians/Nightingale.html. Retrieved February 14, 2005.
4. Kopf EW. Florence Nightingale as a statistician. *J Am Stat Assoc.* 1916;15:388-404.
5. Nuttall P. The passionate statistician. *Nurs Times.* 1983;28:25-27.
6. Baly ME. *Florence Nightingale and the Nursing Legacy.* London: Croom Helm; 1986.
7. Baly ME. *Nursing and Social Change.* London: Routledge; 1995.
8. Cohen IB. Florence Nightingale. *Sci Am.* March 1984:128-136.
9. Small H. The "coxcomb"—Florence Nightingale's most famous statistical diagram (1858). Available at: http://www.florence-nightingale-avenging-angel.co.uk/Coxcomb.htm. Retrieved February 21, 2005.
10. Small H. *Florence Nightingale: Avenging Angel.* London: Constable; 1998.
11. Nightingale F. *Notes on Nursing. What It Is and What It Is Not.* London: Blackie & Son Ltd.; 1974 (originally published 1859).
12. Office for National Statistics. *Childhood and Infant Mortality—England and Wales.* General information. London: Her Majesty's Stationary Office; 2003. Available at: http://www.statistics.gov.uk/StatBase/Analysis.asp?vlnk=15&More=Y. Retrieved January 5, 2005.
13. Office for National Statistics. *Mortality Statistics: Childhood, Infant and Perinatal. Review of the Registrar General on Deaths in England and Wales, 2002.* London: Her Majesty's Stationary Office; 2004. Available at: www.statistics.gov.uk/downloads/theme_health/Dh3_2002/DH3_35.pdf. Retrieved January 5, 2005.
14. Bishop WG, Goldie S. *A Bio-Bibliography of Florence Nightingale.* London: Dawsons of Pall Mall; 1962.
15. Goossen WTF. Nursing information management and processing: a framework and definition for systems analysis, design and evaluation. *Intl J Biomed Comput.* 1996;40:187-195.
16. Nightingale F. *Introductory Notes on Lying-in Institutions together with a Proposal for Organising an Institution for Training Midwives and Midwifery Nurses.* London: Longmans, Green and Co.; 1871.
17. Seymer L. The writings of Florence Nightingale. An Oration Delivered by Mrs. Lucy Seymer before the Ninth Congress of the International Council of Nurses, Atlantic City, NJ, USA, 1947. London: The Cornwall Press Ltd. (no date).
18. Loudon I. *Death in Childbirth.* Oxford: Clarendon Press; 1992.
19. Macfarlane A. Appendix 3, Enquiries into maternal deaths during the 20th century. In: Lewis G, ed. *Why Mothers Die. Report on Confidential Enquiries into Maternal Deaths in the UK. 1997–99.* London: RCOG Press; 2001.
20. Lewis G, ed. *Why Mothers Die. Report on Confidential Enquiries into Maternal Deaths in the UK. 1997–99.* London: RCOG Press; 2001.

CHAPTER 23

Translating Knowledge-Based N
Referential and Executable Appl
Intelligent Clinical Information

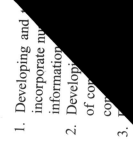

By Norma M. Lang, PhD, RN, FAAN, FRCN; Mary L.
Mari E. Akre, PhD, RN; Tae Youn Kim, PhDc; Karen Be
Sally P. Lundeen, PhD, RN; Mary E. Hagle, PhD, RN; a

This chapter describes the work of a unique collaboration of a health care organization (Aurora Health Care in Wisconsin), a university school of nursing (University of Wisconsin-Milwaukee) and a software company (Cerner Corporation, Kansas City, Missouri). The partnership originated from discussions about the near total absence of evidence-based nursing content for use in clinical information systems (CIS). Aurora identified the gap as it began to implement plan of care documentation for its acute care team. Seeking answers, Aurora invited Cerner and the University of Wisconsin-Milwaukee to join in a collaborative effort. From the exploratory discussions emerged a proposal to conduct an applied research initiative to discover best practice content for the major nursing practice categories that are unique in the care of patients.

Collaborating to Transform Health Care

Several visionary leaders from all three partnering organizations worked to build the terms and conditions that allowed the three-way partnership to become a reality. The nurse leaders identified a window of opportunity in the near invisibility of nursing care and outcomes in CIS today. Specifically, the enabling tools of electronic clinical information and health record systems can now support a codified and standardized nursing terminology, a plan-of-care documentation solution, and a repository for data storage and analysis of outcome data. The partners recognized that discovering the requisite nursing knowledge and building it into a successful system required the expertise of researchers, practitioners, informaticians, and technology experts. Thus, the three organizations forged an industry-first partnership to take advantage of the opportunity made possible by this alignment of interests, vision, and state-of-the-art technological readiness—including advances in evidence-based nursing, terminology standards, and electronic clinical information and health record systems.

The vision guiding the collaboration is defined as follows:

> To create a paperless clinical decision support and documentation system accessible to all health care providers, and their patients, across various settings in an integrated health care system; able to prompt, collect, store, aggregate and report data so as to provide accurate, easily retrievable information to both providers and consumers that promotes the delivery of accessible, acceptable, efficient, high quality health care across the continuum of care and the attainment of the healthiest possible outcomes for all.

The Aurora, Cerner, University of Wisconsin-Milwaukee (ACW) Knowledge-Based Nursing Initiative was launched in July 2004. Project aims include:

...testing innovative clinical decision support and documentation systems that ...sing data elements, based on evidence-based nursing knowledge, into integrated ... technology (IT) solutions

...ng and testing models of transformational change in the adoption and implementation ...prehensive, integrated clinical software applications in practice settings across the care ...tinuum, with special emphasis on the critical roles of the nurse in system implementation

...Exploring the expansion of clinical software applications to provide support for health-focused and community-driven models of health care delivery, rather than continued use of the relatively limited illness-focused and institutionally-driven models

4. Developing and testing the research applications of data derived from clinical software as mechanisms to improve the quality of care and to measure clinical outcomes according to a comprehensive set of indicators

The ultimate goal of the University of Wisconsin-Milwaukee Knowledge-Based Nursing Initiative is to determine and improve nursing's contribution to patient outcomes through the use of an intelligent CIS.

The remainder of the chapter describes the conceptual framework for representing knowledge, as well as the process used to generate evidence-based nursing knowledge, to convert it to referential and executable knowledge, and to embed it in point-of-care decision support and documentation solutions. Because this collaborative initiative was in the early stages at the time of writing, the chapter details (1) the schema for incorporating knowledge into the nursing process, (2) the representation model developed for nursing knowledge to support decision making and evidence-based best practice embedded in the documentation solutions, and (3) the evidence-based knowledge development methodology.

Incorporating Evidence-Based Knowledge into the Nursing Process

There are many ways of knowing, and nurses use many kinds of knowledge in practice. There is practical knowledge, gained through practicing skills, and there is theoretical knowledge that Benner et al[1] describe as "know-how" and "know that." The ACW Knowledge-Based Nursing Initiative aims to enhance nurses' decision making and recording by making both kinds of knowledge more accessible and usable, especially at the bedside or patient side. It is important to point out, however, that an intelligent system will never replace human reasoning and the skilled know-how of experienced nurses.

Evidence-Based Decision Support in Practice

Numerous efforts have been made to fill the quality chasm stemming from wide variations in practice patterns and access to health care providers. Efforts to develop and apply the best possible science to inform health care delivery has been intense.[2,3] Surprisingly, although nurses are thought to be knowledge workers, much of what they do remains essentially invisible in most CIS and there are few examples of decision support for nurses.[2] So what is the best science and knowledge that will enhance nurses' ability to affect patient outcomes and health care delivery? Evidence-based practice (EBP) and IT are regarded as two means of changing the quality of care positively in the long term.[4-6] Whereas research utilization, a subset of EBP, emphasizes putting new empirical findings from a set of studies to practical use by health care professionals,[7] EBP judiciously employs the best current evidence in making decisions about patient care.[8,9] Importantly, EBP also empowers patients and families to make more informed decisions about the treatment and management of their health conditions and includes them as partners in care decisions. A view that is probably more compatible with holistic views often held by nurses is offered by Eddy,[10] who suggests the term *evidence-based individual decision making* to reflect the need to consider the preferences and values of the individual patient.

EBP begins with a search for the best available evidence from a variety of sources.[11] Although controversies still exist concerning what constitutes evidence, the term has evolved to include research findings (randomized controlled trials, meta-analyses, systematic reviews, and quality studies), scientific expertise, patient preferences and values, existing resources, and evidence-based theories.[9,12-14] As a means to improve the quality of care, evidence-based decision making[3] is therefore based on sound evidence and on an individual patient's condition within a specific context in which health care professionals deliver quality care.

A variety of barriers impede health care professionals, however, in obtaining and applying the best evidence, including a lack of clinician competency for conducting literature searches, evaluating studies, and translating results into EBP, unfavorable attitudes toward EBP, and relatively non-supportive external environments.[15-18] According to Balas,[19] seventeen years, on average, are needed to fully use study findings in clinical practice. Considerable gaps have also been reported among research findings, nurses' awareness, and the practical implementation of the resultant knowledge.[20-25]

Decision support using IT is a powerful way to fill the gaps between practice and knowledge.[26,27] Concomitant with the increasing implementation of CISs, a growing body of literature, along with expert opinion in the CIS field, strongly favors the development of clinical decision support systems and their embedding in electronic health records (EHR) systems.[27,28] In other words, when equipped with artificial intelligence, information systems can facilitate change in clinicians' behavior by linking clinical best evidence (i.e., knowledge) to patient health information and then generating timely reminders or alert messages. The effectiveness of clinical decision support, therefore, relies on the generation of recent, high-quality, useful, and actionable *best knowledge.*[29,30] From a practical standpoint, it is imperative to determine how to continually generate the best knowledge and to use such knowledge concurrently to support clinician decision making in the work flow.

The Knowledge Representation Model

Conceptual Architecture: Evidence-Based Decision Support Using Information Systems

The purpose of the collaborative partnership is threefold: (1) to discover and generate the evidence-based nursing knowledge related to major clinical conditions; (2) to define a framework for representing that knowledge to clinicians, who can then apply it in clinical practice using a CIS; and (3) to provide the essential nursing data for quality measurement and research. Specifically, the goal is to discover the most effective way to represent the knowledge in the context of a CIS and a care delivery process so as to support the ongoing analysis of outcomes.

Figure 23-1 shows the "big picture" description of this evidence-based initiative in the applied context of a CIS and health care delivery organization. The upper left box indicates the integrated health care system and the capture of clinical information as a by-product of care delivery. These clinical data are stored in the clinical data repository (CDR) and data warehouse (DW), shown in the lower right corner. The CDR is a comprehensive database that stores all health information gathered from care delivery and that clinicians use as the transactional database to deliver care. The DW serves as the summarized data storage area for patient-related data from multiple sources that can be used for aggregate analysis, trending, reporting, and research.[31]

The middle four diamonds in Figure 23-1 represent the conceptual framework used to guide the research team's process for discovering and organizing the EBP content. The nursing process (assessment, diagnosis, intervention, and outcome) is also used to represent the knowledge to clinicians in the CIS. The end deliverables involve (1) translating the EBP content into *referential interdisciplinary knowledge* to inform and guide clinicians in their work flow and (2) providing a centralized expert database. The knowledge content used to define criteria for triggering an action in the system is termed *executable interdisciplinary knowledge.*

The summarized referential knowledge is organized in a centralized database according to clinical conditions within the four nursing process categories. The evidence-based knowledge is embedded in the work flow of the clinical decision support and documentation solutions to support the process of developing patient-specific plans of care. In addition, the ongoing evaluation of outcomes against interventions for a given problem generates new findings and knowledge that in turn are used to inform clinical practice. This concept is shown in Figure 23-1 by the two-way arrows between the care delivery system and the data warehouse.

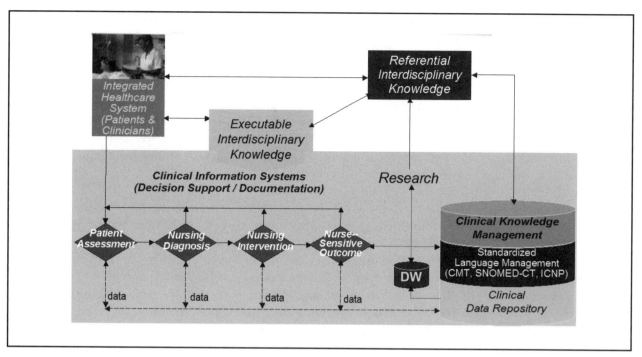

Figure 23-1. *Conceptual Architecture: Evidence-based Decision Support Process Using Information Systems.*
Source: © ACW Knowledge-Based Nursing Initiative (July 2005).

As shown in Figure 23-1, the conceptual architecture depicts that the CIS captures patient health information and supports clinician decision making based on evidence-based knowledge in both the referential and executable contexts. Further, the CIS is designed to sustain a cyclical nursing care process of patient assessment, nursing diagnosis, nursing intervention, and nurse-sensitive outcome. Dotted lines, broken lines, and solid lines with an arrowhead illustrate, respectively, the flow of data, information, and knowledge necessary in clinical practice.

Methodology for Creating Evidence-Based Nursing Practice

In the ACW Knowledge-Based Nursing Initiative methodology, the *phenomenon of concern* is the starting point for the EBP search strategy. A huge challenge in establishing nursing knowledge is that there is no general agreement on, or taxonomy for, the phenomena of concern for nursing practice. This holds true for nursing care related to a medical diagnosis as well as for care related to nursing problems and diagnoses in general. Therefore, drawing on the domain and classes of nursing practice from Docheterman and Jones,[32] the team asked expert clinicians, nursing managers, and nurse executives to advise them on how to prioritize the selected phenomena of concern for development. As EBP knowledge for nursing phenomena continues to be built, nursing frameworks may become more universally embraced. The next section includes a detailed discussion of the discovery, synthesis, translation, and design process along with the use of standardized language.

The Discovery Process

Once a phenomenon of concern is identified, literature searches are conducted using established search strategies. The findings from selected literature are analyzed and classified into detailed evidence tables. The next step is to *discover* the useful knowledge by synthesizing the evidence by topic according to the following appraisal and synthesis protocols.

Clinical and research findings are translated into knowledge by means of a critical appraisal of the evidence obtained from a systematic search. Craig and Smyth[33] define *critical appraisal* as the "systematic evaluation of evidence to assess its quality, importance, and applicability." The methodology consists of (1) the critical appraisal process (asking answerable questions), (2) searching the literature for the best evidence, and (3) identifying the best research design to fit the question.[34] The steps we used in discovering, organizing, and applying the evidence-based knowledge for clinician use are depicted in Figure 23-2.

As illustrated in Figure 23-3, the discovery process generates evidence pertinent to the selected phenomenon. That evidence is then analyzed according to a critical appraisal process, which is enhanced by summarizing the evidence and drawing out the study findings relevant to patient assessment, nursing diagnosis and problems, nursing interventions, and nurse-sensitive outcomes. The findings are summarized into comprehensive evidence tables according to a structured schema.

Passing this initial high-level screen moves the article forward for abstraction into the evidence table using a structured evidence abstraction process. The criteria used to rate the evidence reviewed (listed in Table 23-1) encompass a broad range of categories, from randomized clinical trials to expert opinion.[13,35] Rating the evidence in the summarized abstraction tables not only keeps the strength of evidence clear but also the kind of research that resulted in the reported findings.

In the evidence appraisal process, a broad array of evidence related to a selected phenomenon of concern is reviewed and analyzed, and key findings across several dimensions are summarized. *Synthesis* is the combination of often diverse conceptions (evidence) into a coherent whole. The process brings together multiple factors that influence the effective management of patient problems (clinical expertise, clinical research evidence, and nationally established guidelines) to generate a more robust synthesis of the evidence. The process and outcome terms and metrics reported by the study authors are also incorporated. To the extent possible, nationally established experts review the evidence synthesis. The citations are sorted by level of evidence. Figures 23-4 and 23-5 provide partial examples of how evidence is synthesized for two selected phenomena of concern (Medication Adherence and Activity/Exercise), as related to the care of patients with heart failure.

The Translation Process: Putting EBP Knowledge into the CIS

The synthesized content is ready for translation into the CIS in two steps. First, a summarized view of the knowledge is prepared. As shown in Figure 23-6, the EBP knowledge is organized by nursing phenomena of concern in the nursing process conceptual framework. In that framework, the findings are systematically outlined according to each of the following categories:

1. Clinical reminder
2. Rationale (evidence summary)

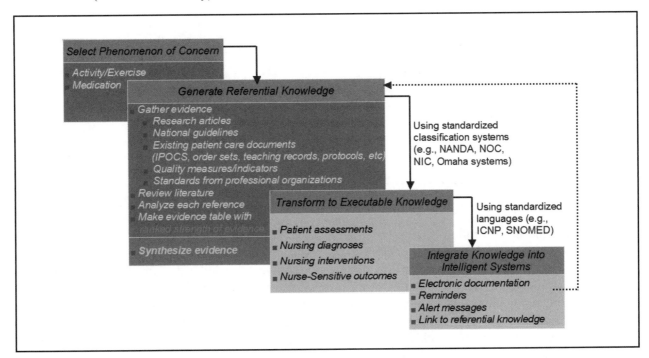

Figure 23-2. *Developing and Implementing Referential and Executable Knowledge for Nursing.*
Source: © ACW Knowledge-Based Nursing Initiative (July 2005).

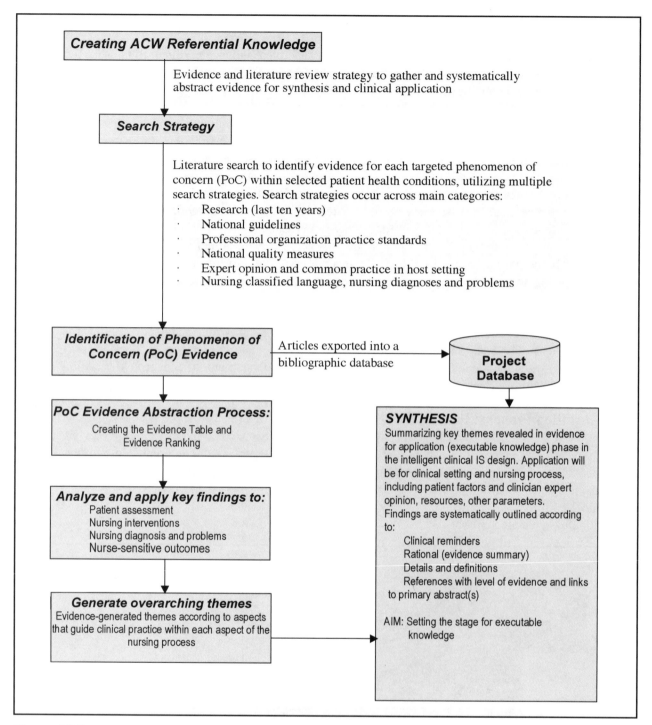

Figure 23-3. *Source: © ACW Knowledge-Based Nursing Initiative (July 2005).*

3. Details and definitions

4. References (including level of evidence and links to abstracts and articles)

The second step is the work flow design process, which includes defining the knowledge content and deciding where to put it in the assessment and plan of care. This step requires close collaboration among clinical practitioners, the research team, and the software design team. The objective is to begin providing the knowledge to be built into the decision support rules and clinical documentation content. Once the work flow design is defined, links to the reference database are embedded at key decision points throughout the clinical documentation.

The reference database is built so that it can be accessed directly, as well as by links in the clinical documentation. The database includes all referential knowledge in the form of original articles,

Table 23-1. Evidence Rating[35]

Level I	Evidence from a systematic review or meta-analysis of all relevant randomized controlled trials (RCTs) or evidence-based clinical practice guidelines based on systematic reviews of RCTs
Level I	Evidence obtained from at least one well-designed RCT
Level I	Evidence obtained from well-designed controlled trials without randomization
Level I	Evidence from well-designed case-control and cohort studies
Level I	Evidence from systematic reviews of descriptive or qualitative studies
Level I	Evidence from a single descriptive or qualitative study
Level I	Evidence from the opinion of authorities and/or reports of expert committees
Source: Reprinted with permission from Blackwell Publishers, Ltd.	

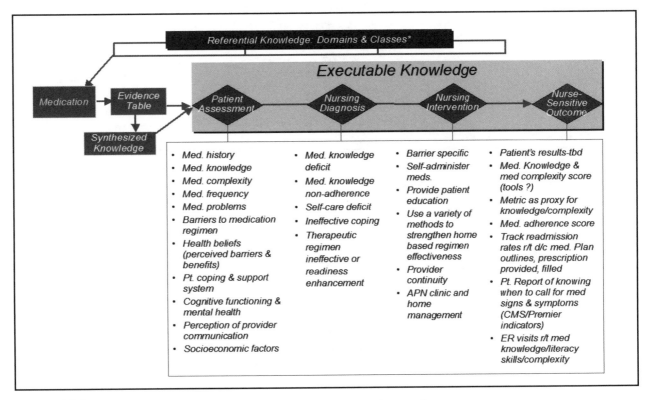

Figure 23-4. *Synthesized Knowledge Related to Patients with Heart Failure: Medication.*
Source: © ACW Knowledge-Based Nursing Initiative (July 2005).

article synopses, tables of evidence, descriptions of key findings, synthesis tables, and selected executable knowledge tables. The referential knowledge information includes a list of supporting publications with links to the actual articles on the Web, in PubMed™ of the National Library of Medicine, or in Adobe PDF formats.

The Design Process: Creating Executable Knowledge

The Institute of Medicine (IOM) has made strong recommendations that initiatives be developed to reduce the gap between knowledge and practice.[36] O'Neill et al,[37] while conceptualizing bedside decision making, emphasized the need to translate knowledge into practice by developing rule-based systems that deliver evidence when complexity increases, data collection decreases, shortcut strategies are taken, and the likelihood of error increases. Chang et al[38] reported that nurses performed poorly in the areas of problem identification and care planning, especially in cases entailing psychosocial problems and patient education.

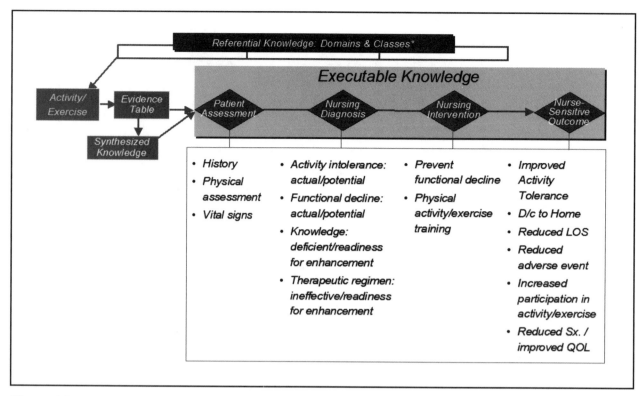

Figure 23-5. *Synthesized Knowledge Related to Patients with Heart Failure: Activity/exercise.*
Source: © ACW Knowledge-Based Nursing Initiative (July 2005).

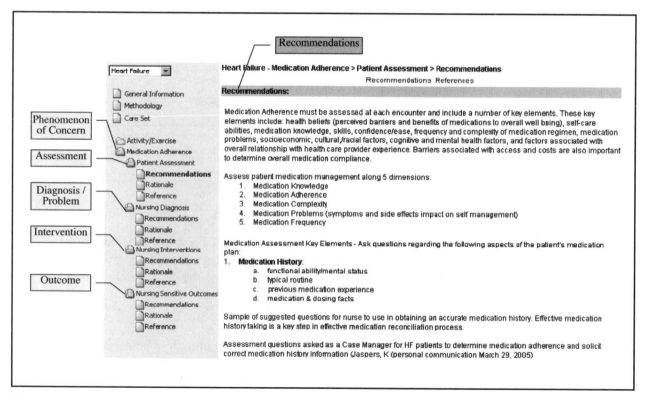

Figure 23-6. *Web-Based Application Presenting Synthesized Knowledge.*
Source: © ACW Knowledge-Based Nursing Initiative (July 2005).

Using the EBP knowledge to support best practice and decision making means taking the difficult step of defining which actions should be made to happen automatically in response to documentation that detects a profile of clinical risk. In the ACW initiative, one of the key deliverables is the ability to embed EBP knowledge content in the rules engine to support clinical decision making. The rules can range from simple actions, e.g., presenting an alert or causing a consult order to be placed, to more complex ones. The most daunting task is to synthesize the incredible knowledge gained in the referential data process into a few carefully selected "actionable" items that support nurses in problem identification, decision making, and care delivery. That means presenting concise evidence at the point of care at key times in the care process.

The knowledge translation framework provides a structured process to manage large amounts of evidence as it is converted to *executable knowledge,* which consists of actionable items in an information system. The content designers on the ACW team extract key data from the referential information that include but are not limited to:

1. Nursing orders and interventions in an order set
2. Interventions and activities that are posted on an activity list for nurses or other disciplines, as appropriate
3. Data elements to be documented on a form by nurses or other care providers (e.g., assessments or treatment delivered)
4. Expected outcomes that are defined for a problem
5. The edited version of the protocol with mark-up language

This actionable information is formatted and embedded in the automated electronic information system by knowledge and content developers from the ACW project team. The executable knowledge includes links to the referential knowledge Web site. The final step is to embed the executable knowledge in a software solution so that it triggers actions in the context of documentation and care delivery. In this collaborative design work, all the team members' skills are brought to bear to ensure that the system provides the right information at the right time and at the right point in the work flow.

There are five design steps to embed actionable knowledge:

1. Describe the future state of automated work flow.
2. Define the clinical content to be available at the point of care for each step in the work flow.
3. Identify and incorporate the outcome-focused data elements to be captured as a by-product of care delivery.
4. Standardize the data elements according to a controlled medical terminology.
5. Maintain the currency of the content through updates and tools to easily integrate the most recent clinical content when updates are identified.

Steps one and two focus on the analysis of the care process to determine how and where knowledge should be applied to affect care positively. The care process (Figure 23-7) entails the assessment of the individual's health care status, identification of problems and risks to health; definition of the plan of care, performance, and documentation of therapeutic interventions; and the assessment of the progress against the expected outcomes. As an individual proceeds through the care delivery process, the cycle recurs, and the clinician continually reassesses the patient, updates the clinical diagnosis and plan of care, and proceeds to deliver and document the care. In the translation of knowledge into software, the goal is to address all components of the care process and to create clinical content templates that capture all the appropriate data elements.

For each care process component, the clinical content developers use the nursing evidence tables to identify the data elements that need to be captured as well as the sequence in which they should be captured. They then display the information consistently so as to optimize usability and enable the work flow. For example, the evidence might indicate that the inability to self-administer medications directly influences the readmission rates of heart failure patients. Delineating the assessment criteria that identify individuals who are unable to manage their medications allows the risk to be linked to a specified plan of care to improve their adherence to a medication schedule. In the ACW initiative, the criteria are embedded into the assessment documentation templates and a rule is built

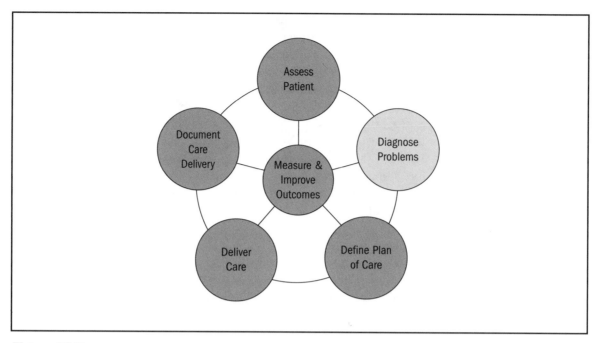

Figure 23-7. *Analysis of the Care Process.*

to capture the risk as a problem with a "suggested" plan of care, which recommends that the nurse educate the individual on medication administration.

Evidence-based clinical content appears in several key formats:

- Key data to be assessed or planned are embedded in templates for documentation and plans of care (e.g., order sets). The data are defined by the evidence and displayed to the clinician at the time of care delivery. The templates are actionable in that the clinician's selection of the template items documents assessment or care delivery; generates notifications or alerts about specified clinical problems or issues; or specifies treatments, assessments, or consults from within the plan of care.

- Data displayed in the documentation and plan of care templates can be linked to the supporting evidence. Icons in the software serve as portals to the up-to-date information housed on the referential Web page.

Nursing standards, policies and procedures, and regulatory agencies require the capture of specified data elements to consistently assess the progress of an individual during a care encounter, as well as to evaluate the patient in the context of a like population. The data elements needed for the consistent evaluation of individuals against expected outcomes and indicators are most effectively captured when the foundation data elements are presented to the clinician at the point of care and captured as a by-product of documented care.

The Use of Standardized Terminology

Consistent and standardized terminology that is shared across all venues of care and that is understood by various disciplines is hugely important. A controlled medical and nursing terminology ensures that clinical information is accurately reflected and understood by all caregivers, regardless of domain preferences on what to call a condition, procedure, diagnosis, or intervention. For example, clinicians readily understand that pulmonary renal syndrome, Goodpasture's syndrome, anti-GBM nephritis, and lung purpura with nephritis are the same clinical condition. However, computer systems and outcome measurement tools must be built with the intelligence and cross-mapping capabilities to discern that these very different terms define the same clinical phenomenon. When provided with the terms to describe the same concept, the system can report accurate results. As another example, nurses sometimes use various terms to describe the same concept, such as "urinary incontinence" and "ineffective voiding." Tying a concept identifier to a hierarchical vocabulary, such as SNOMED CT, provides the underlying framework for accurate outcome reporting and efficient rules and reports. Advanced clinical decision support, reporting, and associated quality improvement measures are virtually impossible unless all clinical concepts are mapped to a standard vocabulary.

The Ultimate Goal: Improved Nursing Practice and Patient Outcomes

Health care information systems and technology with embedded knowledge hold the potential to transform health care. Matching a person's health information with the right medical and nursing knowledge will place up-to-date, evidence-based, patient-specific information at the clinician's fingertips at the optimal time and place in the care process to positively influence pending decisions. Such a capability—that is, knowledge-driven care or knowledge-based nursing—can yield measurable improvements in health outcomes.

The translation of the referential knowledge into knowledge-driven care or a knowledge-based nursing model is a design-intensive activity that views research and EBP as an organizational process. It is organizational in that the implementation of knowledge-based nursing requires a supportive work environment as well as a commitment to a multidisciplinary team. The knowledge development and application process described in this chapter is time-intensive and demands strong organizational and system supports. Most organizations cannot afford to do this work. The ACW initiative aims to construct and test the framework and the system that allows us to put best knowledge into practice. Because of the complexity of nursing practice, the work is hard and requires collaboration among researchers, practitioners, informaticians, and software and hardware developers.

More to Come...

There has been a dramatic increase in nursing and health research over the past two decades. Major work has focused on the clinical management of patients, on the management of the enterprise, and on the organizational characteristics in which nursing practice takes place, as well as on basic biomedical research and the behavioral responses of people. An incredible amount of knowledge has been amassed regarding phenomena of care, including pressure ulcers, sleep, fatigue, exercise, treatment adherence, comfort, pain, health beliefs, anxiety, fear, oxygen deprivation, and dyspnea. Add this evidence to that derived from medical, biological, and psychological research affecting the practice of nurses, and the magnitude of the requisite knowledge is huge. Studying what is done in medical and nursing practice becomes the next source of new knowledge.

With more than a half million new articles and results from thousands of research studies published annually, the need to filter and synthesize information is essential to help clinicians keep up with the pace of health care discovery and to apply such information in the clinical setting.

Connecting the findings of relevant research to practice is a continuing challenge. As the content is embedded in a new generation of software, an ongoing process to review and update the information must be in place. As new knowledge is defined, it is essential to have knowledge management systems and tools to notify clinicians of the new information, as well as to furnish continual updates to the referential and actionable or executable content. IT has opened a new avenue of making knowledge accessible to practicing nurses in ways not available in the past. Just how does that useful knowledge get to the bedside? The translation of the results of published studies into clinical action deserves to be given the highest priority by all stakeholders in quality patient care.

The ACW Knowledge-Based Nursing Initiative described in this chapter provides a model for identifying and synthesizing knowledge, and embedding it in intelligent information systems so as to enhance clinical decision making and to improve nurse-sensitive outcomes for individuals and families in all health care settings. The conceptual architecture presented can guide the intelligent information system to directly help clinicians to:

1. View patient care consistently across the continuum of care
2. Customize care plans according to patient conditions and provide sophisticated, optimized quality care, based on the best evidence and specific care contexts
3. Communicate more precisely with other care providers by improving documentation practice in

connection with care processes

4. Further improve quality care through the auditing of health outcome and care process, feedback, and interactive online education

5. Conduct subsequent research that generates new evidence to inform practice.

Embedding evidence-based nursing knowledge in CIS holds the promise of leapfrogging the seventeen-year delay[19] between new knowledge discovery and its application to practice. With the new IT and standardized terminology, nurses are in a position to identify what constitutes the practice of nursing, to recognize the contributions nursing makes to patient outcomes, and to build the nursing knowledge base in support of best practice.

References

1. Benner P, Hooper-Kyriakidis PH, Stannard D. Clinical wisdom and interventions. In: *Critical Care: A Thinking-in-Action Approach*. Philadelphia: Saunders; 1999.

2. Clancy CM, Cronin K. Evidence-based decision making: global evidence, local decisions. *Health Affairs*. 2005;24:151-162.

3. Institute of Medicine Committee on Quality Health Care in America. *Crossing the Quality Chasm: A New Health System for the 21st Century*. Washington, DC: National Academy Press; 2001.

4. Swan BA, Lang NM, McGinley AM. Access to quality health care: links between evidence, nursing language and informatics. *Nurs Economic$*. 2004; 22:325-332.

5. National Committee for Quality Assurance. *The State of Health Care Quality: 2004*. Available at: http://www.ncqa.org/communications/SOMC/SOHC2004.pdf. Accessed October 17, 2004.

6. The Leapfrog Group. *Leapfrog Fact Sheet (2004)*. Available at: http://www.leapfroggroup.org/about_us/leapfrog-factsheet. Accessed October 10, 2004.

7. Titler MG, Herr K, Schilling ML, et al. Acute pain treatment for older adults hospitalized with hip fracture: current nursing practices and perceived barriers. *Applied Nursing Research*. 2004;16:211-227.

8. Polit DF, Beck CT. *Nursing Research: Principles and Methods*. 7th ed. Philadelphia: Lippincott; 2004.

9. Sackett DL, Rosenberg WM, Gray JA, Haynes RB, Richardson WS. Evidence based medicine: what it is and what it isn't. *BMJ*. 1996;312:71-72.

10. Eddy DM. Evidence-based medicine: a unified approach. *Health Affairs*. 2005;24:9-17.

11. Swan BA, Boruch RF. Quality of evidence: usefulness in measuring the quality of health care. *Med Care*. 2004;42:Suppl.II-12-II-20.

12. Jennings BM, Loan LA. Misconceptions among nurses about evidence-based practice. *J Nurs Scholarship*. 2001;33:121-127.

13. Melnyk BM, Fineout-Overholt E. *Evidence-based Practice in Nursing & Health Care: A Guide to Best Practice*. Philadelphia: Lippincott, Williams & Wilkins; 2005.

14. Rutledge DN, DePalma JA, Cunningham M. A process model for evidence-based literature synthesis. *Oncol Nurs Forum*. 2004;31:543-551.

15. Cabana MD, Rand CS, Powe NR, et al. Why don't physicians follow clinical practice guidelines? a framework for improvement. *JAMA*. 1999;282:1458-1465.

16. McColl A, Smith H, White P, Field J. General practitioners' perceptions of the route to evidence based medicine: survey questionnaire. *BMJ*. 1998;316:361-365.

17. Pravikoff DS, Pierce S, Tanner A. Are nurses ready for evidence-based practice? a study suggests that greater support is needed. *AJN*. 2003;103:95-96.

18. Solberg LI, Brekke ML, Fazio CJ, et al. Lessons from experienced guideline implementers: attend to many factors and use multiple strategies. *Joint Commission J Quality Improvement*. 2000;26:171-188.

19. Balas EA. Information systems can prevent errors and improve quality. *JAMIA*. 2001;8:398-399.

20. Brett JL. Organizational integrative mechanisms and adoption of innovations by nurses [doctoral dissertation]. Philadelphia:University of Pennsylvania; 1986.

21. Bostrom J, Suter WN. Research utilization: making the link to practice. *J Nurs Staff Dev*. 1993;9:28-34.

22. Coyle LA, Sokop AG. Innovation adoption behavior among nurses. *Nurs Res*. 1990;39:176-180.

23. Michel Y, Sneed NV. Dissemination and use of research findings in nursing practice. *J Professional Nurs*. 1995;11:306-311.

24. Rutledge DN, Greene P, Mooney K, Nail LM, Ropka M. Use of research-based practices by oncology staff nurses. *Oncol Nurs Forum*. 1996;23:1235-1244.

25. Rubin GL, Frommer MS, Vincent NC, Phillips PA, Leeder SR. Getting new evidence into medicine. *Med J Aust*. 2000;21:180-183.

26. Bates DW, Kuperman GJ, Wang S, et al. Ten commandments for effective clinical decision support: making the practice of evidence-based medicine a reality. *JAMIA*. 2003;10:523-530.

27. Safran C, Rind DM, Davis RB, et al. Effects of a knowledge-based electronic patient record in adherence to practice guidelines. *MD Computing*. 1996; 13:55-63.

28. Bates DW, Cohen M, Leape LL, et al. Reducing the frequency of errors in medicine using information technology. *JAMIA*. 2001;8:299-308.

29. Perreault L, Metzger J. A pragmatic framework for understanding clinical decision support. *J Healthcare Information Manage*. 1999;13:5-22.

30. Sim I, Gorman P, Greenes RA, et al. Clinical decision support systems for the practice of evidence-based medicine. *JAMIA.* 2001;8:527-534.

31. Uthurusmy R. From data mining to knowledge discovery: current challenges and future directions. In: Fayyad UM, Piatetsky-Shapiro G, Smyth P, Uthurusmy R, eds. *Advances in Knowledge Discovery and Data Mining.* Cambridge, MA: AAAI/MIT Press. 1996;561-569.

32. Docheterman JM, Jones DA, eds. *Unifying Nursing Language: The Harmonization of NANDA, NIC, and NOC.* Washington, DC: NursesBooks.Org; 2003.

33. Craig JV, Smyth RL, eds. *The Evidence-Based Practice Manual for Nurses.* Edinburgh: Churchill Livingston; 2002.

34. DiCenso A, Ciliska D, Marks S, et al. Evidence based nursing. In: Sackett DL, Richardson WS, Haynes B, eds. *Evidence-Based Medicine: How to Practice and Teach EBM.* 2nd ed. Edinburgh: Churchill Livingston; 2000.

35. Melnyk BM. Evidence digest. *Worldviews on Evidenced-Based Nursing.* 2004; 1(2):142-145. Available at: http://www.nursingsociety.org/worldviews/wv_article.pdf. Accessed December 1, 2004.

36. Institute of Medicine. *Keeping Patients Safe: Transforming the Work Environment of Nurses.* Washington, DC: National Academy Press; 2003.

37. O'Neill ES, Dluhy NM, Fortier PJ, Michel HE. Knowledge acquisition, synthesis, and validation: a model for decision support systems. *J Adv Nurs.* 2004;47(2):134-142.

38. Chang BL, Lee JL, Pearson ML. Evaluating the quality of nursing care: the gap between theory and practice. *J Nurs Adm.* 2002;32:405-418.

CHAPTER 24

The International Nursing
Minimum Data Set (i-NMDS)

By William T.F. Goossen, PhD, RN; Connie White Delaney, PhD, RN, FAAN, FACMI;
Amy Coenen, PhD, RN, FAAN; Virginia K. Saba, EdD, RN, FAAN, FACMI;
Walter Sermeus, PhD, RN; Judith J. Warren, PhD, RN, BC, FAAN, FACMI;
Heimar F. Marin, PhD, RN, FACMI; Hyeoun-Ae Park, PhD; Alain Junger, MHS, RN;
Evelyn J.S. Hovenga, PhD, RN, FACHI, FCHSE, FRCNA, MACS;
Karl Øyri, MNS, MS, RN; and Anne Casey, MSc, RN, FRCN

*The International Council of Nurses (ICN) and the International Medical Informatics
Association–Nursing Informatics Special Interest Group (IMIA-NI SIG) cosponsor the International
Nursing Minimum Data Set (i-NMDS) project, which seeks to describe nursing care around the
world. This chapter (1) provides a brief historical overview of nursing data collections, (2) describes
and analyzes the essential data set initiatives around the world, (3) identifies the needs and purpose
for the i-NMDS and (4) discusses the results of a pilot study related to the i-NMDS. It concludes
with a view into the future in which the i-NMDS can be used to make nursing's contribution to health
statistically visible.*

Historical Overview of Nursing Minimum Data Sets

Florence Nightingale is considered the first health scientist because she initiated the process of documenting care for the individual and aggregating data systematically on the group level for statistical analysis.[1,2] Obviously, the need for these types of data collections are still valid today, with clinical data documented by nurses supporting the care of and the decisions for individual patients and grouped data supporting the care of families and communities. Further, selections of clinical data can be aggregated to support decision making by management, researchers, and policy makers across all settings of nursing care delivery. Two countries are considered the pioneers of the aggregate use of nursing data: the U.S. and Belgium.

In the U.S., several nursing researchers identified nursing practice standards or concepts that could be aggregated as nursing data.[3-8] The current American Nurses Association (ANA) definition of nursing, which reflects the contemporary and dynamic practice of registered nurses, affirms the nursing process as the organizing framework for practice: "Nursing is the protection, promotion, and optimization of health and abilities, prevention of illness and injury, alleviation of suffering through the diagnosis and treatment of human response, and advocacy in the care of individuals, families, communities, and populations."[9] To support the documentation of the nursing process, ANA has recognized numerous standardized languages that also support the aggregation of nursing data.[10] Moreover, nursing has consistently recognized information technology's potential for documenting and improving nursing practice.[11-14]

Harriet Werley was among the first nurses who identified the need for a nursing minimum data set (NMDS) in the early 1970s. Since that time, the NMDS has been promoted as an instrument to help in the selection and aggregation of nursing data.[15-17] Belgium began research on a national NMDS in 1985,[18] and the Belgian government mandated the collection of data on a national scale in 1988.[19]

A *nursing minimum data set* is defined as a minimum data set of items of information with uniform definitions and categories concerning the specific dimension of nursing that meets the information needs of multiple data users in the health care system.[15] An NMDS provides a minimum, but essential, core number of data that are maximally useful for different purposes.[15]

In Europe, "telenursing" which is a European Union-funded initiative of the Concerted Action in Nursing Informatics Project began disseminating the concept of an NMDS in 1994.[20,21] Telenursing had as a main goal the advancement of nursing informatics (NI) in Europe. The project focused on investigating the use of nursing languages, NMDS, the use of standards, nurses' use of electronic patient records, and NI education.[20] It included a short test involving a simplified nursing minimum data collection to which the Belgian methods for analysis and feedback were applied. The pilot test illustrated that there are many practical problems associated with the multinational collection of nursing minimum data.

At the IMIA NI 1997 conference, discussions among experts working on NMDS projects all over the world led to the idea of a coordinated international approach to NMDS development.[22] During the 1999 ACENDIO (Association for Common European Nursing Diagnoses, Interventions, and Outcomes) Conference, a European nursing data set was discussed.[23] This was followed by a presentation given at the 1999 ICN conference that proposed an international approach to NMDS development.[24] The i-NMDS ideas and experiences were brought together in a panel discussion at the NI 2000 conference.[25] During the official IMIA-NI meetings in Auckland, it was formally decided that the IMIA-NI SIG would accept the development of i-NMDS as an official project. The ICN immediately agreed to cosponsor (with IMIA-NI SIG) the development of the i-NMDS. The preparations for a pilot started at the NI 2000 conference, a proposal was discussed at Medical Informatics Europe (MIE) in 2002, and further planning occurred at the NI 2003 in Brazil.[26] Outcomes of the NI 2003 meeting included confirmation of the need for the i-NMDS, the beginning formulation of nursing data items, and the description of goals for a pilot project. The i-NMDS Steering Committee decided to test the methodology through a retrospective study, collecting and comparing existing data across countries. The results of the pilot were discussed at the Medinfo 2004 conference,[27-29] and decisions about how to continue i-NMDS development resulted in plans for a prospective international study.

An International Look at National Nursing Minimum Data Set Initiatives

The i-NMDS project builds on work in individual countries. In a review of national NMDSs, four countries (the U.S., Belgium, France, and Australia) had an NMDS in use (see Table 24-1).[15,18,19,30-33] Further, the Netherlands and Finland had tested an NMDS in the general hospital setting.[27,33] Switzerland had tested an NMDS in hospitals and other settings.[34,35] Other countries (Thailand, Iceland, Canada, Sweden, Japan, and Brazil) are developing NMDSs of different kinds and for different purposes,[36-41] whereas Portugal is in the definition and pilot testing phase.[42] The countries listed in Table 24-1 use an NMDS in one stage of development or another.[26]

Belgium has collected MVG (Minimale Verpleegkundige Gegevens) NMDS on a national scale since 1988.[18] Currently, twenty-three nursing interventions form the minimum set.[19] Besides nurs-

Table 24-1. Stage of Development of NMDS by Country

Stage of Development	Country
In use nationally	Belgium,[18,19,29] France[30,31]
In use locally	United States[15]
In use on state level for community health	Community Nursing Minimum Data Set Australia (CNMDSA)[32]
Implementation phase	Iceland[37]
Pilots	Netherlands,[27] Telenurse for Europe,[20, 21] Finland,[33] Switzerland,[34] Portugal[42]
Definition phase	Canada,[38] Sweden,[39] Thailand,[36] Japan,[40] Brazil[41]
Research phase	Ireland[43]

ing intervention data, data about patient demographics, medical diagnoses, hospitalization, and caregivers are collected. These data are recorded four times per year during a fifteen-day period. Out of the fifteen days, data from five random days are sent to the Ministry of Public Health. Graphical presentation techniques are used for transforming data into information to bridge the gap between clinical nurses' and policy makers' understanding of the data.[29] Currently, approximately three percent of the budget for health care on the national level is based on the Belgian NMDS.[29] The Belgian NMDS is now being updated to include the use of the Nursing Interventions Classification (NIC) as the framework for interventions, to achieve full integration in the hospital discharge data set, and to improve the use of data.[44]

The French NMDS, called *Resumé de Soins Infirmiers* (RSI, meaning summary of nursing care), was established in 1987 as an addition to the French hospital minimum data set in order to better understand nursing and the composition of costs per the Diagnostic Related Group.[30,31] The RSI, defined as "the syntheses of the nursing process as written in the patient record,"[30] consists of nursing diagnoses, nursing interventions, nursing outcomes, and nursing intensity. For the measurement of nursing intensity, a patient classification system, *Méthode des soins infirmiers individualisés à la personne soignée* (SIIPS), was tested in thirty-five French hospitals from 1984 to 1986. Three categories of care were identified: (1) basic care, (2) technical and diagnostic care, and (3) educative, supportive care. The SIIPS is now in use in France.

The U.S. NMDS includes nursing diagnoses, nursing interventions, nursing outcomes, and an indicator of nursing intensity,[15,16] which adds to health care statistics that typically are limited to illness and disease. Ryan and Delaney[45] reviewed research on the NMDS and reported on its ability to describe nursing practice. They argue that evidence of variance in nursing diagnoses associated with medical diagnoses and surgical procedures exist, that relationships between nursing diagnoses and interventions could be established, and that nursing diagnoses sometimes are the only significant predictor variables for utilization measures. They further describe other uses of the NMDS.

Other countries are developing national NMDS systems as well. In Australia, the objective of the Community Nursing Minimum Data Set Australia (CNMDSA) is to introduce standardization and comparability into the collection of a minimal set of data to describe community nursing.[32] Although ongoing tests and data collections have taken place on a regular basis, no reports from Australia on the use of CNMDSA are available in the literature. Following Anderson and Hannah's[38] assertion of the need for an NMDS in Canada, the Alberta Association of Registered Nurses suggested the inclusion of nursing components in the Hospital Medical Records Institute database under the heading of "Health Information: Nursing Components."[46] This work is ongoing within and across provincial and national health information initiatives.

The Nursing Minimum Data Set for the Netherlands (NMDSN) has been developed[47] and was tested during the spring of 1998.[48] The goals for the NMDSN are twofold. First, the NMDSN should describe the diversity of patient populations from different wards and hospitals, as well as the variability of nursing care in terms of the prevalence of nursing phenomena (diagnoses, patient problems), nursing activities, and nursing outcomes.[47,48] Second, the nursing care information is intended to assist nursing managers in personnel allocation and to assist policy makers in decision making on issues involving resources.

In Switzerland, the need for an NMDS was recognized also[34,35] and the key components of a Swiss NMDS were identified during the 1998–2000 study period.[34] In the first phase, a theory was developed that built on existing workload systems (see http://www.hospvd.ch/public/ise). Currently, the nursing data project is in its second phase.

All these examples confirm that national efforts to develop, pilot, implement, and use national NMDSs are expanding. Clearly, leaders are examining other established NMDSs, thereby fostering a discussion of the philosophical and policy underpinnings, the commonalities and differences in definition, and the strengths and limitations related to data collection, management, analyses, and interpretation. These professional scholarly critiques contribute to the development and use of an i-NMDS.

Commonalties and Differences

Existing NMDSs can be compared with respect to their purpose and scope, data elements, methods of data management, analysis, feedback methods, benefits, and problems. In general there are many commonalities that are important for the consideration of an i-NMDS. Most NMDSs share a common purpose of description and comparison of nursing care and may be used to facilitate research and management. Further, the information from NMDS systems can influence policy making with respect to nursing care budgets and staff allocation. Table 24-2 compares the purposes of various NMDS systems.

NMDS Data Elements

The commonalities and differences among the NMDS systems reflect variations in financials structures linked to workload, reimbursement schemes, and management of population health. Table 24-3 presents an overview of data elements used in several NMDSs, based on a review by Goossen et al.[49] All NMDSs obviously have several items in common, but there are differences as well. The main commonalities are the nursing care data items (e.g., the nursing diagnosis, nursing intervention, and nursing outcome) and the demographic data items (about the patient, nurse, and institution). However, the Belgium MVG does not include nursing diagnoses and outcomes at this stage. The Australian CNMDSA, when compared with other systems, includes several additional items, e.g., dates of first contact, referral, and first visit because of its focus being home and community nursing.[32]

Methodology

Another aspect of the comparison of NMDS conducted by Goossen et al[49] concerned the processes of data collection, sampling size, analysis, and feedback (see Table 24-4). In some NMDS systems, the nursing care data are collected electronically, whereas others use paper-based systems or a combination of both. Sample sizes vary from approximately 100 to 15,000 patients per study in the U.S., to a 5.4 percent sample of all inpatient days, giving 1.2 million nursing records per year for a random sample of approximately 400,000 patients per year in the Belgian B-NMDS national database since 1988. Analysis of the data varies by study. In the U.S., data generation is dependent on indi-

Table 24-2. Comparison of the Purposes of Various NMDS Systems

NMDS (United States)	Belgium-NMDS (MVG) (Belgium)	CNMDSA (Australia)	Health Information: Nursing Components (HI:NC) (Canada)	Netherlands
Describe and compare nursing care	Bridge the gap between nursing practice and policy making	Comparison of performance of institutions	Deliver information that reflects nursing care	Describe the diversity of patient populations and the variability of nursing care
Demonstrate and analyze trends in nursing care	Describe health status	Allocation of budgets	Demonstrate the unique contribution of nurses to the health of Canadians	Relate to workload
Support nursing research	Allow for clinical nursing research	Monitor and compare the health status of the population		
Support policy based on data	Determine costs and effectiveness of nursing care	Deliver information		
	Determine the intensity of nursing care			
	Determine hospital budgets and staffing			
	Contribute to appropriate evaluation protocols (AEPs)			
	Produce nursing care profiles per diagnosis-related group (DRG)			

Table 24-3. Common and Different Elements in Selected NMDSs

Country	United States	Belgium	Australia	Switzerland	Netherlands
Name	Nursing Minimum Data Set	Minimale Verpleegkundige Gegevens	Community Nursing Minimum Data Set Australia	Nursing Data	NMDSN (Nursing Minimum Data Set the Netherlands)
Patient demographics	5 items	3 items	5 items	3 items	6 items
Medical care items	None	ICD-9-CM: linking to hospital discharge data set	Medical diagnosis	ICD-10 code surgical intervention	Medical diagnosis Medical condition items
Nursing care elements	Nursing diagnosis Nursing intervention Nursing outcome Intensity of nursing care	Nursing interventions ADL	Nursing diagnosis Goals of nursing care (7 types) Nursing intervention (8 types) Client dependency Discharge (4 items)	Nursing phenomena (56*3), Nursing intervention (51*4) Nursing outcome (indirect) Intensity of nursing care	24 Nursing diagnosis 32 Nursing intervention 4 Nursing outcome (fixed lists)
Variables about service elements: Agency provider	Unique service or agency number Unique health record number Unique nurse identifier	Unique hospital code Code specialty Code ward Number of beds	Agency identifier source of referral	Geographical location, unique institution code (hospital, nursing home, home care agency) type of ward	Five hospital related items, including: Type institution Type of ward
Variables about service elements: Episode	Episode or encounter date Discharge/ termination date	Admission date Length of stay Day of stay Discharge date	Date first contact Date of referral Discharge date from hospital Date first visit Discharge date Date last contact	Admission date and hour Discharge date and hour Intermediate movement date (transfer)	Moment of stay (admission, discharge)
Variables about service elements: Resources		Number of nursing hours available Number of nurses available Qualification mix	Resource utilization	Data by function for each caregiver, level of education, role, total amount of time worked by year, and percentage by function	Nursing's time for particular interventions
Variables about service elements: Other	Disposition of Patient Expected payer of the bills.		Other support services	Data collection linked with other health statistics	3 complexity of care items 10 nursing process items

Source: Updated from Goossen et al.[49]

viual research projects. Appropriate statistical analyses are selected based on research questions, and there are no national comparisons. Belgium has applied specific statistics for ordinal data, along with a multivariate approach, because no single indicator can measure all aspects of patient care. Almost all NMDS use is reported in the literature and in research reports, as well as at conferences, including international conferences.

Table 24-4. Data Collection, Sample, Aggregation, Analysis, and Feedback of Selected NMDSs

Name	NMDS (United States)	Belgium NMDS/Reference Information Model (RIM)	CNMDSA
Means of data collection	From electronic and paper records, based on inclusion criteria for study	Surveys during 15 days 4 times a year: paper, bar codes, or electronic records	Electronic records
Sample size	Sampling of about 100 to 15,000 patients per study and larger	1.2 million nursing records per year About 20 million nursing records since 1988	Not reported
Analysis of the data in the database	Dependent on every research project Appropriate statistics are selected based on research question No national comparison currently	Statistics for ordinal data Multivariate approach; no single indicator can measure all aspects of the complex process of patient care Cross-sectional approach to many interactions in nursing care	Not described in literature
Aggregation levels	Patient, unit, institution, and several institutions	Patient day, patient stay, patient, unit, hospital, and national	Patient, institution, national, international
Feedback Information	Reported in literature and/or research reports. Reported on local, regional, national, and international conferences	Fingerprints for ward, institution, and nation All wards and medical specialties Sent back to all hospitals on CD-rom and Internet (http://www.health.fgov.be/vesalius/devnew/NL/prof/regsys/mvg/index.htm)	Not described in literature Goes to the institutions that participate, and others that have an interest

Source: Based on Goossen et al, 1998.[49]

Strengths and Limitations of NMDS

Delaney and Moorhead[50] discuss the advantages of including nursing data in health care statistics for the health care community and for patients. They argue that nursing information provides added views of patients that were never before accessible, including, for example, the patient's health problems related to life processes, the costs of nursing care, and outcomes measurements, e.g., functional status and quality of life. Thus, an NMDS would have benefits for nursing and for health care delivery. On the other hand, problems associated with NMDS have also been reported. Goossen et al[49] summarized the potential and actual benefits, as well as the problems of NMDS. The benefits of an NMDS include the abilities to:

- Describe patient problems, nursing interventions, nurse-sensitive patient outcomes, and nursing resources across settings, clinical populations, geographic areas, and time.
- Compare nursing practice at different levels, offer testimony on nursing issues, develop databases, assess the cost effectiveness of nursing interventions and the costs of nurse resources, and provide data to influence health policy making.
- Share data with various health providers and researchers.

    There is empirical evidence that an NMDS offers additional benefits, specifically the abilities to:

1. Make the clinical contributions of nursing visible in figures and graphical representations (Belgium).[29]
2. Perform clinical, quality assurance, and epidemiological studies (Belgium)[51]
3. Finance nursing care at the national level (Belgium) or the institutional level[19,29,52]
4. Predict the intensity of nursing care and the necessary allocation of staff (United States)[53]
5. Abstract data in a cost-effective manner, and produce patient profiles (United States)[52]
6. Compare the prevalence of nursing diagnoses for several medical diagnoses and surgical procedures (United States)[54]
7. Visualize the differences in patient populations and variations in nursing practice (Netherlands)[48,55]

Problem areas and limitations of NMDS also exist. These include:

a. The lack of comparability of NMDS data items and inconsistent definitions[49]
b. The lack of relationships among nursing diagnoses, interventions, and outcomes in stored data[49]
c. Differences in the specificity and detail of vocabularies (granularity)
d. The inability of one vocabulary to fit all purposes[56]
e. The inhibition of the use of standards because of the ownership of definitions
f. The need to address informed consent issues and to take measures to protect privacy. (Ryan and Delaney[45] argue that approval from committees for the protection of human subjects should be obtained prior to the abstraction of nursing minimum data.)
g. The need to assess the reliability and validity of the database
h. The expense of updating an NMDS and upgrading existing data collections; of changes in the methodology, instruments, or classifications; of changes in information systems; and of the ongoing education of (new) users
i. The paucity of electronic patient record systems that allow users to directly retrieve nursing minimal data[17]

Commonalities and Differences in NMDSs in the World

We find the following common categories and items across countries: (1) service, setting, and provider items; (2) patient demographics; (3) medical condition; (4) nursing diagnoses and nursing phenomena; (5) nursing interventions; (6) nursing outcomes; and (7) intensity of nursing care. However, there are also differences across countries. Some countries use a unique patient identifier, whereas others do not because of privacy issues. Most NMDSs include nursing diagnoses and outcomes; however, Belgium MVG does not, but national quality indicators are currently being defined. The granularity of items differs, as do the record formats. For instance, the U.S. records all nursing diagnoses that might be present, whereas the Netherlands asks whether a patient has pain, which is answered yes or no. This difference involves the issue of the fixed versus the variable set of items in the NMDS. There are also differences in sampling and design. The U.S., for example, uses multiple designs (e.g., retrospective or prospective data collection) and all cases or sampling cases, with variation in sample size. Sampling and design are dependent on the research questions. Belgium uses a single design that evolves over time. To use nursing data across countries, we must tap into the benefits of national nursing minimum data projects, focus on the commonalities, and find ways to eliminate the differences. Given the earlier research illustrating both commonalities and differences in existing NMDSs, there clearly needs to be consistency both in the data set and in the research design for the collection and analysis of data.[42-44]

The Need for and Purpose of i-NMDS

There is a need to provide nursing data for several purposes.[15,18,19,47,57,58] Among these purposes are those affecting clinical, managerial, research- and policy related responsibilities and work. The nursing profession is in the process of developing and testing designs and methods for the collection and analysis of an i-NMDS in order to compare nursing care over time, populations, providers, locations, and nations.

The collecting of the i-NMDS can be justified by the fact that health care systems are influenced by many developments. All health systems and nursing services in particular are required to adjust and adapt. Changes in health care result from developments that include but are not limited to the following conditions:

1. The world population is aging, and there is a growth of individuals with chronic diseases, requiring more health care resources.
2. Funding for health care is limited, and expenditures have to be justified.
3. Consumers are increasing their demands, and they want transparency and evidence that they receive the appropriate and quality care to which they are entitled.
4. Innovations in practice and the growing application of technology are leading to increased demands for the management of patient data.

5. There is a need to continuously monitor the health status of the population and the effectiveness and quality of care.
6. The growing interest in evidence-based health care requires the availability of current research knowledge at the point of care in a format suitable for immediate use and analysis of variations.

Information Needs in Nursing

Nursing needs to collect data on the international level to make improvements in care delivery. Arguments can be found in Roemer's[59] reasons to study and compare health systems at large. Roemer advocates the use of comparison to best understand how to achieve health equity under different circumstances. Roemer maintains that through comparisons one can learn how to achieve efficacy and efficiency in relation to existing values and variables that influence health needs and health status of populations, and to support generalizations. Learning through comparisons can be done only when data are collected and managed in a manner that generates information and new knowledge.[60]

Roemer (1991) identifies three major areas of data that need to be available: (1) the health needs of the population (e.g., aggregates of nursing diagnoses and patient problems); (2) the service delivery system (e.g., nursing intervention and organization); and (3) the results or outcomes of care for the population that would include nursing outcomes based on risk adjustment and other corrections for known differences.[59]

According to the ICN, the continuous developments and changes in health care are of concern for nursing worldwide.[58,61] Clark argues that the value of nursing is no longer self-evident; it must be demonstrated to those who do not have the understanding derived from practice but who do have the power to affect or to determine the nature of nursing through policy determination and resource allocation.[61]

The Purpose of i-NMDS

There is a growing need for nursing data in electronic format for different purposes.[58] These needs span the continuum of care for the client (individual, family, and community) and reach across time-frames and health care delivery settings. Given the recognized challenges and the needs for nursing information at several levels in the organization of health care, there is a need for an i-NMDS. The general purposes of an i-NMDS can be derived from the challenges, the needs, and the advancement of an ICNP®.[58] The goals of the i-NMDS are to:

1. Describe nursing care
2. Enhance nursing documentation, clinical decision making, and continuity of care
3. Use measurable, comparable data and summaries to estimate the need for care
4. Monitor the quality of care, and evaluate quality improvement efforts
5. Measure the effectiveness of care provision, and improve the costing of nursing services
6. Share data with health providers, nurse educators, and researchers
7. Demonstrate trends
8. Develop and refine (electronic) clinical record systems
9. Support health policy based on nursing data and epidemiological studies, cost-benefit studies, the determination of the health status of populations, and studies of the contribution of nursing practice to multidisciplinary-based health care[58,60]

Tools

The tools needed to fulfill nursing's information needs include terminology standards, e.g., ICNP® and the International Classification of Functioning (ICF)—both ANA-recognized terminologies. Also needed are messaging standards (e.g., HL7), documentation and reporting tools (such as electronic health records), and mechanisms for decision support (DSS). From the perspective of the i-NMDS, such tools are essential. Other tools are necessary to aggregate nursing data from the individual to group levels. The i-NMDS can assist in this process. The Nursing Information Reference Model (NIRM) serves as a guide to determine more specific nursing information that is needed for decisions at different levels in health care[62,63] (Figure 24-1). The hierarchy in the multilayer model is consistent with earlier work in the U.S., e.g., ANA's nursing information pyramid.[17]

However, there is an added focus on the types of decisions (clinical, managerial, and policy-related) and on the contextual variables that influence them. The original NIRM figure, developed by Goossen, Epping, and Dassen (1997),[63] depicts four layers of nursing data and the decision support at different levels of data. Atomic data about the individual in the primary care process (layer 1) are transformed into conclusions (layer 2) by professionals by means of clinical decisions, resulting in nursing diagnoses, interventions, and outcomes, for which standardized terminology can be used. On the third level, institutional data sets can be defined to support nonclinical decisions, including those on staffing, budget, quality programs, education, and research. On level 4, the national use of an NMDS is placed to support health statistics and policy decisions on nursing care. The decisions on levels 3 and 4 usually do not require detailed information that can be traced back to an individual person. Therefore layers 3 and 4 allow adequate privacy protection. Moreover, a review of the data elements of several national NMDSs, as well as of the ANA-recognized Nursing Management Minimum Data Set (NMMDS), reveals valuable foundation work in the definition and measurement of key contextual variables needed to be responsive to the NIRM.

The NIRM initially was developed for national use. For the purpose of the i-NMDS, a fifth level can be added. This layer would include international policy and inform ICN and the World Health Organization (WHO), among other international organizations. The NIRM implies the use of several health care informatics standards, regulations, and systems, including, of course, standardized terminologies such as ICNP® and ICF.

The i-NMDS has to be based on clinical data. Also important for aggregate information is the context in which the care is delivered and thus where clinical data were collected. Context data are needed to interpret a quality benchmark, to adjust for fluctuations in staffing, to control for bias and confounders in research, and to balance policy. In brief, it is necessary to interpret the clinical data adequately. Data on workforce are collected at the national levels in many countries and by ICN, WHO, and other international organizations.

The NIRM model is based on the principle of documenting data at the point of care through the EHR and making data available for different uses and purposes. One such reuse of data is for decision

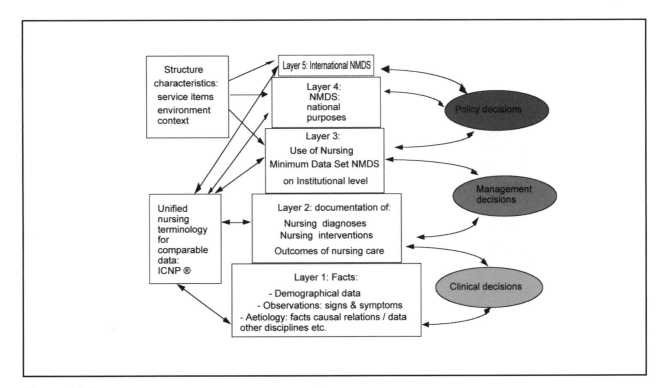

Figure 24-1. *The Nursing Information Reference Model,*[63] *adapted for i-NMDS.*

making, which requires additional information management (e.g., reliability and validity checks), comparisons, and analysis needs, to assure that the information is meaningful at the higher levels. Thus, the collection of nursing data, the development of nursing information systems, and the development of aggregated nursing information are represented on the NIRM, as depicted in Figure 24-1.

The Design and Results of the Pilot i-NMDS Study

Over several IMIA-NI meetings, a pilot i-NMDS was suggested and formally accepted by the board and general assembly at MIE 2002. The pilot work consisted of several activities. An extensive review of the literature was completed and still in process is the creation of a comprehensive data bank of all individuals in the different countries who were interested in participating in the project. Also, a survey was developed and administered on the purposes, the items, and the possible methodologies of an i-NMDS.

During the NI 2003 conference, the panel decided that it was too early to pilot the implementation of an i-NMDS on an international level because several issues related to specific international data set variables were not resolved. The panel decided that a better start would be to analyze existing recent nursing data sets from three or four countries that were ready for a comparative analysis. The other course of action was to further work on the conceptual definition of the i-NMDS.

The Medinfo 2004 panel discussed the initial results for the pilot of an i-NMDS, which was based on retrospective analyses of the Swiss, U.S., Dutch, and Belgian NMDSs.[27] These NMDSs had been collected for different purposes and at different levels and scales, and consequently, they were not easily comparable. Dealing with the issues and differences across countries became critical to the ongoing i-NMDS project.

The pilot study tested a method for the collection and analysis of potential variables of an i-NMDS, using the ICNP®. The research questions included:
• Can nursing diagnoses and corresponding interventions be reported?
• Can nursing diagnoses and corresponding interventions be related to each other and mapped to the ICNP®?
• What data collection methods are feasible?
• What data analysis procedures are valid and reliable?
• What are the most effective and appropriate reporting mechanisms?

Data from the Swiss test of the NMDS were to be compared with recent data from the U.S. and Belgium. In addition, the NMDSN data from the Netherlands were used. However, the preceding research questions proved to be too ambitious at that stage, mainly because of the retrospective nature of this kind of comparison. It was found that:
1. Gathering the data files and coding lists proved to be time-consuming and problematic.
2. The differences in languages and the lack of standard codes required the data sets to be translated into English.
3. The four example NMDSs were all developed for slightly different purposes.
4. Differences existed in the organization of the four data sets.
5. The levels of abstraction in the data varied: One serves a whole population, the other a state, and still others serve various local levels.
6. Periods of the samples did not match (1998 compared with 2000, 2001, and 2003).
7. There were differences in the granularity and coding used. Although this issue was foreseen and the ICNP® was selected as the basis for the reports, recoding proved again to be too time-consuming due to the need for manual operations.
8. Interventions and outcome are not always linked to nursing diagnoses.

The results of the data analysis from retrospective convenience samples of the U.S., Switzerland, the Netherlands, and Belgium revealed that there are too many differences in the details of the data for adequate statistical analysis, even for simple descriptions of prevalence. However, this pilot offered insight into specific methodological details to be tackled, suggested a beta version for the i-NMDS data elements, and supported the decision that the prospective approach might be more feasible for the i-NMDS development and testing.[27,66] Dealing with these issues from a variety of approaches in four countries was an important part of the panel discussion. Thus, the pilot, although it did not result in the statistical analysis of data, provided valuable insight for future research. The decision to work further with prospective studies (including the necessary prospective data selection, collection, and analysis) moved the work in a new direction.

This decision led to a discussion among the Steering Committee members about the purpose of the pilot. Although it is possible to carry out the plan, it was essential to clarify the i-NMDS's purpose, variables, and uses by ICN and WHO. Finally, the pilot study resulted in the following proposal for the variables in the i-NMDS.

Proposed Variables and Research Designs Resulting from the i-NMDS Pilot

The 2004 pilot i-NMDS led to consensus on the conceptual model of the i-NMDS and on three essential areas for the data: (1) nursing care, (2) client, and (3) setting. In August 2005, the ICN supported the i-NMDS–Beta as a working data set (Table 24-5). A validation study of the proposed variables will occur in 2005–2006.

Further, the i-NMDS should include the following characteristics about the data set:

- Start and stop dates of the i-NMDS collection
- Country code (ISO)
- Responsible person for collection
- Responsible agency of collector

Table 24-5. i-NMDS–Beta Version

1. Nursing Care Data*
Patient/client diagnoses/focus of care
Nursing interventions
Patient/client outcomes
Intensity of care
2. Patient/Client Data*
Start date of care episode
Stop date of care episode
Country of residence
Discharge status
Year of birth
Gender
Reason for admission (medical diagnoses, if applicable)
3. Setting Data†
Agency location
Ownership of agency
Country system of payment
Clinical service type
Clinical service capacity (number of units of service)
Care personnel: nurse gender
Care personnel: nurse training and education
Care personnel: quantity
Ratio of patients or clients to care personnel
* *Collected for each client for each encounter through care documentation.*
† *May be collected by management or retrieved from other paper or computer systems, files, or records.*

- E-mail and phone contact
- Medium of submission
- Unit of measurement (e.g., individual patient or client, family, group, community)
  Guidelines for all data collection related to the i-NMDS will:
1. Identify the specific purpose(s).
2. Assure linkage among the patient/client diagnoses and focus of care, nursing interventions, and client/patient outcomes.
3. Use prospective design when possible.
4. Assure the data set for the collection specifies data variables, codes, and values, applying the international standard for "Specification and Standardization of Data Elements" (ISO/IEC 11179–2003 version).
5. Allow local terminology to be used and mapped to ICNP®.
6. Use terminology from ICNP®, equivalent reference terminologies, or project-endorsed classifications.
7. Be prioritized by ICN's and WHO's strategic goals for nursing and midwifery.
8. Contribute to evidence-based nursing practice.
9. Disseminate results to the global community.

Linking to WHO's and ICN's Strategic Goals

The need for data to describe health is crucial. It is imperative to prioritize the work of the i-NMDS to maximize its service to and its impact on ICN and WHO priorities initiatives and requirements.[64] The linkage between the WHO objectives for nursing and the i-NMDS project is illustrated by the abstract in Table 24-6.[65] For example, as an excellent priority for initial work, the ICN and WHO workforce-related strategic goals were taken into account as a starting point for prospective studies. The ICN and WHO have set several priorities for projects with particular patient categories (e.g., tuberculosis and HIV). Therefore, in addition to understanding the nursing workforce, there is an interest in collecting information about nursing care for particular patient categories. The studies would include focused research questions and the development of questionnaires in which select i-NMDS variables are included.

Beyond the institutional and national uses of the i-NMDS work, applications support international health care priorities on both the clinical and the workforce agendas.

Future Directions

The i-NMDS project has evolved over the last eight years since the NI conference discussion in 1997. The work has now come to focus on the future use of the i-NMDS.[66] The 2004 pilot and the Medinfo 2004 panel discussion proposed future directions for the i-NMDS, that is, to identify spe-

Table 24-6. Examples of the Interrelatedness of the i-NMDS and WHO Strategic Planning for Nursing

Key Result Area	Objective	Expected Results—Direct Relationship
1. Health planning, advocacy and political commitment: National development and health plans provide for adequate nursing and midwifery services and expertise.	1. To strengthen those mechanisms relating to human resources policy intervention and planning in order to contribute to the maintenance of adequate levels of nursing and midwifery personnel so that health systems may function more effectively. 2. To mobilize policymakers, the general public, partners, and health care practitioners to support changes designed to strengthen nursing and midwifery services and to enhance their contribution to health system performance and outcomes.	1. Models developed on causes of workforce shortage and migration within and between countries. 2. Uniform indicators and systems established for monitoring human resources levels, shortage, and migration. 3. Evidence developed and disseminated to policymakers on success stories of the nursing and midwifery contribution to health system goals.

cific purposes, variables, and the use of a prospective design. Because the purposes of the i-NMDS will help guide the actual use of the data items, we will summarize its definition and purposes.

The Definition of and Purpose for i-NMDS Collection

After the pilot and discussions, the following recommendations can be proposed for future work on the i-NMDS.

- The *definition* of the i-NMDS is based on Werley's[15] and Sermeus'[18] definitions of NMDSs: "The International Nursing Minimum Data Set is a minimum but essential data set of items of information with uniform definitions and categories concerning the specific dimension of nursing internationally that are maximally useful for different purposes, and which meets the information needs of multiple data users in the health care system worldwide."
- The *purposes* of an i-NMDS are to meet information needs at the international level and to provide direction for data standards at the national level.

To achieve its identified purposes, the i-NMDS should:

1. Refer to ICN and WHO strategic goals for nursing and midwifery
2. Select desirable and feasible goals for one study
3. Formulate research questions
4. Focus on concrete and operational objectives
5. Institute a prospective design
6. Layout a data set for collection (data variables, codes, values, applying the international standard for "Specification and Standardization of Data Elements" [ISO/IEC 11179–2003 version] to ensure a consistent application of the nursing data elements
7. Formalize the collection method
8. Identify the requirements for collection
9. Allow local terminology to be used and mapped to ICNP®
10. Use terminology from ICNP®, equivalent reference terminologies, or project-endorsed classifications
11. Analyze data
12. Present results and disseminate them to the international community
13. Contribute to evidence-based nursing practice; allow for global comparisons

Work to Be Done

At the time of this writing, preparations are under way for a Web-based validation survey on the i-NMDS goals, the data elements, and the methodological principles for collection and use of the i-NMDS. Further discussions are taking place on specific research projects and operational goals. Please refer to the i-NMDS Web site for further information: available at www.inmds.org.

The suggestions for the future i-NMDS pilot study were presented to the ICN and WHO in October 2004. ICNP® committees met with Jean Yan (chief nurse scientist, WHO–Nursing and Midwifery), Miklos Zrinyi (technical officer, WHO), and Alain Junger (Institute of Health Economics, Switzerland) to discuss the i-NMDS and the ICNP®. The group discussed the importance of collaboration between ICN and WHO, specifically with respect to standards (e.g., nursing data sets and the ICNP®) and ICF classifications. It was decided to link the developments and to see where in the near future cooperation for specific research studies or surveys would be feasible. WHO and ICN thus confirmed the importance of the work and collectively encouraged the identification of the priority health populations and health conditions to study. Plans to target specific patient populations and specific nursing concerns were discussed with ICN and WHO. The ICNP® Strategic Advisory Group suggested the need for an i-NMDS to examine the linkages among nursing resources, clinical practice patterns, and patient outcomes within select patient populations. These condition-specific core data sets could evolve as information needs are defined by ICN and their members. The framework of an i-NMDS would be used to develop condition-specific surveys or data collection tools to be used at the national level for reporting to ICN or WHO.

The IMIA-NI SIG, as a cosponsor of the project, fully supports the initiative, facilitating the process through the Nursing Concept Representation Working Group. IMIA-NI SIG congregates expert nurses from more than thirty-two countries and organizes a worldwide conference every three years. For the last eight years, at every conference, its members have worked hard to include the subject on the scientific program. In this way, attendees might be stimulated to participate in the project. To IMIA-NI SIG, the development of an i-NMDS is fundamental to better understand our similarities and differences, share resources and information, and provide better-quality nursing care. Before the results of this project can be applied in real practice, the challenge for everyone is huge. However, we know that the findings will lead to more universal nursing care, equally available to the world population.

Summary

This chapter provides a brief historic overview of nursing minimum data sets around the world. Many countries are using or developing NMDSs, and the relevance of nursing data is growing. There are sufficient commonalities in NMDS to support building on the national initiatives. However, the differences in systems must be tackled to get meaningful information on the international level. The need for an i-NMDS has been identified, which has led to discussions, ongoing review, and pilot testing. A 2004 pilot resulted in important recommendations for the future.

A set of nursing data items in three areas of concern could be established, and they are open to further consensus, standardization, and application. Also, the i-NMDS can support prospective studies. Fundamental to achieving the goals for the i-NMDS is the ability to document nursing data at the point of care, ultimately possible only through efficient electronic health records.

In the future, with work in this area linked to the international work of ICN and WHO, it will be easier to identify the priorities for patient groups to be studied with the i-NMDS and to engage nurses all over the world to visualize their work and improve patient care. Also, educators, researchers, managers, and policy makers will be able to base decisions pertaining to nursing care on information.

References

1. Nightingale F. *Notes on Nursing*. New York: Dover Publications: 1860.
2. Nightingale F. *Notes on Hospitals,* 3rd ed. London: Roberts & Green: 1863.
3. Henderson V. *The Nature of Nursing*. New York: MacMillan: 1996.
4. Abdellah F, Beland I, Martin A, Mathney R. *Patient-Centered Approaches in Nursing*. New York: MacMillan: 1960.
5. Gebbie KM, ed. *Summary of the Second National Conference: Classification of Nursing Diagnosis*. St. Louis: National Group for Classification of Nursing Diagnosis: 1976.
6. North American Nursing Diagnoses Association. *NANDA: Nursing Diagnoses Definitions & Classifications: 2005–2006*. Philadelphia: NANDA International: 2005.
7. American Nurses Association. *Standards of Clinical Nursing Practice*. Washington, DC: ANA Publishing: 1973.
8. American Nurses Association. *Standards of Clinical Nursing Practice*. Washington, DC: ANA Publishing: 1998.
9. American Nurses Association. *Nursing's Social Policy Statement* (2nd ed.). Washington, DC: nursesbooks.org: 2003.
10. McCormick AK, Lang N, Zielstorff R. Toward standardized classification schemes for nursing languages: Recommendations of the American Nurses Association Database Steering Committee to Support Nursing Practice. *J Am Med Inform Assoc.* 1994; 1:422-427.
11. National League for Nursing. *Management information systems for public health / community health agencies: Report of the conference*. New York: NLN: 1974.
12. Saba VK, Levine E. Management information systems for public health nursing services. *Public Health Rep.* 1978;93:1:79-83.
13. Saba VK, Levine E. Patient care module in community health nursing. In: Werley HW and Grier MR, eds. *Nursing Information Systems*. New York: Springer Publishing Co.: 1981.
14. Saba VK, McCormick KA. *Essential of Computers for Nurses*. Philadelphia: J.B. Lippincott Co.: 2000.
15. Werley HH, Lang NM. *Identification of the Nursing Minimum Data Set*. New York: Springer Publishing Co.:1988.
16. Werley HH, Devine EC, Zorn CR, Ryan P, Westra B. Nursing minimum data: abstraction tool for standardized, comparable, essential data. *Am J Publ Health.* 1991;18:421-426.

17. Zielstorff RD, Hudgings CI, Grobe SJ. *Next-Generation Nursing Information Systems, Essential Characteristics for Professional Practice.* Washington, DC: American Nurses Publishing: 1993.

18. Sermeus W, Delesie L. The registration of a nursing minimum data set in Belgium: six years of experience. In: Grobe SJ and Pluyter-Wenting ESP, eds. *Proceedings Nursing Informatics '94. Nursing Informatics: An international overview for Nursing in a Technological Era.* Amsterdam: Elsevier North Holland; 1994:144-149.

19. Sermeus W. Variabiliteit van Verpleegkundige verzorging in Algemene Ziekenhuizen. *Leuven: Dissertatie Fac. der Geneeskunde,* school voor de Maatschappelijke Gezondheidszorg: 1992.

20. Mortensen R, Mantas J, Manuela M, Sermeus W, Nielsen GH, McAvinue E. Telematics for health care in the European Union. In: Grobe SJ and Pluyter-Wenting ESP, eds. *Proceedings Nursing Informatics '94. Nursing Informatics: An international overview for Nursing in a Technological Era.* Amsterdam: Elsevier North Holland; 1994:750-752.

21. Nielsen GH, Mortensen RA. *TELENURSING Nursing Minimum Data Sets in Europe* (vol. IV). Copenhagen: Danish Institute for Health and Nursing Research; 1994

22. International Medical Informatics Association, Nursing Informatics (IMIA-NI). The impact of nursing knowledge on health care informatics. *6th International Congress on Nursing Informatics NI'97.* Stockholm, Sweden; 26 Sept.-Oct. 1, 1997.

23. Goossen WTF. A European nursing minimum data set [plenary abstract]. In: Abstract book 2nd European Conference of the Association for Common European Nursing Diagnosis, Interventions and Outcomes (ACENDIO). Venice, Italy; 1999:7-8.

24. Goossen WTF. Can we compare nursing care internationally with the current Nursing Minimal Data Sets? [lecture]. *ICN Centennial Celebrations Conference: Celebrating Nursing's Past, Claiming the Future.* London; June-1 July 1999.

25. Clark J, Delaney C. Conceptualization and feasibility of an international Nursing Minimum Data Set (i-NMDS). [abstract] In: Saba V, Carr R, Sermeus W, and Rocha P, eds. *One Step Beyond: The Evolution of Technology & Nursing, Proceedings of the 7th International Congress on Nursing Informatics.* 2000:865.

26. Delaney C, Goossen W, Park H, et al. Seeking international consensus on elements of the international Nursing Minimum Data Set (iNMDS) [abstract]. In: Marin H, Marques E, Hovenga E, and Goossen W, eds. *Proceedings of the 8th International Congress in Nursing Informatics.* 2003:74-75.

27. Goossen W, Delaney C, Sermeus W, et al. Preliminary results of a pilot of the international Nursing Minimum Data Set (i-NMDS) [abstract]. In: *Proceedings of Medinfo 11th World Congress on Medical Informatics of the International Medical Informatics Association.* 2004:S103.

28. Ford Y, Rukanudding R, Thoroddsen A, Jones J, Delaney C. The CIC Nursing & Health Informatics Consortium: A new model for NI research & education—an examination of the proposed international Nursing Minimum Data Set (iNMDS) [abstract]. In: *Proceedings of Midwest Nursing Research Society 28th Annual Research Conference.* 2004:81.

29. Sermeus W, Delesie L. Development of a presentation tool for nursing data. In: Mortensen RA, ed. *ICNP in Europe: Telenurse.* Amsterdam: IOS Press; 1997:167-176.

30. Ministère des Affaires Sociales de la Santé et de la Ville, Direction des Hôpitaux. *Le Résumé de soins infirmiers RSI.* France: Minestère; 1995.

31. Duboys Fresney C. *Le Résumé de Soins Infirmiers.* Paris: Maloine; 1997.

32. Gliddon T, Weaver C. The Community Nursing Minimum Data Set Australia: From definition to the real world. *Proceedings of the Fifth International Conference on Nursing Use of Computers and Information Science.* 1994:163-168.

33. Turtianen AM, Kinnunen J, Sermeus W, Nyberg T. The cross-cultural adaptation of the Belgium Nursing Minimum Data Set to Finnish nursing. *J Nurs Manag.* 2000;8:281-290.

34. Berthou A, Junger A. *Rapport Final Nursing Data 1998–2000.* Lausanne: ISE; 2000.

35. Weber P. An instrument for better dealing with costs: minimal data for nursing care. *Krankenpfl Soins Infirm.* 1996:89:4:13-17.

36. Kunaviktikul W, Anders RL, Srisuphan W, Chontawan R, Nuntasupawat R, Pumparporn O. Development of quality of nursing care in Thailand. *J Adv Nurs.* 2001;36:6:776-784.

37. Haraldsdottir S, ed. Minimum Data Set in hospitals in Iceland [Lagmarksskraning vistunarupplysinga a sjukrahusum]. Reykjavik: Directorate of Health; 2001.

38. Anderson B, Hannah KJ. A Canadian nursing minimum data set: a major priority. *Can J Nurs Admin.* 1993;6:7-13.

39. Elo S. The Public Health Nursing Minimum Data Set: Development, application, and use. *Vard I Norden.* 1995;15:3:9-16.

40. Shimanouchi S, Uchida E, Kamei T, Sasaki A, Shinoda M. Development of an assessment sheet for home care. *Int J Nurs Prac.* 2000;7:3:140-145.

41. Filho JR. The complexity of developing a nursing information system: A Brazilian experience. *Computers in Nursing.* 2001;19:3:98-104.

42. Paira A, Pereira F. Nursing Minimum Data Set in Portugal. ESEnf.S.João, College of Nursing. http://www.fnaee.pt/index.php?set=links-esenfs

43. Scott A, et al. Irish NMDS as part of research project [website]. 2003. Available at: http://www.dcu.ie/nursing/decision_making.shtlm. Accessed February 22, 2005.

44. Sermeus W, Van de Heede K, Michiels D, et al. A nation-wide project for the revision of the Belgian nursing minimum dataset: from concept to implementation. In: Roger France FH, De Clercq E, de Moor G., van der Lei J, eds. *Health Continuüm and Data Exchange in Belgium and in the Netherlands.* Proceedings MIC 2004. Amsterdam: IOS Press; 2004:21-26.

45. Ryan P, Delaney C. The Nursing Minimum Data Set: Research findings and future directions. In: Fitzpatrick JJ and Stevenson JS, eds. *Annual review of nursing research.* New York: Springer Publishing Co.; 1995:13:169-194.

46. Hannah K, Duggleby W, Anderson B, et al. The development of essential data elements in Canada (health information: nursing components). MEDINFO; 1995:Pt 2:1375-7.

47. Goossen, WTF, Epping PJMM, Van den Heuvel WJA, Feuth T, Frederiks CMA, Hasman A. Development of the Nursing Minimum Data Set for the Netherlands (NMDSN): Identification of categories and items. *J Adv Nurs.* 2000:31:3:536-547

48. Goossen WT, Epping PJ, Feuth T, van den Heuvel WJ, Hasman A, Dassen TW. Using the nursing minimum data set for the Netherlands (NMDSN) to illustrate differences in patient populations and variations in nursing activities. *Int J Nurs Stud.* 2001;38:3:243-257.

49. Goossen WTF, Epping PJMM, Feuth T, Dassen TWN, Hasman A, Van den Heuvel, WJA. A comparison of Nursing Minimum Data Sets. *J Am Med Inform Assoc.* 1998:5:2:152-163.

50. Delaney C, Moorhead S. The nursing minimum data set standardized language and health care quality. *J Nurs Care Qual.* 1995:10:16-30.

51. Evers G, Viane A, Sermeus W, Simoens-De Smet A, Delesie L. Frequency of and indications for wholly compensatory nursing care related to enteral food intake: a secondary analysis of the Belgium National Nursing Minimum Data Set. *J Adv Nurs.* 2000:32:1:194-201.

52. Delaney C, Mehmert M, Prophet C, Crossley J. Establishment of the research value of nursing minimum data sets. In: Grobe SJ and Pluyter-Wentign ESP, eds. *Nursing Informatics: An International Overview for Nursing In a Technological Era. Proceedings of Nursing Informatics 1994.* Amsterdam: Elsevier North Holland; 1994:169-173.

53. Saba VK, Zuckerman AE. A home health care classification system. In: Lun KC, et al, eds. MEDINFO '92: 334-348.

54. Ryan P, Coenen A, Devine EC, et al. Prevalence and relationships among elements of nursing minimum data set. In: Grobe SJ and Pluyter-Wentign ESP, eds. *Nursing Informatics: An International Overview for Nursing In a Technological Era. Proceedings of Nursing Informatics 1994.* Amsterdam: Elsevier North Holland; 1994:174-178.

55. Griens AMGF, Goossen WTF, van der Kloot, WA. Exploring the Nursing Minimum Data Set for the Netherlands using multidimensional scaling techniques. Koudekerk and den Rijn, eds. *J Adv Nurs.* 2001:36:1:89-101.

56. Hoy D. Managing expectations: Users, requirements and the International Classification for Nursing Practice. In: Mortensen RA, ed. *ICNP in Europe: Telenurse.* Amsterdam: IOS Press; 1997:207-215.

57. Renwick M. National minimum data sets: the Australian experience. *Inf Tech Nurs.* 1992:4:3:4.

58. Clark J, Lang NM. Nursing's Next Advance: an International Classification for Nursing Practice. *Int Nurs Rev.* 1992:39:109-112.

59. Roemer MI. *National Health Systems of the World, Vol 1: The Countries.* New York, Oxford: Oxford University Press; 1991

60. Goossen WTF. Digitizing health information: Why and how? Nursing's contribution to better health outcomes [keynote address for: APAMI - HIC 97 Joint Conference, HISA, Sydney, Australia]. In: Hannan T, McGhee S, Symonds I, eds. *Conference Proceedings APAMI – HIC'97: Managing Information for Better Health Outcomes in Australia and the Asia Pacific Region.* Sydney: HISA; August 1997:8 (abstracts), 142-162.

61. Clark J. An international classification for nursing practice. In: Henry SB, Holzemer WL, Tallberg M, Grobe SJ, eds. *Informatics: the infrastructure for quality assessment and improvement in nursing.* Austin, TX: IMIA; 1994.

62. Epping PJ, Goossen WT, Dassen TWN, Hasman A. Towards congruence in nursing information provision in the Netherlands [review in Dutch]. *Verpleegkunde.* 1996:11:4:215-227.

63. Goossen WT, Epping PJ, Dassen T. Criteria for nursing information systems as a component of the electronic patient record: An international Delphi study. *Comput Nurs.* 1997:15:6:307-315.

64. Mortensen RA, ed. *ICNP in Europe: TELENURSE.* Amsterdam: IOS Press; 1997.

65. World Health Organisation. (2005) *Nursing and Midwifery Services: Strategic Directions 2002–2008.* Geneva: WHO; 2005. http://www.who.int/health-services-delivery/nursing/index.htm. Accessed February 15, 2005.

66. Goossen WTF, Delaney C, Coenen A. Lessons learned for the international Nursing Minimum Data Set (i-NMDS). In: Oud N, Sermeus W, Ehnfors M, eds. *Proceedings of the ACENDIO 2005 conference, Bled, Slovenia.* Bern: Hans Huber Verlag; 2005:31-35.

SECTION V

The Electronic Health Record Initiatives Across the Globe

SECTION V

Introduction

Robyn L. Carr, RGON

Section V ambitiously attempts to give an around-the-world glimpse of the current state for uses of information technology (IT) in health care and specifically, the status of electronic health record (EHR) initiatives among a wide sampling of nations. The move toward EHRs is nearly a worldwide phenomenon, driven by governments' search for more effective and efficient mechanisms to manage their populations' health and the escalating costs associated with care delivery. Over the past decade, the consumer public has been shocked by publications documenting the high level of error, waste, inefficiencies, and quality deficits across western medical systems. Spurred by the growing evidence that health care systems around the world are marked by extensive variance in treatment approaches, surgical procedure rates, outcomes, and costs, governments have begun pushing for the use of IT to better structure coordination of care against best practices. This transition to using IT in the clinical processes of care delivery is happening at an explosive rate. As a result, nurses are increasingly being recruited to work as members of project teams, as team leaders, as leaders in strategic planning, and as leaders of major organizational- and government-level initiatives.

As our health care systems struggle to achieve transformation, at some point along the journey it is being discovered that the need for significant and lasting change requires full engagement of nursing. This demand translates in two ways. Nurses are engaged to help make change happen. Then nurses are asked to change their own culture and work practices to make transformation happen, and in the process they bring along the other disciplines. These EHR initiatives present both challenges and great opportunity for nursing as a profession, for the discipline of nursing informatics, and for the career path options that nursing informatics creates. Section V aims to capture the effects EHR initiatives have on nursing in all their variation. It is important that we not miss this snapshot in nursing's evolution and that we pause to document these developments for our own understanding and for our history.

Section V is organized into five chapters, according to their geographic areas: the Americas; the United Kingdom and Ireland; Europe: Western, Central, and Eastern; Africa; and Australasia and the South Pacific. Grouped under these major geographic sections are seventeen case studies that provide rich descriptions of the role and status of nursing, the level of development of nursing informatics and the impact of EHR initiatives on nursing within their given countries. Even countries in which health informatics has been active for more than three decades and that have national EHR strategies in process, extensive variation in nursing's involvement, inclusion, and integration, as seen in these case studies. For more about these contrasts, read the Norway, Finland, Sweden, and Germany case studies.

Countries whose entry into the nursing informatics (NI) surge is more recent, but who are rapidly moving toward full professional engagement in regard to nursing and nursing informatics in integrated EHRs, are described in the case studies of Ireland, Spain, Italy, Korea, Australia, and New Zealand. It is obvious from reading the case studies from the United Kingdom, Canada, and the United States that even in those countries that are investing heavily and are fully committed to implementing an EHR nation wide, that initial steps have only been taken and that the end point is a decade or more away. And finally, leaders in nursing informatics in nations just beginning to introduce IT into health care services have stepped forward to ensure that their countries are represented in this overview. These include Africa, Brazil, Chile, and the Central and Eastern European countries. Despite differences in economic and political structures, as well as geographic variations across these seventeen case studies, there are also many similarities and common themes to be found in their stories. These contrasts and similarities provide remarkable insights into the correlation between nursing education and professional status and to inclusion in EHR initiatives within a given country.

CHAPTER 25

The Americas: Overview of EHR National Strategies and Significance for Nursing

By Connie White Delaney, PhD, RN, FAAN, FACMI; Jorge Gonzales Vivo, MD; Lynn M. Nagel, PhD, RN; and Heimar F. Marin, PhD, RN, FACMI

Although the global impact of national electronic health record (EHR) initiatives has yet to be realized, there is growing evidence that the work of international standards and informatics organizations, e.g. International Medical Informatics Association (IMIA) are crucial for leveraging knowledge and learning. This chapter is an overview of the state of the science for nursing and EHR initiatives across the Americas. This is a daunting task given the diversity and variation across this massive geographic area and thus this overview chapter begins with a sampling rather than an in-depth description for all countries in this geography. Following this overview, a brief description of Canada, the U.S., and Brazil is presented as nations with formally defined EHR strategies in various stages of implementation. Three geographic areas in Latin America and the Caribbean, as well as two countries in South America (Argentina and Chile) are reviewed as examples of emerging EHR initiatives and development of professional nursing.

Overview of the Americas

Geographically, the Americas consist of forty-five nations and territories across four major areas, as depicted in Figure 25-1.[1] The geographic expanse of the Americas is enormous. North and South America alone include more than 42 million square kilometers (29.5 percent) of all land in the world. Adding the land mass of the Caribbean and Central America extends this total by more than 20 million square kilometers, giving an approximate total land mass of more than 60 million square kilometers. Canada is ranked by land as the second largest country in the world when volume and area are measured (which includes water); Brazil ranks eighth in total land. To provide a more detailed health context for examination of EHR initiatives, each component of the Americas, including geographical composition and health-related statistics, follows.

North America includes Canada, the U.S., Mexico, and Greenland[2] (see Figure 25-2). Table 25-1 summarizes health-related statistics for the four countries comprising North America.[3] Although English is the predominant language spoken, French is spoken in parts of Canada, Spanish in Mexico, and Greenlandic in Greenland. A review of the health statistics indicates wide variation in most dimensions, including population, gross domestic product (GDP) and both infant and adult mortality. Across the gradient of developing, developed and industrial countries, health expenditures are used as a key indictor to reflect a population's health status and health care quality. However, the U.S. is an exception to this statistical correlation, having the highest healthcare expenditures per GDP in the world (see Figure 25-3) but ranking far below other industrial countries on most quality indicators. The Pan American Health Organization provides an excellent two volume analysis and comparison of health systems, population health statistics, and health care access across this diverse geopolitical aggregate in their 2002 edition of *Health in the Americas.*[4]

As shown in Figure 25-4, Central America encompasses eight countries, and the Caribbean includes 23 nation states and islands.[5] The socio-economic status across these nations ranges from considerable affluence throughout many of the Caribbean countries (e.g., Aruba) to the most dire (e.g., Haiti). This marked variation in economics, health expenditures, and health status indicators across the countries within this geography is outlined in Table 25-2.[3] Finally, the South American

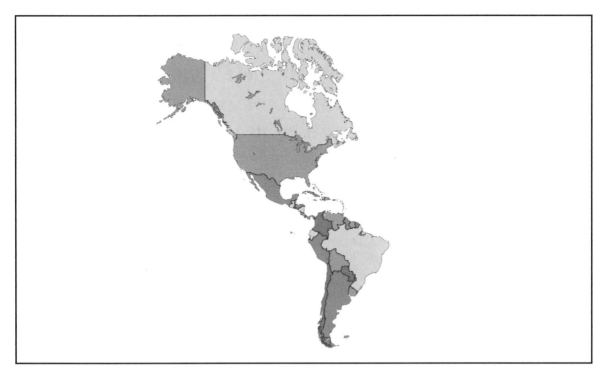

Figure 25-1. *Map of the Americas.*

continent encompasses Argentina, Bolivia, Brazil, Chile, Colombia, Ecuador, Guyana, Paraguay, Peru, Suriname, Uruguay, and Venezuela as depicted in Figure 25-5.[6] Culturally, in land mass and through language, Brazil stands apart from its Spanish-speaking neighboring countries, and its uniqueness is addressed in Marin and del Sasso's following Case Study 25C. Table 25-3 outlines key health statistics for the larger countries comprising South America.[3]

Many variances in statistical reporting occur, making even simple comparisons such as land mass, population, and economic indicators difficult. In other circumstances, particularly in emerging countries, statistics simply do not exist. However, Figure 25-3 is included to depict at least one example of comparisons possible with World Health Organization data—a bar graph illustrates money spent on health care per country in Central and South America compared with the U.S.[7]

Electronic Health Record Progress
The complexity of developing EHRs within countries as well as the challenges of interoperability across countries and continents is massive. The following section describes EHR initiatives in Canada and the U.S. in North America and Brazil in South America, as nations with formally defined EHR strategies in various stages of implementation. Following these summaries, examples of emerging EHR efforts are discussed. Three geographic areas in Latin America and the Caribbean as well as two countries in South America (Argentina and Chile) are reviewed.

Canada
Canada established an aggressive, proactive agenda to provide the information infrastructure to support health care delivery in the 1990s, as noted by Nagle and Shaw's Case Study 25A following this chapter. Canada's information infrastructure movement was in response to the findings of virtually every health services study since the 1960s that emphasized the importance of accurate and adequate information to manage the system and that highlighted major concerns about system inefficiencies. Federal and provincial reports were permeated with recommendations for relevant information and data to be consistently captured in information systems initiatives. The creation of the Canadian Institute for Health Information in 1992 resulted in a coordinated effort to provide access to data that increases understanding and improvement of the health system.

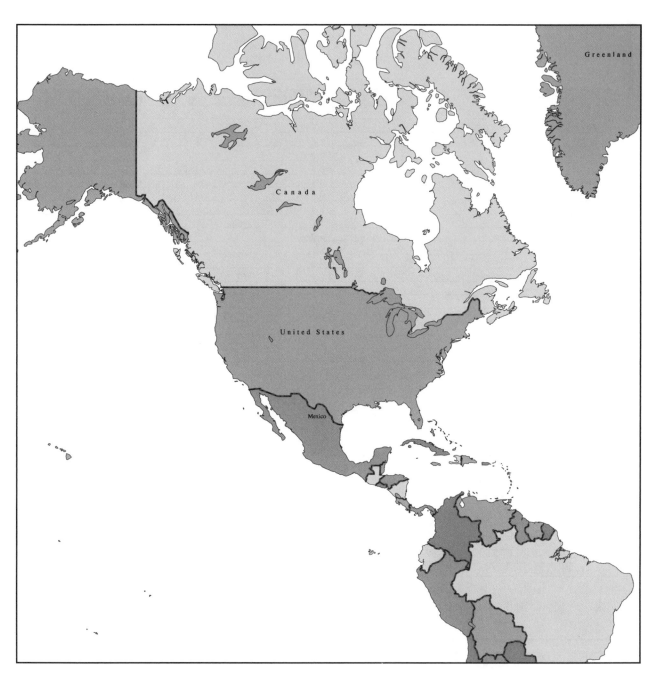

Figure 25-2. *Map of North America.*

Table 25-1. North American Country Health Statistics

Country	Total Population	GDP per capita	Life expectancy at birth m/f years, 2002	Healthy life expectancy at birth m/f years, 2002	Child mortality m/f (per 1000)	Adult mortality m/f (per 1000)	Total health expenditure per capita (Int; $, 2002)	Total health expenditure as % of GDP (2002)
Canada	31,510,000	30,429	78.0/82.0	70.1/74.0	6/5	93/57	2,931	9.6
USA	294,043,000	36,056	75.0/80.0	67.2/71.3	9/7	139/82	5,274	14.6
Mexico	103,457,000	8,979	72.0/77.0	63.4/67.6	31/25	166/95	550	6.1
Greenland (no data available)	55,000							

Country	Ordered by **Total expenditure on health as % of GDP, 2002**
United States of America	14.6
Uruguay	10.0
Canada	9.6
Costa Rica	9.3
Argentina	8.9
Panama	8.9
Suriname	8.6
Paraguay	8.4
Colombia	8.1
El Salvador	8.0
Brazil	7.9
Nicaragua	7.9
Haiti	7.6
Cuba	7.5
Bolivia	7.0
Bahamas	6.9
Barbados	6.9
Dominica	6.4
Honduras	6.2
Dominican Republic	6.1
Mexico	6.1
Jamaica	6.0
Saint Vincent and the Grenadines	5.9
Chile	5.8
Grenada	5.7
Guyana	5.6
Saint Kitts and Nevis	5.5
Belize	5.2
Saint Lucia	5.0
Venezuela	4.9
Antigua and Barbuda	4.8
Ecuador	4.8
Guatemala	4.8
Peru	4.4
Trinidad and Tobago	3.7

Figure 25-3. *Total expenditure on health as a percentage of the gross domestic product, by country.*

The Canadian Health Infoway, Inc, is important in the continued development of the EHR.[8] This emerging EHR in Canada is compatible with national and international standards and communication technologies. The strong positioning of nurses and the clear voice of nursing informatics (NI) expertise have resulted in the design of an EHR that incorporates both nursing data and information requirements. The nursing data, succinctly described as the Health Components of Health Information (Goossen et al in Chapter 24) clearly builds on the Nursing Minimum Data Set (NMDS) work from the U.S. and increases nursing's capacity for implementation of evidence-based practice in Canada.[9]

The United States
The EHR initiative in the U.S. gained a focus and national commitment with the creation of the Office of the National Coordinator for Health Information Technology (ONC).[10] Created under the

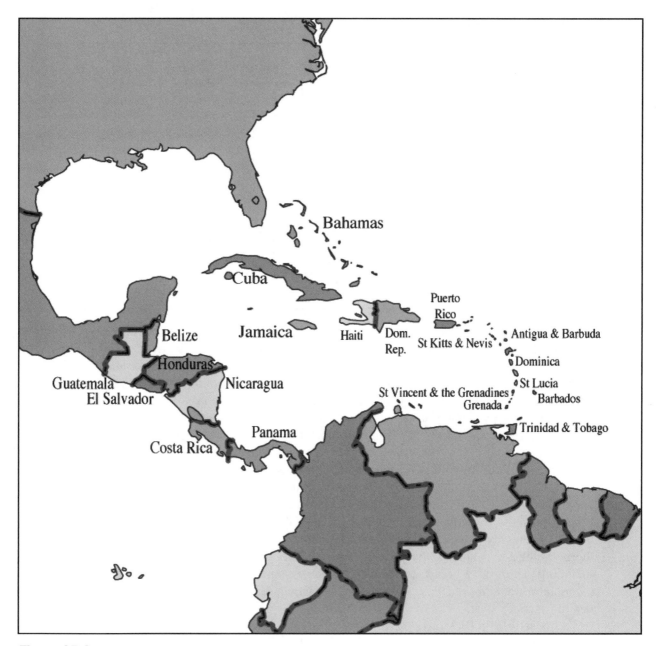

Figure 25-4. *Map of Central America.*

Secretary of Health and Human Services, the ONC Office provides leadership for the development and the nationwide implementation of an interoperable health information technology (HIT) infrastructure to improve the quality and efficiency of health care and the ability of consumers to manage their care and safety. The EHR effort in the U.S. is focused on four key goals:

1. Informing clinicians
2. Interconnecting clinicians
3. Personalizing health
4. Improving population health

First, "*informing clinicians*" focuses on adoption of the EHR across all settings and among all clinicians. Strategic actions include (1) creating shared investments between the clinicians and others in the health care system; (2) EHR certification to support the selection of software vendors based on a minimum set of functions or capabilities; and (3) access to EHRs in rural and underserved areas.

Table 25-2. Central America Selected Country Health Statistics

Country	Total Population	GDP per capita	Life expectancy at birth m/f years, 2002	Healthy life expectancy at birth m/f years, 2002	Child mortality m/f (per 1000)	Adult mortality m/f (per 1000)	Total health expenditure per capita (Int; $, 2002)	Total health expenditure as % of GDP (2002)
Guatemala	12,347,000	4,145	64.0/69.0	54.9/59.9	50/44	289/165	199	4.8
Honduras	6,941,000	2,511	65.0/69.0	56.3/60.5	42/40	248/181	156	6.2
Nicaragua	5,466,000	2,590	68.0/73.0	59.7/63/1	41/35	209/138	206	7.9
Costa Rica	4,173,000	7,966	75.0/80.0	65.2/69.3	11/9	129/76	743	9.3
Panama	3,120,000	6,471	73.0/78.0	64.3/68.0	26/22	146/84	576	8.9
Cuba	11,300,000	3,166	75.0/79.0	67.1/69.5	8/6	137/87	236	7.5
Jamaica	2,651,000	3,917	71.0/74.0	64.2/65.9	21/19	165/123	234	6.0
Dominican Republic	8,745,000	4,802	65.0/72.0	57.2/61.9	38/32	250/147	295	6.1

The second goal of "*interconnecting clinicians*" focuses on supporting the portability of patient information. Interoperable systems based upon a common architecture are a critical foundation strategy for reaching this goal. Three strategies being implemented to support the portability of patient health information include (1) fostering regional collaborations among health care entities (Regional Health Information Organizations); (2) use of a common set of standards so that systems and clinicians can communicate with one another by using the National Health Information Network (NHIN); and finally (3) using common standards and architecture within the government.

The third goal of "*personalizing health*" focuses on creating the personal health record, maximizing use of the Internet, and increasing informed consumer choice. Toward the goal of an informed consumer public, all federally funded clinical research must be published on the Internet and made available to the tax-paying public.[11] In addition, a number of government sponsored and private business initiatives are in process that makes the quality performance information on health systems by geographic locations available to consumers in formats easily understood by the lay public.[12,13] Finally, the goal of "*improving population health*" uses numerous strategies including (1) unifying public health surveillance systems; (2) streamlining quality and health status monitoring; and (3) accelerating the pace at which scientific discoveries are disseminated into health practice.

As described in Bickford's Case Study 25B that follows this chapter, the strong voice of nursing has informed the national EHR agenda in the U.S. Similar to Canada, the decades of work that nursing has done to define vocabulary standards, to identify data sets that reflect nursing specific data, and to develop information systems (IS) standards that support essential nursing data are serving as key contributions to the development of the national EHRs.

Brazil

Development of the EHR in Brazil is highlighted as an example for South America. In Case Study 25C on Brazil, Marin and Dal Sasso describe the challenges that EHR initiatives present in a developing country. As noted in the Canadian and U.S. examples, the development and organization of nursing informatics (NI) have a clear relationship to nursing's role in participating in a nation's EHR design and deployment. Brazil is making great strides in addressing the NI specialty capacity. For example, NI education is developing, and a clear integration of NI experts into existing health-focused informatics organizations is occurring. Marin's leadership in affecting IT development beyond Brazil is exemplified in her leadership within the Pan American Health Organization. Under Marin's leadership, standards for building the nursing information component within EHR systems have been defined and placed in the context of strategies for increasing the EHR capacity across Central and South America.[14]

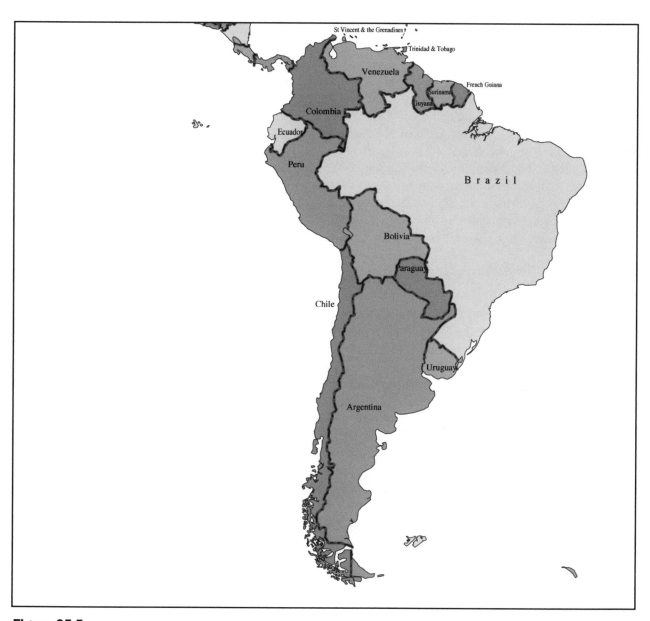

Figure 25-5. *Map of South America.*

Table 25-3. South America Selected Country Health Statistics

Country	Total Population	GDP per capita	Life expectancy at birth m/f years, 2002	Healthy life expectancy at birth m/f years, 2002	Child mortality m/f (per 1000)	Adult mortality m/f (per 1000)	Total health expenditure per capita (Int; $, 2002)	Total health expenditure as % of GDP (2002)
Brazil	178,470,000	7,762	66.0/73.0	57.2/62.4	39/32	240/129	611	7.9
Argentina	38,428,000	10,781	71.0/78.0	62.5/68.1	19/16	176/90	956	8.9
Chile	15,806,000	11,086	74.0/80.0	64.9/69.7	10/9	133/66	642	5.8
Venezuela	25,699,000	5,587	71.0/77.0	61.7/66.7	24/19	181/97	272	4.9
Columbia	44,222,000	6,622	68.0/77.0	57.8/66.3	25/18	231/97	536	8.1
Peru	27,167,000	5,101	68.0/73.0	59.6/62.4	36/32	193/133	266	4.4
Bolivia	8,808,000	2,568	63.0/67.0	53.6/55.2	68/64	247/180	179	7.0

In summary, the EHR initiatives within Canada, the U.S., and Brazil are the most advanced in the Americas. Also within these three countries, nursing has been integral in leading standards development for both vocabulary and nursing system requirements. Consequently, in these three countries, nursing is contributing to the core foundation of the interdisciplinary EHRs. These three examples demonstrate the strong interdependency between the level of NI practiced and the professional status of nursing in a given country. It is evident that the elevated status of nursing creates the foundation for the emergence of NI. As forward and leading edge as the Canadian, Brazilian and U.S. EHR initiatives are, the success of any nation's EHR strategy ultimately depends on interoperability and connectivity. As challenging as these dependencies are proving to be for the most developed nations, they do not convey the same picture for the emerging efforts toward EHR development within the Americas. The next section highlights the current state in Latin America and the Caribbean, with a specific focus on Argentina and Chile. These summaries will provide a preview of additions to EHRs with capacity to extend beyond national boundaries.

Emergent EHR Initiatives in the Americas

Latin America and the Caribbean

Latin America and the Caribbean is a heterogeneous region with diverse social, economical, and political structures. In those countries with political and economic stability, purchase and implementation of clinical information systems is occurring, but not always linked to an EHR national strategy. There may also be health care organizations within developing countries that have the economic resources to purchase and implement electronic medical record systems, but these tend to be organization specific rather than a part of a country-wide strategy. Nationwide IT health strategies across this region can be found in varying developmental stages. And importantly, there is a shared vision among health care leaders of the function of EHR systems and a commitment for their adoption to transform health care systems.[15] Targeted goals include improving health system accessibility; reducing inequity; providing high quality and integrated services; and orienting health care delivery toward primary care centered on people. Structurally, change is being promoted in the areas of health care systems roles, new insurance and payment methods, and human resources' needs with new workforce competencies, legal framework, and the organization of work processes with an emphasis on teamwork.[16]

Within Latin America and the Caribbean, there is movement toward becoming more involved in global health care initiatives. The Internet supports these new trends of using information internationally. Companies that operate internationally have introduced technology and related standards, which are consistent with international strategies and activities supported by the International Medical Informatics Association, International Standards Organization (ISO), and the European Community.[14]

As with Canada, the U.S., and Brazil, there is a clear relationship between the status of nursing and nursing's involvement in informatics. Of particular note in Latin America and the Caribbean region, 60 percent of care is provided by the nursing workforce. Nursing in Latin America has strong management and support roles and a well-developed emphasis on client education.[17-18] There is high interest in continuing education and progress toward developing a professional curriculum that is homogeneous throughout Latin America and the Caribbean. Significant nursing initiatives include using information technology (IT), standardizing nursing terminology based on the International Classification of Nursing Practice (ICNP v.1) for nursing documentation, and identifying and using quality indicators.[14]

Professional challenges within nursing that span across Latin America and the Caribbean include inequities between educational programs with wide disparity in the levels and quality of nursing education. Additional impediments include the shortage of nurses with informatics education and job skills, dissatisfaction with working conditions within the nursing workforce in general, and lack of professional recognition. Too often, nurses define their work status through wage earning, rather than as a profession with a career path.

Combining the strengths and challenges in Latin America and the Caribbean creates opportunities to establish new information system requirements, new delivery models, mechanisms for monitoring resources, and benchmarking of care. Multinational companies and globalization may further facilitate addressing these opportunities by sharing knowledge and experience from other countries. As with many developing countries with emerging EHR strategies, budget limitations and political priorities often run counter to investing in health care infrastructure and reform. Because many of the countries that make up Latin America and the Caribbean are small nations without a mechanism such as that in the European Union, wide disparity in financing policies for continuous education, bureaucracy in public system decision making, and limited availability of technology exist. Moreover, language barriers are pervasive among the Latin America and Caribbean countries.

Nurses are the largest single group of health professionals who directly influence the quality of most health services provided, as well as their outcomes. Looking to the future, as a result of the introduction of IT, nursing professionals will be able to provide better services and to evaluate the nursing process, thus making a greater contribution to population health.

Argentina

Challenges to advancing the EHR agenda in Argentina are many.[17] There is lack of understanding of the importance of data and information and potential system and care efficiencies, e.g. innovations such as disease registries and time saved in using IT. Fear of identification of users and other confidentiality and security issues complicates system implementation. The legal stability of the EHR is another barrier to progress. The lack of health care personnel and physical resources also complicates the development and adoption of the EHR.

Moreover, several issues specific to nursing hamper the advancement of EHRs. Today, Argentina's lack of advanced education degrees and health care systems structures combine to limit the development of nurse leaders. This lack of nursing leadership in practice, research, and education is directly reflected in limited nurse involvement in informatics. This is further complicated by the absence of informatics courses or programs in the health professional schools that would allow for a broader base of informatics activities, organizations, and knowledge-base.[18] The informatics leaders that are active in the country today are largely organized around the Argentina Association of Medical Informatics, and nursing is not yet a participant in this professional organization.[16,18] These leaders in informatics are pushing to progress EHR development so that they address professional values, preserve ethical principles, and meet professional responsibilities.

Additional barriers to the advancement of the EHR and health and NI include the lack of medical director interest in implementation of IT that address health care delivery. There is a major focus on the cost of such systems but little attention given to the health care benefits from IT, e.g. lower costs of care, increased productivity of personnel, increase health care quality, and lowered risk of adverse events.

Despite these challenges, numerous actions currently are advancing the EHR agenda. There is support for learning about the EHR and informatics in the form of congresses and symposia. The diffusion of health information and health informatics knowledge to the public through health magazines, radio, and television are occurring. The success of these activities is highly dependent on exceedingly low or no cost and the ability to show immediate benefit and cost savings.

Continued development of the EHR in Argentina is dependent upon addressing organizational control issues and establishing a visionary orientation to the EHR. This will necessitate achieving professional autonomy, conquering challenges, and identifying risk. Most importantly, visionary leadership must emerge to facilitate the technological transformation affecting the profession.

Chile

EHR development in Chile is dependent upon developing a cadre of trained professionals knowledgeable in the area. Sirebrenik[19] conducted a study in 2003 to describe the state-of-education in meeting this goal. This work focused on the amount of computer science provided at the level of predegree of infirmary (health care) in Chile. The following findings were identified in a study of 26 schools of infirmary. Thirteen schools of infirmary responded to the questionnaire, resulting in a response rate of 50 percent. Eighty percent of the infirmary (health care) schools had some level of computer science, or component of computer science, e.g. methodology, statistics, epidemiology and biostatistics.[19] Because computer science is the responsibility of the faculty of mathematics, physics and engineering, there is a need for a bridging of this expertise to the science of health care. Interestingly, 85 percent of the infirmary schools teach computer science to their students. Within the infirmary schools that teach computer science, 46 percent require computer science, 38 percent designate it as an elective, and only one university designates it as totally optional. When students are exposed to computer science independent of the health care field, there is a dearth of knowledge related to the applicability of computers and IT to health care.

Sirebrenik[19] also examined the content and skills included in the computer science courses. Hardware, software, and operating systems were addressed. Applications and skills included the Internet, electronic mail, spreadsheets, and online literature searches, while database was not taught. Course content included computer security and confidentiality. By formal agreement among all the universities, no content or skill included the more mobile technologies, e.g., the personal pocket computer or palm handheld device.

Because e-learning, or education at a distance is just being implemented, course content currently is not available in this format. All students have full access to the use of computers and the Internet, either through computer laboratories or the libraries. Moreover, Sirebrenik's study showed that although 80 percent of the students own computers, only 60 percent have connection to the Internet.[19] For faculty, clinicians, and students, understanding computer science in health care and the use of the technology in information and communication and in the education and medical care required a holistic focus. Finally, the study acknowledged the critical need for more faculty trained in informatics.

Summary

This chapter has summarized the most progressive, as well as the newly emerging EHR agendas within the Americas. It is readily acknowledged that further progress, or at the least, fast adoption in all countries is dependent upon increasing the availability of informatics specialists. It also is clear that independent of country, there is a critical need for training for all clinicians in IT, the EHR, and in all of the transformative potential of these technologies.

References

1. World Health Organization. Available at: http://www.who.int/about/regions/amro/en/index.html. Accessed November 7, 2005.
2. World Health Organization. Available at: http://www.who.int/about/regions/amro/en/index.html. Accessed November 7, 2005.
3. World Health Organization. World Health Report 2005. Available at: http://www.who.int/countries/en/. Accessed November 8, 2005.
4. Pan American Health Organization. Health in the Americas, 2002. Pan American Health Organization / World Health Organization, Division of Health Systems and Services Development. Washington, DC: Pan American Health Organization, 2002.
5. World Health Organization. Available at: http://www.who.int/docstore/peh-emf/EMFStandards/who-0102/Central_America/Central_America.JPG. Accessed November 8, 2005.
6. World Health Organization. Available at: http://www.who.int/docstore/peh-emf/EMFStandards/who-0102/South_America/South_America.JPG. Accessed November 8, 2005.
7. World Health Organization. Available at: http://www3.who.int/whosis/country/compare.cfm?language=english&country=ecu&indicator=strTotEOHPctOfGDP2002. Accessed November 8, 2005.
8. Canada Health Infoway, Inc. About Infoway: Vision & Mission. Available at: http://www.canadahealthinfoway.ca. Accessed November 4, 2005.
9. Hannah K. Health Informatics & Nursing in Canada. *HCIM&C*. 2005, Fall: 45-51.
10. Health and Human Services. Available at: http://www.hhs.gov/healthit/. Accessed November 8, 2005.
11. National Institutes of Health. Available at: http://publicaccess.nih.gov/. Accessed November 8, 2005.
12. Hurtado MP, Swift EK, Corrigan, eds. "Designing the National Health Care Quality Report", In: Envisioning the National Health Care Quality Report. Washington, DC: National Academy Press, 2001, pp 139-158.
13. Leap Frog Group. Available at: http://www.leapfroggroup.org/cp. Accessed November 8, 2005.

14. Marin H, Rodrigues R, Delaney C, Nielsen G, Yan J. (Eds). *Building Standard-Based Nursing Information Systems.* 2000. Pan American Health Organization/World Health Organization, Division of Health Systems and Services Development. Washington, DC: Pan American Health Organization.

15. la Asociación Argentina de Informática Médica. Available at: http://www.aaim.org.ar/ and on-line informatics journal, available at: www.emis.de/journals/SADIO/editorial.htm. Accessed November 8, 2005.

16. Pan American Health Organization. Special Issue on Health Sector Reform. *Pan Am. J Pub Hlt* 2000;7(1-2). Also available at: http://publications.paho.org/english/backissues/backissues.cfm?Product_ID=803 #Contents. Accessed March 12, 2005.

17. Personal communication with CB Lorena. Department of Clinical Information, Associate Professor of Nursing School. Faculty of Medicine—Pontificia Universidad Católica de Chile. 2005. lcamus@med.puc.cl, March 12, 2005.

18. Pan American Health Organization. 1999. La enfermeria en las Américas: Nursing in the Americas. Pan American Health Organization/World Health Organization, Division of Health Systems and Services Development. Washington, DC: Pan American Health Organization.

19. Sirebrenik JW. Computer science in the Pre degree of Infirmary in Universities of Chile. 2003. sanitary info@webmastersanitario.cl. http://publications.paho.org/english/backissues/backissues.cfm?Product_ID=803#Contents.

Case Study 25A

Canada's Journey toward an EHR and Nursing's Role

Lynn M. Nagle, PhD, RN, and Nicola T. Shaw, BSc(Hons.), PhD, MBCS

Introduction

The Country

Canada is the second largest country in the world. It encompasses 3.9 million square miles and has approximately thirty-two million residents. Canada's geography is extremely diverse, including mountains, prairies, badlands, sand dunes, boreal forests, rain forests, tundra, parkland, aspen forest, and the Canadian Shield.[1] It borders three oceans, shares the world's largest lake with the U.S. (Lake Superior), has the world's largest freshwater island (Manitoulin), has land access to the North Pole, and encompasses seven time zones. Canada is made up of ten provinces (Alberta, British Columbia, Manitoba, New Brunswick, Newfoundland and Labrador, Nova Scotia, Ontario, Prince Edward Island, Quebec, and Saskatchewan) and three territories (Northwest, Nunavut, and the Yukon).

Canada is a member of the British Commonwealth and as such recognizes Queen Elizabeth II as monarch, although the Crown's presence is purely that of a figurehead. Canada received independence from Britain on July 1, 1867. Paul Martin, elected leader of the Liberal Party of Canada, was sworn in as Canada's twenty-first prime minister on December 12, 2003. Canada is officially bilingual, its population speaking English and French.

Canada's Health Care System

Canada's health care system is made up of socialized health insurance plans that provide coverage for all Canadian citizens. It is publicly funded and administered on a provincial or territorial basis, within guidelines set by the federal government. The Canada Health Act[2] is federal legislation that puts in place conditions by which individual provinces and territories in Canada may receive funding for health care services.

Under the health care system, citizens receive preventive care and medical treatments from primary care physicians, and have access to hospitals, dental surgery, and additional medical services. With few exceptions, all citizens qualify for health coverage regardless of their medical history, personal income, or standard of living.

Moving Toward a National Electronic Health Record (EHR)

As in other countries, Canada's health care industry has been viewed as lagging behind other industries in terms of the adoption of information and communication technologies (ICTs). Based on a 2003 study of information technology (IT) in Canadian hospitals, IT consumes just 1.43 percent of the total operating budget for the average hospital or health region (Figure 25A-1).[3] In an earlier study, which examined the overall expenditure on computerized systems in Canadian hospitals and physician practices, researchers suggest that IT spending approximated $622 million in 2001. Furthermore, chief information (or informatics) officers claimed to need two to three times more than the current funding allocation to function effectively.[4]

Business and operations systems account for the highest degree of installations, followed by admission-discharge-transfer and materials management applications, as well as core departmental systems, e.g., pharmacy, laboratory, and radiology information systems. The least emphasis has been placed on the implementation of systems to support direct patient care delivery.[3] Given the costs associated with deploying clinical information systems and the nature of health care funding in Canada, the pace of systems implementation has been slow over the last few decades. Nonetheless, in recent years, there has been increased attention to the use of ICTs in health at the federal, provincial, and local levels. Recent findings indicate that electronic patient records constitute the top IT priority (36 percent) for Canadian hospitals (see Figure 25A-2).[3]

Further review of these data demonstrates that only 28 percent of Canadian hospitals have already fully implemented electronic health records (EHRs). This figure might be somewhat inflated because of the variable interpretations as to what constitutes an EHR. The extent to which they have been implemented in other sec-

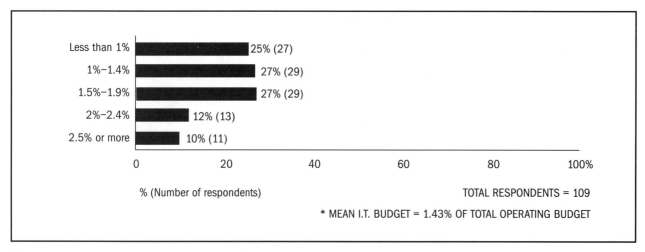

Figure 25A-1. *Hospital IT Budgets as Percentage of Total Operating Budget*[3]

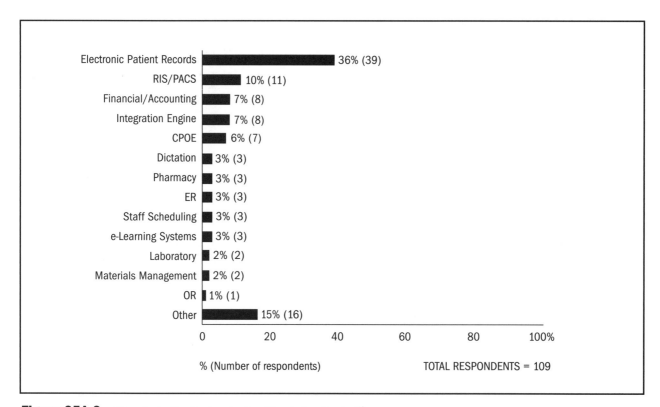

Figure 25A-2. *What Is the Top Project in Your Hospital or Region?*[3]

tors (e.g., community care) is unknown, but it is presumed to be even lower.[3] Computerized provider order entry (CPOE) was found to have the lowest level of implementation among systems studied (13 percent).[3] These findings suggest that the Canadian hospital sector needs considerable IT maturation in the clinical care arena.

Canada Health Infoway

In 1999, the Advisory Council on Health Infostructure stated that "...health information is an essential public good which should be readily available and accessible to all Canadians as a component of Canada's publicly funded health system."[5] With the support of federal funding, Canada's Health Infoway (CHI) was established as a not-for-profit corporation and given a mandate to deploy the infrastructure and systems components to support the concept of a "pan-Canadian health record." In the view of CHI, investments in key aspects of "infostructure" will have direct benefits, improving the quality, accessibility, portability, and efficiency of health services delivery across the continuum of care.[5] CHI's mandate includes (1) strengthening and integrating health services through EHR; (2) empowering the public by increasing health information access; (3) addressing issues of privacy; (4) developing and implementing standards, and (5) assuring the adoption of emerging technologies through private and public sector collaboration.[5] CHI has already distributed substantial funding to several jurisdictions to support numerous initiatives that align with CHI's core objectives.[6]

In 2003, the CHI business plan outlined a three-year investment plan to address the following elements: (1) infostructure (e.g., standards, interoperability), (2) registries (e.g., patient, provider, and location), (3) interoperable drug information systems, (4) regional diagnostic imaging systems, (5) laboratory information systems, and (6) "telehealth." Further details of each of these investment programs can be obtained from the CHI Web site: http://www.infoway-inforoute.ca/. Today CHI has $1.1 billion in investment capital to direct to partnerships for the development, replication, and deployment of reusable interoperable EHR solutions.[6]

Canadians Online

A 2002 Ipsos-Reid report[7] showed that Canadians looking online for health information supersedes all other online activity (e.g., electronic banking, e-commerce). The survey found that two-thirds of Canadians who visit sites to access health information do so on a regular basis, at least monthly. Most commonly, online Canadians are interested in sites that provide information about reducing threats to their own health, including nutrition, prescription drug information, exercise, and support group Web sites.[7] Consequently, many Canadian citizens are much more knowledgeable about health care and seek to be active participants in managing their health. Today's ready access to online resources will imminently lead to consumer expectations of also having online access to their personal health information from anywhere in the country. Realistically, meeting this expectation in the near term will necessitate accelerated investment and deployment of the Canadian EHR.

Clinical Information Systems

The term *electronic patient record* has been adopted widely in reference to the aggregate of modules or applications that constitute computerized clinical information. Instances of "best of breed" and "turnkey" system environments continue to exist in health care organizations across Canada. Additionally, a wide array of vendor solutions continues to be adopted. However, in many of the smaller jurisdictions, e.g., Nova Scotia and Prince Edward Island, the trend in recent years has been to adopt a single vendor solution to cover most of the entire region or province. This strategy of a common platform eases the integration of information and offers economy-of-scale benefits. The least evidence of this approach can be found in the province of Ontario, which to date has the least regionalization but the largest and most complex health system. In some areas, e.g., the Capital Health region in Alberta, portal solutions have been deployed to support access to an individual's health information from disparate vendor solutions and across care delivery settings.

In response to CHI's investment strategies, several efforts are also underway across the country to develop unique provider and client identifiers and registries to support the concept of a regional, provincial, and national health record for all Canadians.[6] In some instances, provinces have banded together to develop solutions collaboratively (e.g., the Western Health Information Collaborative includes the provinces of British Columbia, Alberta, Saskatchewan, and Manitoba).[8]

As is evident in other countries, Canadians are focused on the anticipated benefits of electronic patient records to enhance patient safety. A recent study found the incidence of adverse events in Canadian hospitals to be comparable to the rates found in other countries.[9] Hence clinical systems are being designed to incorporate alerts and reminders to clinicians. The greatest benefit will be derived when these are integrated into a CPOE system. For example, during the ordering process, the system could alert clinicians about potential drug-to-drug interactions, patient allergies, or abnormal blood values that may be problematic for patients receiving specific medications or drug dosages. Other useful decision support tools that could be integrated include direct links to evidence in the form of reference databases, current research, and relevant literature. Applications such as CPOE also provide opportunities for the broader deployment of standardized protocols, order sets, and best practice guidelines. The integration of these tools will facilitate more consistency in the use of diagnostics and therapeutics for patients with like diagnoses.

Human Resources

In general, there is recognition that the successful implementation of CIS requires significant human resources, including individuals with informatics skills and knowledge of clinical care processes who can support projects before and after implementation. Thirty percent of Canadian IT leaders find that the resources for maintenance, support, and training are extremely inadequate.[3] If the benefits of these solutions are to be realized, more attention needs to be given to the human factor, yet in many instances projects continue to be under-resourced, ultimately compromising success.

Overall, Canadian health IT leaders are well aware of what needs to be in place to realize the vision of a "pan-Canadian" EHR. The slow progress is not caused by a lack of will or vision but rather by the lack of requisite financial and human resources. In light of the fact that nurses constitute the single largest health profession in the country, engaging nurses in this work is critical.

Nursing Informatics in Canada

The term *informatics* is now consistently applied to the work of Canadian nurses engaged in the use of ICTs in all settings and sectors. Historically, Canadian nurses have had limited education and involvement in the area of informatics. However, there is an emerging recognition of the significance of ICTs to support the work of nurses and the advancement of nursing knowledge. There are increasing efforts to engage nurses in activities, e.g., system selection, design, implementation, and evaluation, but most practicing nurses lack core informatics competencies. Based on the findings of a 2003 national study,[10] few Canadian schools of nursing have integrated core concepts of informatics within their basic nursing curricula. At the time of this writing, there is also a considerable lack of faculty capacity and expertise to facilitate this integration. Yet it is clear that the heightened focus on and profile of CIS in Canada necessitate attention to the informatics education of nurses.

Nursing Informatics Leadership

Many nurses have embraced informatics as a new area of nursing specialization, and the number of nurses in informatics roles has been gradually increasing over the years. This increase can be attributed to the recognition of a need to converge nursing expertise with the knowledge of informatics to better inform systems design, implementation, education, and evaluation. Nevertheless, there is still much work to be done to initiate all nurses into the world of informatics as it relates to their practice and to educate them appropriately. We are now confronted not only with a demand for nurse informaticians but with an entire workforce that needs to be much more knowledgeable about the capacity and use of information and IT.

In 2002, the Canadian Nursing Informatics Association (CNIA) was established as an interest group of the Canadian Nurses Association (CNA). The CNIA's mission is to provide a voice for Canadian nurses on issues of health and NI. The intent of the CNIA is to engage nurses in all sectors and in all the roles related to informatics practice, administration, education, or research. The CNIA membership comprises primarily registered nurses, but is also open to vendor and non-nurse participation. The board of directors comprises NI leaders representative of each provincial and territorial region. The CNIA has leveraged its position and formalized linkages with regional NI interest groups previously in existence and is working to support the emergence of new regional groups. The CNIA seeks to:

1. Provide nursing leadership for the development of nursing and health informatics in Canada
2. Establish national networking opportunities for nurse informaticians
3. Facilitate informatics educational opportunities for all nurses in Canada
4. Engage in international NI initiatives
5. Act as a nursing advisory group in matters of nursing and health informatics
6. Expand awareness of NI to all nurses and the health care community

In 2004, the scope and growth of CNIA's national membership and its compliance with the CNA criteria granted CNIA Associate Group status. This status brings further credence to the CNIA as well as opportunities to review and influence relevant national nursing policy and strategic directions. The establishment of the CNIA was also strongly supported by the Canadian Organization for the Advancement of Computers in Health (COACH), Canada's health informatics organization. The two organizations established a formal strategic alliance at the outset, which facilitated the appointment of a Canadian nurse nominee to the

International Medical Informatics Association–Nursing Informatics Working Group (IMIA NI-WG). The IMIA NI-WG provides an opportunity to collaborate and network with international NI colleagues.

CNIA is also participating in a collaborative forum designed to engage key Canadian health informatics and health professional organizations in discussions regarding the national ICT strategies supported by Canada's Health Infoway. Members of this collaborative include CHI, COACH, the CNA, the Canadian Medical Association, the Canadian Health Information Management Association, and the Canadian Telehealth Society.

Nursing Informatics in Practice

There are currently numerous efforts underway to weave informatics into the fabric of every nurse's daily practice. Nurses are becoming increasingly engaged in the design, implementation, and evaluation of CIS. Yet to date, Canada's national health data repository includes no specific data and information related to nursing clinical services. National and provincial nursing organizations are beginning to take action to advance the adoption of a consistent nursing data set and reporting structure that will reflect nurses' contributions to the health care services provided to Canadians.

Over the past decade, the extension of nursing services and expertise beyond urban centers has been made possible through the use of ICTs. Given Canada's vast geography and numerous remote communities, applications of telehealth are among the earliest and most significant success stories of informatics in Canadian nursing practice.

Nursing Data. The significance of timely access to valid and reliable data has become more important as providers are increasingly accountable for sustaining quality care in a financially constrained environment. With the looming shortage of nurses, investments in nursing need to be cost-justified. Since the late 1990s, the Canadian Institute of Health Information (CIHI) has managed centralized national health data reporting. To date, the core data set reported to CIHI by health care provider agencies includes little to no data reflective of nurses' contributions to clinical care.

Nursing workload systems have been the predominant application used by nurses in Canadian practice settings. These systems are typically used to proxy the cost of nursing care to the health care system. However, the limitations of the systems have been extensively researched over the past decade and have been demonstrated to fall short of consistently and comprehensively capturing nursing workload. Efforts are currently underway to develop new methodologies that more accurately reflect the intensity of nursing resources being brought to bear on patient care.[11,12] Without adequate measures of nursing workload, nurse leaders in an already constrained fiscal environment find it difficult to cost-justify nursing resource requirements.

Since the early 1990s, the CNA has been engaged in discussions regarding a nursing minimum data set (NMDS). Originally formulated as health information: nursing components (HI:NC), this data set includes information on client status, nursing interventions, nursing resource use, and client outcomes. The intent of capturing HI:NC was to assist and support clinical, administrative, educational, research, and policy development decisions.[13] In addition, linking these data elements to measures of nursing intensity and unique nurse identifiers has been proposed as a means to represent nursing contributions in the broader context of client-centered health information.[14] In 2000, a CNA discussion paper provided an overview and comparison of major nursing classification systems and promoted the testing of the International Classification of Nursing Practice (ICNP®).[15] The following year, a position statement was developed endorsing the adoption of nursing data in a manner consistent with the approach of the ICNP.®[14] CNA advances the position that registered nurses should be advancing and leading efforts to collect, store, and retrieve nursing data at the national level. Although national data are available on the numbers and location of nurses, limited information is available about the nursing care delivered, the use of nursing resources, and related health outcomes. The existence of a national reporting repository (CIHI) provides Canadian nurses with an opportunity to influence the future directions of clinical data reporting.

In the province of Ontario, an important initiative is currently under way for the collection of clinical outcomes within different clinical care settings. The Nursing and Health Outcomes project is an effort to collect standardized clinical outcomes data across the health care system. The data set includes measures of functional status, symptoms (pain, nausea, dyspnea, and fatigue), therapeutic self-care, falls, and pressure ulcers.[16] In 2003, a feasibility study was completed in four regions of the province within acute, long-term care, complex continuing care, and community care settings.[17] Recommendations for system-wide implementation of outcomes data collection by nurses have been given high priority on the provincial health ministry's agenda.

Consequently, work is in progress to develop the data collection methodologies for gathering a core set of outcome data from specific clinical settings (e.g., acute care, community care, long-term care, complex continuing care) throughout the province. This initiative is funded and wholly supported by the provincial Ministry of Health and Long-Term Care. Future work will focus on applying the methods to remaining care sectors and including the related contributions of allied health professionals. This project will provide information about health outcomes that will assist in evaluating whether investments in full-time nursing positions are resulting in better patient outcomes.[16] In the long term, information about specific clinical outcomes from all care settings will guide decisions about the appropriate care setting and caregiver mix for specific patient populations.

Although the CNA supports the inclusion of nursing data in health information systems as critical for supporting evidence-based decision making by registered nurses,[18] there is still a need for the development of a national system to collect, store, and retrieve nursing data in Canada. The advancement of nursing knowledge and health human resource planning would be facilitated by such a system. Moreover, understanding nursing's contributions to health outcomes will further substantiate its position as core to the delivery of Canadian health services.

Telehealth. A wide variety of nursing services are provided using "telehealth" methods. In Canada, nursing *telepractice* is a "nursing-specific application of telehealth that includes all client-centered forms of nursing practice and the provision of information, conferences, and courses for health care professionals occurring through or facilitated by the use of telecommunications or electronic means."[19] "Telepractice" is recognized to be within the scope of nursing practice by all Canadian jurisdictions. Given the vast geographic regions and numerous remote communities, nurses need to be able to reach out to and from isolated areas of the country. With the emergence of more sophisticated ICTs, the use of telepractice is growing rapidly across the country. In many locales, nurses are the only health care providers and rely on such tools as videoconferencing to relay vital clinical information (e.g., electrocardiogram data). The technology has facilitated the early discharge and return to home for many individuals whose recovery can now be monitored remotely by means of ICT tools. In this regard, Canadian nurses using telehealth technologies are leading the way in the adoption of ICTs to improve patient access to services.

Nursing Informatics and Education

Over the past decade, there have been a couple of key national initiatives focused on the need for nurses to develop informatics competencies. Specifically, in 1999, several nursing groups submitted a collaborative report to the CNA on the National Nursing Informatics Project.[20] This report addressed (1) informatics competencies for entry-level nurses and specialists, managers, educators, and researchers, (2) curriculum implications and strategies for both basic and continuing nursing education, and (3) priorities for implementing national NI education strategies. The nursing groups that developed this report by building on previous related works set the foundation for national discussions of nurses and informatics.

In May 2002 the CNIA secured funding from the federal Office of Health Information Highway (OHIH) to undertake a national study of Canadian schools of nursing. This study sought to better understand the informatics curricula provided in basic nursing education programs across the country. In particular, the study focused on the availability of informatics expertise among nursing faculty, informatics content within core curricula, and the state of technology infrastructure to support informatics in schools of nursing. Completed in 2003, the study findings highlighted the significant gaps in the informatics knowledge of nursing faculty, the lack of informatics integration into core curricula, and the need for ICT investment in Canadian schools of nursing.[10] Recommendations have been directed to a number of professional nursing organizations, but particularly to the Canadian Association of Schools of Nursing, the Association of Canadian Executive Nurses, the Office of Nursing Policy, CNIA, and the CNA. A copy of the final report is posted at http://www.cnia.ca/research.htm. Several presentations have been made to a number of nursing groups, and the study findings have been published.[21]

CNIA is currently focused on addressing the need for education and communication on issues of NI using a variety of media, including workshops, e-rounds, and a national NI conference. In total, each of these initiatives has and will contribute to the further advancement of the national NI agenda in Canada.

Similar to other countries, there is much opportunity to advance the basic and expert levels of understanding within Canada's nursing community. The rapid evolution of Canada's e-health agenda underscores the criticality of addressing this need immediately.

Summary

This case study has provided a brief overview of the Canadian health care system and highlighted nursing's role in our journey toward a pan-Canadian EHR. As with many countries, we have a long way to go. However, we hope to have demonstrated that Canadian nursing is part of this process and that Canadian nurses are taking a highly active role in helping to shape and direct the route we take.

References

1. Canadian shield. Available at: http://talmud.epsb.ca/regions/north/lz/csi/csi.html. Accessed February 21, 2005.
2. Health Canada. Available at: http://www.hc-sc.gc.ca/medicare/chaover.htm. Accessed February 21, 2005.
3. Irving R, ed. *2003 Report on I.T. in Canadian Hospitals: Top Issues, Applications, & Vendors.* Thornhill, Ontario: Canadian Healthcare Technology; 2003.
4. Irving R, ed. *2002 Report on Information Technology in Canadian Hospitals.* Thornhill. Ontario: Canadian Healthcare Technology; 2002.
5. Advisory Council on Health Infostructure. *Canada Health Infoway: Paths to Better Health, Final Report;* 1999:7. Available at: http://www.hc-sc.gc.ca/hcs-sss/pubs/ehealth-esante/1999-paths-voles-fin/index_e.html. Accessed September 6, 2005.
6. Canada Health Infoway. Building momentum: 2003/04 business plan. Available at: http://www.infoway-inforoute.ca/. Accessed February 18, 2005.
7. Mossop, S. Two-thirds of all online Canadians have visited a health Web site, up from 55% in 2000. *Electronic Healthcare.com.* 2003;2(1):47-48.
8. Noseworthy T, McAllister J, Bader D. A provincial strategy in the development of Canada's health infostructure. *Electronic Healthcare.com.* 2001;1(1):23-32.
9. Baker GR, Norton, PG, Flintoft V. Canadian Adverse Events Study. *Canadian Med Assoc J.* 2004;171(8):829-834.
10. Clarke H. Assessing the informatics education needs of Canadian nurses. Project G3-6B-DP1-0054 report to the Office of Health Information Highway. Available at: http://www.cnia.ca/research.htm. Accessed February 18, 2005.
11. Hernandez C, O'Brien-Pallas L. Validity and reliability of nursing workload measurement systems: review of validity and reliability theory. *Canadian J Nurs Leadership.* 1996; 13(2):32-50.
12. O'Brien-Pallas L, Irvine D, Peerebroom E, Murray M. Measuring nursing workload: understanding the variability. *Nurs Economics.* 1997;15(4):171-182.
13. Canadian Nurses Association. International classification for nursing practice: documenting nursing care and client outcomes. *Nursing Now: Issues and Trends in Canadian Nursing.* 2003:14. Available at: http://www.cna-nurses.ca/CNA/resources/bytype/corporate/now/default_e.aspx?y=2003. Accessed September 6, 2005.
14. Canadian Nurses Association. Position statement: collecting data to reflect the impact of nursing practice. Ottawa: Canadian Nurses Association; 2001. Available at: http://www.cna-nurses.ca/CNA/issues/position/research/default_e.aspx. Accessed September 6, 2005.
15. Canadian Nurses Association. Collecting data to reflect nursing impact: a discussion paper. Ottawa: Canadian Nurses Association; 2000. Available at: http://cnanurses.ca/CNA/resources/bytype/papers/default_e.aspx?y=2000. Accessed September 6, 2005.
16. The Nursing and Health Outcomes Project. Available at: http://www.health.gov.on.ca/english/providers/project/nursing/nursing_mn.html. Accessed September 6, 2005.
17. Doran D. An evaluation of the feasibility of instituting data collection of nursing sensitive outcomes in acute care, long-term care, complex continuing care and home care. Report to the Ministry of Health and Long-term Care, Government of Ontario; 2004.
18. Canadian Nurses Association. Evidence-based decision making and nursing practice. Policy statement of the Canadian Nurses Association; November 1998. Available at: http://www.cna-nurses.ca/CNA/issues/position/research/default_e.aspx. Accessed September 6, 2005.
19. Canadian Nurses Association. The role of the nurse in telepractice. Position statement of the Canadian Nurses Association; November 2001. Available at: http://www.cna-nurses.ca/CNA/issues/position/practice/default_e.aspx. Accessed September 6, 2005.
20. Hebert M. A national education strategy to develop nursing informatics competencies. *Canadian J Nurs Leadership.* 2000;13(2):11-14.
21. Nagle LM, Clarke HF. Assessing informatics in Canadian schools of nursing. In: Fieschi M, Coiera E, Yu-Chuan, JL, eds. *Proceedings of the 11th World Congress on Medical Informatics,* San Francisco; 2004 [on CD-ROM].

Case Study 25B

United States: Electronic Health Record Initiative

Carol J. Bickford, PhD, RN, BC

Today's legacy health care clinical documentation systems, both paper- and computer-based versions, reflect a medical model that focuses on an individual's disease and pathology. The computer-based documentation systems, in particular, originated to address the financial aspects of health care, billing, and the associated coding methodologies, e.g., the Current Procedural Terminology® (CPT-4) and the International Classification of Diseases, Ninth Revision, Clinical Modification (ICD-9-CM), which are deemed necessary for the reimbursement of physician services. Such an approach does little to support the systems of care and health and the wellness perspective of registered nurses and other similarly focused health care providers.

In 2003, the American Nurses Association (ANA) published a new definition of nursing that reflects the contemporary and dynamic practice of registered nurses, the largest group of U.S. health care professionals: "Nursing is the protection, promotion, and optimization of health and abilities, prevention of illness and injury, alleviation of suffering through the diagnosis and treatment of human response, and advocacy in the care of individuals, families, communities, and populations."[1] This practice focus includes concepts and terms (e.g., family coping [diagnosis], mutual goal setting [intervention], and dignified dying [outcome]) that are foreign to the frameworks of ICD-9-CM and CPT-4.

Registered nurses most often rely on the nursing process as a framework for critical thinking and decision making in evidence-based practice within all practice settings. The process includes the iterative steps of assessment, diagnosis, outcomes identification, planning, implementation, and evaluation. Such systematic thinking and problem solving mandate documentation mechanisms that reflect and communicate the transformation of data into information and of information into knowledge.

Nursing practice occurs in clinical, administrative, educational, and research domains, which in turn demand significant diversity in record-keeping mechanisms and communication strategies to support safe, quality health care. The focus of nursing concern may be individuals, families, communities, populations, health promotion and wellness, outcomes associated with quality improvement and risk management initiatives, systems (e.g., the health care enterprise or an educational facility, nursing services administration, information systems), or other nonpatient entities.

Nursing's Vision for Clinical Documentation

Nursing's demands for support of the nursing process and a systems view for decision making can finally become the long-awaited reality with the development and refinement of an interdisciplinary electronic health record (EHR). However, success can begin to be measured only after certain key characteristics are integrated into the design of the EHR. A fundamental requirement is expressed by the well-known principle, "Write once and read many times." In the acute care setting, nurses must provide twenty-four-hour services that involve significant patient care coordination efforts and innumerable references to diverse components of the clinical documentation. Redundancy in data entry requirements creates opportunities for errors, causes the expenditure of precious minutes spent finding and verifying information, and raises data integrity questions when different values for the same question, measure, or test are discovered.

Confidentiality and the associated security measures must also be integral characteristics of the information systems (IS) supporting the EHR. Nurses are especially concerned about this aspect because of nursing's long tradition of patient advocacy. The *Code of Ethics for Nurses with Interpretive Statements* holds nurses accountable for such thinking and appropriate actions, including specific mandates related to protecting patient information.[2]

The EHR has to support a patient-focused and holistic systems perspective. Such an expansive and longitudinal view must include the capability to document and then present content related to the context of the patient's health and the use of health care services. Data linkages and displays of those relationships must be present to assist the clinician in decision making and care management activities. If the patient is identified as a family, community, or population, today's legacy IS cannot yet adequately support such a focus.

Nursing's Preparatory Work for the EHR

Early on, nursing leaders identified a framework based on research and the development of standards that has contributed for many decades to the vision and creation of the EHR. Central to the framework has been the definitional work related to:

1. Describing the content of practice to populate the EHR and help drive its design
2. Creating structures and processes to promote thinking about the EHR
3. Participating in the interdisciplinary initiatives to establish the EHR

The ANA and its members, the Congress on Nursing Practice and Economics, and numerous other councils, committees, task forces, and workgroups have been instrumental in all three areas, fostering development of the EHR to support nurses' decision making and evidence-based practice.

Content of Practice to Populate the EHR

Werley and Lang[3] described the development of the nursing minimum data set (NMDS) as "an important first step" toward the creation of comparable data and reliable, uniform, and standardized data sets to describe nursing practice. The NMDS established the focus for significant standardized nursing language initiatives to identify, describe, and link diagnoses, interventions, and outcomes of patient care. As Lang has stated: "If you can't name it, you can't control it, finance it, research it, teach it, or put it into public policy." This quotation reflects not only the continued, but the heightened importance of standardized terminologies in today's health care delivery system.[4]

Concurrent research efforts initiated during the 1980s and 1990s fostered the development of standardized terminologies to describe clinical nursing practice: the Omaha System (for visiting nurses), that of the North American Nursing Diagnosis Association (NANDA), the Nursing Interventions Classification (NIC) and the Nursing Outcomes Classification (NOC). Other development efforts culminated in the original version of the Home Health Care Classification, which is now named the Clinical Care Classification, and the Patient Care Data Set. One nursing specialty organization, the Association of periOperative Registered Nurses (AORN), financed the research and development work to establish the perioperative nursing data set, a specialty data set incorporating select NANDA, NIC, and NOC terms that can be used in all perioperative settings. Although these terminologies were developed by nurses to represent the concepts of interest to nurses and include nursing within the title, other health care professionals have discovered and embraced the patient-centric focus and terminologies for their practices.

Alternative Link uses another approach for the development of ABC codes, a standardized terminology supporting nursing practice. The ABC codes identify complementary and alternative medicine therapies, including nursing interventions, coupled with the legal scope of practice information and relative value units to support appropriate reimbursement for health care providers engaged in integrative health practice. Another terminology initiative, the nursing management minimum data set, has gained increased importance as it focuses on the context, resources, and environment of care, rather than on the description of clinical practice content and linkages of terms.

Nurses continue to be key participants in the development of LOINC® (Logical Observation Identifiers Names and Codes) and SNOMED CT (SNOMED International Clinical Terminology) to ensure that these terminology efforts incorporate content pertinent to the patient-centric view of clinical practice, a necessary perspective to support nursing and other health care provider practices. The challenges presented by the complex use cases provided by nurses have stimulated heated discussions and new thinking in the development of standardized health care terminologies.

To this point, the discussion of the terminologies for nursing has been oriented toward U.S. initiatives, e.g., the U.S. federal government's efforts toward the EHR and National Health Information Infrastructure (NHII). However, because nurses think of the bigger picture and regularly engage in international discussions about nursing practice and health care systems, much of the research and development work for NANDA, NIC, NOC, and other terminologies has helped provide frameworks and lessons learned as foundations for the development of the ICNP® (International Classification Nursing Practice). The ICNP® is a combinatorial terminology for nursing practice that facilitates cross mapping of local terms with existing vocabularies and classifications. The development and maintenance of the ICNP® is a long-term effort of the International Council of Nurses to establish a common language to describe nursing practice worldwide and to improve communication among nurses and between nurses and others. As this terminology advances and its use becomes more global, perhaps the NHII and EHR initiatives will need to address the inclusion of ICNP® as a standardized terminology.

Structure and Processes to Promote Thinking About EHR

In its role as the professional organization representing all U.S. nurses, the ANA, among its many activities, maintains the Code of Ethics for Nurses, establishes standards of practice, and lobbies for and promotes legislative and regulatory actions important for nurses, patients, communities, populations, and health care. The ANA House of Delegates has over the years passed resolutions addressing issues, needs, and concerns related to clinical documentation, standardized terminologies, and IS.

The ANA Board of Directors has in turn ensured appropriate organizational initiatives to support those mandates. The ANA established two programs in the 1990s to evaluate, recognize and promote the emerging standardized terminologies for nursing. First, the ANA established the Steering Committee on Databases to Support Clinical Nursing Practice. The expert members of the Committee defined the specific review criteria to evaluate and recognized voluntarily submitted standardized nursing terminology. Thirteen standardized languages have received ANA recognition.

The committee name has been changed to the Committee for Nursing Practice Information Infrastructure to reflect its expanded charge to develop and implement a strategic plan for managing and preserving nursing's information legacy. Oversight for the terminologies recognition program remains the Committee's responsibility. The Committee members continue to conduct research, publish articles and papers about the criteria and other topics related to standardized terminologies, and to advocate for continued funding of the terminologies efforts; they have refined the review criteria as the science has evolved. Other ANA efforts have involved participation in the development of the Pan American Health Organization's publication, *Building Standard-Based Nursing Information Systems* (2001) and continued support for the International Minimum Data Set and ICNP.®[5]

To be of value to clinicians, standardized nursing terminologies need to be ubiquitously available in the practice setting. The ANA established a second program, Nursing Information and Data Set Evaluation Center (NIDSEC[SM]), to encourage that availability. The NIDSEC[SM] developed standards, scoring guidelines, and a voluntary recognition program for IS vendor products that incorporate nursing terminologies within their clinical IS solution. Three products have met the established NIDSEC[SM] standards:
- Pathways Care Manager, HBO (1998–2001)
- Lastword®, IDX (2000–2003)
- CareNet® Solutions, Cerner Corporation (2003–2006)

The NIDSEC[SM] standards have been used internationally and are currently under revision.[6]

The ANA also engaged in parallel efforts, many of which continue today, to promote standards, IS solutions, and the preparation of nurses who can develop, implement, evaluate, and use IS that include some or all of the components of an EHR. NI was recognized as a nursing specialty in 1992. The ANA published the *Scope of Practice for Nursing Informatics* in 1994 and the *Standards of Nursing Informatics* in 1995 to guide the specialty practice.[7,8] The most current resource, the Scope and Standards of Nursing Informatics Practice, is due for revision within the next year and is expected to include a discussion of nursing's significant contribution to the development of the EHR and NHII.[9]

Although increasing numbers of nurses defined NI as their practice specialty, formal and informal networking organizations emerged to promote continuing education and shared learning, to create connections for problem solving, and to establish mentorship and professional support resources. The American Medical Informatics Association's (AMIA) Nursing Informatics Working Group (NI-WG), CARING (Capital Areas Roundtable on Informatics in Nursing), the American Nursing Informatics Association, the Minnesota Informatics Nursing Group, and others began as local, regional, or national NI groups but very quickly evolved to include international members. Discussions began in early 2003 about a proposal to establish a more formal collaboration of NI specialty groups. This entity would leverage the numbers and expertise of a consolidated membership to respond nimbly and with one voice for nursing to pertinent public policy and industry issues.

The informal collaborative garnered significant publicity and recognition with its written response and oral testimonies submitted to the President's Information Technology Advisory Committee (PITAC) on April

13, 2004 and June 17, 2004. The prepared statement responded to specific PITAC questions on how IT can transform America's health care system. Six months later, AMIA and the Healthcare Information and Management Systems Society (HIMSS) announced formation of the Alliance for Nursing Informatics, with an original organizational membership of eighteen NI organizations. CARING and the ANA were instrumental in the formation of the alliance, which is currently jointly resourced administratively by AMIA and HIMSS.

Nursing's leadership and responsiveness related to establishing structures and process to advance informatics support of healthcare are dependent on all nurses demonstrating competencies related to computer literacy and information literacy. That means faculty must be adequately skilled to create curricula and select clinical experiences to ensure adequate preparation of undergraduate and graduate nursing school students. Research has established that extensive work is necessary to remediate deficiencies in this domain, for the preparation of both faculty and students.[10-12]

The federal government's focus on the confidentiality and security of patient information through the privacy rules of the Health Insurance Portability and Accountability Act of 1996 (HIPAA) has provided nurses with many opportunities to contribute within their facility or enterprise, at the local and state level, and in national and international environments. This law protects personally identifiable patient data and information transmitted in electronic, written, and spoken transactions. Such protections for oral and written communications have been part of nursing's long tradition of advocacy for and protection of the patient, and they can be easily transferred to the EHR environment. Nurses have often been the key risk management officials in health care organizations and now have expanded opportunities to assume the role of privacy officer for HIPAA compliance.

Interdisciplinary Efforts

Either nurses must be the consummate collaborators, or patient care suffers. Such collaboration includes active participation in interdisciplinary efforts related to the EHR and NHII. In fact, Standard 11 and the associated measurement criteria of the Standards of Professional Performance in *Nursing: Scope and Standard of Practice* require that nurses partner with others to enhance health care and patient care through interdisciplinary activities, e.g., technological development.[13] Such collaboration fosters successful outcomes but often garners little public recognition of the significant professional commitment and contribution of nurses and nursing.

The Institute of Medicine's (IOM) publication of *The Computer-based Patient Record: An Essential Technology for Health Care* in 1991 received significant accolades and at that time was considered the necessary impetus to move U.S. health care forward to promptly integrate IS architecture across the industry.[14] Although the recognized panel members did not include a registered nurse, ANA staff and many of its members provided significant testimony and comments during the book's development.

One IOM recommendation called for the development of a public-private venture to establish a Computer-based Patient Record Institute (CPRI). The CPRI's purpose is to facilitate development, implementation, and dissemination of the computer-based patient record (CPR), defined *as the electronic patient record resident in a system supporting users with access to complete and accurate data, alerts, reminders, and clinical decision support tools and resources.* The CPRI was established in 1992 to coordinate national efforts for widespread implementation of electronic clinical documentation. Nurses worked tirelessly in committee and work group efforts to ensure that the CPR solution would meet the needs, not just of physicians and financial entities, but of all stakeholders, including patients. The IOM's revised edition of *The Computer-based Patient Record: An Essential Technology for Health Care* in 1997 could not shore up the flagging support of the CPRI.[15] Eventually the CPRI merged with other organizations and disappeared.

Even the earliest visioning discussions about the CPR identified the critical role of standards in the development and implementation of an EHR. ASTM's consensus-based standards development process has benefited from strong nurse participation on the Health Informatics Committee E-31 and its numerous subcommittees that address the multiple EHR issues needing standards solutions, including the recent continuity of care record initiative.

When the Health Level Seven (HL7) standards organization moved from developing packet and messaging standards for the transmission of health care data to discussions about the format of actual message content, a nursing presence became even more critical. The use case for the content of everyday, routine nursing messages challenged the previous financial and medical services models. Nurses have become more active HL7 members and have assumed committee leadership roles, e.g., for the recent development of the HL7 draft EHR Functionality Standard.

Similar challenges confront the standards work being done within LOINC® and SNOMED CT. Each organization relies heavily on the nurse staff members designated to coordinate the specific standards efforts incorporating nursing terminologies content. Again, nurses continue to challenge the thinking and proposed standard development process with examples of routine use cases, as well as more complex and unusual scenarios found in nursing practice.

Increasing numbers of nurses have become active participants in the international standards initiatives, especially within the International Organization for Standardization/Technical Committee 215 (ISO/TC 215) and the U.S. Technical Advisory Group. Of particular note, nurses spearheaded the collaborative effort culminating in the passage of ISO 18104:2003, Health Informatics—Integration of a Reference Terminology Model for Nursing. These interdisciplinary activities strive to develop standards that create the best models for data representation, transmission, and storage to permit seamless application to practice and integration within IS throughout the world. This work, like that creating the ICNP®, involves careful articulation of the multiple views and issues surrounding health care delivery. Such productive interdisciplinary discussions prove enlightening for U.S. participants who discover that other health care concepts, models, terms, and solutions permeate the globe.

Government and Private Initiatives

The U.S. government's commitment, under the Clinton and Bush administrations, to create a national information network has now thrust health care initiatives, such as the establishment of the NHII, the EHR, and the personal health records (PHR), into frontline discussions. The recent focus by the Department of Health and Human Services (DHHS) to coordinate and consolidate its health information initiatives involved the fast track work of the Consolidated Health Informatics (CHI) group. This group was chartered to review which IS standards—including standardized terminologies—were in use within all DHHS agencies, e.g., the Centers for Medicare and Medicaid Services (CMS), the Centers for Disease Control and Prevention (CDC), the Indian Health Service (IHS), and the National Institutes of Health (NIH). The CHI then provided recommendations about which standards should be mandated throughout the DHHS. The group's work also included collaboration with other government representatives from the Department of Defense (DoD) and the Department of Veterans Affairs (VA). Such standardization was intended to end the existing problems associated with incompatible data and different messaging formats that prevented interagency, and even intra-agency, communications about patient care. Nurses were instrumental in coordinating and leading this effort. During the same period, the National Library of Medicine (NLM) completed negotiations to put the previously proprietary SNOMED-CT within the public domain to increase the likelihood of its integration into IS solutions, thereby moving toward standardization in the language of health care.

The announcement by President Bush in May 2004 of the establishment of the Office of the National Coordinator for Healthcare Information Technology (ONC) created a stimulus for action. The short timelines, characteristic of the operations of this office, are reflected in announcements about ONC assessment, planning, implementation, and evaluation activities related to the NHII and EHR. Nurses serve as staff of the ONC and have provided comments to formal and informal requests for information.

Collaborative groups have been created to harness and then focus organizational, financial, and human resources to facilitate the development and implementation of the NHII and EHR. For example, in reply to the recent ONC request for information about the National Health Information Network (NHIN), the following organizations responded collaboratively: the American Health Information Management Association, AMIA, American National Standards Institute—Healthcare Informatics Standards Board, Center for Information Technology Leadership, Connecting for Health, eHealth Initiative, HIMSS, HIMSS' EHR Vendor Association, HL7, Integrating the Healthcare Enterprise, Internet2, Liberty Alliance, and National Alliance for Health Information Technology. Nurses have been active members in these organizations for many years and now are reaching sufficient numbers to be recognized as important contributors in the special interest groups and work group structures, as well as at the board of directors level. Even the federal government has finally named a registered nurse to the membership of the National Committee on Vital and Health Statistics, the advisory board to the secretary of the DHHS.

The contributions of nurses in the design, development, implementation, and evaluation of the NHII and EHR go far beyond the advocacy, requirements definition, policy, and regulation spheres. Nurses, ever present in health care practice settings, strive at all times to optimize the operations of existing IT solutions to provide the right information at the right time to the right person for the right reason. Nurses in the vendor community have moved beyond implementation responsibilities to influence the development of information system solutions that are integrated, patient-centric, and supportive of all care providers. The nurses in the positions of senior leadership, e.g., the chief nursing officer, along with those in research and development positions, can effect such product changes.

Summary

Federal funding has helped establish and then foster the development efforts for the EHR vision and the supporting NHII, but much work remains. International and national standards initiatives have provided tools to facilitate the actual creation of viable solutions and to ensure that interoperability and communication methodologies are in place to allow everything to work together. Organizations are beginning to commit financial resources to meet the challenge of focusing on real-world technology applications to improve health care through the implementation of the EHR. The key point to remember is that the most effective EHR and NHII systems must include and value the people committed to arriving at the best outcome possible. Nurses will continue leading this effort through their undeterred persistence to collaborate and then share the solution through national and international networks of users and colleagues.

References

1. American Nurses Association. *Nursing's Social Policy Statement.* 2nd ed. Washington, DC: nursesbooks.org; 2003.

2. American Nurses Association. *Code of Ethics for Nurses with Interpretive Statements.* Washington, DC: American Nurses Publishing; 2001.

3. Werley HH, Lang NM, eds. *Identification of the Nursing Minimum Data Set.* New York: Springer Publishing Company; 1988.

4. Oyri K. Workload measurement in the ICU. In: Gerdin U, Wainwright P, Tallberg M, eds. *Studies in Health Technology and Informatics.* 1997;46:512-517.

5. Pan American Health Organization. *Building Standard-based Nursing Information Systems.* Washington, DC: Pan American Health Organization; 2001.

6. American Nurses Association. *NIDSEC Standards and Scoring Guidelines.* Washington, DC: American Nurses Publishing; 1997.

7. American Nurses Association. *Scope of Practice for Nursing Informatics.* Washington, DC: American Nurses Publishing; 1994.

8. American Nurses Association. *Standards of Practice for Nursing Informatics.* Washington, DC: American Nurses Publishing; 1996.

9. American Nurses Association. *Scope and Standards of Nursing Informatics Practice.* Washington, DC: American Nurses Publishing; 2001.

10. McNeil BJ, Elfrink VL, Bickford CJ, Pierce ST, Beyea SC, Averill C, Klappenbach C. Nursing information technology knowledge, skills, and preparation of student nurses, nursing faculty, and clinicians: a U.S. survey. *J Nurs Educ.* 2003;42(8):341-349.

11. Pravikoff D, Pierce S, Tanner A. Are nurses ready for evidence-based practice? *Am J Nurs.* 2003;105(5):95-96.

12. Tanner A, Pierce S, Pravikoff D. Readiness for evidence-based practice: information literacy needs of nurses in the United States. In Proceedings of the 11th World Congress on Medical Informatics, Volume 107 Studies in Health Technology and Informatics, M. Fieschi, E. Coiera and Y.-C.J. Li (Editors), Amsterdam, The Netherlands: ISO Press, 2004.

13. American Nurses Association. *Nursing: Scope and Standards of Practice.* Washington, DC: nursesbooks.org; 2004.

14. Dick RS, Steen EB, eds. *The Computer-based Patient Record: An Essential Technology for Health Care.* Rev. ed. Washington, DC: National Academy Press; 1991.

15. Dick RS, Steen EB, Detmer DE, eds. *The Computer-based Patient Record: An Essential Technology for Health Care.* Washington, DC: National Academy Press; 1997.

Case Study 25C

Brazil as a Case Study to Discuss Technology Capacity in Developing Countries: The Starting Point

Heimar F. Marin, PhD, RN, FACMI and Grace T.M. Dal Sasso, DNs, RN

The Nursing Profession in Brazil

Brazil is one of the most important countries in South America because of its geographical size, population, economy, and recent industrial improvement. This tropical nation has 183 million people in an area of 8,547,403 square kilometers. Its territory borders all the countries of South America except Chile and Ecuador. Brazil maintains diplomatic relations with every country in the world, and most short-term visitors do not need a consular visa. Brazil, like other countries in South America, presents a wide diversity of health, education, and economic levels. Some of its regions enjoy a standard of living similar to that of developed countries. Unfortunately, it also has conditions of poverty similar to those found in underdeveloped countries.

The first school of nursing in Brazil was created on September 1890 in Rio de Janeiro. In 1937, the School of Nursing Anna Nery was incorporated into the University of Brazil. The school developed the North American–Parsons Model, which became the prototype for other nursing schools created in the country. This model, based on the Nightingale paradigm of the scientific principles of hygiene and public health and a feminist perspective, addressed the political, regulatory, and economic concerns of the profession.[1]

The 1990s brought a great advance in the nursing profession; correspondingly, the number of nursing journals increased from two in 1970 to eleven in 1990, master's programs from eight to fifteen, and doctoral programs from three to eight. In 1996, 107 nursing schools awarded baccalaureate degrees to 3,300 nurses.

Since then, several nursing schools were established, and the profession has evolved in all care settings. Brazil has 95,542 hospitals and health care centers, 292,732 physicians, and 107,207 nurses. In addition, as of December 2004, there were 335 medical schools and 484 nursing schools. Yet, despite the fact that Brazil has nearly 500 nursing schools, its nursing education programs cannot meet the demands for providing nursing care to the population.

Nursing Informatics in Brazil

Nursing informatics (NI) in Brazil began around 1985. By this time, some hospitals had developed and installed computer systems. In step with the international experience, these early systems supported the finance and administration concerns of hospitals. Consequently, nurses working in administration or in clinical practice began to be involved with the health informatics field, initially using computers to schedule staff and to control material resources in the nursing unit.

In 1990, the Nursing Informatics Group at the Federal University of São Paulo (NIEn/UNIFESP) was created. The first task of this group was to prepare students and faculty to use computers. Since its creation, members of NIEn/UNIFESP have been working in the clinical practice, administration, education, and research areas of NI. Currently, similar groups at other universities across the country and several schools of nursing have established the discipline in the nursing curriculum. Moreover, many hospitals are including NI issues in their continuous education programs. Although NIEn/UNIFESP was not a pioneer group in NI, it can be considered a leader, actively collaborating with professionals from different universities and hospitals in the country.

In 2002, the Brazilian Health Informatics Society (SBIS) granted the creation of the Nursing Informatics Working Group (SBIS-NI), integrating nurses from several states of the country, e.g., Rio Grande do Sul, Santa Catarina, Rio de Janeiro, and São Paulo.

The established goals of the SBIS-NI are (1) to develop a national strategy for NI education, research, and clinical practice; (2) to determine priorities for implementing NI education programs; (3) to develop by consensus a definition of NI according to Brazilian education and professional regulations; and (4) to recommend NI competencies for clinical nurses, managers, faculty, and researchers.

Currently, several nursing schools have established the discipline in the nursing curriculum. A recent national survey showed that NI is a discipline in eighteen undergraduate, twelve graduate (6 master's degrees and 6 doctorate studies), and two specialization programs.

In November 2003, the SBIS-NI founded the TeleNursing Department at the CBTMS–Brazilian Telemedicine and Telehealth Council. The main goals of this group are (1) to increase and promote the use of telecommunications for distance learning education, (2) to use "telemedicine" technologies to provide care to the minorities, (3) to increase access to medical and nursing care centers, thereby decreasing health care costs, and (4) to provide continuous education programs for nurses and nursing students to enhance public health care in rural and urban communities.

Education, Research, Practice, and Management

Technology has changed nursing practice, training, and education models. With the introduction of computers in health care, nurses are now primary users, responsible for data input. Consequently, they have had to become computer-literate to effectively utilize computer technology. After considering educational and training needs, nursing schools and hospitals initiated programs to prepare nurses to use computers in all the areas of their expertise.

The adoption of a new culture—to accept and use IT—has been an important initiative in education and NI practice.[2] Grobe[3,4] and Herbert described the competencies in NI, focusing on three levels: basic, intermediate, and advanced. Further, each category comprised levels of complexity, e.g., technicality, usefulness, and leadership.

The description of competencies is fundamental if the faculty and leaders in Brazil are to facilitate the access to information and are to provide skills (1) to identify, collect, and record relevant data to the nursing care of patients; (2) to analyze, organize, and integrate information to redesign nursing practice; and (3) to analyze nursing care according to the sectors and needs of the country. Considering competencies, the Nursing Informatics Working Group implemented strategies in education, practice, research, and administration to enhance NI deployment in nursing activities.

The increased development of IT has had an impact on all domains of nursing. Consequently, it is necessary to prepare nurses to be knowledgeable participants in the process of selecting, developing, implementing, and evaluating IT and health information systems to produce data, use information, and generate knowledge.

Therefore, the most important strategy to develop competencies in IT and NI is to train nurses in the workplace, that is, to provide access to the Internet and continuing education programs that offer distance education resources, discussion lists, and newsgroups, as well as the use of Intranet systems to provide updated information at the point of need. However, the considerable barriers to accomplishing the competencies in NI in Brazil are the restricted access to adequate technology, few faculty with skills in NI, and the small number of studies that support the outcome of nursing practice in patient care. On the other hand, in the last twenty years, NI faculty and researchers have influenced the education, practice, research, and administration of the nursing profession.

Education

Three major activities are being developed in NI education and training: (1) continuous education programs; (2) undergraduate and graduate disciplines; and (3) patient education. The barriers to advancing NI in the nursing curriculum are (1) the need to set up a nursing culture to encourage the acceptance and use of ITs as basic tools for information management; (2) the definition of appropriate technical resources; (3) a plan to deal with the rapid changes in technology; and (4) insufficient human and material resources in some regions of the country.

Research

The focus of NI research in Brazil has been on studies about the development of (1) nursing information systems, (2) vocabularies and standards, (3) modeling for clinical decision support systems, (4) nursing education systems, and (5) patient health education. Nurse informaticians need to actively participate in the development, evaluation, and selection process of IT; they need to contribute to the growth of nursing knowledge and search for resources that could make daily activities easier in the process of caring for people. The barriers to advancing such research include nurses' unsatisfactory use of informatics resources to advance nursing science and improve patient care. The challenges are related to the development of studies to demonstrate that the use of technology can improve patient care and optimize financial and material resources.

Practice

NI has been focused mainly on computerizing the nursing process. However, health care centers are much more aware of the need to develop standards-based nursing information systems integrated into the computer patient record (CPR). The barriers to expanding NI practice include (1) the small number of nurse informaticians, (2) the fact that most nursing care is delivered by nursing assistants, (3) the need to develop measures to evaluate nursing care outcomes in daily practice, (4) a resistance to using computers as a result of negative perceptions, (5) a shortage of nursing professionals, (6) a lack of integrated automated health information systems in health organizations, and (7) the absence of nursing documentation as a component of the EHR.

Administration

The challenges of nursing in Brazil are related to the need for developing systems that can measure nursing care outcomes according to patients' needs. An additional requirement is to implement automated systems to prevent errors in patient care. For this reason, a national strategy in NI education, practice, research, and administration should address methods to evaluate the effectiveness of nursing care according to regional demands. The strategy should also review nursing competencies and educational methods for ways to make them more effective and efficient.

What Has Changed in the Nursing Profession Because of Informatics?

Technology is a powerful, impelling force in the growth of developing countries. Knowledge acquired through access to IT is vital to improving the quality of life. Correspondingly, the use of IT has changed how nurses perform nursing care, and they are now seeking to enhance the quality of their care by facilitating documentation, education, and research. However, in general, most automated EHRs are limited to registering financial and administrative data, and, although nursing process documentation is mandatory, according to the National Council of Nurses, most of it is done manually.

Although technologies on their own cannot achieve organizational change, they can act as catalysts. Accordingly, national initiatives to implement a national health card across the country are promoting discussions about implementing EHR systems in private and public institutes. Today's nurses seek involvement with the NI or health informatics area, searching out tools that could be useful in identifying what change needs to occur and how to get better results at lower cost. At the last health informatics conference organized in Brazil and hosted by the Brazilian Health Informatics Society, for example, nurses constituted 40 percent of the total attendance.

Ongoing Challenges

An urgent need brought about by the use of computers is for a national health database. The database issue was recognized by nurse informaticians across Brazilian states, as well as in European countries, the U.S., Canada, Australia, and many others that have been developing their database for many years and already have significant results. Yet, making the National Data Base for Nursing Practice a reality in Brazil is challenged by social, cultural, and regional differences. Of these, the major problem is deciding what data are essential for nursing practice. The data elements must reflect information nurses use for clinical judgment and management decision making in *any* practice setting, regardless of regional and technological differences.

In addition to concerns about required data and information issues related to systems requirements as well, a national project is being conducted to establish the requirements for certification of software in the health care area. The Brazilian Health Informatics Society is leading the process with the assistance of the Ministry of Health and the Federal Council of Medicine.

Lessons Learned

Over the last twenty years, several major accomplishments were achieved in NI. From experience, we know that technology is a means and not the final product of nursing care. Education is a continuous demand in the country of Brazil; people living in geographically distant rural regions especially need access to up-to-date health information. Moreover, studies are necessary to optimize resources and to demonstrate nursing's contribution to the health care population.

Education, research, and practice have to be integrated. Otherwise, there will never be enough resources and the quality of patient care could be compromised and become even more expensive. Research using data from nursing practice can help us to evaluate our profession and further enrich our capabilities.

The EHR must contain nursing components that support the data elements related to the nursing process, and it must permit more efficient data entry and retrieval than pre-existing manual and even current automated systems. The nursing components should have the capability of transforming data into information and, from there, information into knowledge. More important is the need to use the information produced by providers to redesign nursing care.

Future Directions

Facing the challenges as opportunities, nurses are working to demonstrate how IT can provide resources to improve practice, education, administration, and research. Schools of nursing are working together to establish the competence of nursing informaticians, the needs for education, and strategies to promote NI education across the country. A National Committee for Telenursing was created, and its members are conducting a research project to identify methodologies to implement and evaluate distance education in the country.

In our history, we have faced many challenges and most of them have helped us to enhance our activities. Caring for the ill or injured will still be an essential part of nursing, but helping people stay healthy and functional will be the primary goal. The most important skill of nursing will still be care. Personal human interaction is vital to recovery, and a computer never gave anyone a hug.

However, for the immediate future, when we are developing systems to support nurses in their practice, we need to collect data at the source and make sure that no patient data that has been collected goes unused. Assuming that the most legitimate source of patient care is the patient, the system must incorporate the needs of the patient to be effective and successful.

References

1. Paiva MS (coord.), Silva MT N.da, Oliveira, I dos RS, et al. *Enfermagem Brasileira: Contribuição da ABEn* [in Portugese]. Brasilia: ABEn Nacional; 1999.
2. Herbert M. National nursing informatics project. Discussion paper; 1999. Available at: http://www.cna-nurses.ca/pages/resources/nni/nni_discussion_paper.doc. Accessed May 20, 2005.
3. Grobe S. Nursing informatics 1997 post-conference on patient guidelines and clinical practice guidelines: the state of our knowledge and a vision. *J Am Med Inf Assoc.* 1998;5(3):315-316.
4. Grobe SJ. Nursing informatics competencies. *Methods Inf Med.* 1989;28(4):267-269.

CHAPTER 26

Information Technology Strategies in the United Kingdom

By Anne Casey, MSc, RN, FRCN

Most nurses in the United Kingdom (U.K.) have a distant relationship with informatics; with a few notable exceptions, they have a limited understanding of information management and little or no experience using computers to support their practice. Many nurses who have used computers generally found the experience negative because they were expected to input data for administrative purposes and saw no benefits for them or their patients. A significant new investment in information technology (IT) for the National Health Service (NHS) across the United Kingdom means that all nurses must begin to integrate information, knowledge management, and IT into their practice. This chapter introduces the context for nurses' engagement with health informatics in the United Kingdom. It also considers the challenges facing the profession as the four United Kingdom governments implement information strategies to achieve their common vision: "a patient-centered service designed around the needs and aspirations of patients ... an NHS which offers patients real choice and involvement and gives them fast and convenient access to high-quality health and social care services."[1]

Context: Devolved Government with Common Goals

Since 1999, government has devolved to each of the four countries that make up the United Kingdom: England, Northern Ireland, Scotland, and Wales (see Figure 26-1). This presents a major challenge to those seeking to influence IT developments on behalf of nursing. Unfortunately, the system of devolution is asymmetric, in that there are different levels of devolved responsibilities. The Scottish parliament has legislative powers and responsibilities similar to those of Westminster, but the National Assembly for Wales and the Northern Ireland Assembly have less autonomy. The U.K. Parliament still legislates in some areas for these countries, including the areas of health and social care.

Despite the different legal and service infrastructures that are evolving, the four countries share common themes in relation to health care. Health services remain free at the point of delivery, but there is increasing use of the private sector. Quality and patient safety have top priority, and standards are being defined centrally for both service delivery and clinical practice. For example, in England and Wales, national service frameworks define the level of service that patients can expect for a number of conditions.[2] The National Institute for Clinical Excellence[3] and the Scottish Intercollegiate Guidelines Network[4] publish evidence-based guidelines that health care professionals are expected to follow. Cross-boundary work between health and social care is encouraged, as are patient choice and public empowerment to participate in service planning. Quality improvement is supported by formal inspection processes,[5] and all health care professionals are expected to participate in clinical governance activities, e.g., audit and performance review.[6] Workforce planning and the development of the health and social care workforce are also being taken forward centrally. The NHS "skills and knowledge framework" applies to most U.K. health workers (doctors are excepted) and creates an improved link between education, career development, and pay.[7] Standard descriptions of the competencies required by health care professionals and ancillary staff include information and knowledge management competencies, because it has been widely recognized that NHS modernization plans can succeed only with the support of better information management and technology (IM&T).

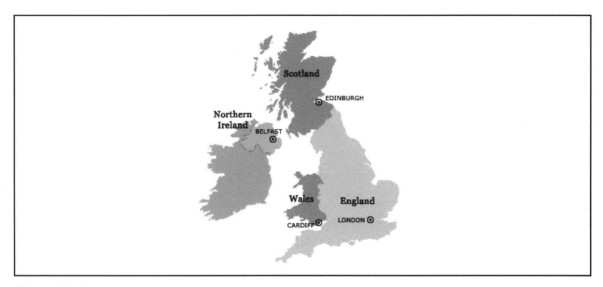

Figure 26-1. *Map of the United Kingdom.*

Context: NHS Information Strategies

Although specific plans and levels of investment vary among the four countries, the IT strategies for the NHS share common themes. First, the single shared patient record is accepted as the best way to ensure communication across the organizational and professional boundaries in health and social care; unidisciplinary, stand-alone systems, e.g., nursing care planning systems, have no place in this integrated future.

Second, budgets for health services are allocated centrally but managed locally so that data about service needs, utilization, quality, and costs are required at each level of management. Providing the data directly from patient-based electronic records when possible has been a central principle of government IM&T plans since 1998, when the NHS produced its "Information for Health" strategy.[8] At this time, the U.K. was already a world leader in primary care computing; enthusiastic general practitioners and a system accreditation/reimbursement plan meant that general practice computing developed rapidly.

The nature of funding arrangements in primary care drove the spread of computers. Yet their widespread use in general practice contrasts markedly with that in the hospital and community health care sectors, where, apart from stand-alone departmental systems, the majority of computer systems still support only administrative and management functions. In this context, the goals of the 1998 strategy remain relevant across the U.K. today:

1. Lifelong electronic health records (EHRs) for every person
2. Around-the-clock online access to patient records and information about best clinical practice for all NHS clinicians
3. Seamless care for patients through general practitioners (GPs), hospitals, and community services sharing information
4. Fast and convenient public access to information and care through online information services and "telemedicine"
5. The effective use of NHS resources by providing health planners and managers with the information they need[8]

Following the publication of the 1998 strategy, the central government provided guidance on the deployment of systems to achieve these goals, but it became clear over time that more central intervention was needed. The pace of change was too slow for the rapidly evolving requirements of the service. In addition, and despite excellent guidance for the education and training of staff in information management, little progress was made in integrating IM&T into professional curricula. Computer literacy is still confused with informatics by many clinical educators, including nurse teachers. A significant investment is now being made to make the most of modern information and

Table 26-1. Sources for NHS Information and Technology Strategies

England	The national program for IT in the NHS: www.connectingforhealth.nhs.uk
Northern Ireland	Information and Communications Technology Strategy: www.dhsspsni.gov.uk/publications/2005/HPSS-ICT-Programme-Summary.pdf
Scotland	National eHealth/IM&T Strategy for NHS Scotland: www.show.scot.nhs.uk/imt/
Wales	Informing Healthcare: www.wales.nhs.uk/sites3/home.cfm?OrgID=365

communications technology in support of quality patient care (Table 26-1 lists sources of information about NHS IM&T strategies). The common approaches across the four countries include the rigorous application of information standards. National standards are being developed, based as much as possible on international standards, to ensure that systems are interoperable and most importantly that the content of patient records can be accurately communicated and stored. Standardization, as well as education at all levels, is vital to ensure the success of these strategies.[9-13]

A well-developed area of informatics in the U.K. is information governance. This brings together data protection, freedom of information, codes of confidentiality, security management, and records management. It also sets standards for how information is held, obtained, recorded, used, and stored. All NHS organizations must have guidelines, processes, and infrastructure in place to ensure the confidentiality and security of personal information. Information governance standards are monitored as a regular part of NHS audit and inspection processes. However, the implementation of such standards is not universal and can be hindered by organizational and professional boundaries.

Recognition that information strategies and developments should not sit apart from other initiatives in health care has resulted in more attention being paid to information as a necessary part of all policy implementation. One example can be found in the information strategies that are produced alongside NHS service frameworks. These service frameworks specify standards of service, treatment, and care that the public can expect for particular conditions (e.g., diabetes and coronary heart disease) or for particular groups (e.g., older people and children). Along with these frameworks, the information strategies are developed with input from the public, clinicians, and informatics experts.[14]

Nursing Informatics: Progress and Challenges

In 2002, the U.K. nursing professions reached an agreement on a set of strategic goals for nursing informatics (NI) that have been the basis for nurse leaders to begin influencing health information policy, educational curricula, and national developments. The five goals are:

1. Nurses, midwives, and health visitors have access to relevant information tools and resources in support of their roles.
2. Nurses, midwives, and health visitors have information and knowledge management skills appropriate to their roles.
3. Nursing perspectives will be appropriately integrated in national and local information developments.
4. There is an informatics career pathway for nurses, midwives, and health visitors.
5. Meaningful, good-quality information about patient care and nursing practice is available to decision makers (including patients and the public).

In 2004, the results of an online survey by the Royal College of Nursing of more than 2,000 nurses and midwives from across the U.K. showed that some progress has been made toward these goals.[15] Areas for further development include evaluations of the impact of systems on patient care/nursing practice and more work on nursing data.

A 2003 systematic review looked at the effects of nursing record systems on nursing practice and patient outcomes and concluded that further qualitative research would be needed to explore the relationship between practice and information use.[16] The experience of designing and implementing care planning systems has given nursing experts a good understanding of the issues that should be addressed during implementations in practice settings. These insights were further expanded during the 1990s through a number of demonstration projects for electronic records that engaged multiprofessional teams across acute, primary, and social care. The "lessons learned" reports[17] from this project form an essential resource for all future NHS informatics developments, to be added to the ongoing lessons from primary care computing.

There is a lack of data to support workforce and educational planning, and it is only now becoming possible to separately identify nurse-led NHS services. The U.K. health services are reviewing and developing resource groupings, data sets, classifications, and other tools to support data collection and analysis. The drive to obtain meaningful data to support planning and quality improvement through clinical data set development is an ideal opportunity to integrate nursing data elements, but they must first be defined and tested. An urgent priority for the nursing profession is to identify, as an integral part of overall NHS information management, suitable indicators that reflect the cost, quality, and performance of the nursing contribution with respect to patient outcome and public health.

One of the barriers to achieving this goal is a general uncertainty among nurses and nurse leaders in the U.K. about the nature of nursing data/information and its uses. Apart from the obvious questions (e.g., how many nurses do we have?), the kinds of information and analyses needed have not been clearly defined. A project undertaken in 1998 considered this question by researching information use and needs in nursing.[18] It explored nurses' requirements to support the activities of finding the right information, making decisions, communicating with others, and aggregating for analysis. Among other recommendations (mainly related to electronic records), the researchers concluded that the NHS needed to undertake a "co-ordinated programme of development and use by the nursing professions of small-scale, focused, purposive classifications." To support this program, there needed to be "a professionally accredited national semantic reference model."[18] Neither of these recommendations was acted on. Much has changed in the intervening years, and the conditions for proceeding with such work are much more positive. It would therefore be useful to repeat the study and to take action on the updated recommendations.

Building on the Past

Despite these challenges, much has been achieved in nursing informatics in the U.K., from active networks through terminology, knowledge provision, "telecare," and information standards developments. U.K. nurses have participated in both European and international informatics projects building on *networks* first established by the British Computer Society Nursing Specialist Group.[19] Involvement in international projects, e.g., Wisecare[20] and the efforts to develop the international standard reference terminology model for nursing[21] have helped U.K. nurses expand their networks, develop new expertise, and participate in new knowledge development.

Nursing terminology development in the U.K. was driven initially by the NHS nursing terms project, which aimed to integrate nursing content into Read Codes, the standard terminology adopted by the NHS in the 1990s. This work has fed into the development of SNOMED® Clinical Terms; U.K. nurses contribute to this global standard terminology through the Systematized Nomenclature of Medicine (SNOMED®) nursing working group.[22] These initiatives ensure that nursing concepts are available for use in electronic records and messages, but, with a few notable exceptions,[23] standard terminologies have not been adopted by U.K. nurses for use in their practice or as part of nursing education programs.

U.K. nursing has been well-served in electronic *knowledge provision,* particularly through electronic libraries and the Nursing and Allied Professions gateway (NMAP) "free access to a searchable catalogue of hand-selected and evaluated, quality Internet resources in Nursing, Midwifery and the Allied Health Professions."[24]

Decision support forms an essential part of teleconsultation services, which are a central part of NHS plans to improve patient access to health care advice. Twenty-four-hour helplines (NHS Direct in England and Wales; NHS 24 in Scotland) complement Web-based information services provided by the NHS. Nurses providing telephone consultation have access to protocol-driven decision support systems in this context,[25] as well as in other settings, e.g., for prescribing medicines in primary care.[26]

As in other countries, nurses in the U.K. have participated in the development and implementation of a number of "telehealth" applications, improving patients' access to clinical expertise at a distance.[27] But as Hibbert et al[27] found in a study of health professionals' response to telehealth care, the integration of technology into daily working practices is not a simple process: "Our work highlights the complex problems that health professionals encounter when they try to integrate new technologies into routine service delivery. The concerns arising from the interplay of new technology with existing professional practices and relationships go beyond simple issues of training."

Summary

The four U.K. countries are embarking on ambitious programs to deploy information and communications technology across the health care fields, integrating appropriately with social care and with the private health sector. If this new technology is to be used effectively to support patient care and improve patient outcomes, the nursing professions must be involved in developments at every level. Equipping nurses with the necessary skills and providing opportunities for them to participate in developments will ensure that local and national developments are appropriate to the care environment and to patient requirements. We must develop more opportunities for nursing careers and for academic leadership roles in health informatics, so that the art and science of nursing can be effectively complemented by the science of health informatics.

In this area, the U.K. still has much to do; a major effort is needed to research and develop the "specific interplay" between nursing and information, not just IT in general. The Royal College of Nursing's online survey revealed that many nurses welcome the development of single shared electronic patient records and other technologies to support the health of patients and the public. However, we lack an evidence base to support nurses' inputs to informatics developments. There is a growing literature from other disciplines, such as primary care physicians,[28] but we know very little about nurses' use of information and technology or its impact on nurse-patient interactions and the quality of care. Nurses need to be sure that systems are acceptable to patients and caregivers and that different systems are both safe and fit for their intended purposes. Nurses need to develop advanced skills in helping patients and caregivers access and manage information themselves. The identification, definition, and validation of data requirements to support planning, delivery, and monitoring of nursing services are urgent priorities.

Nevertheless, the nursing professions in the U.K. are well-positioned to take advantage of the opportunities provided by the current NHS programs. Increasing, the engagement of nurse leaders and nurses in practice in the informatics agenda will enable us to build on the excellent work of the past. Overcoming the current informatics challenges will ensure a future in which nurses:

1. Reach for information tools as readily as they reach for the pen, telephone, and reference book
2. Help their patients manage information and knowledge effectively
3. Use information and knowledge to support the delivery of accessible and evidence-based nursing services

References

1. Department of Health. The NHS plan: a plan for investment, a plan for reform. Available at: www.dh.gov.uk/PublicationsAndStatistics. Accessed February 20, 2005.
2. Department of Health. National Service frameworks. Available at: www.dh.gov.uk/PolicyAndGuidance/HealthAndSocialCareTopics. Accessed February 20, 2005.
3. National Institute for Clinical Excellence. Welcome to the National Institute for Health and Clinical Excellence Web site. Available at: www.nice.org.uk/. Accessed February 27, 2005.
4. Scottish Intercollegiate Guidelines Network. SIGN: Scottish Intercollegiate Guidelines Network. Available at: www.sign.ac.uk/. Accessed February 27, 2005.
5. Healthcare Commission. Healthcare Commission: Inspecting Informing Improving. Available at: www.healthcarecommission.org.uk. Accessed February 27, 2005.
6. Royal College of Nursing. Clinical governance: an RCN resource guide. 2003. Available at: www.rcn.org.uk/publications/pdf/ClinicalGovernance2003.pdf. Accessed February 20, 2005.
7. Royal College of Nursing. Agenda for change: information and guidance. Available at: www.rcn.org.uk/agendaforchange/. Accessed February 20, 2005.
8. NHS Executive. Information for Health: an information strategy for the modern NHS. Available at: www.nhsia.nhs.uk/def/pages/info4health/1.asp. Accessed February 20, 2005.

9. Information Standards Group (Scotland). Available at: www.show.scot.nhs.uk/isdonline/index.htm. Accessed February 27, 2005.

10. NHS Information Standards Board (England). Available at: www.isb.nhs.uk. Accessed February 27, 2005.

11. Murphy J, Stramer K, Clamp S, et al. Health informatics education for clinicians and managers—what's holding up progress? *International Journal of Medical Informatics.* 2004;73(2):205-213.

12. UK Council for Health Informatics Professions (UKCHIP). Available at: www.ukchip.org/. Accessed February 27, 2005.

13. National Occupational Standards—Health Informatics. Available at: http://www.skillsforhealth.org.uk/ view_framework.php?id=48. Accessed August 20, 2005.

14. Department of Health Information supporting NSFs and NCASP Available at: www.dh.gov.uk/ PolicyAndGuidance/InformationPolicy/Information SupportingNSFAndNCASP/fs/en. Accessed August 22, 2005.

15. Royal College of Nursing. Nurses and NHS IT developments. Available at: www.rcn.org.uk/downloads/ research/nurses-it-devs-survey.doc. Accessed February 20, 2005.

16. Currell R, Urquhart C. Nursing record systems: effects on nursing practice and health care outcomes. *Cochrane Database Systematic Review.* 2003; 3:CD002099.

17. Sanderson H, Adams T, Budden M, Hoare C. Lessons from the central Hampshire electronic health record pilot project: evaluation of the electronic health record for supporting patient care and secondary analysis. *BMJ.* 2004 Apr 10;328(7444):875-8.

18. The Nomina Group. The Nursing Information Research Project report. 1998. Available at: www.nhsia.nhs.uk/pdf/nirp.pdf. Accessed February 20, 2005.

19. British Computer Society Nursing Specialist Group. The nursing specialist group Available at: www.bcsnsg.org.uk. Accessed February 27, 2005.

20. Kearney N, Miller M, Sermeus W, et al. Multicentre research and the WISECARE experience. Workflow information systems for European nursing care. *J Adv Nurs.* 2000;32(4):999-1007.

21. ISO TC 215 Working Group 3. Work item on nursing terminology model. Available at: www.tc215wg3.nhs.uk/ pages/nursterm.asp. Accessed August 20, 2005.

22. SNOMED® nursing working group. Available at: www.snomed.org/clinical/nursing.html. Accessed February 27, 2005.

23. Clark J, ed. *Naming Nursing: Proceedings of the First ACENDIO Ireland/UK Conference.* Bern: Verlag Hans Huber; 2003.

24. Nursing Midwifery and Allied Professions (NMAP) gateway. Available at: http://nmap.ac.uk/. Accessed August 20, 2005.

25. O'Cathain A, Sampson FC, Munro JF, et al. Nurses' views of using computerized decision support software in NHS Direct. *J Adv Nurs.* 2004;45(3):280-286.

26. Robinson G. Using a clinical decision-making support tool to enhance practice. *Nurs Times.* 2004;100(40):32-34.

27. Hibbert D, Mair FS, May CR, et al. Health professionals' responses to the introduction of a home telehealth service. *J Telemedicine and Telecare.* 2004;10(4):226-230.

28. Booth N, Robinson P, Kohannejad J. Identification of high-quality consultation practice in primary care: the effects of computer use on doctor-patient rapport. *Inf Primary Care.* 2004;12(2):75-83.

Case Study 26A

Taming the Tiger: Ireland

Rita Collins, MEd., RGN, RM, RNT and Fintan Sheerin, BNS, PGDipEd, RMHN

It may seem improbable to talk of tigers in Ireland, the most westerly country in the European Union (EU). However, the tiger in this case is a virtual tiger—"the Celtic Tiger." This is the name given to the economic boom that Ireland has experienced for the past seven to eight years. This boom has raised our expectations about health care. It has also allowed us to consider an investment in technology to support health care.

This case study will explore the emergence of an electronic health record (EHR) in Ireland's health care sector, along with the debate on its purchase and development. Key elements, e.g., record-keeping and the professional development of nurses, will be explored against the backdrop of this electronic format. Finally, future possibilities and trends will be outlined.

Background to the Irish Health System

The Department of Health and Children is responsible for planning health services and developing health policies for Ireland's four million people. Its mission statement sets out its aims:

> To support, protect, and empower individuals, families, and their communities to achieve their full health potential by putting health at the center of public policy, and by leading the development of high-quality, equitable and efficient health, and personal social services.[1]

People living in Ireland are entitled to a range of health services that are free through the public health system. Other services, e.g., general practitioner visits, are means tested, and people classified above a certain income threshold pay the full cost of these services. A private health system also exists with approximately 40 percent of the population as members.

Health Care Informatics

Currently in Ireland, there is an ever-increasing use of technology for data collection. Hospital information systems are in widespread use and have developed considerably over the past number of years. Information and communication technology (ICT) has become central to delivering fast, comprehensive information to managers. Human resource management has benefited from the implementation of PPARS (Personnel Payroll and Related Systems), an integrated system comprised of a number of business modules that support personnel management and shift planning within the Irish health services. Laboratory data and imaging are among many of the specialties that share data and information pertaining to patient care. However, this is mainly site driven; depending on the application in use, it can be difficult for systems to share information. What is required is a national system that can interface with all areas where data is collected and shared that, in turn, will be of benefit to the delivery of quality patient care.

This framework for future development lies in the launch of the National Health Information Strategy (NHIS), which focuses on the EHR and an Internet-based health information portal. Both are intended to provide a rich information base for health professionals, the public, research, and policy makers.[2] NHIS consolidates the previous initiatives on health reform as directed in "Quality and Fairness: A Health System for You," a government report that identified health information as an area in need of significant improvement.[1] This is a positive step forward and builds on the ICT already in existence in many of our health care settings. The focus on health information will provide both decision support in clinical settings and provide a more standardized, comprehensive basis for health surveillance and promotion. It is envisioned that the EHR will be implemented in the next two to five years.[2] This will bring together global, integrated, up-to-date health care information on patients/clients and will incorporate a sophisticated communications system.

The responsibility for implementing this program lies with the Health Information and Quality Authority. The implementation will be incremental, involving appropriate health care staff for the development of specialized modules. Already we have seen the introduction of phase one, the European Health Insurance Card, issued in June 2004, a smart card that replaces the paper form E111.

Nursing Records

The health care setting is one of the most knowledge-intensive environments.[3] Nurses collect perhaps the largest volume of information per patient during a hospitalization, compared with other personnel. Nurses are also the largest group of professionals employed in the health services.[4] Within a health care environment, information is health oriented and outcome driven. Hospitals, by virtue of their nature are hubs of information activity. In health care, many key decisions concerning data pertain to what information to collect and to having that data available to the right people, at the right time, and in the right form.[5] The use to which nurses put information and the sharing of information between members of the multidisciplinary team will determine the value of the information and its contribution to the outcome of patient care. The nursing profession needs to recognize the value of information that is available to the nurse as well as the value of a documentation system for capturing that information.[6] Patient-focused data from the clinical environment provides nursing management with the information needed to determine workloads and to execute the accounting tasks of nursing administration.[7] To ensure that the nursing content of the EHR represents the extent and the quality of care delivered, nurses need to be actively involved in the development of nursing systems.[8]

Although many nursing administration systems are in use throughout the country, within the community and hospitals, little work is done on electronic clinical nursing records. Extensive work has been carried out within nursing on skill mix, duty rostering, and dependency levels. Intensive care units have integrated technology into nursing notes, thereby providing up-to-date information on patients, and a myriad of disease-focused systems are used to manage specific client groups. However, the clinical nursing record (particularly the care plan) needs considerable work before it is integrated into the EHR. Below we examine the nursing record and its history to gain an understanding of the problems that may be encountered when adapting the nursing record to electronic format.

In the 1980s, there was a new focus on the nursing record, as the individualized nursing care plan developed. It may be argued that the nursing care plan became paramount, generating a document that demonstrated clear links between problem identification, setting of goals, interventions, and evaluation. The problem was that this record often described the ideal and bore little relevance to the reality of care.

The 1990s saw major developments in nursing education in Ireland. The hospital-based certificate programs, although regularized under the Irish Nursing Board (An Bord Altranais), had their origins in the old nurse training apprenticeship model. During this period, they became associated with third-level institutions in the short-lived diploma program. The move from nurse training to nurse education reached its zenith in 2002 when Irish nursing became a graduate-entry profession. In the run-up to this, many qualified certificate and diploma nurses returned to education and completed their bachelor degrees, whereas others, who were suitably qualified, commenced master degrees.

In 2000, An Bord Altranais issued a final report, "Review of the Scope of Practice for Nursing and Midwifery," which recognized that the practice was expanding and that a framework was required to support the complex diagnostic decisions nurses were increasingly making.[9] Allied to this was the development of clinical nurse specialist and advanced nurse practitioner roles. This report was followed by An Bord Altranais guidelines that laid down parameters for nursing documentation.[10] These guidelines were mainly concerned with legal matters, e.g., legibility, completeness of the document, and signatures for entries. There is a need for more direction if the nursing profession is to develop standards for their records. To this end, a national project on nursing terminology and classification is needed.

An examination of the nursing record—its structure, content, and quality of measurements—needs to be conducted in light of impending computerization. This move to automation will also have implications for quality improvement, professionalization of nursing, and the value nurses place on the documentation of care. The role of information in nursing needs to be considered.

As yet, there has been no move to formally adopt nursing classification systems and common terminologies. The North American Nursing Diagnosis Association (NANDA) diagnoses are used sporadically in areas such as intensive care, and one community is using the OMAHA classification system. There is a concerted move among Healthcare Informatics Society of Ireland members to get NI content prioritized for inclusion in undergraduate nursing curricula throughout the country.[11] Nursing classification systems and terminology need examination in light of European and U.S. developments, and a decision needs to be made on how data, information, and knowledge are represented within nursing documentation.

Developments within these areas will also facilitate the computerization of nursing records. For this to occur and be widely accepted, the nursing profession needs to formally recognize the value of information to nursing care.

The Clinical Decision Making Study, a major national move toward nursing input into the EHR, involves the construction of an Irish nursing minimum data set. This project—begun in 2002 and scheduled to run until 2007—is a partnership between Dublin City University and University College Dublin. Funded with one million euros awarded by the Health Research Board, the project is focused on providing a basis for clinical applications to support evidence-based practice within the clinical area. It explores areas such as decision making with the intention of maximizing effectiveness in the clinical area.

In the past few years, nurses have increasingly asked: what are the key components of nursing? The issue of exploring language as a means of describing the foci of the profession has become the subject of research studies.[12] It is arguably more difficult to assign shared conceptual meaning to terms now that nursing, in Ireland, has become multicultural. This is, however, what must be done, and leaders in Irish NI from the Healthcare Informatics Society of Ireland and the Association for Common European Nursing Diagnoses, Interventions, and Outcomes (ACENDIO) Ireland/UK Group are driving this work.

Special Olympics Project

Both the potential of and the expertise to implement an EHR was tested in 2003 when Ireland hosted the Special Olympics. Through the use of HEALTHone,[13] an EHR application, there were 4,800 consultations, and a database of 10,000 screenings on 3,600 athletics was complied. Many of the entries were made using conventional personal digital assistants (PDAs). The PDA users were volunteers trained each morning on using the PDA. This event demonstrated that not only could valuable information be collected systematically through a simple electronic piece of equipment, it was also easy to use. The real task facing nursing is to ensure that the data and information that nurses enter is both evidence-based and standardized so it can be used for research and quality improvement purposes.

Standards

The ultimate aim of nursing care is quality patient care as measured by standards because care is dependent on the quality of information available.[14] To be useful, this information needs to be formally recorded so that it may be communicated accurately on an ongoing basis to other nurses and to the multidisciplinary team.

The value of the information depends upon its reliability, validity, accessibility, comprehensiveness, and accuracy.[15] Information gathered and the toll for gathering and processing this information will need to conform to measurable standards. Two areas—technical standards and quality standards—need consideration when implementing an EHR. The Health Information and Quality Authority (HIQA), in cooperation with health service agencies and national and international experts, will put a framework in place for adopting and implementing data.

In 2004, the National Standards Authority of Ireland (NSAI) established a new committee to consider standardization in health care informatics. Through NSAI, which is allied to the European Committee on Standardization (CEN) and International Standards Organization (ISO), national concerns in relation to standards will be represented. Global perspectives from the work of CEN TC 252 and ISO Committee 215, as well as Health Level 7, will also influence Irish informatics work.

Much of the value of information can be ascribed to "people power."[16] In other words, the ultimate success of any system depends on the people who interface with the system. The user will determine how the information is used to generate knowledge.

Security

The primacy of protecting patient data needs reconsideration when inputting data into electronic format, as the data are now capable of being accessed remotely, in addition to on-site. Steps to protect this data are addressed within the NHIS. It has been suggested that the personal identification numbers already allocated to people for public services be used or that a new health sector national identifier be used for each client/patient. Other security measures, e.g., personal identification numbers, encryption, and audit trails, will also be considered. Within existing legislation, the Data Protection Act 1988 and the Freedom of Information Act 1997 combine to provide security for records contained within paper and electronic format.[17,18]

Summary

Back to the Celtic Tiger. It is hoped that economic growth will continue and allow the NHIS to be fully implemented over the coming decade. By that time, the ICT strategy recommended by the NHIS to direct areas such as "telehealth," support for primary care and a national waiting list will have been published and will give further impetus to the EHR. One of the welcome recommendations by the NHIS is allocating funding for change management programs to support implementation of the EHR strategy. This is considered integral to its successful adoption. Meanwhile, the nursing profession needs to take ownership of nursing records to make clear the nursing contribution to patient care.

References

1. Government of Ireland. *Quality and Fairness: A Health System for You.* Dublin: Stationary Office; 2004.

2. Department of Health and Children. *Health Information— A National Strategy.* Dublin: Stationary Office; 2004.

3. Drucker P, Garvin D, Leonard D. *Knowledge Management: The Definitive Resource for Professionals.* Harvard: Harvard Business School Press; 1998.

4. Simpson, R. Why nursing needs informatics and informatics needs nursing. In: Clarke J, ed. *Naming Nursing.* Bern: Verlag Hans Huber; 2003.

5. Smith J. *Health Management Systems.* Buckinghamshire: Open University Press; 2000.

6. Casey A. Naming nursing in the UK: goals and challenges. In: Clarke J, ed. *Naming Nursing.* Bern: Verlag Hans Huber. 2003.

7. Murnane R. Empowering nurses, improving care: introducing an integrated nursing information system in an acute teaching hospital in Ireland. In: Clarke J, ed. *Naming Nursing.* Bern: Verlag Hans Huber; 2003.

8. Kurtz C. Accurate documentation equals quality patient care. *Insight.* 2002;27:8-10.

9. An Bord Altranais. *Review of the Scope of Practice for Nursing and Midwifery.* Dublin: An Bord Altranais; 2002.

10. An Bord Altranais. *Recording Clinical Practice: Guidelines for Nurses.* Dublin: An Bord Altranais; 2002.

11. Collins R. Development of a common language for nursing. In: *Proceedings 2nd Healthcare Informatics Society of Ireland Annual Conference and Scientific Symposium.* Dublin: Healthcare Informatics Society of Ireland; 1997.

12. Sheerin F. Employing NANDA and NIC in identifying the key components of intellectual disability nursing in Ireland. Paper presented at: 2nd Biennial Conference of NANDA, NIC and NOC, 2004; Chicago.

13. Health Ireland Partners Limited. Case study: the special olympics. Available at: www.healthone.ie/ case_studies_ enterprise.html. Accessed February 25, 2005.

14. Currell R, Wainwright P, Urquhart C. Nursing record systems: efforts on nursing practice and health care outcomes. *Cochrane Database of Systematic Reviews.* 2002;2.

15. Oppenheim C, Stenson J, Wilson R. Studies in information as an asset 11: repertory grid. *J Inf Studies.* 2003;32:601-611.

16. Introna L. *Management, Information and Power: a Narrative of the Involved Manager.* London: Palgrave Macmillan; 1997.

17. Government of Ireland. *Data Protection Act.* Dublin: Stationary Office; 1988, 2003.

18. Government of Ireland. *Freedom of Information Act.* Dublin: Stationary Office; 1997.

Case Study 26B

A Scottish Perspective on Issues Surrounding the Electronic Record

Charles Docherty, PhD, RNT

Against the backdrop of massive information technology (IT) developments now under way in the National Health Service (NHS) throughout the United Kingdom, collaboration between the Greater Glasgow NHS Board and Glasgow Caledonian University (GCU) provides strategic direction for nursing locally. This case study identifies specific issues in relation to Scottish developments, but a wider perspective is taken on nursing's influence and engagement, philosophical conflict, and the implications for the education of nurses, all with particular reference to the development of the electronic health record (EHR).

Background

Since political devolution in 1999, four separate NHS structures have formed within the UK. Particular focus has been on the English National Program for IT (renamed "Connecting for Health"), which has been recognized as the largest civil IT project in the world, projected to cost as much as £30bn by 2010.[1,2] The Connecting for Health project scope includes EHR, appointment booking, prescribing, picture archiving, and communications.

Although Connecting for Health has received international attention, equally ambitious developments have been proceeding throughout the other UK countries on a smaller cost scale. In Scotland, the challenge of meeting the differing needs of urban, rural, and remote communities has contributed to the development of a flexible eHealth and Information Management and Technology (IM&T) strategy.[3] The scope is similar to Connecting for Health, yet less well-funded per-capita. Scotland's eHealth strategy also differs significantly in its implementation; for instance, clinicians have been involved from the beginning, legacy systems have been retained, and local development has been encouraged. Central to this is the Scottish Care Information Program that aims to provide software applications suitable for use throughout the fifteen Scottish health boards.[4] Many of the developments are pragmatic; for example, an emergency summary containing information, e.g., drug therapy and allergies is planned for every man, woman, and child to improve the efficiency and safety of out-of-hours and Accident and Emergency (A&E) care.[5]

The locally controlled, incremental approach in Scotland, although beneficial in some regards, has disadvantages. For example, the rollout of a unique patient identifier (the Community Health Index or CHI number), ubiquitous in some regions, has been hindered in others because legacy systems have been unable to make the transition.[4] Similarly, the generic clinical records "tool-kit" at the national level requires a lengthy and complex tendering and procurement process that invites preemptive local developments and the consequent proliferation of smaller-scale records projects. The system currently being piloted in the Managed Clinical Networks (MCN)—stroke and cardiac care in Glasgow—serves as an example. This system uses a suite of applications within a portal supplied by Orion. Although these developments have been motivated by a desire to deliver advantages quickly, major issues can be given little time for resolution. Representing nursing information in a standard way is a major challenge because we find that these decisions are being made locally with no formal consultation with the wider profession nationally.

Scotland has historically invested in good primary care systems, and 85 percent of General Practitioners use the same system—the General Practice Administration System for Scotland (GPASS). Currently, an electronic community health information project is under way to develop multidisciplinary health records. Major advances are being made to create nationwide access to local data repositories and enable the secure transmission of data between primary and secondary care providers, between the health and social care sectors, and indeed between Scotland and the rest of the UK.[4,6] This infrastructure is paving the way for the introduction of ambulatory care and diagnostic units in Glasgow by 2008. Both will require high-quality communication systems between primary and secondary care and ruthless standardization for their effective functioning.[7] However, major gaps are evident within secondary care, particularly in nursing, where there has been little recent development. In 2002, the director of nursing for a large acute NHS trust in Glasgow expressed dismay that the local IM&T strategy did not have a nursing focus. Noting that professions such as medicine and pharmacology were well represented in the IM&T strategy, this nursing leader called attention to the absence of nursing. To address this challenge, the local NHS trust and GCU formed a collaborative partnership. The overall aim was to develop informatics in nursing practice and to create a supportive educational infrastructure. The group developed a white paper defining the local nursing IT strategy and defined a work plan. Initial work involved raising awareness and delivering quick wins, while establishing how education and training could best contribute to the final phase—delivering value and enhanced patient care. What follows is an account of the context and achievements of this strategy in its initial years.

Glimpsing the National Strategy in Scotland

A challenge to health professionals in Scotland is to keep up-to-date with current, local developments in IT, as it is difficult to discriminate between Scottish and English developments within UK media. The spotlight is fixed firmly on England, where the majority of the UK population lives. For example, a special informatics edition of the *British Medical Journal* focused exclusively on the English National Program for IT, while failing to make explicit how this varied throughout the UK.[8] The Scottish strategy differs considerably in direction and timescale. For instance, the UK media and Westminster politicians broadcast the importance of patient choice in booking consultant appointments and treatment, but in Scotland this is not an immediate priority. Scotland is instead introducing a system to remind patients of clinic appointments in order to reduce the number of those not attending.

Because of this sublimation, nurses have difficulty discerning a clear strategic direction in the Scottish NHS. As a result of being poorly informed, nurses risk missing opportunities to actively contribute to decision making in IT matters. In turn, this leads to crucial decisions being made on behalf of the nursing profession without its full consultation. One such example is agreeing on having a nursing minimum data set (NMDS). As a basic in the support of professional nursing practice, the use of an NMDS ought to be a high-level consideration to facilitate the aggregation of data for management and research purposes. However, nursing stands to lose this opportunity as local electronic records are developed with little or no regard to the secondary use of nursing data.

In addition, when nurses are asked to contribute to projects, they are usually invited for their clinical expertise or their management position. Unfortunately, few UK nurses are experienced in informatics, therefore the distilled wisdom of decades of nursing involvement in these matters is underutilized. Such important issues as data security, confidentiality, and sharing as well as charting by exception need to be fully discussed within the profession because they cannot be developed in increments.

The development of electronic records requires a balanced input from all disciplines to allow access to tacit and domain knowledge, to dispel stereotypical views of professional roles, and to facilitate change.[9,10] Given the intricate relationship between system design, its use, and consequent changes to practice, nurses ought to be engaged at all levels and in all stages of development, from design through to implementation. However, in a UK-wide online survey by the Royal College of Nursing in 2004, only 2 percent of nurses (N = 2,020) felt they had "fully adequate information," whereas 26 percent had not heard of planned national IT programs.[11] Within Scotland, the Executive Health Department holds regular national strategy meetings for clinicians and IT professionals. In November 2004, of the more than 90 delegates attending the national IT strategy meeting, there were no nurses. This lack of nursing engagement has serious consequences: When users lack motivation to become involved, system implementations inevitably fail, a fate that befalls 50 percent of such projects.[10]

Much more, therefore, needs to be done in communicating with and engaging nurse clinicians. In Glasgow, this has been a central feature of the nursing IT strategy, and the group continues to be inclusive, representative, and outward looking, actively seeking involvement in strategic planning and local initiatives. Recent IT conferences have witnessed presentations from care assistants, IT professionals, data controllers, lecturers, librarians, and nursing management.

Keeping Connected

Conscious of the dangers of working in isolation, an element of the nursing IT strategy in Glasgow has been to network with nurses locally, nationally, and internationally. Thus, a presence has been established in the British Computer Society Health Informatics Scotland and nursing specialist groups, the Scottish Nurses' eHealth

Forum, and the Association for Common European Nursing Diagnosis, Interventions, and Outcomes (ACENDIO). Participating actively within these groups is time-consuming but has the potential to influence developments, a vital activity if nurses are to take control and not merely be subject to events. As part of this networking process, groups such as GCU Research Forum and the Society for Computing and Technology in Anaesthesia have attended seminars, and these group's activities have been presented at national and international conferences.[12,13,14] The participative processes in these professional forums allow for discussion, debate, and peer review of developments that have been invaluable in providing direction for the ACENDIO group.

Practice Development: Sharing and Learning with Others

Focus groups with nurses on a local level uncovered a desire to use technology to reduce the bureaucratic burden of clinical nursing. Based on these results, the nursing strategy group commissioned a project to establish parameters, politically and professionally, for developing electronic nursing records. This involved an extensive review of literature, consultation with experts, and site visits, and resulted in a strategy document disseminated locally to inform nurses of relevant issues. This work was invaluable preparation for subsequent pilot projects to develop electronic records for local Managed Clinical Networks in stroke and cardiac care. It was decided to focus the strategy group's resources on one project. The project's goal was the development of a standardized approach to represent nursing using forms and templates that could be implemented, not just in a cardiac context, but in any context. This is important because nurses are fundamentally holistic in the provision of 24-hour care. Other members of the multidisciplinary team are time limited in their contact with patients, more focused on their professional role, and more specific in their information needs. This contrast requires nurses to develop a record to address all aspects of holistic care, and not simply to produce the cardiac nursing component. IT professionals initially did not understand this.

This standardized documentation work is only in progress, yet it already has the full commitment from nurses locally. Despite the consideration of culturally alien terminology systems, e.g., North American Nursing Diagnosis Association International (NANDA), efforts to structure templates in the record are progressing well. The term *nursing diagnosis,* considered divisive, has been politically resisted since the 1980s.[15] In practice, nurses place higher value upon unstructured patient narratives in a postmodern tradition, compared with a "tick-box" or menu-driven approach to documentation consistent with positivism. The result is that there are few documented examples of the successful use of NANDA in the UK.[16,17] However, the Anglicized version as used in the Chelsea and Westminster Hospital in London appears promising and provides a useful starting point for representing nursing information within the MCN pilot.[18]

Education for Practice

If nurses are to contribute and not just be consulted in the specification, design, procurement, and implementation of IT systems, then a knowledge of health informatics theory is as important as acquiring IT skills or receiving training on a clinical system's use. Providing effective education and training in such a rapidly changing field is a major challenge, with the result that many undergraduate health care curricula in the UK have neglected informatics teaching.[19,20] In contrast with the innovative use of technology to enhance the experiences of health care students,[21-23] those with the skills and knowledge to teach health informatics are in short supply and undervalued both in practice and higher education contexts.[19,20] This is compounded by a historic lack of demand for informatics knowledge and skills and the absence of professional and political drivers to influence health care curricula. The result is stasis. Education institutions do not provide courses for which there is no demand, and students do not demand courses for which there is no apparent workplace application. Attempts have been made in Glasgow to break this deadlock.

Following several unsuccessful years of speculatively offering an NI module to students, the course was revamped and renamed. The first offering of the new eHealth module at degree level in GCU in 2005 thus attracted a full complement of students. This module explores concepts of eHealth and informatics from a health care provider's perspective. Using the application Blackboard as a virtual learning backdrop, students transition from face-to-face to an online environment within a few weeks, maximizing the complementary nature of the medium and the message. Students present seminars on fieldwork exercises, such as a visit to the local hospital to interview an IT professional about his or her role. Students have praised the module, making such comments as:

"I feel the module is expanding my learning capabilities. I feel my brain creaking and groaning into action, similar to first-year experience. It's like learning a new language that can be applied to the working environment. It's a positive learning curve and one which I'm embracing. It helps to open your mind to new ways of working and thinking."

The NHS in Glasgow and GCU collaborated to find the funding necessary to help strategically placed nurses take this module as part of their continuous professional development. It is also hoped that contractual arrangements between the NHS and higher education move toward ensuring that nursing undergraduate students have opportunities for acquiring the European Computer Driving License as part of their degree. This qualification is gaining recognition as the IT skill level for employment within the NHS and is consistent with GCU's commitment to ensuring graduate employability.[24]

Conclusion

The phrase "necessity is the mother of invention" neatly sums up the approach to IM&T in the cash-strapped Scottish NHS. The famous eighteenth-century Scottish economist and philosopher Adam Smith would have been proud of the way prudence, pragmatism, and imagination have worked to our advantage. However, there is a danger of missing out on the full benefits of health system reengineering when instead we incrementally automate Byzantine processes, pander to custom and practice, and avoid politically sensitive issues. At some point, radical change in Scotland will be required, and nurses need to be educated and primed in order to participate as change agents rather than stand on the sidelines in awe of technology.

Issues surrounding the use of technology in nursing are long-standing. Understanding the potential clinical benefits of electronic records—increased efficiency, effectiveness, and safety in patient care—may be insufficient incentive to win the hearts and minds of nurses. Successful adoption requires that nurses are willing to undertake additional education and training and temporarily assume an increased workload as they learn to deliver care using new clinical systems. This willingness to assume an additional learning workload may have philosophical roots in the area of nursing theory where positivist technology can be considered intrusive in a postmodern world. In Scotland, increasing emphasis has been placed on clinical engagement in the change process, but this has not yet extended to every nurse in every ward. Such a change must occur in order to change the culture, but is a challenge to the traditional approach of involving nurses at strategic levels to represent the profession. What is needed is transformational leadership, complementing the introduction of recognizable NI roles within education and practice at all levels, from strategic to operational. There is some optimism that this is beginning to happen in Scotland, but it has yet to be formalized and consolidated.

This case study demonstrates the importance of nurses, as professionals, working together to transcend the false dichotomy between education and practice that has plagued our profession. Nurse educators and practitioners working cooperatively can provide a much more powerful force in collaborations with IT, with medical professionals, and while serving on multidisciplinary teams. This is important if we are to dispel stereotypical views, align the educational preparation of nursing students with the expectations of practice, and ensure that nursing philosophies are represented within Scotland's clinical information systems.

References

1. Guenier R. England's National Programme for IT: a personal view. *Br J Healthcare Computing Inf Manage.* 2005;22(2):24-5.
2. Carvel J. NHS faces £15bn black hole. *The Guardian.* October 12, 2004.
3. Scottish Executive Health Department (SEHD). *National eHealth/IM&T Strategy.* Edinburgh: The Scottish Executive; 2004.
4. Silverman A. Progress by increments. *Smart Healthcare* 2005;2(2):16-17.
5. Robertson K. The Scottish approach to clinical information. In: Kay S, ed. *HC 2005: Shaping Sands, Shifting Services.* Harrogate, England; 2005:21-23.
6. Editor. News. E-Health Insider Primary Care 2005;14. Available at: support@e-health-media.com.
7. Feachem RGS, Sekhri NK, White KL. Getting more for their dollar: a comparison of the NHS with Kaiser Permanente. *BMJ.* 2002;324:135-43.
8. Smith R (ed). Can IT lead to radical redesign of health care. *BMJ.* 2004;328(744): theme issue: 1136-1158.
9. Keenan G, Stocker J, Geo-Thomas AT, et al. The HANDS project: studying and refining the automated collection of a cross-setting clinical data set. *Comput Inf Nurs.* 2002;20(3):89-100.
10. Lorenzi N. Transformational change. In: Kay S, ed. *HC 2005: Shaping Sands, Shifting Services.* HC 2005 Harrogate, March 21-23. 2005, 11-13.

11. Royal College of Nursing. *Nurses and NHS IT Developments.* London: Royal College of Nursing; 2004.

12. Docherty C, Kellagher M. Missing in UK nursing: a structured conceptualisation of nursing care as a pre-requisite to electronic records. In: Oud N, Sermeus W, Ehnfors M, eds. *Acendio* April 7–9, 2005. Bled, Slovenia: Verlag Hans Huber; 2005:297-304.

13. Docherty C, Kellagher M. Moving toward the electronic record: issues for nurse education and practice. In: Kay S, ed. *HC 2005: Shaping Sands, Shifting Services.* Harrogate, England; 2005:21-23.

14. Kellagher M, Docherty C. The Scottish eHealth and IM&T strategy: a clinician's view. In: *National developments in eHealth;* May 6, 2004; Glasgow Caledonian University; 2004.

15. Walker P. Problems with the Process. *Nursing Times,* 83(2), 12-13, 1987.

16. Coiera E. *Guide to Health Informatics.* 2nd ed. London: Hodder Arnold: 2003.

17. Walsh SH. The clinician's perspective on electronic health records and how they can affect patient care. *BMJ.* 2004;328:1184.

18. Westbrook A. Incorporating nursing diagnosis into a hospital information system. In: Clark J, ed. *Naming Nursing.* Swansea: Verlag Hans Huber; 2003:225-30.

19. Murphy J, Stramer K, Clamp S, et al. *Health Informatics Education for Healthcare Professionals.* London: DOH; 2002.

20. National Health Service Information Authority (NHSIA). Health informatics education and development for clinical professionals: making progress? Available at: http://www.nhsia.nhs.uk/informatics/pages/resource_informatics/ItmPart1.PDF. Accessed May 10, 2005.

21. Docherty C, Hoy D, Topp H, Trinder K. Using eLearning techniques to support problem based learning within a clinical simulation laboratory. In: Fieschi M, Coiera E, Li YJ, eds. Proceedings of the 11th World Congress on Medical Informatics, Vol. 107. Amsterdam, The Netherlands: ISO Press, 2004: pp. 224-227.

22. Docherty C. The Instructional Design and Evaluation of a Multimedia Program to Help Mentors Develop Skills in Assessing Student Nurses' Clinical Performance [PhD thesis]. Glasgow: Glasgow University; 2002.

23. Hoy D, Docherty C, Topp H, Trinder K. Learning systems: supporting curriculum change in nursing education. In: 6th International Congress of Nursing Informatics. Auckland, New Zealand; 2000.

24. National Health Service Information Authority. Health informatics skills and competencies—a framework to support NSF implementation. Available at: http://www.nhsia.nhs.uk/nhid/pages/resource_informatics/Informatics.pdf. Accessed May 10, 2005.

CHAPTER 27

Electronic Health Initiatives: European View

By Patrick Weber MA, RN, MA

This chapter explores the impact of electronic health record (EHR) initiatives on nursing across Europe and is supported by nine case studies from the following countries: Iceland, Finland, Norway, Sweden, Netherlands, Germany, Italy, Spain, and countries in Central and Eastern Europe. The case studies show extensive variation at the national government level of health policy, the extent to which EHRs are used in health services delivery, the role and status of nursing, and nursing education programs. Not surprising, the degree to which nursing informatics (NI) is included as a basic skill competency in nursing education, practice, and research is closely correlated with the professional and educational evolution of nursing within a given country. Across these nine case studies there is a clear trend between the degree of NI activities found in a given country and the maturation level of their university-based nursing education programs and professional status. In those countries where nursing education is just being established as university-based, the tendency is for nursing to be excluded from participating in electronic health record (EHR) initiatives.

Fortunately, standardization of nursing education with full degree offerings, from baccalaureate to PhD, is being promoted by the standardization effects of the 1999 Bologna Declaration. Signed by 29 ministers of education and supported by the European Union Commission, this declaration defines six action strategies for achieving standardization across European higher education programs by 2010.[1] This declaration is credited in a number of these case studies as the impetus for higher education programs being created for nursing and owned by nursing faculty.[1]

As shown in Figure 27-1, Europe is composed of 48 countries covering a little more than 10 million square kilometers and where 20 official languages are spoken.[2]

Law and health policy emerge as important themes across these nine case studies for the ramifications and obstacles that they can present for an integrated EHR that supports all clinicians in all venues. For instance, Swedish law forbids the transfer of patient health data between providers without the patient's consent. As Enhors and Ehrenberg point out in Case Study 27D, not only does this act to discourage health information exchange between clinicians and disciplines, it also acts to block clinicians from sharing health data with a patient over the Internet. In the Germany case study (27F), Hübner et al outline the central role that the health card plays in their EHR strategy as the mechanism for embedding health data by approved clinicians. Hübner et al. explain that the German Health Modernization Act defines only three categories of health professionals permitted access to patients' health care data: physicians, dentists, and pharmacists. The health card system is to be deployed in 2006 and, as the authors predict, unless these restrictions change, German nurses will be excluded from accessing the EHR, and nursing data will be not be included in the EHR.

Case Study 27C, which focuses on Norway, presents an example of the way that legal precedent can structure a country's efforts to achieve an EHR. Given Norway's legal mandate that health care delivery must be documented to show planned and delivered care, Moen et al relate that stand alone documentation systems emerged as the first clinical information systems and tended to be discipline-specific. The challenge that follows in moving to an EHR is cultural and structural. The task becomes one of cooperation and coordination in being able to standardize documentation across the disciplines to avoid redundancy and to achieve an integrated record. Moen et al capture the work involved for all disciplines as they move away from their historical traditions of communicating within their own domains to respond to the opportunities that an integrated EHR makes possible.

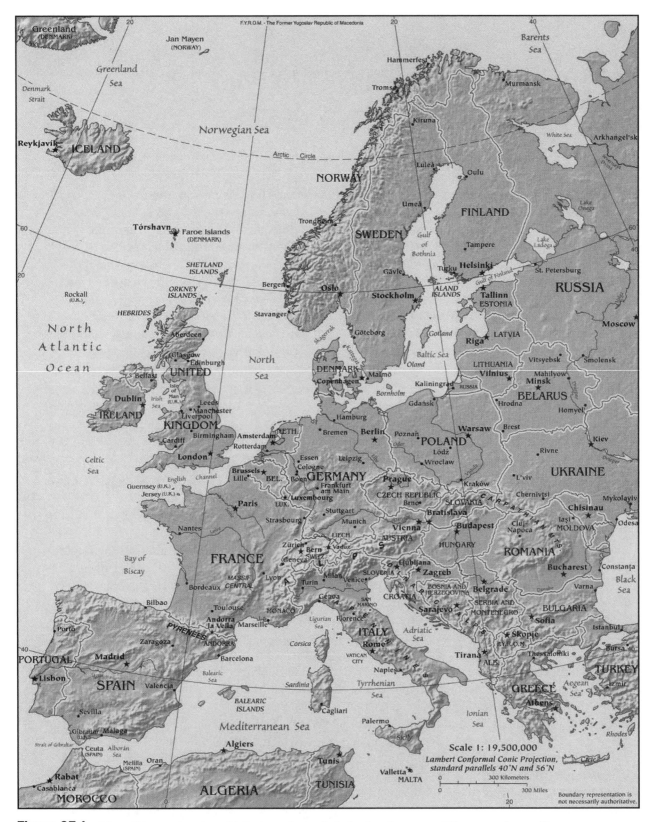

Figure 27-1. *Map of Europe (starting with Spain to the south, Iceland to the west and Norway to the north).*

The final case study (27I) in this section includes a look at Central and Eastern Europe. Because the countries in Central and Eastern Europe have not been included in previous works, Ioana Moisil has organized with her NI colleagues within these countries to provide an overview into the current state and developments for Romania, Bulgaria, Turkey, Poland, and Lithuania. Although the summaries are brief, it is evident from their descriptions that these authors are pioneers who are pulling actively from international networks to interject rapid learning and change for nursing, health care, and patient services within their countries.

Prior to reading these case studies, it is good to have a sense of the financial variation that occurs across these nations' health care systems. Figure 27-2 contrasts the expenditures for the European and the Eastern European countries. The trend shows a steady decrease in spending going from Western Europe to Eastern Europe. Germany ranks highest in spending while the United Kingdom ranks next to lowest for European countries, with Finland last. Azerbaijan and Switzerland represent another stark comparison. With health care as 0.9 percent of their gross domestic product (GDP), Azerbaijan spends the least of industrial countries compared with Switzerland who ranks at the top with 10.7 percent of their GDP for health care. In marked contrast, the U.S. has the highest health care expenditures in the world with 13.2 percent of their GDP (value 2000) going for health care.[3]

The World Health Organization ranks countries' health care systems according to indicators of health status, services, personnel and expenditures.[4] Table 27-1 presents these indicators for most of the countries included in this section. Germany again ranks highest costs with Romania ranking lowest, but Germany's health status indicators are lower than Finland who has the lowest expenditures of the Western European countries. Health care expenditures are presented in relation to the country's population, GDP per capita shown as a ratio to purchasing power of a country's currency, for example, the rate of currency exchange that equalizes the cost of a fixed representative basket of goods and services in the home country.

Case Studies

There are 48 countries in Europe, therefore, clearly the case studies included in this section only represent a sampling from this total. The authors for each case study discuss the current state of the EHR in their country, nursing's involvement in these initiatives, and health policy developments relevant to these endeavors. Combined, these case studies provide excellent contrasts and show how their unique historical backgrounds shape current nursing practice today. Fortunately, two case studies from the "Latin countries," Italy and Spain, are included. These countries have had difficulty reporting in the past because of the barrier of having to report in English. Additionally, Central and Eastern Europe are represented, adding even more breadth to this current state overview.

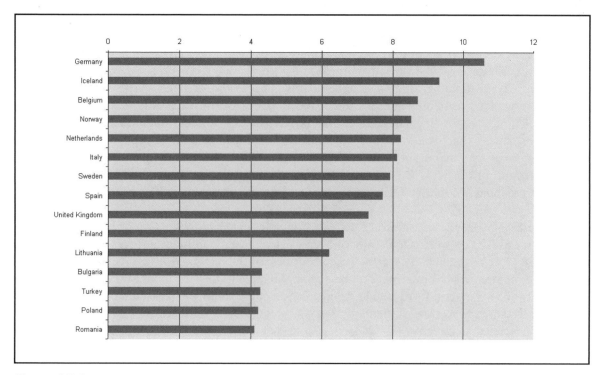

Figure 27-2. *Health expenditures for European and Eastern European countries.*

Table 27-1. Data from WHO 2000–2001[3]

	Life expectancy							
	Health expend. in % of GDP	Population in 1,000	GDP per capita PPP*	Women	Men	LOS† Acute hospital	Number of nurses per 100,000[4]	Number of physicians per 100,000
Germany	10.6	82'349.9	26'427.9	80.8	74.8	10.7	973	358
Iceland	9.3	285.1	29'294.3	81.4	77.6		898	336
Belgium	8.7	10'26.4	27'745.9	81.4	75.1	8.7		414
Norway	8.5	4'513.8	36'678.5	81.5	76.2	6.0	2'055	470
Netherlands	8.2	16'043.7	29'456.0	80.6	75.5	7.7	1'328	322
Italy	8.1	57'844.0	26'3457.4	82.9	76.7	7.1		567
Sweden	7.9	8'896.0	26'156.8	82.1	77.5	5.5	975	
Spain	7.7	40'265.5	21'577.4	82.9	75.6	8	367	329
United Kingdom	7.3	59'755.7	25'894.2	79.7	75.0	5.0		
Ireland	7.2	3'838.9	30'088.4	78.5	73.0	6.5	1'676	249
Finland	6.6	5'188.0	26'587.3	81.5	74.6	4.3	2'166	307
Lithuania	6.2	3'477.8	8'539.0	77.9	67.6	8.3	775	380
Bulgaria	4.3	7'951.6	6'366.0	75.3	68.2	10.7	362	337
Turkey	4.3	67'612.2	5'901.1	72.5	66.8	5.4	240	127
Poland	4.2	38'641.0	9'843.7	78.0	69.7	9.3		226
Romania	4.1	22'408.4	6'973.8	74.2	67.0	8.9	418	189

* GDP per capita at current prices and current PPP

† LOS Length of stay

EHR in Europe

Each country is making an effort to integrate the EHR into the health care system. EHR implementations are mostly done for medical purposes and less for nursing. Nurses still have to find their place in this implementation process and take the lead on behalf of nursing implementation concerns. At the EU (European Union) level, a number of projects aim to explore how public authorities may use EHRs for public health purposes, e.g., collecting data on the health status of the population.[5] To fulfill this goal, the use of standards is necessary. For many years, European countries have organized to build standards under the auspices of the CEN, the French acronym for European Committee for Standardization, and TC251, is the technical committee responsible for health informatics. Many standards and beta standards are available. With regards to the development of the EHR, two main standards are under development: HISA (Health care information system architecture pre ENV 12967)[6] and EHR (Electronic health care record ENV13606 1to4).[7-10] Many other standards could be taken into account when developing an EHR but will not be cited here.

The HISA[6] prestandard establishes general principles for the architecture of health care information systems (IS), as well as the scope of a set of Healthcare Common Services, provided by the middleware layer of the health care IS. These services are fundamental in any generic IS for supporting the requirements of information management related to the treatment of the subject of care.

EHR 13606[7-10] is a multipart standard and consists of the following parts, under the general title *Electronic Healthcare Record Communication:*

- Part 1: Extended architecture
- Part 2: Domain term list
- Part 3: Distribution rules
- Part 4: Messages for the exchange of information

International standards, e.g., ISO and HL7, which may not readily be compared with the CEN standards, are also needed to enhance the communication capacities. Some of those standards are well-known by the developers, some are not; but the implementations rarely take into account the recommendation made in the standards' documentation. This is a subject of discussion, especially in Europe when initiating automatic translations, language—such language always being a barrier to information sharing.

The EU stimulates joint strategies and initiatives with other health-related policy areas. These are important tools to ensure that health concerns are being properly addressed from the beginning. Such joint approaches have been developed, e.g., on health and the environment, health and social policy, health "telematics," research on life sciences, and health policy or health and pharmaceutical policy.[11]

Combined, these case studies paint an amazing and powerful picture of the depth and duration of these countries' nursing leaders efforts to use IT to promote improvements in health care services and patient outcomes. These nurse leaders contributions have directly resulted in moving the industry and profession forward on achieving standard health information that will support an EHR, nursing science and practice, and optimum patient care.

References

1. Bologna Declaration. Convened in Bologna, Spain, June 19, 1999. Available at: http://www.crue.org/decbolognaingles.htm. Accessed October 17, 2005

2. Europe: *Wikipédia L'encyclopedie libre.* Available at: http://fr.wikipedia.org/wiki/Europe. Accessed July 2, 2005.

3. UNECE Statistical Division and Health for All database, 6.15 *Total health expenditure as a percentage of GDP, 2000* WHO Regional Office for Europe. Available at: http://www.unece.org/stats/trends/register.htm. Accessed July 2, 2005.

4. European Health for all Database. WHO Regional Office for Europe. Available at: http://www.hfadb.who.dk/hfa/. Accessed July 2, 2005.

5. European Programmes. Available at: http://europa.eu.int/information_society/qualif/health/index_en.htm. Accessed July 5, 2005.

6. Medical Informatics Healthcare Information System Architecture Part 1 (HISA) Healthcare Middleware Layer CEN/TC251/N97-24. Final Draft 2. prENV 12967-1:1997.

7. Health informatics - Electronic healthcare record communication - Part 1: Extended architecture CEN prENV 13606-1:2000.

8. Health informatics - Electronic healthcare record communication - Part 2: Domain term list CEN ENV 13606-2:2000.

9. Health informatics - Electronic healthcare record communication - Part 3: Distribution rules CEN ENV 13606-3:2000.

10. Health informatics - Electronic healthcare record communication - Part 4: Messages for the exchange of information CEN ENV 13606-4:2000.

11. Available at: http://www.europa.eu.int/comm/health/ph_overview/other_policies/joint_action_en.htm. Accessed May 6, 2005.

Case Study 27A

Clinical Informatics for Quality of Care and Patient Safety: The Icelandic Garden

Asta Thoroddsen, MSc, RN; Vilborg Ingólfsdóttir, BScN, MPH; and Maria Heimisdóttir, MD, PhD, MBA

Preparing the Soil

Infertile soil may yield a lush garden when given time, nurturing, and care. Careful tilling, appropriate moisture, and the right minerals can create hospitable ground for even the most delicate plants to grow and blossom. This hypothetical scene depicts the elements that help facilitate growth, much like the elements that facilitated the changes in health care that occurred in Iceland in the 1970s: a series of developments occurred that affected health care, particularly nursing, for years to come.

First, the University of Iceland launched a baccalaureate degree program in nursing in 1973. Prior to that time, only diploma schools offered nursing education. Achieving academic status was a major boost toward nursing flourishing as a profession.

Second, the Health Service Act transferred the responsibility for all nursing care to the nursing profession.[1] This transfer of responsibility, and the resulting power and greater autonomy on the part of nurses to determine professional decisions, led to greater expectations both within and outside the profession and increased the independence of nurses. This empowerment, in turn, gradually led to changes in the profession itself, as nurses called for more educational opportunities and improved documentation of care for evaluation, quality control, and research. The patient was brought into focus.

In the 1970s, primary health care centers were established throughout Iceland. In one of these centers in 1976, a problem-oriented medical record (POMR) system for primary care—*The Egilsstadir System*—was developed in 1976.[2] It was based on Laurence Weed's theories, in which patients and their problems are the focus of care.[3] Although the system did not address nursing, it was adopted by most centers in the country. The response was generally favorable; the system was thought to improve quality of care, support teaching and served as a useful source of information for research and report preparation.[2]

Seeding

By the 1980s, the time had come for some seeding based on the groundwork laid in the 1970s. In 1986, the Directorate of Health (DOH) established a consultant team on documentation in nursing (CTDN) in response to a proposal by directors of nursing in health care centers. The goal was to create a nursing information system that would be useful for clinical practice, quality assurance, promotion of nursing research, and policy-making at a national level.[4] Vilborg Ingólfsdóttir, chief nursing information officer at the DOH, was selected as chair. Participation was on a voluntary basis; many of the nurses working on the team have since become Iceland's nursing informatics (NI) experts.

The team identified the nursing process as a common conceptual framework and began working on the basis for systematic nursing care, the nursing assessment. They moved to identify a nursing diagnosis classification system that would serve to coordinate the documentation of nursing care. The North American Nursing Diagnosis Association (NANDA) classification system was chosen as it was widely recognized and its coding system was, at the time, found to be applicable for computerized records. In 1991 the first handbook with a tool for assessing patients' needs, based on Marjory Gordon's Functional Health Patterns (FHP) and 1997 NANDA nursing diagnoses, was published in Icelandic.

Over time, consensus was reached on using the FHP and the NANDA diagnoses nationwide. Several factors played a role in this accomplishment. Although the initiative originated with nursing directors themselves, the project was run by the DOH, which gave it a heightened status and momentum. The nurses involved were deeply engaged and were credible leaders in the eyes of their colleagues. The project was intensely publicized to nurses in the workplace, and nursing programs included preliminary translations of the FHP and NANDA in their curricula.

The implementation effort met some resistance, however, not the least in relation to the translation. The criticism centered on lack of cultural sensitivity, awkward wording, detachment from clinical nursing, and stereotyping patients. Some also found the translated diagnoses inflexible and difficult to learn.[5] Nevertheless, a retrospective audit of 1,103 charts from 1993 to 1994 showed that 58.5 percent of all nursing diagnoses were documented according to NANDA.[6]

At this time, nursing documentation was still paper-based. However, because standardized terminologies are a prerequisite for capturing and retrieving clinical data from an electronic health record (EHR), the dissemination of NANDA later bore fruit.

Moreover, although CTDN started out as a nursing documentation effort, it helped health authorities and nursing leaders gradually realize the importance of creating an interdisciplinary EHR where all relevant patient data could be collected and used.

Weeding

In 1991, four computerized health records systems were in use in Iceland: the Egilsstadir System POMR launched in 1976; Medicus, a PC DOS, Clipper dBase system established in 1985; Starri, a COSTAR based (MUMPS) system developed in 1989; and Hippocrates, an Apple Macintosh system established in 1991.[7] All were pioneered by physicians, but none addressed nursing specifically. The size of the Icelandic market clearly did not allow for four competing systems and, although each of them had their strong points, their growth and development were severely limited. Weeding became necessary. Five owners of the old systems merged into a new software company, Gagnalind, in 1992.

The Garden Grows

Several types of plants sprouted but grew at different rates. The Ministry of Health and Gagnalind signed a contract in 1993 to develop an EHR—the SAGA system—for the eighty primary health care centers in Iceland. The goal was to build a common user-oriented, integrated system that supported patient-focused care, patient safety, and quality of care. Gagnalind created a task force of physicians and representatives from the two national nurses associations to work on development of the system.

They emphasized work-flow analysis and gathered information through interviews with users, site visits, and videotaping of care processes. Patients were also considered users, hence they were included in the data collection. Nursing care was addressed from the outset and integrated into the health record.

In 1996 the CTDN and Gagnalind received a grant from the Icelandic Research Council for further development of nursing documentation in SAGA. The grant enabled Gagnalind to hire a project manager, Asta Thoroddsen, CTDN member and an assistant professor in nursing at the University of Iceland. The aim was to create interest in the project and eagerness to start using SAGA. Motivated users from a variety of settings, such as home care, school nursing, well-baby care, emergency medicine, and psychiatric nursing, were considered necessary participants for pilot testing. The first pilots took place in 1996; implementation in primary health care centers and hospitals commenced in 1997.

Currently, all but two health care centers use SAGA. A few hospitals and several physicians in private practice also use the system. SAGA, now owned by TM software, is in continuous development.

The Importance of Natural Fertilizer

All gardening and growth of the plants require attention and fertilizer or booster for growth. Several projects had a great impact on the development of NI and supported the role of nurses in the future world of informatics. Policy, practice, education, and research were the natural fertilizers. In 1996, the Minister of Health delegated maintenance and coordination of documentation in all nursing care to the CTDN. The team then incorporated representatives of the various nursing services and educational programs and policy.

In 1997, the Icelandic government provided a clear boost to the development and use of information technology (IT). The government promulgated a policy on the use of IT in health care. The main objectives were to increase the quality and efficiency of services, to ensure data protection and personal privacy, and to improve access to health care and communication between the public and the health sector. The policy defined several means by which to reach the objectives: a "healthnet" interlinking all places of health care, further development of an integrated EHR, and "telehealth."

At this time, the SAGA system was ready for pilot and required a standardized language for nursing treatments and interventions. CTDN chose the Nursing Interventions Classification (NIC) project language vocabulary developed at the University of Iowa, and translated its labels and definitions into Icelandic. A feasibility study subsequently confirmed NIC's applicability in Iceland. The results were used to further improve the translation.[10]

The DOH holds the user licenses for NANDA and NIC. Licensing for the Nursing Outcomes Classification is under way. These classification systems thus hold the same status as those used for similar purposes by other professions, such as the ICD-10 and Nordic Classification of Surgical Procedures. The substantial support of health authorities and the enthusiasm of the CTDN and its user contacts made the growth of the terminologies easier than expected.

Unfortunately, the pace of these initiatives has been slower than expected. A new government IT policy was issued in 2004, reemphasizing the healthnet (to be operational in 2005) and system-wide implementation of an EHR.[8,9]

Pruning

Proper pruning is required to maintain healthy plants. The paper version of NANDA turned out to be unsuitable for use in an EHR. Although the labels and definitions could be used, as well as the codes for the diagnoses, the defining characteristics and the etiologies were too broad and lacked terms to describe signs and symptoms of specific patient populations, e.g., neonates. Because they needed considerable work (these items are still not coded by NANDA), internal codes were developed and maintained within SAGA. Many inconsistencies within NANDA were discovered, e.g. different terms were used for the same concept, and the long sentences and lists used to describe a defining characteristic were inapplicable.

The CTDN and Gagnalind also participated in the Telenurse project from 1996 to 1999. The goal was to promote consensus in Europe on the use of the International Classification of Clinical Nursing Practice (ICNP).

Translation of the alpha version of ICNP was completed in October 1996 and presented widely in Iceland. A prototype to demonstrate the use of ICNP was developed in SAGA and tested in Icelandic hospitals.[11] This early work may provide additional insight into adapting nursing vocabularies for the EHR.

Nurturing

All gardens require nurturing. Standardized languages of nursing care have long been nurtured in teaching and nursing care plans. This is part of the Icelandic nursing profession's common ground via their homogeneous education. Until recently, standardized languages were not addressed to the same extent in the education of other health professionals. In 2003, the DOH reminded health science educational programs nationwide to increase their emphasis on clinical coding systems. DOH stressed the importance of quality documentation by health professionals and the role of the programs in preparing students to take on that responsibility. The universities were already equipped with a practical teaching tool as each had been granted a user license to the SAGA system.

The DOH is responsible by law for the collection, processing, and dissemination of health statistics in Iceland. The directorate then issued a mandate for a (nursing) minimum data set (MDS) in health services in 1997. The MDS contains information on health institution (identification number, service area/specialty, and physician/nurse responsible for the patient treatment); patient (ID number, gender, age, nationality, residence, marital status); admission and discharge (date, time, where from, where to, etc.); diagnoses (ICD-10, NANDA); treatment (NCSP, NIC), and waiting lists. Nursing elements, such as nurse ID number (active since 2004), nursing assessment, nursing diagnoses, and interventions, were first presented in a 2001 edition of the MDS.[12]

A set of general, minimum requirements for the EHR, based on the IT policy from 1997 and the MDS mandate, were issued by the MOH in 2001.[13] The requirements address hardware and software standards, user interface, data and databases, coding, security issues, content, and communication standards.

Following the MDS mandate, a nursing working group was appointed at Landspitali University Hospital (LUH) to develop a new hospital policy on nursing documentation. LUH serves as Iceland's sole tertiary care center and university hospital but is also the community hospital of Reykjavik. The new policy was implemented in 2002 and reflected traditions and elements important in the information age, as well as the new governmental mandate and law on patients' rights. It was also intended to advance nursing as a profession. The implementation of the policy was followed in 2003 by a year-long educational initiative on nursing documentation (paper and electronic). Comparative studies before and after the initiative revealed great improvements in documentation in general, including the use of nursing classifications.

While SAGA is being further developed, LUH has implemented a small, homegrown software application to prepare nursing care plans with NANDA and NIC. Although this system is clearly a temporary solution, it gives nurses time to get accustomed to electronic documentation based on classifications. Furthermore, to prepare for translation and implementation of nursing outcomes in clinical practice, pilot projects and studies are being conducted.[14] Moreover, several projects in smaller health institutions have served as natural fertilizers for the garden of clinical informatics by preparing the institutions for IT development in one form or another.

Beginning in 2000, with a grant from Nordplus, the faculties of nursing at the University of Iceland, Örebro University in Sweden, University of Oslo, Norway, and the University of Iowa, Iowa City, U.S., have collaborated on a nursing and health informatics course. This initiative won the Education Technology Award in 2001, given by Sigma Theta Tau International for international NI education collaboration for computer-based professional education.

In fall 2004, an interdisciplinary health informatics master's program was launched at the University of Iceland in close collaboration with the health informatics program at the University of Iowa. This brings together five faculties: engineering, medicine, nursing, pharmacy, and social sciences.

Expansion of the Garden

The extensive work described here laid the ground for expansion of the informatics garden, including further development at LUH. Formed in 1999 as the product of two successive mergers, LUH combined three hospitals, each with its own organizational culture, infrastructure, and information systems. Each hospital had acquired some clinical applications, mostly for support services, such as labs and imaging services. Other clinical data were stored in unstructured format, either on paper or in first-generation EHRs (some homegrown) resembling word processors rather than true information systems. Computerized data existed as islands because systems were not integrated. A common patient administration system was in place, but this legacy application was faltering and no longer up-to-date with demands. In summary, the organization was starving for electronic data to support its clinical services, research, teaching, and administration. The lack of structured clinical data became even more obvious with the introduction of the Diagnostic Related Groups (DRGs) system in 2002. Swift action was needed.

In the spring of 2003, the executive committee of LUH appointed an interdisciplinary committee to tackle the situation. The nature of the group led to a meeting of the minds by the various professions, allowing them to learn from each other. The group (led by a physician/epidemiologist, along with two other MDs, two RNs, and one computer scientist) immediately identified three principles as the basis of the project. In time, these principles became LUH's vision for its EHR.

First, the EHR should be patient-centered, bringing the patient, rather than the caregivers or the organization, to the forefront. Thus, all clinical data, whether a lab result or a written consultation, should be accessible within a single-user interface, or what soon was dubbed "the face" of the EHR. Second, this aim should be realized via a modular approach, making use of "best of breed" applications, each designed to support certain areas of the care process (e.g., surgery or inpatient wards), rather than aiming for a single hospital-wide system. This approach requires standard interfaces of all modules but it also provides the organization with the ability to select the optimal tool for each task and to protect its investment by replacing one module at a time without disrupting the functional entity. The third dictum was that the task of building an EHR is in fact without an end. There is no such thing as a complete EHR; there is always room for improvement, and the needs of patients and users are ever-changing. The EHR must evolve with them.

Given these principles and the informatics landscape of the organization, two tasks were identified as top priority. First, all three hospital campuses had to agree on a common basic EHR, the future face of the integrated EHR. The SAGA system, long in use on one campus, was chosen for this role and is being further developed for hospital use. Second, in order to maximize the utilization of data and leverage the value offered by the systems already in place, a major integration effort was launched in which, one by one, specialized modules were integrated with SAGA.

Thirty years have passed. The pioneer work done at a remote health center in the 1970s tilled the ground for the budding garden just starting to bloom and bear fruit. Research endeavors abound and harmony has been reached between policy, practice, and education. Soon it will be time to harvest—harvest data, preserve the information, and create new knowledge in the field of health informatics.

References

1. *Lög um heilbrigðispjónustu.* [Health Service Act]. No.57/1978; No. 97/1990.

2. Sigurdsson G, Einarsson I, Josafatsson JI, et al. A medical record and information system for primary health care in Iceland: the Egilsstadir project. *Scand J Prim Health Care.* 1984;2:159-161.

3. Weed LL. Medical records that guide and teach. *MD Comput,* 1993;10(2):100-114.

4. Directorate of Health. *Skráning hjúkrunar—handbók* [Nursing Documentation Handbook]. Reykjavík: Directorate of Health; 1991.

5. Thoroddsen Á. ed. *Skráning hjúkrunar—handbók* [Nursing Documentation: Handbook]. Reykjavík: Directorate of Health in Iceland; 1997.

6. Thoroddsen Á, og Hrund Sch. Thorsteinsson. Nursing taxonomy across the Atlantic Ocean: congruence between nurses' charting and the NANDA taxonomy. *J Adv Nurs,* 2002;37(4):372-381.

7. Sigurdur Örn Hektorsson. *The Icelandic success, SAGA.* Reykjavík: Directorate of Health in Iceland; 1996.

8. Ministry of Health. *Stefnumótun í upplysingamálum innan heilbrigðis-kerfisins* [Policy on information technology within health care.] Reykjavik: Ministry of Health; 1997.

9. Ministry of Health. *Auðlindir í allra págu. Stefnumótun í upplysingamálum* [Resources for the Benefit of All: Policy on Information Technology]. Reykjavík: Ministry of Health; 2004.

10. Thoroddsen Á. Applicability of the nursing intervention classifications (NIC) to describe nursing. *Scand J Caring Sci.* 2005;19:128-139.

11. Thoroddsen Á, Víglundsson TI. *Feasibility Study for ICNP and NMDS incorporation in EDDA.* Telenurse: Project No. HC1113, Deliverable: D.04.09. Telematics for Health Care European Commission DGXIII. 1997.

12. Sigríður Haraldsdóttir. *Lágmarksskráning vistunarupplysinga á sjúkrahúsum* [Minimum Data Set in Hospitals]. Reykjavík: Directorate of Health; 2001.

13. Ministry of Health. *Almenn kröfulysing fyrir rafræna sjúkraskrá* [General Requirements for an Electronic Health Record]. Reykjavík: Ministry of Health; 2001.

14. Gudmundsdottir E, Delaney C, Thoroddsen A, Karlsson T. Translation and validation of the nursing outcomes classification labels and definitions for acute care nursing in Iceland. *J Adv Nurs.* 2004;46(3):292-302.

Case Study 27B

Finland's National Health Project and the EHR

Pirkko Kouri, MNSc, PHN; Kaija Saranto, PhD; Kristina Häyrinen, MSc;
Jari Porrasmaa, MSc; Jorma Komulainen, MD; and Martti Kansanen, PhD, MD

The Structure of the Finnish Health Care System

The population of Finland is 5.3 million. Its welfare state is a combination of social services and health care work with health care services funded mainly from tax revenues. Integration between these fields needs strengthening, however, to clarify division of tasks and to avoid duplicating services. The responsibility for organizing health care services lies with the local authorities, i.e., municipalities across the country. These can either provide primary health care services independently or form joint municipal boards with neighboring municipalities and then set up joint health centers. They can also buy health care services from other municipalities or from the private sector. Municipalities are also responsible for organizing specialist medical care for their residents. In addition, hospital districts organize and provide specialist medical services for the populations in their areas. Public health is supplemented by private health care services, which are primarily concentrated in the larger municipalities. Further, there are some private hospitals in Finland.[1] At the end of 2003, private health services employed 27,000 people. At the beginning of 2004, there were 39 different registered professions in the field of health care.[2] Table 27B-1 represents the main occupational groups in the public sector.[3]

The public (first) sector forms the main basis for health care, and the private (second) sector supplements it. The role of the third sector, volunteerism, is to complement public and private health care services, too. Volunteer roles in Finland comprise a variety of activities, e.g., unpaid voluntary work; visiting friends; voluntary rescue services; support person services; providing first aid; hosting youth, cultural, and sports events; and common neighborly help. Voluntary work is widely accepted locally, regionally, nationally, and even internationally. Moreover, businesses are increasingly taking the third sector into account by giving financial support or use of facilities, e.g., hosting health education seminars; some researchers have started to speak about societal responsibility of businesses under corporate citizenship. In the future, as the costs of health care services grow, it is crucial to take into account the meaning of volunteerism and citizen empowerment.[4,5]

For more than thirty years, the main strategic goals of the Ministry of Social Affairs and Health (MSAH) have been promoting health and functional capacity; making work more attractive; preventing and alleviating social exclusion; and guaranteeing functional services and reasonable income security. During the past decade, an interest in building up an operational network for health services in Finland emerged. In 2001, the Council of State initiated a national project to ensure the future of Finnish health care. Based on the health-related needs of the population, the aim of the project is to ensure the availability, quality, and sufficiency of care throughout the country, irrespective of the residents' economic abilities. To reach this goal, reform of the functions and structures of the health care system will be required.

One part of the national health project is development of a national electronic health record (EHR). In Finland, the paper-based patient record has evolved in the form of longitudinal (continuing) content. In hospitals, different health care professionals, e.g., physicians, nurses, physiotherapists, and social workers, have used the same record for several decades. Over the years, this mutual patient record led to more and more multidisciplinary work. An EHR is needed to better support such multidisciplinary communication and cooperation in health care. Ideally it should also tie together data from the private, social, and volunteer sectors. This goal has been acknowledged at the national level. Because the social sector has its own national project, i.e., the Development Project for Social Services in Finland (2003 to 2007),[6] cooperation between the health and social sector should increase in the future. This case study will focus on how the Finnish EHR is being developed and used to improve health services.

Table 27B-1. Employees by Occupational Group in the Finnish Public Sector[3]

Number of employees	1995	2000	2002	2003
Medical doctors	9,650	10,940	11,030	11,290
/10,000 inhabitants	18.9	21.1	21.2	21.6
Dentists	2,180	2,320	2,380	2,410
/10,000 inhabitants	4.3	4.5	4.6	4.6
Social workers	4,300	4,500	4,800	4,970
/10,000 inhabitants	8.4	8.7	9.2	9.5
Nurses	21,900	27,800	31,800	34,400
/10,000 inhabitants	42.8	53.7	61.0	64.1
Social work instructors	4,000	5,100	5,600	6,480
/10,000 inhabitants	7.8	9.9	10.8	12.4
Practical nurses	21,800	24,600	28,200	30,500
/10,000 inhabitants	42.6	47.5	54.2	58.4
Assistant nurses and hospital ward assistants	21,000	16,600	14,500	12,300
/10,000 inhabitants	41.0	32.1	27.9	25.4
Home care assistants	14,400	14,500	13,800	12,300
/10,000 overs-75s	481	426	385	334
Pre-primary education teaching professionals	8,500	10,100	10,600	10,640
/10,000 children aged 1–6	217	279	304	310
Childminders and kindergarten assistants	15,500	17,500	17,450	17,600
/10,000 children aged 1–6	395	482	501	512
Private childminders	17,700	17,500	16,100	15,550
/10,000 children aged 1–6	452	481	463	453

The Evolution of Patient Records

The history of patient care documentation is long. Documentation has evolved from physician's notes into a multidisciplinary paper record, following the changes in the health service system. As more health care practitioners took part in patient care, the need for collecting data from these different professionals grew. In response, the different professional groups developed their own forms for documenting care. The lack of unified documentation led to proposals for a unified national manual patient record (MPR). Both the specialized medical care[7] and primary health care[8] sectors formed their own MPRs and used them for more than thirty years. The structure of MPRs consists of three levels (see Figure 27B-1).[7] The first level is an index that summarizes the patient's risk factors and diseases. The second level summarizes care episodes by different specialists. It includes information about planning, executing, and assigning patient care. The third level includes all patient care data, e.g. nursing documentation, medication, laboratory test results, and radiology imaging reports. The summary of care episode refers to aggregated information from the third level. The patient record continues to act as a tool for setting objectives, planning patient care, delivering care, and assessing outcomes.

The first EHR system, Finstar, was introduced in 1982, and is still in use today. In primary care, 93.6 percent of health centers, 62 percent of hospitals, and 82 percent of private sector organizations used EHRs in 2003.[9] However, over the years, a number of different software applications have been built, which have developed in heterogeneous ways. Moreover, there are different versions of the same software application used in various organizations. Most of the current EHR applications are only for storing the paper form in the computer system. Additionally, they are passive, inflexible, and do not automatically support education, statistics, quality assessment, health care management, or continuity of care. Furthermore, the develop-

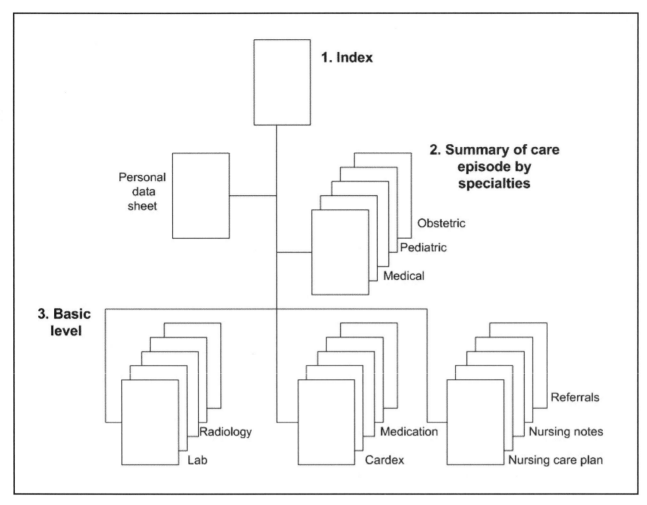

Figure 27B-1. *The three levels in the structure of MPRs.*

ment of the EHR systems has taken place under the control of commercial software producers and has been directed only toward immediate practical solutions.[10]

The nursing care plan is usually a part of the EHR systems. In the 1990s, nurses were active in developing electronic nursing documentation. The application was separate from the electronic hospital information system and was used only by nurses. The nursing care plan, using an application named Florence, followed the nursing process model as a structure, and the Swedish VIPS (this acronym stands for, in Swedish, well-being integrity prevention, and safety) model[11] was used as a standard. Despite the positive attitude of the nursing facilities toward the adoption of this software, it was used in few organizations. Thus, the vendor did not continue to maintain the software after the year 2000.

The Finnish Strategy Toward a Modern EHR

According to the Government Decision in Principle of April 11, 2002, on Securing the Future of Health Care, a national EHR will be introduced by the end of 2007. The MSAH has set up a working group to steer the introduction of EHR documents. One of the tasks is to create a strategy for promoting the introduction of structurally and functionally compatible information systems within various health care organizations. The goal is that the most essential patient information in regard to the provision and monitoring of care will be recorded in a uniform electronic form and that the information can be used with the patient's consent by different health care organizations. The EHR project includes many subprojects (see Figure 27B-2)[13] that address different issues, e.g. the core data elements, open interfaces, data security, document metadata, national code, terminology server, architecture, and documentation of nursing care. The different actors, e.g., the National Research and Development Center for Welfare and Health, the Association of Finnish Local

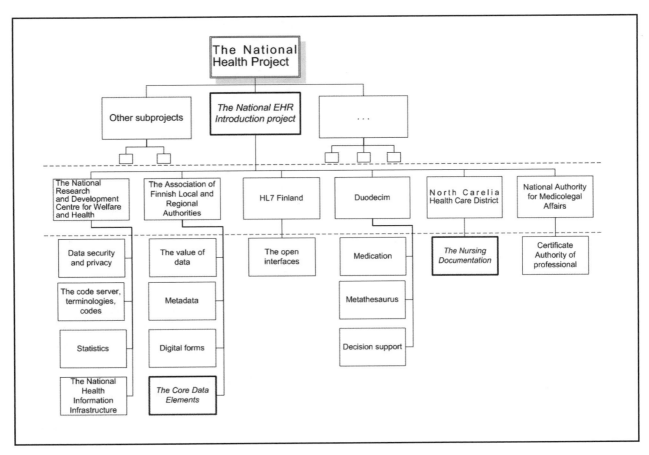

Figure 27B-2. *Subprojects within the EHR project.*

and Regional Authorities, HL7 Finland, Duodecim, the North Carelia Health Care District, and the National Authority for Medicolegal Affairs, are responsible for various tasks. The different subprojects are coordinated, and the results of subprojects will be crossutilized in other projects.[12]

It is assumed, in addition, that the EHR system will produce the information required by the access monitoring system electronically, as required by a National Research and Development Centre for Welfare and Health project on statistical data transfer. In the future, the goal is to extend the data transfer to all national data collected via the basic system (a standardized EHR).

The Role of Nurses in EHR Development

As the biggest group of health professionals, nurses have been involved in the national EHR development work in many ways. At the national level, nurses have networked under the auspices of the MSAH and the Finnish Nurses' Association. They also have a nursing representative in the EHR implementation working group of MSAH. MSAH has organized seminars and meetings to inform and involve directors of nursing in the national development of the EHR. The Finnish Nurses' Association has also organized workshops as well as an international symposium to share knowledge about nursing classifications and terminologies. The association has also published a guide book for electronic nursing documentation. All of these activities are critical in reaching the goal of national developmental work.

In the North Carelia Health District, electronic documentation development has a long history, and nursing documentation there is based on standardized terminology and the nursing process model. The Finnish translation of the Clinical Care Classification (CCC, formerly the Home Health Care Classification) has been used since 2001. The use of CCC started with the use of care components in nursing referrals and discharge summaries between primary and specialized health care.[14]

In the nursing documentation development project, the classifications for nursing diagnosis and interventions have been implemented and tested in an EHR system and also used for nursing documentation. The results have been rewarding, and the electronic model for care planning and daily notes is highly appreciated by the nurses.[15] Educating nurses to use a standardized terminology has also been a part of the nursing documentation project. In 2004, an outstanding sign of the progress toward a national EHR was reaching consensus on the data requirements, including the nursing minimum data set, i.e., diagnoses, interventions, outcomes, and nursing intensity. By spring 2005, a nationwide terminology project began to achieve the objectives of a nursing minimum data set. The ultimate goal is to implement a unified nursing language system within the Finnish EHR.

The Basis of Secure Health Care Services in the Information Society

Today, health care is strictly regulated, both externally through legislation and internally by the practitioners themselves via ethical guidelines and professional codes of conduct (see Figure 27B-3). Equity as a part of patients' rights has been considered a central objective in the Finnish health policy during recent decades. The Constitution of Finland (Act 731/1999) is the legislation under which important issues related to basic human rights in the information society are described. The legislation follows international development on these issues and adapts them into national laws. One of the most important norms is the EU Directive 95/46/EC, also known as the "The Data Protection Directive." Its objectives are to protect individual health care data and to ensure the free movement of such data.[16]

As the health care sector enters the era of knowledge management, it must have security as the foundation of the transition. With secure practices based on the law and seeking to avoid or mitigate the effects of these risks, e.g., patient data misuse, health care organizations can ensure that health-related knowledge is attained, stored, distributed, used, destroyed, and restored securely. The challenge in creating ethical guidelines for systems of health informatics is connected to the multiprofessional teams involved. The ethical principles relevant in the context of health informatics are the following: justice, efficiency, autonomy and respect for privacy and avoiding causing harm toward others. The right to privacy means that everyone's privacy is guaranteed. In Finland, the Personal Data File Act came into force in 1988 as the first national law concerning data protection and best data processing practices. In 1999, the Personal Data Act was

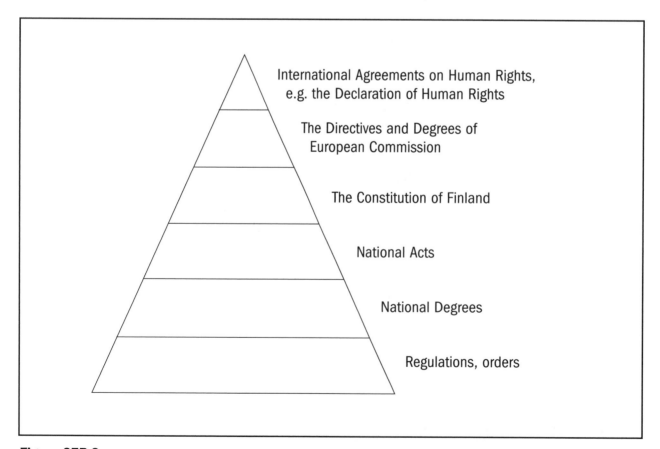

Figure 27B-3. *Hierarchy of legislation and norms in Finland.*

introduced. This act accommodates the constitutional reform and the EU Data Protection Directive (1995) and Data Protection Act (2003), both of which aim to protect personal data and the free movement of such data. All those using personal health data must be able to show a legitimate purpose for collecting and processing such data. The access to personal health data by legitimate users requires the explicit informed consent of the data subject. Furthermore, the patient/customer should have the right to participate in the design of the information and communication technology systems in health care, and appropriate procedures for achieving this must be developed.[17]

Summary

A national EHR system is a very demanding objective that includes several risks. However, the atmosphere toward the developmental work in Finland is very positive. The software vendors, experts, authorities, and end users are working in networks toward implementing a national EHR system by 2007. As of spring 2005, the standardization of the data elements was in progress. This standardization means that each data element will be defined through terminologies, e.g., codes, classifications, nomenclatures, or vocabularies. All accepted terminologies will be delivered through a national code server. The goal is to enhance the transfer of data between health care providers, to manage resources, and to maintain the quality of care. For health authorities and professionals, this standardization also yields advanced possibilities to collect comparable data at the national and international level. Electronic administration of patient consents, delivery of information, and production of log information concerning the use and transfer of patient data according to national recommendations are keys to successful EHR adoption.

References

1. The Ministry of Social Affairs and Health. *The National Project on Safeguarding the Future of Health Care Service.* Working Group Memorandum; 2002:3.

2. Kauppinen S, Niskanen T. *Private Provision of Social and Health Care Services* [summary in English]. The National Research and Development Centre for Welfare and Health (STAKES). Report 288. Helsinki;2005.

3. The National Research and Development Centre for Welfare and Health (STAKES). Facts about Finnish social welfare and health care 2005. Available at: http://www.stakes.info/files/pdf/Raportit/Facts_2005.pdf. Accessed March 12, 2005

4. Kaunismaa P. Transformations in associational life in the rural Finnish localities in 1990s. Paper presented at: ISTR Fourth International Conference; July 5–8, 2000; Dublin, Ireland. Available at: http://www.jhu.edu/~istr/conferences/dublin/abstracts/kaunismaa.html. Accessed March 12, 2005.

5. Zadek S. *The Civil Corporation. The New Economy of Corporate Citizenship.* London: Earthscan; 2001.

6. Sahala H. *Project Plan for Promoting the Use of Information Technology in Social Services* [in Finnish]. Stencils of the Ministry of Social Affairs and Health; 2005:1.

7. Sairaalaliitto. *Terveys ja Sairauskertomus Erikoissairaanhoidossa* [in Finnish]. Printel Oy; 1991.

8. Suomen K. Terveyskertomusjärjestelmä: Ohjekirja [in Finnish]. Suomen Kunnallisliitto: Helsinki ; 1982.

9. Kiviaho K, Winblad I, Reponen J. *The Information Systems which Support Health Care Processes in Finland: Survey and Use Analysis* [in Finnish]. Publications of the Network of Excellence Centers; August 2004.

10. Hartikainen K, Kuusisto-Niemi S, Lehtonen E. *Survey of Social and Health Care Information Systems 2001* [in Finnish]. Publications of the Network of Excellence Centers; January 2002.

11. Ehrenberg A, Ehnfors M, Thorell-Ekstrand I. Nursing documentation in patient records: experience of the use of the VIPS-model. *J Ad Nurs.* 1996; 24:853-867.12.

12. The Ministry of Social Affairs and Health. *Final Report of the Working Group Steering the Implementation of Electronic Patient Record Systems.* Working Group Memorandum; 2004:18.

13. Häyrinen K, Porrasmaa J, Komulainen J, Hartikainen K. *The Core Data Elements of EHR: Final Report* [in Finnish]. Publications of the Network of Excellence Centers; May 2004.

14. Ikonen H, Ensio A, Saranto K, Keskisärkkä P. The development of an electronic nursing referral system. In: Marin H, Marques E, Hovenga E, Goossen W, eds. *eHealth for all: Designing a Nursing Agenda for the Future.* Proceedings of the 8th International Congress on Nursing Informatics. Rio de Janeiro: Adis International Limited; 2003:716.

15. Ensio A, Saranto K. The Finnish classification of nursing interventions (FiCNi) – development and use in nursing. In: Clark J, ed. *Naming Nursing. Proceedings of the First ACENDIO Ireland/UK Conference.* Bern: Verlag Hans Huber; 2003:191-195.

16. Ylipartanen A. *Tietosuoja terveydenhuollossa: potilaan asema ja oikeudet henkilötietojen käsittelyssä* [in Finnish]. Helsinki: Tietosanoma; 2004:34.

17. The European Group on Ethics. The European Group on Ethics adopts for the first time an opinion on the ethical aspects of the information society. European Commission Secretariat-General. Directorate C. Secretariat of the European Group on Ethics in Science and New Technologies. 1999. Available at: http://europa.eu.int/comm/european_group_ethics/docs/cp13_en.pdf. Accessed March 11, 2005.

Case Study 27C

Transition to the Integrated EHR— Impact on Nursing Documentation in Norway

Anne Moen, PhD, RN; Torunn Wibe, MNSc, RN; Torun Vedal and Eva Edwin, MNSc, RN

Integrating appropriate solutions for representation of nursing practice into an electronic health record (EHR) will provide valuable clinical and strategic information resources that support care delivery and will reflect nurse-patient interactions. In Norway, different systems, conceptual structures, formats, and methods of documentation have been suggested to improve and ease nursing documentation. The national guidelines align with the problem-oriented nursing process,[1] as do the proposed national standards for a common information model to represent clinical practice in the EHR.[2]

At the same time, however, nursing documentation is viewed as time-consuming, lacking in comprehensiveness, and non-representative of the actual complexity of nursing practice.[3] Most studies, audits, and reviews of nursing documentation also point out problems related to incomplete and imprecise charting,[4,5] poor overview,[6] and lack of standards to ensure the documentation's consistency and comprehensiveness.[7]

Ongoing efforts to improve nursing documentation coincide with the introduction of EHRs to improve the quality and efficiency of health care services, and the newly introduced legal mandate to document planned and delivered care.[8] Design of any EHR calls for a formal, systemized representation of clinical practice. Introduction of this new technology also requires contextually sound implementation strategies.[9] Nursing documentation will be part of the EHR. However, that implementation should involve more than the straightforward transfer of current care plans, nurses' notes, and progress reports from a paper-based to a digital medium.

At the Ullevål University Hospital, there has been a long-time effort to improve nursing documentation, partly in the belief that this will ease the transition from paper-based to EHR-supported charting. This case study will present Ullevål's hospital-wide, endorsed approach to systematize nursing documentation, discuss experiences from the transition process, and share findings from repeated audits that indicate how nursing documentation fared during introduction of the EHR system.

Systematization of Nursing Documentation

Although there are different approaches to systematize documentation of assessment, problems, goals, resources and needs, interventions, and evaluations/reports, the most common information model for EHR integrated documentation is the problem-based nursing process.

In our hospital, the VIPS (acronym for Swedish spelling of well-being, integrity, prevention, and safety) approach was recommended to structure the documentation, improve paper-based nursing documentation, and prepare for EHR-integrated nursing documentation.[10] The VIPS model defines documentation components as (1) nursing history, (2) nursing status, (3) problem statement or nursing diagnosis, (4) nursing goal, (5) nursing intervention, (6) nursing outcome(s), and (7) nursing discharge note or transfer report. Keywords are provided to structure nursing history, nursing status, and nursing interventions.[7]

The structuring keywords of the VIPS model are more detailed than the components of the nursing process. The information is written as free text, which is a low-level standardization of documentation, but provides some structure. In transition to the EHR, general templates based on the VIPS keywords were introduced to structure the notes and to ease charting. Capitalizing on similarity to existing VIPS approaches allowed a smoother transition to EHR-integrated nursing documentation.[11]

The VIPS keywords provide structure to admission notes, shift reports, and discharge notes, with the information charted as free text.[12] To offer more support and ease charting, units have also started to systematize clinical pathways, i.e., commonly expected problems, goals, and interventions related to the common patients cared for in the unit. These pathways will become templates with standardized text in the EHR-integrated nursing care plan. This is a step toward standardized representations, which will be recommended for use in the institution as guidelines to ease charting of patient status, as outcome measurements, as standardized care plans, and as templates for information sharing.[13]

Documentation that started at the lower level of standardization is moving to a higher level following requests from health care providers for incorporation of standardized text. The standardized texts are largely local expressions. Some terms and concepts, however, were derived from the North American Nursing Diagnosis Association (NANDA),[14] the Nursing Interventions Classification (NIC) system,[15] and the Clinical Care Classification (CCC) system.[16] NANDA and CCC are available in Norwegian, and a NIC translation to Norwegian is in progress.

Implementation and Transition to EHR

To prepare for EHR integration and to deal with some of the nursing documentation problems, the choice of approach and level of standardization were important. To ease challenges, Ullevål chose an incremental transition toward EHR-integrated nursing documentation.[17]

The first unit began using EHR-integrated nursing notes in September 2001. The hospital continued adding units and expanding EHR functionality. As a result, the somatic sector now uses the EHR to chart all nursing notes. Figure 27C-1 shows the increasing use of EHR functionality for nursing documentation, as reported over a twelve-month period.

These measurements began being recorded when all units in the medical division were instructed to use the EHR as a requirement. The increased use can be viewed as a result of visible and articulate leader commitment, exemplified by stating clear expectations, challenging reluctance to use the EHR, and supporting staff in the transition.[12,17] User problems, e.g., time constraints or lack of computers, were eased by training courses and instruction made available to personnel on and off site. And as EHR-integrated notes accumulated, the positive experiences of improved access to information reduced the perceived barriers.

Improvements and Change in Nursing Documentation

Integrating nursing documentation in the EHR, starting with structured free text, and gradually incorporating standardized terms, required systematization and discussions about the current documentation practices. At Ullevål, this resulted in increased professional attention to nursing documentation and vigorous discussions of professional and ethical concerns about the documentation, including appropriateness, embedded

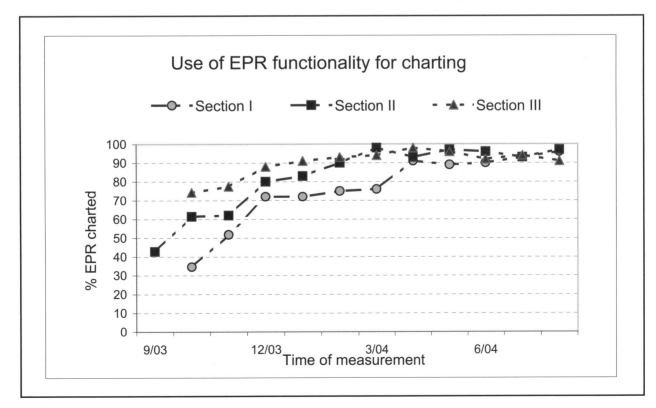

Figure 27C-1. *Increasing use of EHR functionality for nursing documentation, as reported over twelve months.*

assumptions, and potential bias. The discussions addressed, in particular, the interplay of a provider's professional accountability and his or her ability to express specific, subjective evaluation in efforts to individualize and personalize the documentation, as well as approaches to systematization and standardization.

Repeated audit of the nursing documentation since the EHR integration started shows some changes in the charted content. To assess and document whether the transition led to changes in the documentation—as a product—we audited a set of the nursing notes from different units using a customized assessment tool of selected indicators.[18] In the medical division, components of the nursing documentation were audited in 2003 and 2004. Figure 27C-2 shows findings from the audits.

This figure shows average findings from the audit of October 2003 (N = 74) and the audit of October 2003 (N = 53) admission notes. Value 2 indicates that information was fully charted, value 1 shows that information was partly charted, and value 0 indicates that the information was absent. The documentation was entered as free text, structured by a general template with keywords. The more explicit structure introduced by the template led to increased comprehensiveness, in terms of nurses carefully writing more information associated with more keywords. Because the EHR offered templates for structure as well as content of the documentation, some of the increase should be attributed to the template, and some should be credited to the EHR system. The templates can be perceived as guidelines or checklists that provide more structure and norms about what to chart. Questions related to the usability of current templates, the appropriateness and relevance of VIPS keywords per clinical speciality, the added documentation burdens from typing the free text notes into the EHR, and the potential to aggregate the charted information are important, but have not been fully answered yet.

Discussion

We have observed increasing computer literacy and EHR proficiency, and there are indications that informatics literacy develops as well when the nurses get hands-on experiences with new clinical information system tools. Requests for standard text and attempts to reuse information in the EHR system are examples of developing informatics literacy.

Taking time to systematize, evaluate, and modify well-known approaches has been important. Because the VIPS approach is similar to the problem-oriented nursing process, it is a familiar information model for nursing documentation.[10] Although started as a structuring exercise, the project is inspiring increased use

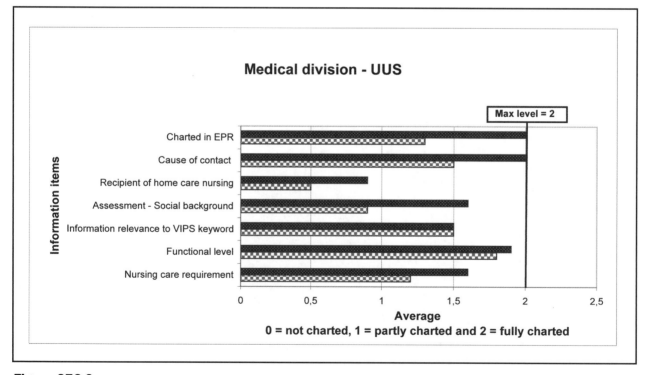

Figure 27C-2. *As audited in 2003 and 2004, components of the medical division's nursing documentation.*

of standardized texts. However, similar to most other efforts to improve nursing documentation, the chosen approach was developed as a stand-alone system aimed at providing comprehensive, coherent pictures of planned or provided nursing care. In an integrated EHR, redundancies and overlaps in the collaborating professions' documentation become very visible. Although introduction of an EHR system per se does not resolve such problems, it inspires an examination of the documentation practice that helps future approaches reflect a more interdisciplinary clinical practice.

Our experience so far indicates that selecting and incorporating predefined or standardized terms and concepts requires more thorough preparation in transition to an EHR. Although an EHR better supports use of standardized text, challenges in linguistic translation of terms and concepts and choosing expressions to reflect contextually bound, clinical practice have been brought to our attention. Concepts and terms in a classification system are not empty vessels, available and ready to be used, but have embedded assumptions, inscribed history, and politics, as well as embedded cultural values—all of which should be subject to careful deliberations.[19] The potential exists for improvements and eased information flow and interaction when the collaborating units use a similar approach to documentation. Common structure contributes to comprehensiveness and overview, eases reuse of charted information, and may facilitate follow-up and continuity of planned care. At the same time, there are issues of interpretation and "buying" embedded assumptions when labeling experiences, judgments, and evaluations with keywords.

The VIPS approach may be viewed as an alternative to using terms and concepts from classification systems to represent nursing content. Narrative representation and free-text entries in the nursing documentation are frequently seen as an underutilization of capabilities in informatics applications.[3] However, integrating templates and predefined text entries in clinical pathways, treatment protocols, or standardized care plans introduces structure and some standardization to documentation. Establishing coherent sets of templates and free text entries are labor-intensive but probably unavoidable to describe or streamline information content in transition to an EHR.

Audits and repeated reviews of nursing documentation facilitate systematic work to streamline information content and improve quality of the documentation. At Ullevål, repeated audits led to discussions and reflections about the documentation's coherence, comprehensiveness, and appropriateness. This should be an ongoing activity, preferably integrated as a quality improvement activity. In addition, such experiences will be important to harmonize and refine requirements and to consider levels of standardization in the EHR-integrated nursing documentation.

Summary

In this case study, we have shared experiences from our work to improve representation of nursing practice in a transition to EHR-integrated nursing documentation. Most reports of EHR introduction share experiences of implementing standardized terms and concepts from classification systems to represent nursing practice. Sometimes the improvements could have been more promising.[3,6] There are fewer reported approaches of lower-levels standardization, representing nursing practice and patient progress in an EHR system as free text. The experiences reported here show that the local processes to systematize nursing documentation are crucial. Our audits demonstrate changes in the comprehensiveness of the documentation. This may be credited with the further development of documentation practices, and the availability of general templates in the EHR system. Audits and accompanying discussions of representations of nursing practice contribute to improved representations of planned and offered care. In this regard, the experiences shared here point to further discussion and potential for synergies in efforts to structure nursing documentation and incorporate formalized terms and concepts from classification systems and terminologies.

Acknowledgement

We acknowledge the great contribution of Ms. Jorun Vego, RN, MNSc(s), past Director of Nursing, Medical Division, Ullevål University Hospital, and the commitment of Senior Nursing Leadership at Ullevål University Hospital to improve nursing documentation in the hospital. We also greatly appreciate editorial assistance from Ms. Kathryn Mølstad.

References

1. Mølstad K, Lyngstad M, Larsson LE, Rønning E. Dokumentasjon av sykepleie i pasientjournalen [in Norwegian]. Oslo: NSF;2003.
2. KITH. Kravspesifikasjon for elektronisk dokumentasjon av sykepleie. Nasjonal standard [in Norwegian]. Trondheim: KITH;2003.
3. Allan J, Englebright J. Patient-centered documentation: an effective and efficient use of clinical information systems. *J Nurs Admin* 2000;30(2):90-95.
4. Ehrenberg A, Ehnfors M, Thorell-Ekstrand I. Nursing documentation in patient records: experience of the use of the VIPS model. *J Adv Nurs* 1996;24:853-867.
5. Stokke TA, Kalfoss MH. Structure and content in Norwegian nursing care documentation. *Scand J Caring Sci* 1999;13:18-25.
6. Boldreghini S, Larrabee JH. Difference in nursing documentation before and after computerization: a pilot study. *OJNI* 1998;2(1).
7. Ehnfors M, Ehrenberg A, Thorell-Ekstrand I. VIPS-boken: om en forskningsbaserad modell för dokumentation av omvårdnad i patientjournalen [in Swedish]. Stockholm: Vårdförbundet; 1998.
8. Moen A, Hellesø R, Quivey M, Berge A. Dokumentasjon og Informasjonshåndtering. Faglige og juridiske utfordringer og krav til journalføring for sykepleiere [in Norwegian]. Oslo: Akribe forlag; 2002.
9. Dick RS, Steen EB, Detmer DE, eds. *The Computer-based Patient Record: An Essential Technology for Health Care.* Rev. ed. Washington, DC: National Academy Press; 1997.
10. Børmark SR, Bjøro K. Klinisk veileder for sykepleiedokumentasjon Ullevål sykehus [in Norwegian]. Oslo: Ullevål universitetssykehus; 2001.
11. Hellesø R, Ruland CM. Developing a module for nursing documentation integrated in the electronic patient record. *J Clin Nurs* 2001;10(6):799-805.
12. Wibe T, Edwin E, Møller E, Moen A. Videreutvikling av elektronisk sykepleiedokumentasjon In: Dale JG, Fensli R, eds. *Proceedings of the Scandinavian Conference in Health Informatics.* Arendal; 2004: 23-25.
13. Børmark SR, Wibe T. Sykepleiedokumentasjon i pasientjournalen [in Norwegian]. *Instruks.* Oslo: Ullevål universitetssykehus; 2005.
14. North American Nursing Diagnosis Association. *Sykepleiediagnoser: Definisjoner & Klassifikasjon, 2001–2002* [in Norwegian]. Oslo: Akribe; 2003.
15. McCloskey JC, Bulechek GM, eds. *Nursing Interventions Classification (NIC).* 3rd ed. St. Louis: Mosby; 2000.
16. Saba VK. Clinical Care Classification (CCC) System. Available at: http://www.sabacare.com/. Accessed February 25, 2005.
17. Hammer SV, Moen A, Børmark SR, Husby EH. A hospital-wide approach to integration of nursing documentation in the electronic patient record. In: Marin H, Marques E, Hovenga E, Goosen W, eds. *E-Health for All: Designing Nursing Agenda for the Future.* Rio de Janeiro, Brazil; 2003.
18. Wibe T, Edwin E, Moen A. Audit and quality improvement of nursing documentation as the documentation is integrated in the electronic patient record. In: Marin H, Marques E, Hovenga E, Goosen W, eds. *E-Health for All: Designing Nursing Agenda for the Future.* Rio de Janeiro, Brazil; 2003.
19. Bowker GC, Star SL. *Sorting Things Out: Classification and Its Consequences.* Cambridge, MA: The MIT Press; 1999.

Case Study 27D

Development of Electronic Health Records to Support Nursing Care in Sweden

Margareta Ehnfors, PhD, RN and Anna Ehrenberg, PhD, RN

Overview of the Swedish Health Care System

Similar to that of other developed countries, the Swedish health care system is facing increasing demands from an aging population. These demands are especially challenging because Sweden has the oldest population in the European Union (EU). In addition, Sweden has reduced its hospital staff by 20 percent over the past decade. In 1992, all responsibilities for care of elderly and disabled individuals, along with 55,000 health care employees, were transferred from county councils to local municipalities. To cope with this dramatic change, improved efficiency in hospital care has resulted in a 25 percent decrease in the average length of stay in hospital. Thus, a greater extent of patient care is now provided in primary and home care. Improved efficiency has enabled hospitals to increase specific procedures, e.g., cataract outpatient surgery, a treatment available in Sweden to more people than in any other EU country. Swedish health care costs are about 50 percent per inhabitant of the costs of health care in the U.S. and lower than in most other EU countries. Sweden also has the lowest proportion of hospital beds per inhabitant in the EU. Nevertheless, the increase in health care costs has been considerable during the past few years, having increased approximately 45 percent (a figure similar to that of many other countries). Cost constraints have had a substantial effect on the working environment and staff conditions, as well as on reduced accessibility to health care services.[1]

Despite their vital importance to keep up with quality of care in a changing health care environment, electronic systems that facilitate care processes and communication of information between care providers are still not in place. Systems for continuous measurement and evaluation of health care productivity, efficiency, and quality are also largely lacking. There are increasing amounts of information in health care. For instance, in 1971, a four-week Swedish hospital stay for hip surgery generated three sheets of paper; in 1984, this same surgery generated eighteen sheets, and, in 1999, a shorter stay of ten days generated thirty-four sheets of record information.[2] Although the amount of clinical data is continuously increasing, the resources or routines to make proper use of this information are limited. The electronic health record (EHR) has the potential to solve some of these problems.

Development of Information Technology in Swedish Health Care

The Swedish government has set goals for establishing a high-speed information infrastructure for all regions of the country within a few years.[3] The government's information technology (IT) policy has three objectives: to develop confidence in IT, to increase levels of competence to use that technology, and to make information about various social services available to all citizens. One goal is that all households and companies throughout Sweden should have access to an IT infrastructure with high-speed connections within a few years. The government supports private enterprises to reach this objective as well as other IT-related goals. Confidence in IT also implies that individuals must trust that when information is retrieved, it is done so in a secure manner, and the data is not available for others to use. The use of electronic signatures will facilitate information security and integrity of the individual data. The ability to have good communication between systems is another goal of the Swedish government.

Because the Swedish health care system is mainly tax-financed, the potential for expansion of standardized IT solutions in health care is relatively favorable. However, several obstacles are in the way for successful development. Although the state has the responsibility for health care policy, local county councils (N = 20) and municipalities (N = 290) are authorized to provide health care for their inhabitants. The extensive decentralized health care system and the division of the management of health care between county councils (hospitals and primary health care centers), and municipalities (care of elderly and of mentally and physically disabled individuals) have resulted in innumerable IT solutions and noncompatible systems. It is estimated that there are anywhere from 600 to 800 IT systems in each county.[4] The resulting lack of compatible systems and integrated health information leads to fragmented patient information, loss of patient data, nonaccessible data, and high risks of errors in health care.

To support cooperation between the independent regions and local actors in Swedish health care, a special organization for the development of the use of IT was founded in 2000 (www.carelink.se). One effect of this development is that the directors of all the regional health care services in Sweden have agreed to develop their hospital systems so that they can communicate with each other nationwide and still adhere to the rules of confidentiality. This is different from the incompatible information systems currently in place in many instances. The first phase of this joint effort is focused on the patient admittance data that could be shared among different health care professionals and geographical areas to enhance security, as well as to adhere to the idea that data, once entered, can be used many times.

Current Situation of EHR in Swedish Health Care

The development of the EHR was first initiated in the 1980s in some Swedish counties. The estimated occurrence of an EHR is 85 percent to 90 percent in primary health care, 40 percent in hospital care, and somewhat less in municipality care.

Despite expected improvements in efficiency in electronic information management, a consumer survey of 2,000 health care units found that users reported serious problems with the EHR.[5] The major critique can be concluded in the following key points:

1. Users are not satisfied with the systems, although they appreciate the shift from paper-based records.
2. Some systems focus on the hospital organization, rather than on the patient.
3. Disruption in health care is caused by many incompatible systems, leading to inefficient use of time and resources by professionals who have to log into different systems to complete tasks.
4. Integrity of the patient/individual obstructs transfer between caregivers.
5. Security log-ins are complicated.
6. Systems are not very flexible.
7. Implementation of systems is often flawed, marked by low end-user involvement.
8. Evaluations of user satisfaction are not conducted.

Accessibility and security issues are crucial factors in the development of an EHR. There are, however, conflicts between the need for security and easy access for professionals and patients. Swedish law prohibits the transfer of individual health data between caregivers without the consent of the patient. But this leads to risks of omissions and errors, particularly in the care of elderly and cognitively impaired patients. Local projects to make patient records accessible to patients over the Internet have been initiated to promote patient participation in care. Until recently, the National Data Inspection Board has only allowed such access in certain projects, referring to regulations that protect the security of an individual's information and the integrity of health care data. This is one example of the conflict between laws and regulations, on the one hand, and the need for shared data to promote patient security and quality of care on the other. Another example of this conflict is the prohibition to data transfer between care providers (the purposes again are data security and protecting a patient's integrity by requiring consent). This regulation hampers the communication of data needed to provide a continuum of high-quality care.

Process Modeling

As a basis for standards and a clear understanding of information and data flow in different situations, there is a need for development of both concept models and process models. This modeling has been carried out in many national and international projects during the past decade. In Sweden, the Structured Architecture for Medical Business Activities model was developed to capture the work flow process when caring for one individual patient. The model is divided into three main components: (1) the core or clinical process; (2) the management process that monitors and evaluates the clinical process based on the mandate to provide health care; and (3) the communication process that deals with information and interacts with the surrounding world via documents or messages. The model seems useful in most health care situations and can be used to describe the enterprise at different levels of detail.[6]

Multiprofessional Work Toward an Integrated EHR

One focus of the Swedish national informatics work has been to identify similarities and differences in headings used for recording patient records as the basis for progress toward a multiprofessional, integrated record.[7,8] Currently, there is no multiprofessional Swedish classification system for health care, although work is under way in this area. Such a classification system is needed to support quality assurance efforts and to capture all types of health care data to ensure appropriate resource allocation. The work of professional groups, e.g., nurses, physiotherapists, and occupational therapists is still partly invisible in patient records. Therefore, an effort was made by the National Board of Health and Welfare to describe a multiprofessional collaborative work on classification development and to provide suggestions for an organizing structure that would capture interventions made by different health care services. The professional groups have reached a common understanding about the use of The International Classification of Functioning, Disability, and Health (ICF) as a unifying framework. This approach was seen as fruitful in overcoming professional differences and supporting consensus about the use of a common language. In the next phase, nursing interventions will be included in the classification.

Development and Research in Nursing to Facilitate EHR Progress

To achieve optimal effects from the implementation of an EHR, it is imperative to outline the process of care, to document outcomes of care, and to ensure records contain valid, reliable information. Because Swedish law mandates nurses as responsible for recording health data, the quality of nursing recording has been the focus of several research projects. Nurses are compelled to record essential information about the reasons for care, the patient's diagnosis, planned and implemented interventions, and outcomes of care, all of which correspond to the five phases of the nursing process.

Development of IT in health care is currently one of five prioritized areas of research, according to the Swedish Society of Nursing. On a national level, expert nurses and researchers have worked together in professional organizations for almost two decades—first to promote the training of the diagnostic reasoning process and, more recently, for the development of the entire nursing informatics (NI) knowledge base. There is a national professional interest organization closely linked to the national nurses' organization, with members throughout the country. Areas of shared interest include networking, decision support, terminology, nursing diagnoses and interventions, education, and the strategic influence of decisions in the health informatics field. Swedish nurses and nurse researchers have contributed considerably to EHR progress by developing terminology and models for documentation and by studying how nursing data are represented in health records.

Terminology

The VIPS Model. In 1986, it became mandatory for registered nurses to keep patient records,[9] which sparked local efforts to apply the nursing process for recording. A research-based model for nursing documentation called *VIPS* (an acronym for the Swedish spelling of well-being, integrity, prevention, and safety) was developed to conceptualize essential elements of nursing care, clarify and facilitate systematic thinking, and capture nursing recording.[10,11] VIPS is based on the structure of the nursing process and focuses on patients' functioning in daily life activities rather than on patho-physiological problems or organ systems. Furthermore, it facilitates a process-oriented, patient-centered approach. Experience from its use has shown that the model has good content validity in many areas of nursing care, including stroke, dementia, geriatric, pediatric, perioperative, and psychiatric care.[11] The VIPS model is used for recording everyday nursing and individual care planning throughout Sweden, as well as in Denmark, Norway, Finland, Estonia, and Latvia. Moreover, the VIPS model has been included in the emerging Swedish national database of terms for health care professionals as the recommended key words for nursing care. Several software applications for computerized patient records have included the model, and it is part of most nursing undergraduate programs in Sweden.

The documentation model consists of key words on two levels (Figure 27D-1). The first level corresponds to the nursing process model with the following key words: Nursing History, Nursing Status, Nursing Diagnosis, Nursing Goal, Nursing Intervention, Nursing Outcome, Nursing Report, and Nursing Discharge Note. The second level of key words consists of subdivisions comprising three categories: Nursing History, Nursing Status, and Nursing Interventions. For every key word, explanatory text and prototypes are given.

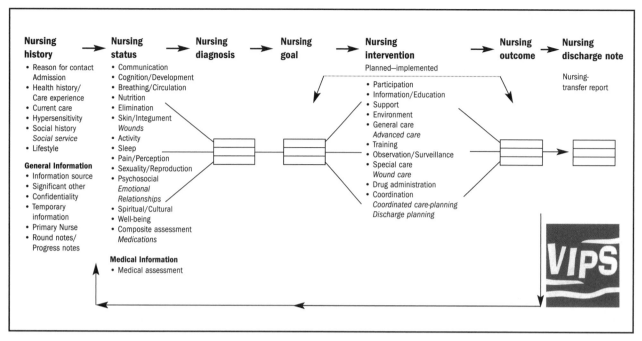

Figure 27D-1. *VIPS Documentation Model.*

The terms used in the model are a compromise or synthesis between clinically oriented everyday nursing language and internationally recognized, professional terms. Well-known terms with distinct meanings in health services were chosen, including Nursing Status and Nursing Diagnosis. The term *Nursing Status* signifies the patient status from a nursing perspective; the term was chosen for practical reasons in that it could be more easily identified when appearing together with medical notes in the EHR.

Testing of the International Classification for Nursing Practice. One international effort aimed at providing terms for nursing practice is the International Classification for Nursing Practice (ICNP®), which was developed by the International Council of Nurses (ICN). Swedish researchers have tested both the content and the use of ICNP® in its early versions. Recommendations for its development and translation in a valid, reliable manner have been forwarded to ICN.[12]

Quality of Nursing Documentation

Concerning relevance of content and adherence to the nursing process, there are a number of Swedish studies on nursing documentation in a variety of areas, such as hospital care,[13] nursing home care,[14] pressure ulcer care,[15] pain management,[16] primary health care,[17] leg ulcer care,[18] and care of patients with chronic heart failure.[19] The findings from these studies reveal several important flaws in the recording of specific assessment and interventions, as well as poor adherence to current clinical guidelines. In addition, questions about the reliability and validity of data from patient records have been studied. For instance, substantial discrepancies have been reported between nursing documentation and care performance in the recording of primary child health care[20] and pressure ulcers.[21] This knowledge forms an important basis in the development of indicators regarding quality of care and decision support in nursing care.

Evidence-based Decision Support Integrated in EHR

For nurses to not only apply evidence to practice, but also to generate evidence from practice, they need easy access to high-quality information from the patient, as well as to have high-quality health knowledge (e.g., research-based clinical guidelines in usable formats). The overwhelming amount of health care information, the increasing time constraints on providers, and the exponentially growing scientific knowledge are obviously too immense for a single nurse to manage. The EHR opens new possibilities for integrating knowledge and decision support so that they are readily available to clinicians when needed. In a small hospital study, unit researchers, in collaboration with a computer software company, developed and tested a computerized decision support system in nursing care planning that was integrated with the patient record.[22]

The prototype system, which allowed a great deal of flexibility in formulating a care plan, consisted of standardized nursing expressions in the areas of skin and nutrition, possible etiologies, interventions, and outcomes derived from literature.[23] The nurses used predefined sentences and natural language equally when writing care plans, and they expressed potential favorable effects of the computerized decision support system. However, the study indicated that nurses were not using the system to the expected extent. Experiences from this study point to the need for more knowledge about the decision processes in nursing care before suitably supportive information systems can be developed.

Implementation of EHR

The implementation of the EHR has been studied in Swedish health care.[24] Findings indicate that the actual use of EHR and its functionalities are not enough to accomplish successful implementation. In many instances, the objective of implementing an EHR is merely to automate the routine documentation of patient care. Instead, the objective should be to understand which basic values in health care can be supported by IT to reach best practice. To fully realize the possibilities in EHR technology, its implementation has to induce organizational transformation, including changes in work flow, process (how actual daily tasks are performed), and the manner in which clinical work and cooperation are organized.

Nursing Education in Informatics

Today, almost all undergraduate nursing programs in Sweden include NI curricula, with the main focus on terminology and documentation. There is only one national university program in medical informatics at the master's level and a few courses in NI at the master's or doctoral level. However, in many health care organizations, nurses participate in shorter NI programs as part of their continuing education. One important aim for the near future is basic informatics training for all health care personnel. To achieve this, there is a crucial need for faculty and leaders trained in NI.[25]

Future Needs in the Development of the EHR in Sweden

In conclusion, Sweden is moving rapidly toward better informatics support for good health care. However, we still need to optimize development of the EHR, including the following prerequisites:

1. Support for health care processes
2. Creation of a standardized common national structure and terminology for patient care data
3. Multiprofessional integration without compromising the unique contributions of each health care profession
4. Development and implementation of computerized decision support systems for bedside use, including the integration of research-based knowledge in patient records
5. Secure communication between information systems
6. The ability to compile and aggregate data without compromising the integrity and security of the individual

References

1. Landstingsförbundet, Kommunförbundet. Swedish health care in transition: resources and results with international comparisons [in Swedish]. Available at: http://uno.svekom.se/brsbibl/kata_documents/doc35570_1.pdf. Accessed February 2005.
2. National Board of Health and Welfare. Omfattningen av administration i vården [The extent of administration in health care] [in Swedish]. Available at: http://sos.se/FULLTEXT/0077-001/0077-001.htm. Accessed February 2005.
3. Socialdepartementet. An information society for all [in Swedish]. Prop.1999/2000;86.
4. Renstig, M. Rätt IT skulle spara miljarder i vården [Proper IT would save billions in health care] [in Swedish]. *Dagens Medicin;* August 25, 2004:28-29.
5. Users Award 2004. Användare och IT-system inom svensk vård och omsorg [Users and IT-system in Swedish health care and social services] [in Swedish]. Available at: http://www.usersaward.com. Accessed February 2005.
6. SFMI 2004. Swedish Association of Medical Informatics. Available at: http://www.sfmi.se/samba/dokument/samba_en_1_8.ppt. Accessed February 2005.
7. Åhlfeldt H, Ehnfors M, Ridderstolpe L. Towards a multiprofessional patient record—a study of the headings used in clinical practice. In: *Proceedings of the American Medical Informatics Association Symposium.* Philadelphia: Hanley & Belfus; 1997:7-11.

8. Ehnfors M, Ehrenberg A, Ridderstolpe L, Åhlfeldt H, Östlinder G. Integrating nursing terminology in the Swedish National Health Care Data Base. In: *Nursing Informatics 2000. One Step Beyond: The Evolution of Technology and Nursing.* Auckland: Adis International Ltd; 2000:363-369.

9. Svensk Författningssamling. Patientjournallagen [The Patient Record Act] [in Swedish]. SFS 1985;562. Available at: http//www.notisum.se. Accessed February 2005.

10. Ehnfors M, Thorell-Ekstrand I, Ehrenberg A. Towards basic nursing information in patient records [Vard Nord Utveckl Forsk] [in Swedish]. *Nurs Sci Res Nordic Countries,* 1991; 21(3/4):12-31.

11. Ehrenberg A, Ehnfors M, Thorell-Ekstrand I. Nursing documentation in patient records: experience of the use of the VIPS model. *J Adv Nurs.* 1996;24,853-867.

12. Ehnfors M, Coenen A, Marin H, Prenkert M. Translating the International Classification for Nursing Practice (ICNP)—an experience from two countries. In: M. Fiesschi et al, eds. *Medinfo 2004.* Amsterdam: ISO Press; 2004:502-505.

13. Björvell C, Wredling R, Thorell-Ekstrand I. Long-term increase in quality of nursing documentation: effects of a comprehensive intervention. *Scand J Caring Sci.* 2002; 16(1):34-42.

14. Ehrenberg A, Ehnfors M. Patient records in nursing homes: effects of training on content and comprehensiveness. *Scand J Caring Sci,* 1999;13:72-82.

15. Gunningberg L, Lindholm C, Carlsson M, Sjoden PO. The development of pressure ulcers in patients with hip fractures: inadequate nursing documentation is still a problem. *J Adv Nurs.* 2000:31(5):1155-1164.

16. Idvall E, Ehrenberg A. Nursing documentation of postoperative pain management. *J Clin Nurs.* 2002;11(6): 734-742.

17. Törnkvist L, Gardulf A, Strender LE. Effects of pain-adviser: district nurses' opinions regarding their own knowledge, management and documentation of patients in chronic pain. *Scand J Caring Sci.* 2003;17(4):332-338.

18. Ehrenberg A, Birgersson C. Nursing documentation of leg ulcers: adherence to clinical guidelines in a Swedish primary health care district. *Scand J Caring Sci.* 2003;17:278-284.

19. Ehrenberg A, Ehnfors M, Ekman I. Older patients with chronic heart failure in home care. a record review of nurses' assessments and interventions. *J Clin Nurs.* 2003;13:90-96.

20. Hagelin E, Lagerberg D, Sundelin C. Child health records as a database for clinical practice, research, and community planning. *J Adv. Nurs.* 1991;16(1):15-23.

21. Gunningberg L, Ehrenberg A. Accuracy and quality in the nursing documentation of pressure ulcers: a comparison of record content and patient examination. *J Wound Ostomy Continence Nurs.* 2004;31(6):328-325.

22. Florin J, Ehrenberg A, Ehnfors M, Wennemyr T. A computerized decision-support system for nursing care planning based on standardized terminology and scientific knowledge. In: de Fatima Marin H, Pereira Marques E, Hovenga E, Goossen W, eds. *Proceedings of the 8th International Congress in Nursing Informatics.* Rio de Janeiro: E-papers Servicios Editorials Ltd; 2003:204-207.

23. Ehnfors M, Ehrenberg A, Florin J. Applicability of the International Classification of Nursing Practice (ICNP) in the areas of nutrition and skin care. *Int J Nurs Terminol Classif.* 2003;14(1)5-18.

24. Nikula RE. Organizational and technological insight as important factors for successful implementation of IT. In: Lorenzi NM, ed. Proceedings of the American Medical Informatics Association Symposium. Philadelphia: Hanley & Belfus, Inc.; 1999:585-588.

25. Ehnfors M, Grobe SJ. Nursing curriculum and continuing education: future directions. *Int J Med Inform.* 2004;73:7-8,591-598.

Case Study 27E

The Netherlands: Getting Nursing Evidence, Terminology, and Data in the Development of EHRs

William T.F. Goossen, PhD, RN

The Netherlands has a long history of development and use of information technology (IT) in health care. Beginning in the 1960s with some national projects, the dissemination of systems grew explosively. However, despite these IT developments, the realization of electronic health records (EHR) is still problematic today. From the perspective of the nursing profession, we have seen few improvements over the past 20 years, although recent developments seem more promising. Since 2000, agreement among health care institutions, professionals, patients, insurers, government, and industry has led to the realization of a safe national IT infrastructure, based on standards for semantic interoperability.

This case study on the use of IT in Dutch health care describes a brief history, the problems of the end of the last century, new plans, and some results. Nursing as a profession in the Netherlands is challenged to step into these developments, contribute, and gain profits to improve nursing care. The reader should not expect a complete historic analysis, or coverage of everything that is going on in Dutch nursing care. Rather, this case study is a status report that highlights only certain examples.

A Brief History on the Use of IT in Dutch Health Care

During the 1960s and 1970s, health care in the Netherlands began applying computers for administrative tasks. This led to the government-funded Nobin-ZIS project in 1972–1976 for an integrated hospital information system (Nobin is the Nederlands orgaan ter bevordering van de informatievoorziening, or Dutch council to support the supply of information; ZIS is ziekenhuis [hospital] information system). The project was a success and led to a cooperation of hospitals developing and exploiting this ZIS. After a successful pilot project in Leiden, the Verpleegkundig Informatie Systeem (VISY) (nursing information system) was marketed and sold commercially to other hospitals as part of the ZIS. This was one of the first Dutch systems with specific nursing components—a nursing assessment module, a care planning module, and sections for recording vital signs and body weight.[1]

Today, there are various health information systems on the Dutch market. The use of health information systems is almost 100 percent, although the types and total number of applications differ for every health institution. Also in home care, nursing homes, and psychiatry, automated systems have become a necessity, mainly for administration and financial purposes. However, some institutions are adopting applications for care planning. General practitioners in the Netherlands are among the first to use EHR in their practices, and now more than 90 percent use such a system.[2]

In the 1990s, reports indicated that integrated hospital information systems had major difficulties in establishing an EHR. Some developments in EHR systems took place in other areas, including psychiatry, nursing homes, care for the mentally disabled, and home care, because these settings were able to invest in newer, cheaper technology, based on modern patient-centered concepts of the EHR and flexible information technology.[3] However, no widespread use has been achieved. Dedicated record software packages were developed that run more or less as stand-alone and single-discipline information systems. Several nursing information systems have been developed in these years, but none of these was able to penetrate the market.[3] (In general, current nursing use of complete EHR systems is estimated at only 1 percent or 2 percent.)[4,5] By the close of the 1990s, the major problems hindering further advancement of the EHR had been identified. Resolving these problems called for an initiative to get all stakeholders around the table to settle the issues.

Roadblocks to Establishing a Dutch EHR

The development of the EHR is often justified by the expectation that it will solve several problems in the use of patient information. But Dutch health care faces numerous other challenges as well, e.g., an aging population; an increase in chronic diseases; the need for information about effectiveness, quality, and efficiency of care; growing use of medical technology; the need for cost containment, and so on. All require intelligent information management and safe exchange of patient-related information. In addition, several organizational and IT problems could be solved by the EHR. The following problems have been identified.[6]

1. Organizational changes and re-engineering of care processes should match automation in health care but are often ignored; thus, improvements are not realized.
2. The need for standardization to the level necessary for the EHR raises professional discussions, and local cultural problems (e.g., habits) stand in the way.
3. Patient care processes often are not conceptualized in detail; therefore, systems offer single-discipline and task-oriented support instead of integrated patient care support.
4. IT is still limited and inflexible; it takes a long time to develop an EHR.
5. Health care data are fragmented; there is no linkage between different medical records and professions. This is exacerbated by the lack of a national unique patient identifier.
6. Traditionally, vendors of clinical information systems prohibited the integration of departmental systems from other vendors. Only recently has a shift toward interoperability happened.
7. The Dutch market is relatively small, which makes it difficult to develop a system that will eventually provide a return on investment for vendors.
8. Developments in seamless care for patients going from hospital to nursing home to their own home again require information flows beyond the borders of institutions and professions.
9. The informatics standards arena lacks coordination, agreement, and application. There have been several years of *laissez-faire* policy, suggesting a free market approach that has, in fact, brought developments in several areas to a standstill.
10. Nursing as a profession did not show much interest in the development of nursing information systems, and what systems were available were not suitable to fulfill professional requirements.[7]

Changing the Trend: Building on Agreement

In early 1999, several parties realized that the problems with IT in Dutch health care called for cooperative action. The "IT platform in the care sector" (in Dutch: IPZorg or IT platform in the Zorg) was set up, involving virtually all parties in health care.[8] IPZorg included representatives of patient organizations and associations of health practitioners, including nursing, hospitals, health institutions, home care, health insurers, and the government. The platform drew up a declaration of intent in September 2000, which all parties signed to establish a secure national IT infrastructure for the EHR.[8] Projects were initiated, and preparations took place to establish the NICTIZ Foundation in December 2001. NICTIZ is the abbreviation of the Dutch name for the National IT Institute for Healthcare.[9]

The Three Major Areas of NICTIZ

NICTIZ supports the creation of a system that will allow an improved flow of information about the patient/client, with a view to raising the quality and effectiveness of health care.[9] NICTIZ has three areas of concern: (1) building the national IT infrastructure for health care; (2) standardizing data for both EHR and electronic messages; and (3) ensuring the security of patient data for broader use. To achieve this progress in these areas, work is under way at the policy level, including dissemination of knowledge, standards development work, and guidance for ongoing and new projects.[9] The national IT infrastructure for the exchange of patient data will be based on linkages between EHR systems, which will allow health care professionals to access patient data from any location at any time. In addition to medical data, the IT infrastructure for health care will facilitate the exchange of logistic and administrative information.

AORTA: The National IT Infrastructure

The NICTIZ's AORTA program provides the infrastructure, including elements, e.g., access, access control, networks, and traffic control, that are indispensable if information is to be exchanged safely and reliably between care professionals.[9] Although not an acronym, AORTA was so named because it will function as the system's "aorta," bringing potentially life-saving information to everyone in health care who needs it and is authorized to access it. It will take into account legislation, regulations, and the level of confidence and trust that exists between various care providers. The AORTA program describes the basic infrastructure that must be created between organizations; infrastructure issues within organizations fall outside the scope of the program.[9] One part of the AORTA will provide a shared data service center, in which health care professionals can find information about their patients reported by other providers. Currently, several regional projects are developing infrastructures, built on the same principles.

Although nurses usually deal with the IT infrastructure within their institutions, they will benefit from the exchange of information via the IT infrastructure. For example, one region's infrastructure is used by nurses for electronic messages, sending care records from the hospital to home care services or to nursing homes, and vice versa.

Safe Exchange of Patient Information

In the area of security, information interchange will require authorization by patients. The actual authorization for data exchange will be based on protocols developed by patient and provider organizations, insurers, and government and will be granted by a to-be-founded Trusted Third Party (TTP).[9] In the EU, directive 1999/93/EC provides a legal framework for the use of electronic signatures, thus reducing security threats to the electronic exchange of information.[10] A public-key cryptography system guarantees the safety of electronic signatures. A pair of related keys is used in such a public-key cryptosystem, one key for encryption for the sender and the other key for decryption by the receiver. "One key, the private key, is kept secret. The other key, the public key, can be made publicly known."[10] Certification Authorities (CAs) issue electronic (public key) certificates that authenticate these keys to prevent misuse and fraud. Electronic certificates establish the identity of a person, company, or Web server on the Internet, thus facilitating secure communication. "Data encrypted with an electronic certificate can only be decrypted with the corresponding private key. Data signed with a private key can only be verified with the corresponding electronic certificate."[10] In this security structure, the CA serves as the TTP in the public-key cryptography system and thus needs to be independent, neutral, reliable, and acceptable for all communicating parties.

Working together with all parties in health care, NICTIZ is developing an identification and authorization policy. Currently, Dutch citizens have a social security number, the use of which is legally limited to income taxes and social security insurances and benefits. For the purposes of identifying patients, a national number will be used, based on the patient's current social security number. However, its legal status will be adjusted to allow this additional use. Also, the name "social security number" will be changed to the Burger Service Number (Civilian Service Number) to acknowledge its use as a unique patient identifier, among other uses. Care professionals and care insurers will also receive unique numbers that will be known as the Unique Care Professional Identification Number (UZI) and the Unique Care Insurer Identification Number (UZOVI). Authorization protocols will determine which care professionals may have access to what, if any, patient information. The UZI numbers for nurses will be based on those assigned to nursing professionals by the National Registered Nurses Administration.

Standards that Support Information Exchange

The uniform exchange of information demands health sector wide use of standards. NICTIZ takes into account several of the international standards (e.g., CEN and ISO) and the Health Level 7 Version 3 (HL7 v3) standard.[11] Currently, HL7 versions 2x are used in almost all Dutch hospitals, and harmonization is taking place between standards organizations, therefore the HL7 v3 standard was chosen for NICTIZ projects.[9] In particular, the HL7 v3 Reference Information Model (RIM), domain and message models, and associated modeling tools are being used.

In the first project, NICTIZ established a domain message information model (D-MIM) for perinatology.[12,13] An electronic message derived from this model was tested with success.[12] This project served as a national pilot to test the applicability of HL7 v3, in particular the RIM.[9,12] The perinatology D-MIM then became the base of what is now the Care Provision Domain Message Information Model in the HL7 v3 standard.[11] Another NICTIZ project focuses on an EHR system for stroke services and has lead to a D-MIM for stroke patients.[14,15] The same methodology was used to develop an EHR with pathways for cardiology.[15]

It has become clear that the D-MIM approach suits many clinical domains, its reusability is high, and, even when information is not 100 percent alike, the same methodology can be used to add specialized content. Thus, the focus is now moving from specific clinical models to mapping the clinical materials to the generic HL7 Care Provision D-MIM, which reduces the time, effort, and costs and improves the reuse and semantic interoperability of clinical information.

In these three projects, nursing played an important role by submitting use cases for perinatology (admission, delivery, and maternity care) and driving the developments of pathways for cardiology. The stroke service model is completely multidisciplinary. The most promising findings of this modeling work is that the same structures can be used for many different patient categories and that they are so powerful they facilitate information management and exchange for all health professionals.[11,15]

Focus on Clinical Domain Analysis, Models, and Messages

The development of domain specific messages now takes place in three phases: (1) the domain information analysis phase; (2) the modeling phase, in which mapping to HL7 Care Provision Domain Message Information Model (D-MIM) is carried out; and (3) the implementation phase. We discuss only phases one and two.

In the domain information analysis phase, distinct products are developed. Care professionals describe prototype cases, i.e., the most frequently occurring care needs. The cases are then organized into story-boards that represent single activities. Thus, the domain is broken down into single data items. Both the interactions and the static aspects are further analyzed. The interactions are used in phase two to determine and model the dynamics of systems sending and receiving messages. The static domain information is used in the second phase to draw the HL7 v3 domain models and HL7 v3 message models for specific content.

The data items are sorted in a spreadsheet then compared with and mapped to the existing classes in the HL7 v3 Care Provision D-MIM, resulting in a mapping table with the detailed domain information on one side and the corresponding HL7 classes and attributes on the other side. Clinicians verify the products of all steps. Nursing information has been included in such tables for perinatology, cardiology, and stroke service.

Nursing-specific Projects Become Relevant to Others

Nursing is challenged to find an answer to such questions as what nursing data should go in the EHR, how nursing-specific information should be exchanged within the IT infrastructure, and how nursing information can be used within the HL7 v3 messages. This requires the involvement of nursing professional organizations that have an interest in standards, IT, and EHR development. In the Netherlands, the General Assembly of Nursing Associations (AVVV) represents the nursing profession[16] and the Netherlands Centre for Excellence in Nursing (LEVV) focuses on developing nursing expertise.[17] Both nursing organizations have declared IT in health care of importance for the profession and participate in or carry out projects in this area. The fact that Dutch nursing organizations have declared IT as important and participate in IT projects is a major achievement because it is the first time in history.

One nursing initiative applies the International Classification of Functioning, Disability, and Health[18] to develop multidisciplinary information tools, e.g., assessments, clinical pathways, and monitoring instruments.[17] This use of an international terminology standard has a positive impact on the exchange of information among professions and institutions and on the development of the EHR. The stroke project especially benefited from work by nurses who identified ICF codes for neurological patient information items.

A project of the national hospital association, with support from LEVV and AVVV, analyzed the benefits of nursing documentation, EHR, IT applications, clinical pathways, and other forms of care documentation.[4,5,17,18] The results show that multidisciplinary approaches with a focus on specific patient problems, clinical pathways, and outcomes are likely to be the most successful and are the key to nurses' information needs.[4,5] Nurses thus can lead and support developments. However, it is of interest to see what nursing as a profession can gain.

What Is In It for Nursing?

The AVVV used a consensus-based approach to determine what nurses expect from the EHR.[19] Building on scientific work in which criteria were set for the nursing part of the EHR,[7] expert nurses achieved consensus about several issues.[19] Motives about why nursing should get involved in IT developments were formulated, as were the goals that should be achieved with IT and the EHR. These include support of care delivery, quality improvement, and professional development. Next, nurses' information needs were made explicit. These include: patient identification; medical investigations, diagnoses, and treatment; nursing assessment, diagnoses, interventions, and outcome indicators; information regarding patient status, e.g., scores on scales for pain and pressure ulcers and scales for activity of daily living, for specific nursing diagnoses; guidelines and protocols; and information for coordination, management, and resources.[19] Several functions of the EHR should support nurses with these information needs and assist in multidisciplinary patient care across the continuum.

Since 2004, projects to develop HL7-based information models that can be used and reused at a national level are under way. An example is the Dutch version of the Barthel Index. The Barthel is a valid and reliable scale to measure different aspects of activities of daily living. The Barthel index can be used on population or individual data to determine outcomes of care.[20,21] The message model for the Barthel index is based on the HL7 v3 Care Provision D-MIM22 (see Figure 27E-1).[22]

The Barthel model specifies the observation class and starts with the naming on top (entry point), under the Barthel Index. Beneath that is the act type observation. This is central for the Barthel model. In this class, the total score of the Barthel Index is shown in the "value" attribute. "Interpretation" shows how the total score should be interpreted (zero to nine for seriously limited, ten to nineteen for moderately limited, and twenty for independent). Further attributes are not discussed here. The Barthel Index consists of ten variables, each of which is another "Observation" class for the score on the variables. The variables are bowels, bladder, grooming, toilet use, feeding, transfers, mobility, dressing, stairs, and bathing respectively.

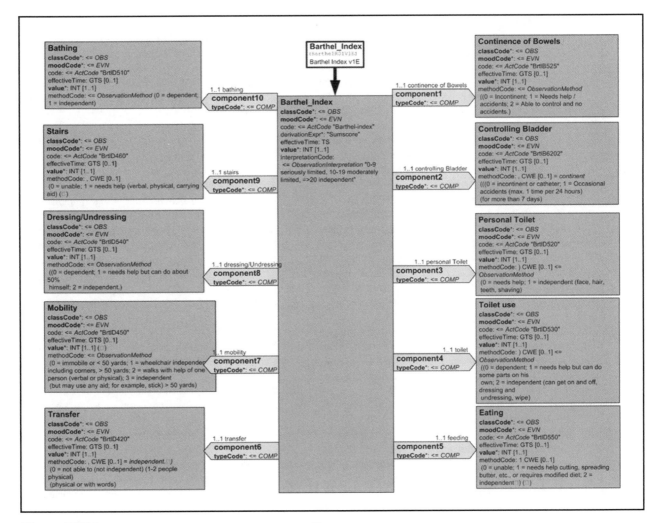

Figure 27E-1. *The message model for the Barthel index.*[22]

Table 27E-1. Detail of Barthel Index Mapping Table from Domain to HL7 Care Provision D-MIM

	DMIM section	Place in HL7 Model	Data type HL7	Cardinality	Vocabulary system used	Code from vocabulary system
Barthel Index total score	OBS	value	INT	1..1	CVA-KIS	Barthel-index
bowels	OBS	value	INT	1..1	"	BrtIB525
bladder	OBS	value	INT	1..1	"	BrtIB6202
etc						

OBS is the observation class of HL7, INT is an integer, a real number for the score, CVA-KIS is the abbreviation for the stroke service continuum of care information system.[21]

The result of each score goes in to the field "value" for each variable. The relationship with the body of evidence, the terminology, and the coding systems are made explicit in the mapping table. A fragment of the mapping table for the Barthel model is presented in Table 27E-1.

In the near future, it is likely that a multitude of clinical models following the example of the Barthel model will evolve internationally. These models, often called *templates* or *archetypes,* integrate the evidence base, terminology developments, information models, standards, and code sets, allowing semantic interoperability on an international level.[23] These clinical models are vendor independent, and their integration into EHR systems and electronic messages will better support nurses in their practice, facilitating their care for patients.

References

1. Pluyter-Wenting ESP, Nieman HBJ. Ontwikkelingen in de verpleegkundige verslaglegging. Tijdschrijft voor Medische Informatica. 1987;16(4):13-17.
2. Van der Lei J, Duisterhof JS, Westerhof HP, et al. The introduction of computer-based patient records in the Netherlands. *Ann Intern Med.* 1993;119:1036-1046.
3. Goossen WTF. Overview of health care and nursing informatics in the Netherlands. *Health Inf.* 1996;2(1):9-20.
4. Hilderink HGM, Epping PJMM, Goossen WTF. ICT in nursing in Dutch hospitals. In: France FH Roger, De Clerq E, De Moor G, eds. E-Health in Belgium and in the Netherlands. *Stud Health Technol Inform.* 2002; 93:83-88.
5. Hilderink HGM, Epping PJMM, Goossen WTF. OVERZORG Een nieuw fundament voor ICT in de Verpleging. Resultaten van een onderzoek naar de stand van zaken en kansen rondom ICT in de verpleging. Leidschendam: NICTIZ; 2002.
6. Goossen WTF. *Electronic Patient Records: A National Agenda in the Netherlands.* Health IT Advisory Report. Newton, MA: U.S. Medical Records Institute. 2002;4(1):4-9.
7. Goossen WTF, Epping PJMM, Dassen TWN. Criteria for nursing information systems as a component of the electronic patient record: an international Delphi study. *Comput Nurs.* 1997;15(6):307-315.
8. IPZorg. Declaration of intent. 2000. Available at: www.ipzorg.nl. Accessed September 2001.
9. Nationaal ICT instituut in de Zorg. NICTIZ Web site. Available at www.nictiz.nl. Accessed August 2005.
10. Workgroup ACT TTP.NL. Scheme for Certification of Certification Authorities against ETSI TS 101 456. Leidschendam, ECP.NL Platform voor eNederland, 2002. Available at: http://www.ecp.nl/publications/TTP-NL_Scheme_version_5_final.pdf. Accessed August 2005.
11. Health Level Seven. Health Level 7, the Netherlands. Available at www.HL7.org and www.HL7.nl. Accessed August 2005.
12. Jonker M, Goossen WTF, Heitmann K, Jongeneel-de Haas I, De Jong, T. Pilotproject 'Modelleren in de Perinatologie met HL7 versie 3. Het Domein Message Information Model Perinatologie (D-MIM Perinatologie) [final report on CD-ROM, in Dutch]. Leidschendam: NICTIZ; 2003. Available at: www.nictiz.nl.
13. Goossen WT, Jonker MJ, Heitmann KU, et al. Electronic Patient Records: Domain Message Information Model Perinatology. *Int J Med Inf.* 2003;70(2-3):265-276.
14. Reuser L, Goossen WTF, Van der Heijden H. Call for ICT within stroke service care. In: Runnenberg J et al, eds. *Health Information Developments in the Netherlands by the Year 2003.* 2003:6:52-56.
15. Goossen WTF. Model once, use multiple times: reusing HL7 domain models from one domain to the other. In: Fieschi M, Coiera E, Jack Li YC, eds. *Proceedings of the 11th World Congress on Medical Informatics Medinfo 2004.* Amsterdam: IOS Press; 2004:366-370.
16. General Assembly of Nursing Associations (AVVV). AVVV Web site. Available at: www.avvv.nl. Accessed February 2005.
17. Netherlands Centre for Excellence in Nursing (LEVV). LEVV Web site. Available at: www.levv.nl. Accessed February 2005.
18. World Health Organization. *International Classification of Functioning, Disability and Health: ICF.* Geneva: World Health Organization; 2001. Also available at http://www3.who.int/icf/onlinebrowser/icf.cfm. Accessed August 2005.
19. General Assembly of Nursing Associations. Digitaal V&V Dossier: Rapportage van de werkconferenties. Utrecht: Algemene Vergadering van Verpleegkundigen en Verzorgenden; 2002.
20. Mahoney FI, Barthel DW. Functional evaluation: the Barthel index. *Md State Med J.* 1965;14:61-65.

21. De Haan R, Limburg M, Schuling J, et al. Klinimetrische evaluatie van de Barthel-index, een maat voor beperkingen in het dagelijks functioneren, Ned Tijdschr Geneeskd 1993;37(18):917-921.

22. Fleurke M, Goossen WTF, Hoijtink EJ, Van der Kooij J, Vlastuin M. Care Information Model Barthel Index. Leidschendam: NICTIZ; 2005. Available at: www.zorginformatiemodel.nl.

23. Goossen WTF. Templates: an organizing framework to link evidence, terminology, and information models in the nursing profession. In: de Fatima Marin H, Pereira Margues E, Hovenga E, Goossen W, eds. *E-Health for All: Designing a Nursing Agenda for the Future. Proceedings of the 8th International Congress in Nursing Informatics NI 2003.* Rio de Janeiro, Brazil: E-papers Serviços Editoriais Ltd; 2003:461-465.

Case Study 27F

Toward Integrating Nursing Data into the EPR: Current Developments in Germany

Ursula Hübner, Dr. Ret. Nat; Carsten Giehoff, RN; Bjoern Sellemann, Dipl-Pflegewirt (FH)

The German Health Care System

The German health care system is based on social health insurance and is controlled by the Federal Ministry of Health and Social Security, which proposes health acts to the parliament and delegates tasks to the health self-governance sector consisting of nongovernmental corporate bodies. In 2003, approximately 87 percent of the population was covered by statutory health insurance. Such coverage, which is based on income, is mandatory for approximately 77 percent of the population and voluntary for 10 percent; the remaining 13 percent are covered by a private health insurance company or by the government.[1] The insurance covers both outpatient and inpatient health care services (German Social Code Book V). Since 1995, long-term care insurance (German Social Code Book XI) has been mandatory for nearly the entire population. It is operated with use of long-term care funds or by private insurance companies. Entitlement to long-term care benefits depends on need, which is assessed according to a three-stage system.

Similar to other industrialized countries, Germany is confronted with steadily increasing health care expenditures (see Table 27F-1),[2-5] and the government has initiated various cost-containment measures. These measures include reductions in the salaries of general practitioners, limited budgets for prescription-drug coverage, decreases in the administrative costs of sickness funds, and increases in beneficiary copayments for certain services.

Because ambulatory care is less costly than inpatient care, government regulations since the early 1990s have been aimed at reinforcing outpatient care and home health care. With the advent of long-term care insurance in the mid-1990s, hundreds of private home health care services were established. There

Table 27F-1. Data on the German Health Care System

Parameter	Number/Percentage
Population of Germany[2] in 2003	82,531,671
Healthcare Expenditures[3] (% of gross domestic product)	
In 1993	10.2%
In 2002	11.1%
Number of Hospitals[4]	
In 1993	2,354
In 2002	2,221
Number of Hospital Beds[4]	
In 1993	628,258
In 2002	547,284
Average Length of Stay in Hospital (days)[4]	
In 1993	12.5
In 2002	9.2
Total number of Physicians[5] in 2003	304,000
Total number of Nurses[5] in 2003	1,001,000

are now approximately 10,000 such services providing either treatment ordered by physicians or nursing interventions within the framework of long-term care insurance.

Inpatient and outpatient services in Germany are only linked loosely if at all. Hospitals interested in building a network of health care providers (integrated delivery networks) can now do so more easily under the Statutory Health Insurance Modernization Act, which allows them to negotiate contracts on behalf of the network with the administrators of sickness funds. Such networks comprise general practitioners, medical specialists, home health care services, rehabilitation institutions, clinics, pharmacies, and other self-employed health care professionals.

Compared with other countries, Germany is known for its high rate of hospital beds per inhabitant and an average length of stay that is higher than that of other EU countries (Table 27F-1). However, there has been a decline in the length of stay over the last few years, a trend that will be further reinforced by the German diagnosis–related group (G-DRG) system that took effect as the mandatory budgeting tool for hospitals at the beginning of 2004. The G-DRG system is an all-patient classification system that was developed on the basis of the Australian DRG system.[6] Patients are grouped into homogeneous categories according to their ICD-10-coded medical diagnoses and the Out Patient Specialist (OPS) procedure codes, a German classification system originating from the International Classification of Procedures in Medicine. Neither nursing diagnoses nor interventions are used for grouping. However, nursing documentation is employed for revealing patient comorbidities and complexities. These data do not contain nursing-specific information but rather represent medical problems that are dealt with mainly by nurses. As shown by Fischer,[7] nursing diagnoses cannot be coded into ICD-10; only a small percentage of North American Nursing Diagnoses Association (NANDA) diagnoses could be expressed in ICD-10 terms. There are proposals for integrating nursing data into the G-DRG system and thereby accounting for heterogeneities and variances within groups.[8] Among clinicians and hospital managers, the adoption of the DRG system has led to an increased awareness about the costs caused by the length of stay and about instruments such as clinical pathways providing a cost framework for patient care and thus helping to decrease costs.

The role of information technology as an instrument for providing transparency and easy communication has finally been acknowledged by the government. Pursuant to the Statutory Health Insurance Modernization Act, the health insurance card containing administrative data will be replaced at the beginning of 2006 by a card containing both administrative and clinical data. The new health card will be integrated in a nationwide health "telematics" infrastructure that will provide security, data management, and administrative and application services. Among the clinical data on the card itself or referred to by the card will be the electronic patient record (EPR).

In summary, the major elements of the German health care framework are health care and long-term care insurance, outpatient and home health care, integrated care delivery networks, DRGs, and the health telematics infrastructure. These forces drive the activities that are integral to the formation of a multidisciplinary patient/health record.

The EPR in German Hospitals

New and more complex financing methods have led to increased investment in hospital information systems, particularly clinical systems that include the EPR. A nationwide survey conducted in 2002 confirmed that management systems are still prevalent in German hospitals but also revealed a tremendous increase in clinical systems (see Table 27F-2).

As shown in Table 27F-2, 19 percent of German hospitals had some type of EPR in use.[9] This figure matches that reported for U.S. hospitals in 2003.[10] Whether the 19 percent rate is construed as significant or modest depends on one's perspective. However, there is no doubt that hospitals that invest in ordering systems (48 percent) and clinical systems (40 percent) are in an excellent position to launch the EPR. Installation rates for nursing documentation systems (seven percent) and care planning systems (six percent) in German hospitals are low. It seems that hospital managers are more interested in nursing documentation than are nursing managers themselves.[11] Perhaps the tools meant to support clinical processes actually support only management tasks by providing data for clinical statistics and controlling. However, one cannot extrapolate from nursing managers' less pronounced interest in electronic documentation that their overall attitude toward the EPR is negative. Nursing managers are well aware of the benefit of other

Table 27F-2. Clinical Modules Implemented in German Hospitals

Module	Rate of Use (%)
Laboratory	69
Surgery (documentation)	68
Anesthesia (documentation)	56
Ordering system (examinations, drugs, material)	48
Patient management (ADT) used on wards	45
Outpatient management	43
Clinical workplace	40
Radiology information system	30
Medical record	19
PACS	12
Care documentation	7
Care planning	6

electronic tools, particularly that of ordering systems for scheduling examinations and for obtaining medical supplies.[11] Their support for ordering systems clearly reflects the importance of tools that can assist in communication and data gathering, both of which are major features of the EPR.

It is hard to predict the speed with which the multidisciplinary EPR will progress, even in the next five years, because the effect of DRGs on the EPR is still unfolding. In addition, other factors, e.g., the telematics infrastructure, have not yet started to leverage clinical applications, most notably, the EPR.

The Electronic Nursing Summary: A Pilot Study

Financial and technical driving forces are important; however, the need to improve the quality of care should be the strongest impetus for sharing patient data, not only within a single institution (EPR) but also among health care providers (electronic health record [EHR]). Deficiencies in providing patients with uninterrupted care when they are moved from one institution to another or when they are discharged to home has spurred nursing leaders from northwest Germany to establish a network named Network for Continuity of Care in the Region of Osnabrueck in 2001. The network comprises an informal group of hospitals, nursing homes, home-care services, and a health care center; it is currently being transformed into a registered association. Its goal is to improve communication among health care providers by means of an electronic nursing summary, sent at the time of discharge to all caregivers involved in the patient's follow-up. The Network receives scientific and technical assistance from the University of Applied Sciences Osnabrueck.

On the basis of input from different types of health care providers, an information model was developed for the nursing summary, which not only reflects the hospital's viewpoint but also allows a comprehensive assessment of the patient's case. The information model builds strongly on the relationship between nursing diagnoses and interventions. This is not new in the context of the nursing process, but it differs markedly from the daily routine in which nursing summaries are hardly more than lists of interventions.[12] The use of nursing diagnoses is uncommon in Germany, as is the use of coded nursing data. Therefore, the network devoted considerable effort to investigating different classification schemes and their usability in Germany. It found that the NANDA[13] and the Home Healthcare Classification (now known as the Clinical Care Classification) systems are highly suitable, despite the fact that they originate from a different nursing culture.

Alternatively, the International Classification for Nursing Practice (ICNP®) system can be employed, particularly when a finite number of clinical expressions has been defined and is made available as a catalogue of diagnoses. Standardized, well-defined expressions—available in all major international classification systems—are of great importance when exchanging information among different health care institutions and different types of institutions. We may assume some sort of mutual understanding among people within one institution, but it is unlikely that nurses share the same vocabulary across institutions. Use of the same terminology promotes better communication among people; this is also the prerequisite for communication among computer systems.

In the case of the electronic nursing summary in Osnabrueck, the informational model and the various classification systems (NANDA and the HHCC, together with the ICNP® as background terminology) were implemented in a Web-based application accessing a central relational database. As shown in Figure 27F-1, confidentiality is ensured by means of a virtual private network provided by Osnatel, a regional telecommunications provider. Systems are authenticated by certificates, and data are encrypted. This system is currently undergoing field tests.

A nursing summary such as the one previously described cannot replace a complete EPR or EHR, but it represents one solution for communicating across institutional borders. In principle, it resembles systems for medical discharge letters, e.g., the one developed by the German project known as Standardization of Communication between Information Systems in Physician Offices and Hospitals Using XML (SCIPHOX),[14] in which an electronic clinical document is sent to physicians providing follow-up care, who often are general practitioners. There are other concepts that build on a common health data repository used by both patients and physicians.[15] One such repository would not only contain summaries of patients' health status, e.g., discharge documents, but would also reflect the continuous course of their health. The repository approach is closer to the idea of a health record than the discharge-document approach, but investigation must be carried out to determine which method better enhances communication for the purpose of better care.

The German Health Card and Health Telematics Infrastructure

No telematics "island" in Germany, whether large or small, can ignore the efforts under way toward implementing the German health card and the telematics infrastructure, which will be introduced in 2006. Proposed as a solution for the electronic prescription and medication record, the concept of a German

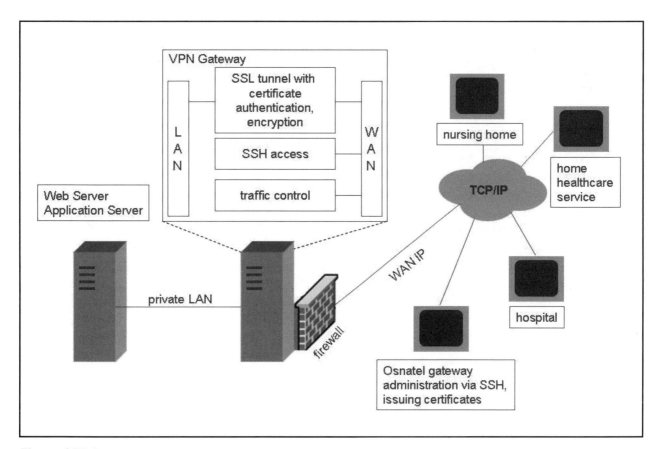

Figure 27F-1. *Security architecture for the Electronic Nursing Summary.*

health telematics platform has broadened and now includes other data sets, e.g., emergency data, medical discharge letters, the EPR, data provided by patients themselves, and electronic receipts given to patients by physicians after each treatment or diagnostic procedure. On the basis of experience in the use of so-called smart cards for about 70 million citizens (although for administrative purposes only), the decision to implement a similar card for health care data was intuitive. However, cards are insufficient as the sole media for health care data, because of their low storage capacity. Thus, the complementary concept of data residing on servers that can be accessed from the card has existed from the beginning, particularly with regard to the EPR and the EHR. Access to all health data is strictly controlled and generally requires an electronic health professional card (HPC). In addition to the 70 million cards to be issued to citizens, 430,000 HPCs are to be issued to health care providers.

This is the point at which the problem starts for nursing. There are two major barriers to German nurses being able to access the data. First, the Statutory Health Insurance Modernization Act restricts such access mainly to physicians, dentists, pharmacists, psychotherapists, and their assistants. Second, there are currently no plans for German nurses to receive HPCs; thus, for practical purposes, they have no access to the data unless they work in a hospital and are regarded as medical assistants. As the electronic HPC and the telematics infrastructure are still under construction, the opportunity for change is much greater than it will be after they have been finalized. From a technical viewpoint, it is important that the system architecture remain open enough to accommodate additional data and applications at a later stage, when the legal issues have been resolved. From an organizational point of view, professional associations for nurses must strongly support the use of HPCs and offer ideas on how to implement them within a short timeframe. The German Council of Nurses is making the electronic HPC a high priority, which is the first step toward change.

Denying nurses full access to data may severely jeopardize patient safety. If timely, complete information is not made available to all health care providers, preventable errors will occur. This concerns first of all data about medications and their administration,[16] as well as emergency data but also includes all data that can be retrieved from the EPR and the EHR, such as information citing risks, diagnoses, treatments, and contraindications to certain interventions.

The electronic HPC and the telematics platform in Germany are unique with regard to their potential for sharing patient information among health care professionals. However, to make it work, additional efforts will be needed that go beyond those required to implement the electronic prescription on the card. These efforts will certainly be required beyond 2006.

Summary

Implementation of DRGs, of integrated care delivery networks, and of the electronic HPC is exerting pressure on all health care providers to increase the use of IT-based methods including the EPR and the EHR, for processing clinical data. The major application of this record is to enable and enhance communication among health care professionals for an efficient, smooth approach to patient care. Supported by nursing managers, German hospitals are optimizing internal communication processes with the help of ordering systems, thereby paving the way for the EPR. However, strong advocacy for inclusion of nursing data in electronic documentation is still needed. Examples such as the Network for Continuity of Care in the Region of Osnabrueck illustrate nurses' awareness of the potential of structured, coded nursing data, and their willingness and efforts to make possible an electronic nursing summary. Using the German electronic HPC as an all-embracing means for sharing health data is a challenge not only for nurses but for all health care professionals. The role of nurses in this undertaking is to ensure that all patient data are represented in the system so that the risk of injury to patients can be minimized and decisions can be made on the basis of an optimal level of information.

References

1. World Health Organization. Country highlights on health, health systems, Germany 2004. Available at: http://www.euro.who.int/eprise/main/WHO/Progs/CHH/DEU/chap4/20041123_1?language=German. Accessed February 16, 2005.

2. Statistisches Bundesamt. Bevölkerung nach Bundesländern. Available at: http://www.destatis.de/ basis/d/bevoe/bevoe_pmtab.php. Accessed February 16, 2005.

3. Statistisches Bundesamt. Entwicklung der Gesundheitsausgaben Anteil am Bruttoinlandsprodukt (BIP). Available at: http://www.destatis.de-basis-d-gesu-gesugra2. Accessed February 16, 2005.

4. Statistisches Bundesamt. Gesundheitswesen Einrichtungen, Betten, Patientenbewegungen Krankenhäuser. Available at: http://www.destatis.de-basis-d-gesu-gesutab29. Accessed February 16, 2005.

5. Statistisches Bundesamt. Gesundheitspersonal nach Berufen. Available at: http://www.destatis.de/basis/d/gesu/gesutab1.php. Accessed February 16, 2005.

6. German diagnoses related groups. Available at: http://www.g-drg.de. Accessed February 23, 2005.

7. Fischer W. *Diagnosis Related Groups (DRGs) und Pflege.* Bern: Huber-Verlag, 2002.

8. Höhenrieder Kreis im Auftrag des Deutschen Pflegerate: G-DRG Änderungsvorschläge des Deutschen Pflegerates. Available at: http://www.fischer-zim.ch/temp/KombiDRG. Accessed February 23, 2005.

9. Hübner U, Sellemann B. Nursing in the information age: status quo and future of ICT use in German hospitals. In: M Fiesschi, et al, eds. *Medinfo 2004.* Amsterdam: IOS Press; 2004:376-380.

10. Healthcare Information and Management Systems Society (HIMSS). 14th annual HIMSS leadership survey. Available at: www.himss.org. Accessed February 16, 2005.

11. Hübner U, Sellemann, B. Current and future use of ICT for patient care and management in German acute hospitals—a comparison between the nursing and the hospital managers' perspectives. *Methods Inf Med.* In press.

12. Hübner U, Giehoff C. Why continuity of care needs computing: results of a quantitative document analysis. In: Surjan G, Engelbrecht R, and McNair P, eds. *Health Data in the Information Society.* Proceedings of MIE2002. Amsterdam: IOS Press; 2002:483-487.

13. Giehoff C, Hübner U, Berekoven B, et al. The interaction of NANDA and ICNP coded nursing diagnoses: an application driven perspective. In: M Fiesschi, et al, eds. *Medinfo 2004.* Amsterdam: IOS Press; 2004: 1615.

14. Heitmann KU, Schweiger R, Dudeck J. Discharge and referral data exchange using global standards—the SCIPHOX project in Germany. *Int J Med Inform.* 2003;70:195-203.

15. Ueckert F, Goerz M, Ataian M, et al. Empowerment of patients and communication with health care professionals through an electronic health record. *Int J Med Inform.* 2003;70:99-108.

16. Ball MJ, Weaver C, Abbott PA. Enabling technologies promise to revitalize the role of nursing in an era of patient safety. *Int J Med Inform.* 2003;69:29-38.

Case Study 27G

Nursing Documentation and Visibility: The Italian Case

Julita Sansoni, PhD and Maria Cristina Mazzoleni, DR Ing

Introduction: General Background

In order to understand the Italian health care system and computerization of health documents, particularly those related to nursing, a brief general background is necessary. It is also necessary to examine the role of nursing within the broader category of health specialists in the context of their education, development and role in health services as well as how data is collected and managed. In Italy, the National Health Service (NHS) guarantees health care to all residents whether they are Italians or not. Nonnationals belonging to the NHS have the right to the same type of care as Italian nationals. Citizens contribute to the cost of health procedures through taxing and payment of a "ticket" that varies according to the cost of the procedure. The role of the regional government in the planning and organization of health care is a basic feature of the NHS. The NHS governance structure gives complete autonomy of both organization and management to the regional health services, leaving national health planning and the establishment of uniform levels of care to the national government.

Health care is still focused on treatment and cure of illness rather than on prevention and wellness. Thus, services are organized toward a model of pathological procedures rather than to the prevention of such. Indeed, health institutions/hospitals are reimbursed by the Ministry and the regional government according to a system based on medical diagnosis (DRGs); whereas, nursing expenditure is part of the general costs and does not have a specific cost or reimbursement. The National Health Plan (2003–2005) takes into account the aims of the European Community and the need for coordination with European programs—Italy being one of its members.

Information plays an important role in communication between the NHS and citizens. In this context, computerization and data collection are fundamental, together with a taxonomic language and system development for continuous monitoring of health care and to render efficient services that must be so. Currently, in our NHS there are several critical situations in the field of computer systems and management control. Most prominently, the level of organization and computerization of the basic health service presents many weak points and in some cases computerization has not been implemented at all.[1] As a result, the use of computer systems is still limited in hospitals. Although there are some situations of excellence and areas of advanced technology (diagnostic imaging etc.), the general level of computerization in hospitals is still not fully developed, and the amount of data that can be collected systematically depends on the individual situation.

Computer and statistical training of health personnel (doctors, nurses, administrative staff) varies considerably although recently these subjects have been included in the training curricula of health professionals. In this climate of sudden, repeated changes, the patient's medical file becomes an indispensable source of information to reach some *strategic objectives in terms of management, organization, and evaluation of the quality of the services provided.* Capturing the patient's medical record data enables the administrative, economic, and qualitative assessment of the services provided and planning for a cost-effective budget. The analysis findings support rationalization and reorganization of the processes to achieve better services, as well as the development of scientific research, both clinical and epidemiological. Bearing in mind this development, nurses also are moving toward the *adoption of computerized instruments capable of documenting not only specific tasks and care but also the entire work process.*[2] Although autonomous professional associations are being formed to promote the electronic health record (EHR), the need for data that can be used from a nursing point-of-view, both to improve care and to professionally enrich nurses, becomes more and more evident.

Some Notes on Nursing Education and Professionalization

The scientific, and therefore professional, evolution of nurses has been slow in Italy. Although there have been encouraging legislative developments, management autonomy is slow both in terms of education and in orienting services. Only since 1990 has nursing education taken place entirely at a University, with programmed admission. At the end of the three years basic training course, the student has a qualification that allows him/her to practice nursing following licensure registration. A further two year course, comparable to a scientific Master, leads to a second-level degree. This type of University education, introduced in 2005 to replace a curriculum dating back to 1965, provides nurses with advanced clinical training. Management, education and research knowledge are taught, enabling them to be responsible for care and high managerial nursing responsibilities along with teaching capabilities.

After both the basic three year degree and the second-level degree, it is possible to attend various professional Master courses lasting one year that have taken the place of the specializations.

The general model of education available is, on the whole, biomedical since doctors in the Faculty of Medicine and Surgery mainly deliver it. To the University, the nursing role is basically one of *coordination* while the doctor is the *president* of the course. This matter is quite difficult to deal with because it has to do with nurse–doctor power and professional awareness of nurses themselves.

The general organization of university nursing professors is still being developed and is, for the time being, controlled by doctors. In fact, within the university, teaching roles are divided into full professors, associates, researchers and contract professors. Generally, the latter do not belong to the University and have annual contracts, often honorary, as a secondary activity. All nurses, with the exception of a very small part, belong to this category. The first Associate Professors of Nursing were nominated in 2000—today, eight associated professors have been nominated along with five researchers.

Patient Documentation and Nursing Training in Terms of Computerization

The documented clinical information takes on importance particularly in interdisciplinary terms and for integration of documentation. In fact, to work in an interdisciplinary manner requires not only mutual respect but also concrete disciplinary definitions. In other words, there must be a substantial acknowledgement of the specific contribution of each professional domain. As far as patient documentation is concerned, the law establishes the elements required for the medical file. Principally, it should be "compiled for every patient and include all personal details, diagnosis on admission, personal and family medical history, general physical examination, routine and specialist tests, diagnosis, treatment, outcome and sequel."[3] Other essential guidelines define how it is filled out, written, and archived.

The medical records law does not specifically refer to nursing documentation. Nurses have always documented their work by means of consignments at the end of each shift. As education and organization of care have improved, so has the quality of documentation. However, once again the method of documentation is influenced by the model of care. In fact, when the model is biomedical, the information collected will regard the situations and needs that originate from the medical diagnosis and that are related to the diagnostic-therapeutic item and the patient's clinical progression (vital signs and symptoms, medical prescriptions) rather than data pertinent to the autonomous and specific field of nursing.

Some advanced organizations have experimented with initiating integrated medical-nursing documentation, especially in environments such as intensive care and emergency. However, even today, there is no legal norm that refers directly to computerization of nursing documentation, even though a law regarding such administration explicitly established the need for computerization of all public files and therefore, indirectly mandated this for medical records as well. In particular, two articles of this law regard "ascertainment of computer competency and knowledge of foreign languages in all public recruitment." This ascertainment includes one's ability to use a computer as well as its most common applications.

In the current nursing education curriculum, computer science is one of the subjects taught at both first level degree and second level degree education and for which each university establishes its own syllabus. In general, computer courses are aimed at providing the student with skills enabling him/her to use a computer in caring and managing all the relative information. Depending on the single course, the syllabus covers the basic concepts of computer technology up to the subject of artificial intelligence. On the whole, the courses enable students to carry out caring activities, using a computer to perform all the operations necessary for creating and managing a document and for creating and employing an electronic calculation chart. Other arguments dealt with are the computer network, institutional computer systems, electronic clinical documents, computer applications for research, (data analysis and presentation of results as well as the instruments used for presentation). Courses are made up of a theoretical and a practical part, using simulations or explaining the use of the specific software.

Computerization

In Italy, for many years now there have been different types of experimentation and utilization of computerized medical and nursing documentation in very advanced settings. However, these sites are the exceptions and do not apply in a general context. Such situations can, in fact, be attributed to the dedication and far-sightedness of a single individual leader or to a convergence of favorable circumstances, rather than to specific planning and investment of the general health service. Several computerization projects exist: some regard the general computerization of health institutions and also include nursing such as the one employed in the Local Health Authority of Caserta.[3]

The computerized system used at Caserta includes three principle subsystems (Health, Administrative-Financial, and Staff) that are interconnected to sustain the managerial and clinical activities of the health structure involved. In the context of the health subsystem, the management procedure "Registry of Patients" and "CUP"—centralized system for information and booking—have been created (Il Melograno–Rome). These procedures control all access to the health structure, specifically the administrative procedures regarding patient admission, emergency admissions, and outpatient examinations. The system also supports the management of health events through the documentation of admissions, as well as through the medical, outpatient, and nursing charts. Functionality extends to the computerization of services provided by radiological examinations, laboratory tests, and ambulatory care. In-patient ward management includes the medical file, anesthetic file, specialist consultations, requested examinations and results, and management of operating theaters. The Melograno system being used at Caserta is just one example, but many other projects are under way, some of which have a nationwide leadership.

Evaluation Shows Benefits for Both Patients and Professionals

Other projects are local, developed by specifically interested groups. One example of this is the S. Pietro Hospital in Rome in which since the year 2000, the entire management of nursing documentation has been successfully computerized in a maternity ward. This project was born during a recurrent educational course concerning nursing documentation, in which a working group consisting of about ten nurses was formed.[4] The working group defined the requirements for the computerized Nursing Chart with the purpose of having available a solution capable of helping in daily activities and facilitating the registration of information for the benefit of the patient. The product of this was integrated in the Melograno operative system. In functional terms, nursing documentation consists of several different display charts for data collection, organization of care, and consultation of nursing procedures. Other specific charts deal with treatment and drug management. Thus, it is possible to have a picture that constantly reflects the status of the information collected and enriched with a nursing discharge file as well as the computerization of some protocols and procedures. The maternity nursing documentation project, in particular, is being met with great success. The evaluations are quite good in terms of resulting in better care, and the project has received the backing of managerial bodies. It will soon be extended to other operative units.

Another important example of computerization is a project that has involved the nurses working in the infectious diseases divisions of several hospitals in the Tuscany region of Italy.[5] Ferri and team 2005[5] describe how a computerized system is used daily and constantly by nurses working in the Infectious Diseases Ward of Prato Hospital. They began in 1997 with just one personal computer and now have eleven computers available around the ward. The initial resistance encountered was the result of prejudice and fear around the implementation, but now several programs are under way for management of preadmission procedures and all the procedures related to hospitalization including nursing documentation. At the beginning in 1997, the program was only used to improve management of antiretroviral drugs given to outpatients, but since then, a flow register has been kept, and the program is now used for the entire management of all information regarding care, both medical and nursing, and including outpatients. Based on the success of the Prato Project and its demonstrated benefits, a nursing expert group has formed and is currently experimenting with the possibility of extending the program to other hospital wards.

Another noteworthy experience concerns mobile computerization of nursing documentation implemented in a Tuscany hospital.[6] Some difficulties were encountered at the beginning because it was necessary to not only prepare personnel but also to change the way in which work was organized. The nurses decided which type of documentation to adopt and which data to memorize. Figure 27G-1 shows the screen for nursing documentation that was designed to cover the main nursing tasks performed in a shift, and Figure 27G-2 shows the screen used to do morning shift rounds by nurses. Today, this nursing documentation system is also used in other divisions besides nursing wards, including the surgical, endoscopic, day surgery, and other wards.

Besides the computerized medical chart, the work-group has also employed or produced standard or flexible care protocols that are monitored electronically. On admission, by means of direct observation of the patient, data are registered using a hand-held computer (PDA) as shown in Figure 27G-3. The PDA is used throughout the work shift and is synchronized on the computer desktop in order to transfer the collected data. This is done via a serial port or USB employing a simple cable connection. It is also possible to employ a wireless Bluetooth or wireless network connection. The advantages of using a hand-held computer for the computerized medical chart are multiple, not the least of which is the possibility of memorizing and having quick access to diagnostic, therapeutic and behavioral protocols, guidelines and procedures, drug registry, diets, and other key clinical information.

Computerization, particularly in day surgery, has made it possible to create a fast system to integrate the collected data; a system to safeguard the privacy of this data has also been created. One advantage that should not be underestimated is the possibility of real-time consultation of pre-, peri- and postoperative nursing protocols. These experiences, although limited in Italy, are examples of an empowerment of the nursing profession in the interest of the patient. In fact, this system has acted as a support for the continuous implementation of nursing protocols. One of its limits is the pre-established number of fields (50). The

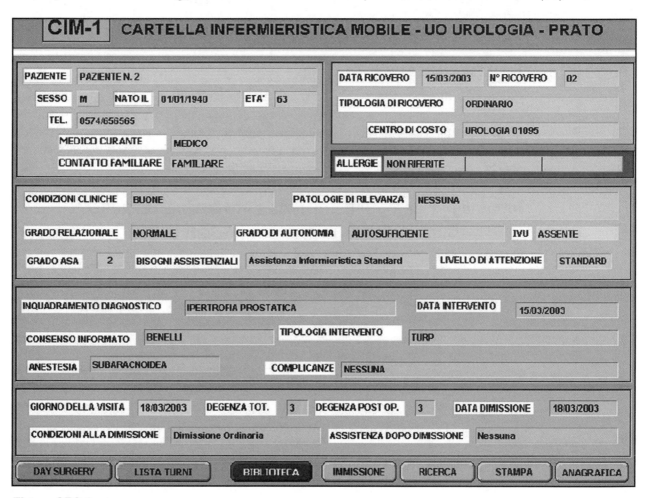

Figure 27G-1. *Computerized nursing documentation: main mask. (Chiti M et al, with permission.)*

CIM-2 CARTELLA INFERMIERISTICA MOBILE TURNO MATTINA

DATI GENERALI

PAZIENTE: PAZIENTE N. 2 | NATO IL: 01/01/1940 | N° RICOVERO: 02

DATA DEL TURNO: 16/03/2003
I.P.: COLELLA CACCAMO

PROFILASSI ANTIBIOTICA: NESSUNA
PROFILASSI ENDOCARDITE: NESSUNA
PROFILASSI ANTITROMBOEMBOLICA: NADROPARINA CALCICA

STATO SOGG.: NESSUNA SEGNALAZIONE
DIETA: SEMILIQUIDA | PURGA: NO
ALVO: 0 | LIQUIDI: NO

TEMPERATURA: APIRESSIA | POLSO: ARITMICO
P.A.: NORMOTESO | RESPIRO: EUPNOICO
DIURESI: 1000 CC | URINE: LAVATURA DI CARNE

FERITA: | TERAPIA LOCALE: | CATETERE: DUFOUR | LAVAGGIO V.: FLUSSO VELOCE
DRENAGGIO: | QUANTITA': | MANOVRE: | SONDINO:
DOLORE: ASSENTE | VOMITO: | MOBILIZZAZIONE: RIPOSO A LETTO

TERAPIA MEDICA: LEVOFLOXACINA 500 MG 1 CP AL DI'
TERAPIA ANTALGICA: KETOROLAC 1 F. OGNI 6 ORE/24 ORE
EMOTRASFUSIONE: NO | OSSIGENO: NO

ESAMI: ROUTINE
ES. STRUMENTALI:
CONSULENZE:

CONSEGNE T.M.: CONTROLLARE IL LAVAGGIO VESCICALE

TURNO POM.-NOTTE | STAMPA

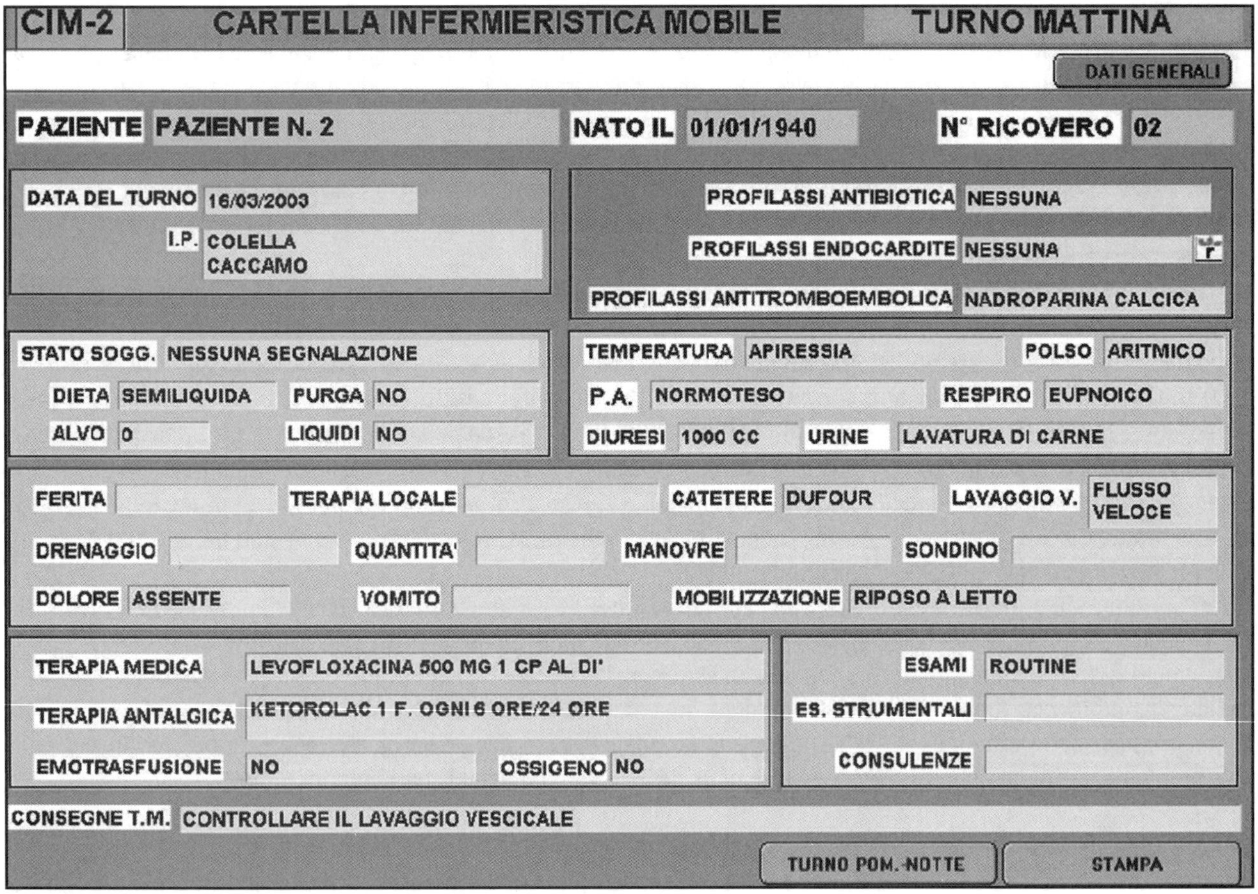

Figure 27G-2. *Mobile nursing chart. Morning shift.*

CIM mobile nursing documentation is structured starting with an analysis of the care requirements of the patients and their registration by means of a preordained number of fields to which a sequence of pre-encoded answers are given, documented by a mere touch of the pen to the PDA. The data collection charts have been submitted to continuous revision to make them more basic and useful.

Terminology and Standardization of Nursing Language: Current State and Future Prospectives

Another major area of interest is nursing's professional attempt to standardize and therefore make uniform a language that can be used for documenting patient care data and for daily use. In the experiences previously described, no specific language was used in taxonomic terms but, looking toward the future, a number of major initiatives are already under way. This initiative involves the Italian translation and validation of the International Classification for Nursing Practice (ICNP® Beta2). This project's aim is to demonstrate the benefits of care using a system that allows nurses to use a common, standardized language.[7,8] This challenge was initiated on world-wide scale by the International Council of Nurses (ICN) and was taken on in Italy by the *Consociazione Nazionale Associazioni Infermieri,* (CNAI):Nursing Societies Association together with the Advanced Nursing Sciences School of Rome La Sapienza University (SDAI).

Today in Italy, several classification systems exist that have been created in different ways and with different aims for documenting and communicating with the health care team; however, none of these completely fill the requirements of a general, uniform language standard.[9] The ICNP®, as described in the Web site of the ICN (www.icn.ch) is made up of a conceptual pyramid gradually subdivided into three main elements: nursing phenomena/principles, nursing tasks, and the outcome of nursing actions. ICNP® is divided

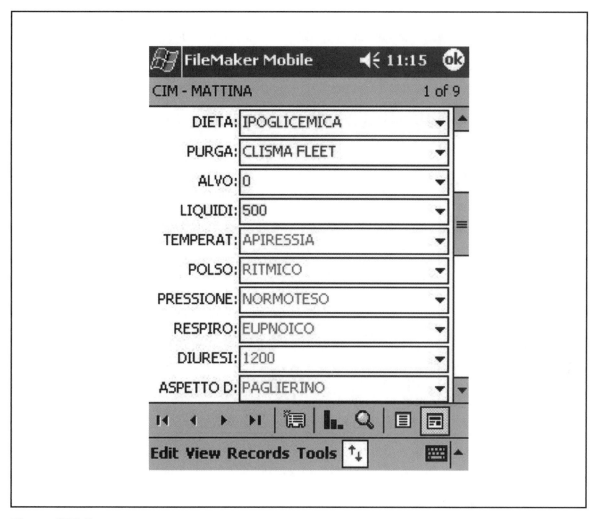

Figure 27G-3. *Palmar input for nursing plan.*

into axes containing the phenomena and procedures that make up nursing, in a tree-like structure. Inside and between the axes, one can find the terms, or labels given to a combination of concepts contained in the axes, that are necessary to identify the nursing diagnoses as defined by the system itself. It is then possible to indicate the nursing actions by identifying the specific axes—the action, purpose, means, benefit, time necessary, and others. By evaluating the course, it is possible to identify the results of a specific nursing task on a single phenomenon and assess its outcome.

The translation of the ICNP® into Italian has presented several difficulties. It was performed in a strictly scientific manner by a system of translation, peer revision, and back translation. Naturally, some problems were encountered regarding conceptual, grammatical, and structural aspects. Even with these limits, we believe that widespread use of the ICNP® represents the first step toward sharing a common nursing language and that this could be used in the future to offer far wider opportunities. The following section describes stages and results of the Italian experimentation with the terminology provided by the ICNP®. The aim of this experimentation was to produce a significant amount of nursing documentation collected in a database so that comparisons would be possible at an international level, as well as to provide a data bank for future research.

One example of translating into the new terminology is that of "arterial pressure measurement," which in the Italian language can be expressed in at least five different ways—all with the same meaning. In ICNP® reference terminology, "arterial pressure measurement" is well identified by a single term that represents and specifies the task performed. The significance of the value of ICNP's specificity and economy of terminology is demonstrated in the findings of a retrospective study on nursing documentation.[10] The study compared the amount of nursing diagnoses extrapolated from the nursing documentation in use and those formulated on the basis of the documentation elaborated using ICNP® terminology. The authors found that in the traditional data collection setting, the greater the number of patient-days, the lower the number of nursing diagnoses. The authors concluded that the accuracy and completeness of nursing documentation is related to the way data are collected. In fact, the caring response was presumably less precise and aware because much of the data was collected in a less relevant manner. In this instance, ICNP® nursing diagnosis, treatment, and outcome concepts and terms were adopted[10] for the creation or revision of protocols with the result that nursing documentation became more precise and explicit.

The aim of this Italian ICNP® translation experiment was to make it possible to put a standardized, coded structure to nursing terminology. With this standardization, it would be possible to produce a significant amount of coded nursing documentation that could be captured and stored in a computer system. This database would then allow comparisons at an international level to support future research. After adequate development, the ICNP® could also be used for management purposes, for calculating the weight of caring tasks and thus attributing a financial value to nursing procedures. Today, this calculation of general daily nursing activities is included in the general budget of the hospital, and there is no specific reimbursement.

In a study conducted by the Advanced Nursing Studies School (SDAI) of the La Sapienza Rome University, nursing activities were simulated in order to assess them in financial terms. The medical reimbursement relative to "cerebral stroke" was compared with the financial entity of the nursing tasks required to fulfil the care requirements of that specific diagnostic related group (DRG). Different scenarios were simulated and calculations made to evaluate nursing tasks, the cost of those tasks and activities, the hourly nursing salary, as well as other parameters. The result of this simulation was that nursing activities accounted for as much as 85 percent of the medical reimbursement. Undoubtedly, although these findings require further study and verification, they will definitely bring benefits to nursing care in terms of gaining recognition of the substantial contributions that nursing care makes in acute care delivery.

Another study conducted by the Advanced Nursing Studies group from La Sapienza Rome University involved an investigation conducted in a pediatric division of a hospital in Rome. The purpose of the study was to register nursing tasks and diagnoses by use of question-sheets specifically created for the purpose of data collection. Data was collected throughout three complete shifts for thirty patients. The grid on the charts allowed data to be recorded according to the multiaxial layout of the ICNP®. The results of this study (see Table 27G-1) made it possible to identify 636 tasks in axis A, 52 percent of which corresponded exactly to the ICNP®classification. Of the terms included in axis B, 74 percent presented an exact fit with the ICNP® classification. This study showed that only 14.3 percent of nursing tasks had an evaluation of the outcome of the nursing diagnosis.

Another interesting finding can be seen in Table 27G-1 where it is evident that in axis A (focus) and axis B (judgement/evaluation), up to 75.3 percent of all nursing activity can be defined by a few terms. The terms employed mainly identify basic needs and confirm that, as mentioned above, Italian nurses are still tied to a biomedical care model.[11]

ICNP® Evaluation of Nurse Electronic Charts and Protocols

In the following section, a project is described in the form of an abstract of a paper[12] presented at a Medical Informatics Europe MIE 2002 conference. Its objective is to demonstrate the attempts made to promote the use of NI and electronic nursing records, in particular, adoption of standard terminology, e.g., ICNP®. The project described is a part of a wider project developed with a grant from the Italian Ministry of Health. In this work, we used the ICNP® to standardize the terminology currently used in both the nursing clinical charts and nursing protocols in a hospital setting. The salient steps of the projects were:

1. Choosing two pilot wards in our hospital and analyzing a sufficient number of nursing documentation charts
2. Developing a nursing information system, using a relational database and a Web-based interface, for distributed access

Table 27G-1. Nursing Documentation Terms Mapped to Italian-translated ICNP®

TERMS	AXIS A—FOCUS	TERMS	AXIS B—JUDGEMENT
8	52.3 %	7	53.3%
15	67.8%	12	66.6%
23	75.3%	17	75.1%

3. Developing an ICNP® browser
4. Integrating ICNP® within both the information system created and an existing electronic protocols editor
5. Tailoring the interface to the specific ward

The User Needs Analysis: Methodology

Twelve and eighteen complete clinical charts were collected from the two wards (Pneumology and Cardiology Rehabilitation) respectively. The mean duration of hospitalization was 19 days in the Pneumology ward and 7 days in the Cardiology Rehabilitation ward, for a total of 354 days analyzed. The initial evaluation of the patient was recorded using the NANDA chart, with the daily nursing activities written in free text format. As shown by analysis, the "most used" sentences that nurses write to document their activity were highlighted and selected for the checklists in the electronic patient record (EPR) interface. The lists are different for the two wards. When possible, an ICNP® code was associated with a sentence. The final result is that nurses continue to fill the records by choosing from a list of sentences they are familiar with, but the EPR only stores codified information.

ICNP within the Electronic Patient Record and Nursing Protocols

For the two pilot wards, a ward-tailored Web-based interface was implemented, whereas the EPR remains the same and relies on a relational Database Management System. Figure 27G-3 shows the form for the nursing care plan. From there, the nurse is allowed to choose sentences and combine them to build a more complex concept. In rare cases, when the concept description is not found within the predefined lists, the nurse can look for it by browsing the complete ICNP® terminology. Using the right panel on the screen, a nurse can choose from a list of terms and also obtain a description of each term. Nurses are allowed to insert free text, but this entry will have no code associated with it. Concerning protocols, GUIDE, a tool for the formal representation of clinical practice guidelines and protocols, was developed.[13] Once they have been computerized, guidelines or protocols may be integrated with the EPR. An example of such integration concerns a pressure-ulcer prevention guideline.[14] GUIDE adopted a terminology server derived from SNOMED but now we also add ICNP®.

Statistical calculations regarding actions and diagnoses were performed and recorded during the 354 patient-days considered in the study, and regarding guideline/protocol tasks, in relation to the possibility of encoding them using ICNP®. Tables 27G-2 and 27G-3 present a summary of the results. It is important to notice that the totally encoded tasks are few.

The results of this project showed, through a text analysis of several nursing clinical charts, that there is an absolute need for standardization of terminology if we want to use data for information exchange and reliable statistics. We have proposed a system that allows, as far as possible, to encode nurse inputs into an EPR, without dramatically changing the nurses' reporting style. It also allows unification of documentation encoding within the EPR and enables capturing and linking of data for guidelines and protocols. Our conclusion is that the continuous improvement of the terminology system and a thorough experimentation could lead to ICNP® becoming a widely used system in Italy.

Summary

In this case study, we present different projects that emphasize how Italian nurses are trying to widen their knowledge, make their work more visible and demonstrate how nursing care benefits patients. The initia-

Table 27G-2. ICNP Encoding of Clinical Charts

	% phenomena totally encoded	% phenomena partially encoded	% actions totally encoded	% actions partially encoded
EPRs	65.38	0.04	80	20

Table 27G-3. ICNP Encoding of Protocols

	number of tasks	totally encoded	partially encoded	not encoded
Central venous catheter	43	11 (25.6%)	23 (53.5%)	9 (20.9%)
Pressure-ulcer prevention	21	10 (47.6%)	8 (38.1%)	3 (14.3%)
Surgical wounds	27	7 (25.9%)	18 (66.7%)	2 (7.4%)

tives reflected in these projects are undoubtedly professional but they also have strong political implications. In fact, we believe that it is necessary to have a nursing director alongside medical directors in both Central and Regional government in order to transmit general policy and to guide the development of nursing care at the local level. The administrators in Italian health care are predominantly physicians, a fact that results in a medical view of health matters that does not leave much room for related professions to rise to equal level and therefore to develop in terms of resources and opportunities. Nursing still has the challenge of gaining a collaborative team member status with physicians in the practice and management of health care. To achieve this professional status in Italy, it is necessary to develop education, management, and research, using a multiprofessional strategy, while respecting each profession's specific requirements and competencies. Only in this way can computerization of each of the aspects of health information be sustained by a specific budget and planned in accordance with national and local standards. Dedication, that must be present even at political level, to the single profession, together with clear general objectives and adequate resources, will lead to the creation of efficient services that fulfill the needs of the public.

References

1. M. Geddes da Filicaia. (2001) La riforma ter, Salute e Territorio, 124-5.
2. Motta PC, (1999) "Cartella infermieristica e personalizzazione dell'assistenza" in Collegio IP.AS.VI. di Sassari (a cura di), La cartella infermieristica come strumento di sviluppo professionale: prospettive di attuazione, atti della 'Giornata di Studio' promossa dal Collegio IP.AS.VI. di Sassari.
3. www.aslcaserta1.it/forum2003/2.htm Produced by ASL Caserta. Accessed on February 10, 2005.
4. Working group–Infermieri professionali reparto UTIR Ospedale S. Pietro FBF Roma: julita.sansoni@uniroma1.it.
5. Working group: E: Livestri - Divisione Malattie Infettive Ospedale Azienda Ospedaliera USL 4 Prato, L'informatizzazione di un reparto di Malattie infettive, da: www.aimi.it/articoli/20040524185253.html. Accessed February 23, 2005.
6. M Chiti, G Sabatini, R Cacciamo, S Cusati, S Nocentini et al. La cartella infermieristica informatizzata mobile (CIM) in day surgery urologia, Nursing Oggi, 2003; 3, 25-28.
7. Sansoni J, L Luzzi, M Degan, G Woinowski, E La Torre et al. Italian translation and validation of the ICNP Beta (International Classification for Nursing Practice) Traduzione e validazione italiana della Classificazione Internazionale per la Pratica Infermieristica (ICNP Beta), Professioni Infermieristiche 2002: 55;2,66.
8. Italian group ICNP translation: Julita Sansoni. (Roma), Lucilla Luzzi (Roma), Elena La Torre (Roma), Gloria Woinowski (Roma). Mario Degan (Mestre), Stesura informatica: Marco Giustini (Roma), Traduzione random: Suzanne Goopy (Brisbane, Australia), 1998, www.icn.ch.
9. Coenen A, Wake M. (1996) Developing a database for an International Classification for Nursing Practice (ICNP). *International Nursing Review.* 1996; 43(6):183-187.
10. Degan M, De Rossi R, Boldrin L (2002) Use of ICNP taxonomy to built nursing protocols: an experience, Un'esperienza applicativa del sistema tassonomico ICNP nella costruzione di protocolli infermieristici, Professioni Infermieristiche. 2002; 55(2):78-118.
11. Sansoni J, Giustini M (2002) Nursing visibility: could the I.C.N.P. help? Visibilità infermieristica: l'ICNP potrebbe aiutare? Professioni Infermieristiche. 2002; 55(2):66-77.

12. Rognoni C, Mazzoleni MC, Quaglini S, Kumar A, Nicola L, Santoro C. Using ICNP for nurse electronic charts and protocols in rehabilitation divisions. *Stud Health Technol Inform.* 2002;90:798-803.

13. Quaglini S, Dazzi L, Gatti L, Stefanelli M, Fassino C, Tondini C. (1998) Supporting tools for guideline development and dissemination. *Artificial Intelligence Medicine* 1998, Sep-Oct; 14(1-2):119-37.

14. Quaglini S, Grandi M, Baiardi P, Mazzoleni MC, Fassino C, Franchi G, Melino S. (2000) Computerized guideline for pressure ulcer prevention. *International J Med Informatics* 2000: Sep; 58-59:207-17.

Case Study 27H

Spain: The Growth and Development of Nursing and Information Systems

Myriam Fernández Martín, PhD Candidate, RN and José Siles González, PhD, RN

Nursing in Spain is currently undergoing major change and professional growth. Nursing achieved university status in 1977, and over the ensuing twenty-five years, it has struggled to find its own academic *raison d'être* and socioprofessional identity. In this case study, the authors focus on the efforts the nursing profession has taken to gain greater recognition of nursing as a science and to implement the use of information technology (IT) to support a standard nursing model and language terminology.

The Path Toward Technological Innovation in the Use of Nursing Records

The massive changes in health care occurring in Europe are driven by standardization initiatives defined by the European Union (EU), as well as by nationally-based electronic health record (EHR) undertakings. National health IT initiatives are currently happening all across Europe, including Spain. These rapid technology innovations are creating the need for changes in countries' educational programs, and Spanish nursing is playing an active role in these processes. The Declaration of Bologna defined the strategy for European higher education programs and set 2010 as the date for having the changes in place. The plan is made up of two-year completion phases, each of which will conclude with a relevant cabinet conference to review what has been achieved and to establish the guidelines for the future. The significance of the initiatives for nursing in Spain is that the Declaration of Bologna is making it possible to establish the first nursing PhD programs in universities across the country.

Nursing in Spain: Background

In contrast to Florence Nightingale's foundations for nursing in the Commonwealth countries and the U.S., nursing in Spain evolved over the past century as a religious-vocational calling. The nursing role derived from the tradition of serving and the belief that, by providing care to those who need it most, one could achieve eternal salvation. As scientific knowledge expanded over the late nineteenth and twentieth centuries, Spanish nursing took on a secular-vocational direction based on social aid and illness and healing modalities. By the 1950s, nursing was clearly defined as an auxiliary to medicine; nurses were able to undertake tasks derived from the practice of medicine, but not to act in any independent capacity. Spain's professional nursing leaders succeeded in elevating nursing education to a university degree level in the late 1970s as part of the effort to raise nursing to a full professional status. In 2005, this professional autonomy stage has culminated in establishing Spanish nursing as a provider of social-medical-scientific services. Nursing practice is based on holistic concepts and is derived from a theoretical-scientific approach to patient care. Nursing's new and evolving identity stems from its sense of being an autonomous profession and discipline.

Undoubtedly, the current state of nursing in Spain comes from the fact that for centuries, care has lacked conceptual systematization. Nursing history in Spain even lacks the documentation or tradition that would allow the rebuilding of the past from primary sources.[1] Because most nurses are women, nursing education suffered the same fate as education for women in general. Educational opportunities for women beyond secondary school is a recent phenomenon, in reality, only a generation deep. As one might expect, the phenomenon of nursing research in Spain has been slow to occur. But with the move to place nursing in university-based programs in the last few years, the nursing research field is expanding rapidly.

As technology and complexity of care exploded from the 1960s onward, nursing education was formalized and expanded to meet the demands. To define the discipline and knowledge base of nursing as separate from medicine, nurse leaders in Spain began searching for theoretical models for nursing care. The first such models were formed in the 1950s and evolved into major schools of thought in the 1970s. For Spanish nurses, the limitation of the later models was that they failed to differentiate nursing from other disciplines.

With the creation of the North America Nursing Diagnosis Association (NANDA) in 1982,[2] however, Spain initiated efforts to adopt diagnostics for nursing. The first attempts to use the Spanish NANDA nursing diagnoses were made with paper charts.[3] The paper-based system proved to be as arduous to use as it was to maintain. Thus, the first effort to develop a nursing clinical documentation solution came as a result of these early efforts. Development focused on using the diagnostic labels from NANDA, with objectives instead of outcome criteria and with activities instead of interventions.

Adopting a Conceptual Model

Modern technology seemed absent from Spain's nursing reality until a very short time ago. Internet use in homes started around 2000, and the first attempts to implement information systems in hospitals started around 1998. However, from these endeavors came the idea to use an electronic nursing record that was based on a conceptual nursing model and that included care planning with a standard language.

Nursing thought leaders in Spain recognized the need for a scientific model to structure the practice of nursing, as well as to support research. Pragmatically, a nursing model was also needed as a reference marker that would allow nurses to differentiate their profession from other health care providers. A professional nurse needs to be able to explain the nature of the job, as well as the underlying nursing management and administration responsibilities, to coworkers and users, in a model that reflects care provisions. Moreover, a model guides activities, helps set professional obligations, and defines a unified goal to which the nurse can refer. It therefore serves as a practical and theoretical instrument that helps nurses to communicate in a clearer, more significant manner, as well as a guide for caring, teaching, and investigating.[4]

The development of the first computerized nursing solution in Spain had a huge impact on nursing across the country. It was the first solution created by nurses for nurses, and in the beginning it used the Virginia Henderson model as the basis for its development.[5] Assessments were made using the fourteen necessities of the model and included a wizard for the diagnostics in the assessment process, suggested objectives, and planned activities. This nursing solution also introduced the use of the bifocal Carpenito model to capture risk for potential complications and to have it included in the patient's plan of care.[6] In addition, it provided the possibility of working with standardized and individual plans and with protocols.

Although this nursing system had large gaps, it represented the first approach to standardized nursing care in Spain. Today, the main nursing model used in Spain for hospital practice is based on Virginia Henderson's model. The Henderson model has become widely adopted across Spain because it is straightforward in its language and concepts, is logical, and has proven easy to use.[4]

Henderson defines the role of nurses as follows: "The unique function of the nurse is to assist the individual, sick or well, in the performance of those activities contributing to achieving good health or recovery, a peaceful death or tasks that he or she would perform unaided if they had the necessary strength, will or knowledge. This must be done in such a way so as to help them gain independence as rapidly as possible."[5] A series of basic concepts and subconcepts of the Henderson model can be extracted from this definition. But its most basic principle is that an individual has fourteen vital human needs that define health, well-being, and independence. Nursing care addresses the actions required to support, meet, or maintain the fourteen needs.

Henderson clearly expressed her intention simply to write a definition without ever hoping to turn it into a model for the scientific community.[7] Other critics believe it cannot be considered a model (in itself) because of the lack of precise definitions of certain essential aspects, thus creating conceptual and professional confusion. For this very reason, some critics are more in favor of Dorothea Orem's model because they consider it to be the only model built on a self-help care concept.[8] Orem's model is not as commonly used because it is more complex. It requires a higher level of training to use, and it adopts a more complicated language that nurses cannot relate to their daily duties. For this reason, considerably fewer hospitals have gone with this model than with the Henderson model.

It must be emphasized that in Spain all critics agree on the importance of using a model, no matter which one. The model must explain what it is doing, what the foundation of the action is, and what results should be expected from the practice. The nursing electronic record must have the capacity to adopt any nursing model that guides its practice; its importance lies in the referent use.

The Use of Standardized Language

The move to use standardized language occurred at the end of the 1980s, with several attempts at implementation on paper. Information systems quickly showed their power to support the use of diagnostic labels in a standardized way. The increasing direction of people toward the European Union (EU) and to a more multicultural society is making the lack of a common nursing language a growing problem in Spain and in Europe in general.

One of the main issues, dealt with at the first European Nursing Forum (1997) and considered essential for professional practice, was the need to use a common language in terms of diagnosis, interventions, and nursing outcomes. The goals for a common nursing language are to enable nursing to communicate their care focus and outcomes; to support the ability to capture and analyze nursing data; to evaluate care outcomes and costs; and to further knowledge development.[9]

Progressive social and technical development, constantly mounting demands, and improved health services point toward a growing interest in basing the profession on scientific criteria. Thanks to World Health Organization (WHO) recommendations, a number of studies and connections have contributed to the international expansion of nursing diagnoses.[10] The NANDA taxonomy (classification) was the first introduced into Spanish electronic records because it is compatible with the Henderson model and is one of the most well-known systems. Moreover, NANDA has been built by nurses from many countries and is ever growing.[11] Although some critics believe that NANDA diagnostics should adopt a cultural change in order to be applied to the clinical Spanish community, all agree that NANDA should be used in spite of this criticism. Importantly, NANDA is also being considered by the WHO for inclusion in the International Classification of Diseases, 10th revision.

The current trend in the Spanish health care system is the demand for the incorporation of the Nursing Interventions Classification and Nursing Outcomes Classification into the electronic nursing records.[12] The demand must be considered as feasible only in the context of using a clinical information system to support documentation, because of the difficulty of achieving the goal on paper media. Most nursing managers throughout hospitals in Spain are in agreement on the requirement for standardized coded language to support nursing documentation.

The Requirements of Spanish Electronic Nursing Records

The initial nursing documentation system introduced in Spain attempted to include nursing language, because this was Spanish nurses' first experience with computerized solutions, and there was a lot left to do. They encountered huge difficulties in practical integration for two major reasons. First, many nurses had not used a computer before (fortunately, this has changed with time). Few were familiar with practical use of the nursing care process and the scientific method, model use, or normalized languages. As a result, the workload in nursing units increased because of time needed for the learning process.

Second, some isolated, relatively inflexible nursing solutions did not allow for a completely paperless documentation system. In addition, the separation of nursing from other members of the care team who had to work in paper did not support the sharing of data and coordination of patient care. The end result was only partial use of the computerized solutions, mostly for graphs, intake/output, and progress comments, which ultimately led to disappointed users.

In designing the next generation of clinical nursing solutions, we can ask Spanish nurses for feedback, refer to what has been published by organizations such as the SEEUE (Spanish Society of Urgency and Emergency Nursing), and consider the ideas developed in forums such as AENTDE (Spanish Association of Nomenclature, Taxonomy, and Nursing Diagnostic). The ideal electronic nursing chart should then be integrated to the unique patient chart and have the following characteristics:

- The nursing documentation record needs to be a legally adopted document, accepted by the institution whose personnel are going to make use of it, because it will be part of each patient's medical record. Essentially, it must identify response patterns and changes in the patient's condition, state the care given, analyze the quality of the care, make certain that the care is continued, ensure understanding of the basic nursing role, justify services rendered, and generate a database.
- The chart needs be designed and structured so that it highlights different stages of the process, because the nursing record is a reflection of the nursing process, i.e., assessment, problems (concerns of the indi-

vidual nursing professional and those that arise because of collaboration with another colleague), outcomes, interventions, and results evaluation.

- The look and feel of the screens must be clear and highly visual, with an attractive design and layout so that the health care professional can easily access essential information. Therefore, it is necessary to use the most advanced technology available in the design phase (with professional advice).
- The nursing record must be founded on a theoretical nursing model that guides design by linking all the sections that must be adopted. The record's contents must be structured according to the principles of the chosen model.
- The nursing record must accommodate standardized nursing language and the nursing process, capturing problems, interventions, and outcomes to enable evaluation of care and evidence-based practice.
- The patient's record should read like a map and, with the appropriate training, to do so quickly and efficiently. Users should be given courses and workshops on the nursing process and nursing records and should be provided with quick reference pocket-sized guides, especially at the beginning.

Discussion and Future Directions

The trend in Spanish nursing is clear. The marketplace is demanding a clinical information system that provides for a unique patient chart, uses a nursing model, and enables standardized language. This level of IT use in care delivery settings requires a considerable commitment to educate and prepare nurses who are not currently practicing in this way or using IT tools to this extent. To gain adoption and a smooth transition to the new state with computer systems, nurse leaders and managers need to provide continuous support. With the use of EHR systems that have a nursing focus and content, Spanish nursing is embarking on a journey. If the right steps are taken, the technology will support its professional practice and identity. The potential is there, and Spanish nurses must embrace this path to ensure that the practice framework for nursing comes from nursing, not from other disciplines.

As Alfaro explains in her book *Critical Thought: A Practical Approach,* the future belongs to those who learn to achieve critical thinking and to maximize their mental power. Alfaro maintains that critical thinking is the key to solving problems and that nurses who do not think this way become part of the problem.[13] Spanish nurse leaders understand that shifting nursing in Spain from a task-based to a critical-thinking based practice has to be done sensibly while keeping a clear objective. The goal is to base nursing practice on scientific principles and methods and to see this reflected uniformly across the country. In other words, the drive is to provide the knowledge base and tools that allow nurses to make judgments based on evidence (facts), instead of on conjecture or tradition.

At this point in the journey, Spanish nursing is at the stage of *aprehender a aprehender,* meaning "learning to learn." The EHR must be the tool that helps nursing move through this stage to full professional maturity and evidence-based practice. Like other EU countries, Spain is embarking on major EHR initiatives that introduce opportunities and support for the advancement of nursing education, research, and practice. Many of the EU's programs are pushing for standardized university degree programs for nursing across all EU countries, and this is accelerating the pace of change in Spain as well as the other EU nations. In addition, these programs are supporting the use of standardized clinical terminology in EHR systems that include nursing practice, documentation, and minimum data sets. With education at the master's and doctoral levels, nurses will have the preparation needed to conduct nursing research. With the structured databases captured from EHR systems, nurses will have the data to support rigorous research to advance nursing knowledge and science. The future for nursing in Spain is very positive. We need only to seize the opportunity and step across the threshold.

References

1. Hernández CJ. *Historia de la Enfermería*. Madrid: McGraw-Hill; 1999.
2. North American Nursing Diagnosis Association (NANDA). Nursing Diagnosis: Definitions and Classification 1995–1996. Philadelphia: North American Nursing Diagnosis Association, 1993.
3. Ugalde M, Rigol A. *Diagnósticos de Enfermería*. Taxonomía NANDA. Barcelona: Masson; 1995.
4. Fernandez FC, Martí N. *El proceso de atención de enfermería*. Estudio de Casos. Barcelona: Masson; 1993.
5. Henderson V. *The Nature of Nursing: A Definition and Its Implications for Practice, Research, and Education.* New York: Macmillian, 1966.
6. Carpenito L. *Manual de Diagnósticos de Enfermería*. 5th ed. Madrid: McGraw-Hill; 1995.

7. Henderson V. *La naturaleza de la Enfermería. Reflexiones 25 años después.* Madrid: McGraw-Hill Interamericana; 1995.

8. Hernandez CJ, Esteban AM. *Fundamentos de la Enfermería.* Teoría y Método. Madrid: McGraw-Hill; 1999.

9. Luis Rodrigo MT, Fernandez FC, Navarro Gomez MV. *De la Teoría a la Práctica. El pensamiento de Virginia Henderson en el siglo XXI.* Barcelona: Masson; 2002.

10. Corrales ME, Muñoz E, Fernández MM, Grijalva UR, Herranz MV. *Contribución de la Unión Europea a la Enfermería.* Madrid: Asociación Española de Enfermería Docente; 2004.

11. North American Nursing Diagnosis Association (NANDA). *Diagnósticos enfermeros. Definiciones y clasificación 2003–2004.* Madrid: Elsevier; 2003.

12. McCloskey JC, Bulecheck GM. *Clasificación de intervenciones de enfermería NIC Cuarta edición.* Madrid: Elsevier; 2005.

13. Alfaro R. *El Pensamiento Crítico en Enfermería.* Barcelona: Masson; 1997.

Case Study 27I

EHR Initiatives in Eastern Europe and Turkey: State of Knowledge and Vision

Ioana Moisil, PhD; Malina Jordanova, PhD; Angelina Kirkova, MSc Eng;
Nedialka Krasteva, DSc Med; Penka Koltchakova, MSc Med; Arvydas Seskevicius, PhD;
Liana Bera, Eng, PhD; Liliana Rogozea, PhD, MD; and Firdevs Erdemir, PhD, RN

Countries in Central and Eastern Europe have experienced, in the last decade, deep social, economic, and political changes. Probably a result of their common history of Soviet dominance and communist systems, they show similar patterns in the development of almost all their domains. These countries also share a long tradition of high-quality nursing care. After World War II, however, there was a slow, but consistent, loss of status for nursing as a profession. At the same time, health care systems also were losing face, meaning that the quality was deteriorating and patients were losing trust in the systems.

But the political changes that began in 1990 have opened new horizons for health care and are having an important, positive impact on nursing in general. The European Union (EU) policy for the development of the Information Society and the eEurope Initiative, which proposes to bring the benefits of the Information Society within the reach of all Europeans by focusing on ten priority areas, including health care, have brought nursing to the attention of information technology (IT) specialists because nursing is the source of more than 80 percent of patient data. These are the driving forces for the nursing revival in Eastern Europe and also in Turkey, as it aspires to become a member of the EU. As we have seen from the previous case studies, nursing education is the domain that reacted the fastest to the required changes and improvements. In clinical settings and especially in reference to electronic health record (EHR) development, change has been slower. All these countries are making a huge effort—financial, political, legal, and managerial—to fill in the technological, economic, and even social gaps between their systems and those of Western Europe but, as mentalities are the last thing to change, nursing is not yet considered a priority.

Romania

Romania has had IT applications in health care since 1989, when the first hospital information system (HIS) was implemented in the small village of Borsa, Maramures. Since then, several experiments for a national standard HIS have been conducted by the Ministry of Health (MoH) without great success. E-health applications are still quite heterogeneous and can be divided into eight major categories: HISs, EHRs (Figure 27I-1), image processing, World Wide Web information centers, "telediagnosis," "teleconsultation," education, and research.[1]

Unifying the existing systems would require development of e-health standards, adequate interfaces, and communication infrastructure. Applications are being piloted for emergency services (e.g., ambulance dispatcher systems), radio links between and within regions, the SMURD (mobile service for emergency and rescue) emergency system and the AMBU (Bucharest Emergency Hospital ambulance dispatcher) project; image processing and transfer; smartcards (diabetes, cardiology, neurology); information desks; general practitioner networks; calling centers; promotion of the International Classification for Nursing Practices for structuring nursing data; health informatics standards; and public health education. There are also some "telemedicine" applications encapsulated in long-distance learning projects. The projects and pilot applications are supported by grants from the Ministry for Education and Research, the Romanian Academy, or by EU research and development programs. Several health portals (interactive consulting and advice, online access to hospital services, discussion forums, etc.) have been implemented, but accessibility is still low. Unfortunately, there are no nursing data in any of the existing IT applications.[2-4]

The health insurance system is operational (Bismark type), but still needs improvement. Nurses do not have a direct contract with the National Public Health Insurance House; they are hired by the general practitioner, the specialist, or the hospital. Hospitals and health units use the International Classification of Diseases (ICD) Version 10 classification and diagnosis-related group (DRG) financial evaluation system. Diagnosis-related group is the quantitative, standard, initial version, with no reference to nursing activity.

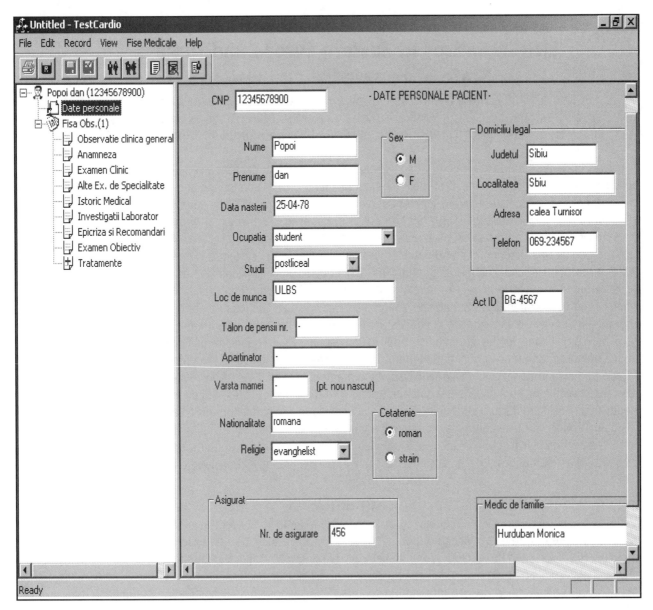

Figure 27I-1. *Image of an Electronic Patient Record in Romania.*

There are two main reasons for this situation: the first derives from the fact that nurses do not use or generate documentation files (not even paper and pencil) in practice settings. There are only two small hospitals that keep nursing records (but not in electronic format). The second reason is linked to the working conditions of the nurses in general and in particular, to the profession's lack of a health insurance contract. One nurse cares for approximately forty patients per shift. There is literally no time to fill in data of any kind in an EHR. Statisticians fill in medical data. Moreover, nurses' competence in IT goes unrecognized, especially in terms of salary. The situation will change when nurses have a direct contract with the Health Insurance House as there will then be a financial interest in evaluating nurses' activity. Change will also come about when European and international bodies, e.g., the World Health Organization ask for reports and statistical data about nursing interventions, practices, and outcomes. The electronic signature is legally recognized but not yet used by the health sector.

Nursing Education

Today, nursing education is undergoing many changes. There are sanitary high schools and post-basic high schools (three-year programs) and, since 1998, university nursing colleges (three-year programs). Recently, the Ministry of Education decided to implement the recommendations of the Bologna Process for restructuring European high-education systems, starting with the 2005–2006 academic year. Any kind of nursing specialty will be structured at the educational level in three stages: bachelor of science (BSc) degree, master's degree, and doctorate level. With the exception of the midwife specialty that requires 240 credits, all nurse specialties will require 180 credits for the BSc degree. There are eight nursing specialties: medical, midwife, radiology and image processing, clinical laboratory, balneo-physio-kineto, dental technique, dental assistant, and pharmacy assistant. In the upcoming academic year, nursing classification terminologies, e.g., the North American Nursing Diagnosis Association system (NANDA), the International Classification of Nursing Practice (ICNP®), etc., and coding systems will be added to the curricula, as will the EHR and health informatics standards.

As a side note, in general, nurses are computer literate, but they do not use IT in their daily work, with the exception of laboratory nurses.

Bulgaria

The Ministry of Health (MoH) is responsible for the overall supervision of the health care system, administered through regional health and emergency care centers and hygiene–epidemiological inspectorates, plus a number of national research centers. Municipalities own polyclinics, small- and medium-sized hospitals, and hospitals providing secondary care. The private sector consists mainly of hospices, pharmacies, dental clinics, laboratories, and specialized health clinics. Bulgaria has implemented a Bismarck-type health insurance fund, the Health Insurance Act, as the legal basis for changing the health care system.

The Health Insurance Act has established the National Health Insurance Fund (NHIF) as a public organization regulating the relationships between NHIF and health care providers. The Health Insurance Act also regulates the signing of the National Framework Contract between NHIF and the professional associations of health care providers. The documentation every health care provider is obliged to keep includes primary and reporting documents. Some of the primary documents are the ambulatory cards (two different forms for outpatient care providers and dental care providers), referral cards for consultations or joint treatments, and referral cards for medical diagnostic activity (hospitalization). Physicians are responsible for filling in and signing these documents, but in many cases the nurses are filling in the electronic or hard copy versions of these forms. NHIF began to accept documentation on electronic media in August 2003. Since January 2005, the MoH and NHIF accepted ICD-10 as a coding standard. NHIF developed classifications and coding systems that make it compulsory for providers to use the registration number of health institutions, the general practitioner code, codes for specialists from the outpatient health care, codes of test packages, and codes of highly specialized medical-diagnostic investigations, nuclear medicine, and immunizations.

Nursing Education

Since 1997, according to the revised law for university education, the complete course of nursing education is three years, and there is a special coordination committee for the requirements and plans in nursing education to keep them in accordance with European standards.

Today, nursing education consists of several levels: medical colleges for graduates of a secondary school (basic computer skills and English language), BSc with a minimum of four semesters, and master's programs (master's degree) with an average duration of three semesters. The BSc graduated nurses receive higher education degrees with specialities, i.e., medical nurses, maternity nurses, X-ray nurses, medical laboratory technicians/nurses, assistant pharmacists, social workers, dental nurses, rehabilitation technicians/nurses, sanitary (public health) inspectors, and masseurs (physical therapists). Since February 2005, the College of Medicine in Plovdiv, a leading school in training nurses, adopted a new pilot curriculum for basic pregraduate nursing training—a diploma with an increased number of academic hours in nursing informatics (sixty academic hours). Doctoral programs (PhD, with an average duration of six semesters) for nurses are uncommon. An attractive doctoral program, Computer Systems and Technologies in Medicine, was recently developed by the New Bulgarian University in Sofia.

In response to the specific demands of some ethnic minorities in the country, specialized educational courses for nurses have been organized during the last four years in the medical college in Blagoevgrad, with the main target being to reach these ethnic minorities.

The EHR and Nursing

With the firm belief that the EHR is the future of medical record-keeping, the MoH expressed its readiness for countrywide implementation of such records. However, there is no systematic governmental policy to support this direction. Neither is there a specific strategy to introduce IT applications for nurses. Special legislation on data protection in health care does not yet exist. The EHRs that are available in other countries cannot be imported because of the differences in language and alphabet (the Cyrillic alphabet is used in Bulgaria). As a result, several Bulgarian companies have developed their own clinical software solutions. Three types of medical records currently are available on the market: patient records, records for emergency care units, and HIS. The EHR includes patient registry, diagnostic coding optimization, anamnesis, details from physical examinations (assessments), laboratory orders and results, appointment scheduling, images such as EKG, X-rays, radiological studies, etc., follow-up, and recall tracking, a medication section that tracks prescriptions and refills—all the information necessary for precise recording of past, present, and future health failures (Figure 27I-2).[5]

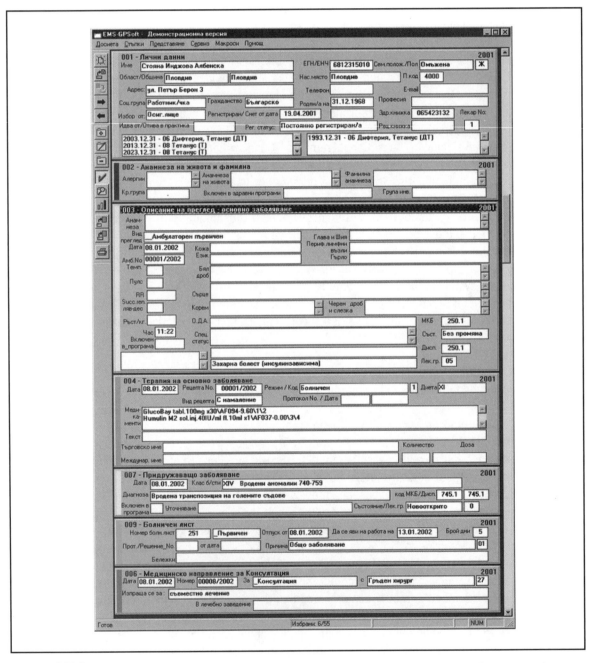

Figure 27I-2. *View of EHR Used by General Practitioners. Source: Danina-G (at http://www.danina-g.com).*

In addition to EHRs, more specialized medical information systems (ISs), especially directed to cardiologists and cardiology clinics, are also available (for example, the MIS2000).[6] An integrated hospital IS is in use in thirty hospitals. This package consists of different subsystems, including a subsystem for registration of inpatients. The electronic inpatients' record is based on formal documents, e.g., a referral card for medical diagnostic activity and disease history, with the second part filled in at the hospital. Neither includes nursing data; doctors are responsible for producing the documentation. The head nurses, however, participate in filling in data along with a computer specialist and a statistician.

The implementation of a health and social security IS using personal information carriers has started as a pilot project with the financial support of the Bulgarian National Science Fund. Experiments so far have been carried out using optical memory cards, e.g., LaserCard®. The project is entirely based on the EU's existing Medical Electronic Data Interchange standards and Health Level 7.

The potential benefits of EHR applications have to be demonstrated in practice. This is one of the tasks of an ongoing pilot project cofunded by Bulgaria and the International Telecommunication Union of Switzerland. The main strategic goals are to test and evaluate the effectiveness of wireless technologies in rural and remote semimountainous areas and to provide a platform for the wide introduction of multimedia services (e.g., "telemedicine," "tele-education," etc.) in ten villages with a total population of about 20,000 inhabitants.

Turkey

In Turkey, studies on the Information Society strategy are in progress, mainly in the frame of the e-Transformation Turkey Project and the e-Europe Action Plan 2005. Important steps have been taken in the area of education to provide such human resources as required by an information society. The core of the e-Transformation project is e-government. In this context, an e-government portal focused on citizens and business requirements is foreseen. Laws regarding electronic signature, the right of access to information, and a draft law on the protection of personal data have been approved.[7]

Health services in Turkey are supplied by a multitude of public and private providers. The Ministry of Health is the major provider of primary and secondary health care and essentially the only provider of preventive health services. The public sector accounts for 92 percent of hospital capacity in Turkey. There are 11,700 health units, 5,700 health centers, and 1,226 hospitals.[7]

Social security and health systems in Turkey are experiencing various structural problems, e.g., low funds and unsatisfactory accessibility (86.4 percent in 2003). The share of the population registered for social insurance programs was established.

EHR in Health Care Units

The Health Reform Project is being carried out jointly by MoH and the Ministry of Labor and Social Security. The project takes into consideration harmonization with the EU regulations. A standard IS is planned for completion in 2005. e-Health and Health Information System projects were to be developed by MoH in the framework of a World Bank project in 1992–1993. Some hospitals implemented EHRs that were compatible with international technical and terminology standards, e.g., ISO 9001 (International Standards Organization) and ICD-10. Use of the Internet and other new digital technologies are also targeted in the Health Reform Project action plan. Nurses and nursing, however, have not been involved in the development of the HIS.

The policy document recommends reorganizing health care delivery so that it is centered in general practitioner offices, and paying physicians for health services via capitation. It also recommends hospital autonomy and decentralization. There are no clear statements concerning quality and needs evaluation systems, e.g., DRGs. Supporting legislation and health information systems are suggested as the necessary anchors for the overall health system.

Nursing Education and Nursing Informatics

Nurses constitute the largest group of health care professionals in Turkey. Unfortunately, nurses and the Turkish National Nursing Association could not be part of e-health projects because of various reasons (heterogeneous educational levels, lack of IT competencies, lack of a common nursing language, and old nursing regulations on nursing professional autonomy and accountability).[7-9]

Turkey has two different categories of basic nursing education and all graduates from these programs are employed as nurses. The first category is the four-year high school-level diploma programs that are run and accredited by MoH. The second type is based on BSc degree programs. The nursing curricula are mostly organized in a manner similar to that of nursing curricula in the U.S. and include computer skills at a beginning level. There have been associate degree programs since the 1970s, and these are standardized by the Council of Higher Education.[10]

Efforts are being made to create and increase the awareness and competencies of nurses, including teaching NI and existing nursing classification systems (e.g., NANDA diagnoses, ICNP®, the University of Iowa Nursing Interventions Classification and Nursing Outcomes Classification) as a prerequisite for using the electronic nursing record.

Poland

The implementation of IT in the Polish health care system has increased continuously from the early 1990s. The first implementations were generally focused on the administrative parts of the health care facilities; however, some homemade applications were also used for EHRs. In 1995, in the World Telecommunication Development Report (Internet availability, PC users/100 inhabitants), Poland was classified on the far end of the ranking among thirty countries.

In 1999, reform of the health care financing system was carried out. This was a critical point for the use of IS in health care. The reform was accompanied by changes in the health care and social insurance systems. The National Health Service was established in every voivodship (county). Voivodship Health Service became the main contractor of medical services delivered by health care institutions. A new reform of the health care system took place in 2004. The main change was based on the establishment of one single National Health Fund with a department in every voivodship.

The continuous changes in the range of information required from health care providers added more pressure on the development of efficient IS in health care facilities. Within the World Bank Project, admission-discharge-transfer and pharmacy modules were implemented in hospitals. Providers of the systems were five large IT consortia consisting mainly of Polish companies. The project resulted in the establishment of IS in most of the hospitals. It can also be seen as the real starting point for the development of EHR in the health care system. Working links between hospitals and IT providers resulted in further investments in IS for health care. However, the unsuccessful reforms of the health care system resulted in the deterioration of the financial status of Polish health care providers and this, in turn, slowed down interest in development of IS in health care organizations.

Currently, most health care providers use IS for recording every day activities. The status of EHR development is, however, highly variable from institution to institution. The standardization process as related to the EHR was also neglected, even after the Center of Information Systems in Health Care, affiliated with MoH, showed some interest in defining the format of electronic message exchange between the main actors in the health care arena.

A new vision of EHR was shaped after Poland joined the EU and developed its ehealth policy for 2004–2006. However, it seems obvious that it can be accomplished only after deep changes to the financing and contracting models of health care services have been made.

The initiatives undertaken by nursing professional bodies are focused on the integration of EHRs kept by nurses. Today, the electronic patient documentation is conducted without significant participation from the nursing staff, although nurses usually have some access to the system. It is expected that the future EHR will have input from all health professionals.

Concerning nursing education, Poland has one of the highest quality academic traditions, with BSc, MSc, and PhD programs implemented in the last century. Today these programs are synchronized with the requirements of the Bologna process.

Lithuania

The implementation of an EHR has recently begun in Lithuania but only in a few hospitals. It is not a complete health information system yet because it is still in the process of being developed. In this EHR, nursing data are also included; e.g., outpatient clinic nurses carry out a vaccination program. Today, one fragment of the EHR has been implemented at the Kaunas University of Medicine Clinic in the module for medicines accounting. Only the Kaunas University of Medicine teaches how to use an EHR.

Most hospitals in Lithuania are in the process of implementing standards for nursing interventions and practices and are using quantitative and qualitative indicators for evaluating nursing activities. The National Health Fund maintains a central database with patients' aggregated data.[11]

For the long term, there are governmental plans concerning a national EHR strategy but the government faces several problems: the lack of funds for computerized systems, a poor IT infrastructure, and no national standards for nursing diagnosis and problems (although these standards are currently being developed).

Nursing Education

Bachelor's degree-level nursing programs were established at Kaunas University of Medicine in 1990. The duration of study is four years. Master's degree and doctoral-level programs started in 1999. In terms of informatics curricula, the BSc program has a course on computerization in nursing. The master's program offers a course on IT in medicine. A distance learning course to teach nursing documentation is also currently being developed.

References

1. National Institute for Research and development in Informatics in Bucharest: http://isv.ascti.ro, http://atlas.ici.ro/ehto/ (05-10-2005).
2. Romanian general information portal Kappa: www.kappa.ro (05-10-2005).
3. Romanian Medical Information Portal: www.romedic.ro (05-10-2005).
4. Tempus Phare Project CME 02555-96 web site for medical information: www.infosan.ro (05-10-2005).
5. Danina-G, 2003. Available at: http://www.danina-g.com Accessed May 10, 2005.
6. MIS2000. Available at: http://www.techno-link.com/clients/demonics.
7. Aksayan S, Cimete G. Nursing education and practice in Turkey. *J Nurs Scholarsh.* 2000;32;(2):211-212.
8. World Bank. *Turkey Reforming the Health Sector for Improved Access and Efficiency (In Two Volumes) Volume II: Background Papers.* Report No. 24358-TU. Human Development Sector Unit Europe and Central Asia Region: World Bank; 2003.
9. Atalay M, Dogan S. Mandating university-based nursing education: Turkey's experience. *Nurs Educ.* 2000; 25(4):166-169.
10. Robertson JF, Lash AA, Okumus H. Nursing education in modern Turkey. *Nurs Outlook.* 1992;40(3):127-132.
11. Lithuanian Health Care Program. Vilnius: Ministry of Health Care (Lithuania) Report; 1998:47.

CHAPTER 28

Nursing Informatics in the African Continent

By Nolwazi Mbananga, PhD

The establishment of nursing informatics (NI) is in a very early stage in South Africa and the rest of Africa. Started only in 2002, efforts have faced many challenges, making the endeavour exceedingly difficult. The concept of NI is new among the very groups that are to take the process forward in the African continent: the government, the tertiary institutions, and the nursing community itself. This novelty raises questions: Why nursing *informatics and not* health *informatics? And, when faced with third-world health problems, can we make NI a priority for certain sectors, e.g., government, health professionals' bodies, and tertiary institutions? Even when these questions are answered convincingly, two other questions arise: Do we have qualified teachers and the required NI educational materials available to us? And, where do we get financial resources to obtain these materials and faculty and to take the process forward? These questions need to be addressed to pave the way for NI in the African continent.*

Historical Background of Nursing Informatics in Africa

In the vast African continent, little has been done in the area of NI, and therefore, the concept remains foreign to the nursing community continent-wide. Several attempts have been made to advance NI in a number of African countries, including Kenya, Tanzania, Uganda, Cameroon, and South Africa. In 2004, the Nursing Leadership Programme in South Africa started an introductory course in NI—organized by Aga Khan University in Nairobi—in which three countries participated (Kenya, Tanzania, and Uganda).[1]

Another attempt was made to start an NI course in Cameroon at the request of Amungwa Athanasius Nche, president of the National Council of Nurses, Midwives, and Health Technicians. The attempt failed, despite interest shown by the nursing leadership in Cameroon, particularly because of the lack of funding support for faculty travel in order to introduce the course. The Medical Research Council of South Africa offered to cover the costs of accommodation and allowances, but it was difficult for the Council to raise the funds to purchase an airline ticket. The World Health Organization was approached for assistance, but none came forth. Simply put, the Cameroon initiative failed in such a cash-strapped community. The Cameroon example illustrates the difficulty of introducing NI in the African continent. Clearly, without an international commitment to this endeavour, very little will be achieved because the concept is new and does not have financial support.

Although South Africa seems to have enjoyed some success in this area, NI development there is also extremely slow, as described later. As a result of the Nursing Leadership Programme course in South Africa, however, the Aga Khan University and other stakeholders decided in 2004 to organize an NI conference and invite speakers from developed countries.[1] It is hoped that the conference will materialize.

Nursing Informatics in South Africa

It is common to refer to South Africa as three worlds in one, that is, containing three developmental categories: underdeveloped, developing, and developed. This description is accurate more so because of a total population of 45 million that is diverse in ethnicity, history, culture, and language. South Africa has eleven official languages and is characterized by uneven socioeconomic development and problems of inequity at many levels. Diversity poses problems, particularly in health care in terms of how health informatics and NI can be developed in a universal format that is acceptable, understandable, and useful to all. Issues of accessibility, literacy, computer literacy, and uneven technological development challenge the realization of the information age's promises.

In 1995, the Department of Health established a national committee to develop a National Health Information System Strategy for South Africa. This is the only committee that has been formally organized by the government in the area of health informatics. Although there have been minimal disjointed efforts toward providing basic skills in health informatics, these represent minimal efforts on the broad scale of health informatics education.

Developmental Stages of Nursing Informatics in South Africa

The concept of NI emerged in South Africa for the first time at a conference presentation given in 2000. The workshop to investigate the new concept, held in 2002, can be regarded as the first step toward the establishment of NI education and research in South Africa. Other attempts have also been made to develop NI groups in South Africa. In 2002, Marion Ball, former president of the International Medical Informatics Association (IMIA), was invited and funded by the Medical Research Council of South Africa to hold a preconference NI workshop in Johannesburg, South Africa. The workshop was attended by nurses from a number of African countries, including Swaziland, Botswana, Tanzania, Nigeria, and South Africa. Later, in 2004, Robyn Carr, founding member of Health Informatics New Zealand and vice chair of the IMIA's Nursing Informatics Special Interest Group (IMIA-NI), conducted a workshop and an introductory course on NI in South Africa, which led to an NI interest group being formed. Even later, the Institute for Health Advancement and the author conducted a similar course in Cecilia Makiwane Hospital in the Eastern Cape province of South Africa, and another NI group was formed in the Eastern Cape. Both NI groups selected official members (chair, vice-chair, and secretary).

Unfortunately, since the establishment of these two groups, no formal activity has taken place; this can be attributed, first of all, to the fact that NI was being facilitated by the Medical Research Council (MRC) which is not the appropriate organization to initiate NI growth in South Africa because it lacks a nursing perspective. The perception among the nursing community is that NI progress can be made only when nurses are linked with nursing academic colleagues and leadership. With this in mind, help in promoting NI growth was requested of the country's two nursing professional organizations, the South African Nursing Council and the Democratic Nurses Association, but to date these alliances have not yet formed.

Second, the lack of activity is a result of financial constraints; even in South Africa, there is a lack of significant support from other organizations. The only support available comes from the MRC. Again, the author, in agreement with the nursing sector, believes that progress in NI needs to be driven by universities and is making attempts to involve the nursing department at the University of Transkei to initiate a suitable course in the subject. The Pretoria University and the University of Cape Town have already been preparing to start such a course. All efforts may fail, however, for lack of funding. Also, it is unclear whether there is a strong demand for formal NI courses at the universities in South Africa.

Hospital Information Systems: A Platform for NI in South Africa

Along with processing modernization and harnessing new health care technologies in South Africa is the pressing and urgent requirement for its health care professionals to be equipped with information and informatics skills, and, importantly, the ability to apply these skills and knowledge in clinical practice and to conduct follow-up research.

South Africa is moving rapidly toward the implementation of integrated hospital information systems in most of its provinces. A classic example is the implementation in 2002 of the total information system for patient care at Inkosi Albert Luthuli Central Hospital in Durban. This system implementation marked an unprecedented shift in patient care and resulted in the first paperless hospital in the country. However, although the hospital's nurses are using electronic systems in the care of patients, they do not know nor do they understand the concept of NI. A number of issues have made it difficult to introduce this concept as a key and formal link in the health care chain. At Inkosi Albert Luthuli, NI is being accepted by default and only to a limited extent. However, there is a need to formalize NI concepts for improved efficiency by nurses in the extended use of the electronic system. This hospital has the same state-of-the-art technology that can be found in developed countries, which provides South Africa with the platform to launch NI to the highest levels in the continent. But this cannot be achieved without the support of appropriate funds and a champion to lead the organizational change required.

Besides Inkosi Albert Luthuli, most hospitals in the country have implemented information systems, working with a combination of electronic and paper components. Use of dual systems will persist in the African continent for a number of reasons, e.g., poor information technology (IT) infrastructure and unreliable power supply. In some locations in South Africa where these clinical systems have been implemented, electricity outages are disturbing the process flows, forcing nurses to switch between systems. Such electrical disturbances cause a high degree of backlogs and double entries, first on paper and later in the computer.[2]

Nevertheless, information and informatics skills and knowledge are now being applied by health workers in South Africa and by nurses in particular. In so doing, nurses are extending the scope of such systems rather than simply computerizing a hospital's processes and are doing it by virtue of their nursing background and problem-solving skills rather than with knowledge of NI concepts as such. However, it is becoming clear that in South Africa, the management of hospitals will be impossible without informaticians (well-trained health professionals capable of running and managing hospital information systems). Applying NI at the point of care is acknowledged as a way forward in some hospitals, further evidence that a sound NI course is needed as a focus area under the umbrella of health informatics.

The Challenges of Nursing Informatics Education in South Africa

NI education and research in South Africa are in their infancy. As a result of this immaturity, NI is a very new discipline in the country, compared with health informatics. It is still unclear what NI is, and why it is so important. These questions become pertinent and difficult to answer—especially the last one—when coming from the nursing fraternity. It is also not clear yet whether these questions result from a lack of distinction between NI and health informatics or as a consequence of the new preference in South Africa for an integrated approach to the education of health professionals.

Whatever the reason, it makes sense to focus on a new program rather than generalizing existing ones. Health informatics is an umbrella concept, encompassing various informatics specialties, e.g., medical, dental, pharmaceutical, etc. The nursing fraternity in South Africa must establish itself first in the NI arena before it can concern itself with health informatics. Particularly in the formative stages of NI, the nursing fraternity needs to develop its own perspective even if that perspective is integrated later. Although no distinct boundary exists between health informatics and NI, it is suggested that nurses in South Africa think about NI first before they enter into the wider arena of health informatics. The international community in NI could assist in their moving to the wider view by spelling out why there is a need for NI education. That remains the question for South African nurses: why NI education and not health informatics education?

Addressing the question of what NI is demands an urgent development of NI education and research in South Africa. Of the number of challenges in meeting these demands, an important one is convincing nursing professionals of the importance of health informatics in nursing practice and of the need for resources to develop NI. Indeed, it is difficult to reach an agreement among nurses themselves on prioritizing NI development and education. A number of questions have been posed, chief of which is how can we prioritize NI while important issues related to third-world health problems remain unresolved? This is a legitimate question in a country where the majority of the population is facing problems related to poverty and underdevelopment and where some areas are characterized by poor infrastructure, both technological and basic.

Although NI might not respond directly to these questions, it has the potential to improve the health of the poor, especially in developing countries in which services are not easily accessible.

There is evidence that home care, "telehealth," and "telenursing" can deliver health care services to people's doorsteps.[3] Yet it is difficult to convince people about what the literature is revealing; to them it is "pie in the sky" and not seen as a concrete solution. The question then is how do we convince nurses in the remote areas of Africa that NI has benefits and will improve practices and services when there is no infrastructure and no resources to prove such a claim? There is no local practical evidence to show the benefits that can be brought about by NI in South Africa or in the developing countries of Africa. (Not all the nurses in South Africa are skeptical about making NI a priority. There is a need to support those positive nurses through funding their endeavours.)

Another challenge facing South Africa and the continent is harnessing NI development in a way that will ultimately narrow the gap between the developing and the developed parts of Africa. Poor coordination and facilitation will be a threat to such NI endeavours in South Africa and the continent, and these problems raise the issue of standardization, that is, standards that will suit the environmental diversities of nursing practice throughout the country. Standards are crucial in adopting and adapting courseware from IMIA. Although IMIA has offered its course ware for international use, much customizing needs to be done before it can be adopted in South Africa and the continent at large. A challenge is to develop course ware that will not discourage nurses coming from rural areas where infrastructure is unavailable. The approach to NI courses should therefore be holistic to include nurses who do not have technological infrastructure. Such an approach, suitable to both South Africa and the continent, involves the adoption of nursing information and informatics course ware with an emphasis on information rather than on informatics.

The approach becomes relevant when informatics as a concept does not depend on technology as an enabling tool. In some parts of the country, nurses have not seen or touched a computer, whereas in other areas, nurses are using computers in their everyday activities. Therefore, when the NI course is ready, the question arises: should we set a technological requirement such as "If you have access to information technology, you can register for the course. If you do not have access, do not register." The 2002 study by Mbananga et al[2] revealed that IT skills are lost when they are not used. Thus, providing such skills for those who cannot use them immediately ultimately fails to be cost effective.

To address issues of diversity, the national stakeholders, especially government, must be lobbied. Although the development of infrastructure and IT might take longer when the government is taking center stage, the approach to facilitating NI can be holistic. In the absence of a national body driving NI in South Africa, disparities, rather than bridges, will be created. The challenge is to organize the NI working group, supported by the IMIA-NI, to become active within the country. Although South Africa has established a number of NI groups in the country, coordination and follow-up are very difficult because of financial constraints. As is always the case when there is no government support, there are no financial resources. The lack of financial resources not only necessitates the need to find sponsors, but also leads to the problem of finding the human and material resources needed to assist in moving the process forward.

Nursing Informatics Educational Material

These challenges may be linked in part to the lack of relevant NI educational material. Although the lack of material might be resolved by substituting Internet information, this is not a plausible solution for all students in South Africa and certainly not for those in other African countries. For students who do have access to the Internet, it is the optimum avenue for obtaining usable educational material. It is problematic, however, for those nursing professionals who should be targeted for NI courses: those who are working already, most of which have no access to the Internet. University students typically have it better because they are more likely to have access to the Internet.

Even given access to the Internet, the information found there presents its own problems in terms of cost, quality, and relevance. Textbooks on health informatics written overseas are very expensive, with a price range of R500 to R1500; prices are inflated further by the rand/dollar exchange rate (e.g., US\$1 = R10). Some of these books need to be screened not only for quality, but also for relevance to situations specific to developing countries. The question posed to the international community in health informatics by this author is how did you resolve these problems?

New Technology, Telemedicine, and Telehealth: An Opportunity for Telenursing

In South Africa today, there are thirty-five telemedicine pilot centers in nine provinces, and the number is expected to increase in the next five years. These centers cover four areas in health care delivery: "telepathology," "teleradiology," "teleophthalmology," and antenatal "teleultrasound." The main aim of the telehealth services is to provide health specialist services in the rural areas of the country. Telehealth is technology-driven; it uses software, terminals, workstations, hardware, e-mail, Internet, and other means in transferring medical images and communicating health messages.

Nurses in South Africa are central to the delivery of health services in rural areas and consequently are also the drivers of telehealth. Today for most such services, there is a nurse on the other end of the technology. With their experience, nurses in the future will use artificial intelligence and decision-modeling systems in their decision-making processes. All these technological advances in health care indicate that, no matter how skeptical or technophobic health workers might be, the health environment is changing into a total information system care environment.

The Future of Nursing Informatics in Africa

NI in Africa will develop slowly because of the challenges discussed in this chapter. Yet it is important that a strategy be developed and implemented with the support of IMIA-NI. The first step is to identify health problems, e.g., HIV/AIDs, malaria, diarrhea, tuberculosis (TB), and many others that are common in the African continent. Nursing practices related to these health problems should be framed with NI principles and disseminated as protocols, developed and tested within the African continent.

NI in Africa will not take the Western IT-centered approach (computers and networks) because such an approach will only engender a lot of negative response from a number of people. There is always the debate between funding bodies of developed and developing countries as to why they should fund computers and networks in the midst of HIV/AIDS epidemics and the prevalence of other diseases. Superficially this is a valid question, but it lacks an in-depth understanding of NI and health informatics. NI can be used to monitor these diseases, especially in Africa where there are low treatment compliance rates.

The effect of tuberculosis is an example of how NI can help in disease control. TB in Africa is a major problem, especially because it coexists with an HIV/AIDs epidemic. In South Africa people do not die of TB because there is no treatment; people die because they do not follow their treatment course properly and because there is poor communication and minimal contact between health workers and patients after patients leave the health facilities. If a directed observed therapy (DOT) strategy for TB can be framed within NI, much will be achieved in controlling the disease. In fact, the MRC in South Africa is engaged in a TB project called TB DOT Plus. The purpose of the project is to enable nurses in the rural clinics to monitor TB patients. Nurses use a handheld device that assists in rural clinics with their analysis and measurements related to disease management. Cell phones are also heavily used rather than land-line telephones because the satellite technology is more readily available throughout the country. Cell phones are key to being able to track patients and do health maintenance for most chronic diseases. With these new technologies, controlling TB in Africa can be easier than it is currently because it can be monitored more closely. This is just one example of how NI can play a major role in disease management and control in the African continent.

Another area that needs consideration is the use of wireless technology. As mentioned above, wireless phones (cell phones) are used throughout most of the African continent by ordinary members of the communities. So the question of funding technology is irrelevant because the people already have the technology. The NI community needs to harness cell phones into their practice in Africa. Wireless technology is good for Africa because it overcomes geographic barriers and is easy to implement. The future of NI in Africa should clearly be wireless-based. The approach should be curative and preventive. Most importantly, the health needs in Africa call for the emphasis to be public health–oriented, not hospital-centered. Africa needs simple technologies with wide impact.

Educational material should be developed that addresses the health and nursing issues prevailing in the continent. NI Web-based education should be encouraged and supported. Telenursing should be a tool used to drive NI education in nursing colleges.

Summary

This chapter has mapped out a number of challenges facing education in NI and the NI field in general in South Africa and the African continent. Currently, these problems seem insurmountable, but with commitment and leadership in Africa in combination with international support, these problems can be mitigated. Nurse informaticians can act as champions, whose endeavors will elicit support. The important issue is the realization that the challenge may not only be facing NI, but also health informatics education in the whole of the African continent. Because this is most likely the case, South Africa has the bigger challenge of being a catalyst in developing NI education and research in the continent.

According to Lun,[4] IMIA has been trying to promote medical informatics in Africa by supporting Health Informatics in Africa (HELINA). This has raised general expectations that HELINA can expand the development of IMIA's fourth regional group (the African region), but such expectations have not been met. Although HELINA is not a success story in Africa, IMIA-NI must promote NI Africa through it, at least its conferences are held in Africa; this means that there should be no HELINA conference without an NI conference. The poor success of HELINA might be associated with challenges similar to those raised in this chapter.

Also, IMIA Working Group 1 on Health Informatics and IMIA-NI should support the initial steps started in South Africa with the aim of expanding to all countries in Africa. Another important step in establishing NI in South Africa is developing an informatics group that enables country membership in IMIA. This step would allow full participation in any of the eighteen working groups of IMIA and particularly of IMIA-NI. A process for joining these groups needs to be planned, and nurses throughout the continent must be encouraged to register.

Despite the challenges and uncertainty, there is no doubt that NI and health informatics education are overdue in Africa. Most countries are implementing some form of integrated hospital information systems. In an evaluation conducted in one South African province, it was found that such systems are bound to fail not because they are bad systems, but only because of a lack of in-depth understanding of how these systems work.[4] Nurses have been identified as drivers of these systems because they do the largest amount of data capturing in the wards. As another case in point, experiences at the new paperless hospital (Inkosi Albert Luthuli Hospital) give an indication that African nurses will be taken by surprise and will lack the necessary skills to cope with the paradigm shift that will be brought about by the information age coming to Africa. The introduction of technology in the health sector in South Africa is moving faster than the necessary health professional educational background.

South Africa, and Africa as a whole, needs to move quickly toward developing nursing education. A major challenge in this regard is that NI education in Africa should not perpetuate or exaggerate the already existing inequities between urban and rural health professionals. NI education should ensure that it takes advantage of technology without creating bigger discrepancies between the rich and poor countries of Africa. As alluded to earlier in this chapter, this can be achieved by an informatics education that emphasizes information rather than technology in places where technology does not exist.

Despite all the challenges to NI education and development in the African continent, clearly the information age is influencing the activities of nurses regardless of prevailing problems. The information age will continue to challenge nursing professional skills in the future, and there is a need to develop NI Africa, with IMIA-NI playing a strong supporting role.

References

1. Dennil K. Introduction to nursing informatics at the East African universities, Uganda, Kenya, Tanzania. Course presented at: Aga Kahn University; 2004; Nairobi, Kenya.
2. Mbananga N. *Evaluation of Hospital Information System in the Northern Province: Report prepared for the Department of Health.* Pretoria; 2002.
3. Ball M, Hannah K, Newbold S, Douglas J. *Nursing Informatics: Where Caring and Technology Meet.* New York: Springer; 2000.
4. Lun KC. Challenges in medical informatics: perspectives of an international medical informatics organisation. *Methods Inf Med.* January 2002;14:1-85.

CHAPTER 29

Nursing and the EHR in Asia, Australasia, and the South Pacific

By Karolyn Kerr, PhD Candidate, MHSc, RGON

Nurses provide holistic care to patients with diverse health care and social requirements in many different types of organizations and geographical locations. This can mean nurses are delivering care in isolation from their colleagues and sometimes in isolation from medical staff support. Access to information, including the patient's previous health encounters, and to intelligent decision support is becoming essential in the modern health care environment for all health care providers.

All of the countries reviewed in this chapter are experiencing nursing shortages, in line with international trends of a nursing workforce that is aging and a profession that is struggling to attract new recruits. By necessity this is leading to innovative ways to improve the efficiency of care delivery. Economic constraints vie with increased expectations from the educated consumer for better health care and more response to the individual's needs and wants. Nursing and medicine need to work together with e-health specialists to meet these expectations. The worldwide developments toward effective electronic health record (EHR) systems to record care delivery and assist with decision making appear to provide some improvement in information management in health care.

The economies of the countries throughout the Australasia region are varied. New Zealand and Australia enjoy considerable affluence, with extended life expectancies and an excellent quality of life. Some countries in the South Pacific, however, have to provide basic health care services to geographically diverse populations with minimal funding and infrastructure. Although the cultures within the region are diverse, they are also actively merging. For example, New Zealand's Asian population has increased by five percent over the past five years through relaxed immigration policies seeking to import people with skills that are locally lacking. Also, there is considerable emigration out of the Pacific Island countries into Australia and New Zealand, leaving ever-decreasing populations to support local infrastructures in the island communities. Further, nurses in this region, including those from the Pacific Islands, are being recruited to work in other countries, predominately the United Kingdom, the U.S., Canada, and Ireland, where nursing shortages are beginning to have considerable impact.

The countries in this region rely heavily on a professional nursing workforce to provide the bulk of hospital-based and primary-care services. Those in Australasia and the South Pacific structure and train their nursing workforce in a similar manner, initially closely aligned to traditional hospital-based three-year courses modeled after the United Kingdom. Most have now moved to a degree program within polytechnics or universities.

Nurses today have raised expectations and are demanding improved work conditions and pay increases to reflect their degrees and specializations. They are often heavily relied on to overlap with the duties of the junior house officer. In addition, several countries have now introduced a nurse specialist qualification that allows nurses to prescribe medications.

To support these changes in nursing practice, knowledge of what nurses do is required. But "what nurses do" is often inexplicit and hard to define, making it difficult for nurses to prove their worth. The EHR has the potential to provide nurses with a medium for recording the effectiveness of the care they deliver in a manner that is transparent and available in a format understood by those outside of nursing.

The trend across the countries in this Asia Pacific region, but in particular Australia and New Zealand, is to move toward a more seamless delivery of health care from hospital to community, thereby minimizing increasing costs and reducing waste. A multidisciplinary health care record would support this change by providing everyone with access to appropriate information about a patient. The danger is in the misinterpretation of information by different disciplines. Nursing language standards are required worldwide to prevent confusion and need to align with other medical languages where appropriate.[1]

Key to achieving language standards are the activities of international standard organizations. Most notable is the international development occurring through the Health Level Seven (HL7) ballot process. HL7 consists of grammar and vocabulary that is standardized so that clinical data can be shared amongst all healthcare systems, and easily understood by all. The HL7 standards will provide much of the world with a direction for EHR developments that will ensure the records are internationally understood in a consistent manner. Many countries of this region are actively involved in the HL7 initiatives, with Australia and New Zealand in particular being early adopters of HL7 standards.

Australia is well advanced in this region in the development of a national EHR strategy. Fortunately, there are many collaborative networks already in place that mean developments in best practice and lessons learned from any country are soon disseminated throughout the region. Below is an outline of the progress of developments in the EHR in Asia, Australia, New Zealand, and the South Pacific, and in particular, the actual and potential nursing developments in the area of EHRs.

Asia

Nursing practice in many Asian countries utilizes both Western and local traditional practices. Education levels are increasing, as is the ratio of qualified nurses to patients. Many Asian countries, such as Singapore and Malaysia, have well-developed nursing informatics (NI) groups that belong to the International Medical Informatics Association's (IMIA's) Nursing Informatics Special Interest Group (IMIA-NI). Members attend international meetings, presenting their latest research findings. Others are just beginning to learn about NI, but are progressing rapidly along with the general increase in the use of technology in Asia.

Hong Kong has an intelligent data network that provides seamless data communications to its forty hospitals and fifty specialist clinics. The network provides a clinical management system that delivers a longitudinal medical history for patients that can be accessed by health care professionals on a need-to-know basis. Telehealth and video conferencing are in use, and multimedia enhancement in the clinical setting with voice recording and imaging now helps to speed up the work process and to strengthen services in the clinical areas.[2]

Singapore is both a city and small nation-state—only 247-square miles including fifty islands that are connected by a causeway to the tip of the Malay Peninsula. However, Lun Kwok Chan, associate professor of medical informatics at the National University of Singapore and past president of IMIA, says Singapore is "probably the only fully wired country in the world."[3] The Singapore Nurses Association has an NI Special Interest Group. Its mission is "to provide networking, education, and information resources that enrich and strengthen the roles of nurses in the field of informatics".[3] This active community provides educational programs and information resources, publishes documents, and facilitates research and publication by its members.

Taiwan's health care services are rapidly improving, with life expectancy rates and a population health status equivalent to that of other industrialized countries. Equal access to health care for all has been an active work program since 1995. The nursing profession actively and effectively uses traditional Chinese medicine in conjunction with Western-style health care. To strengthen the competence of the nursing profession, the Nurses Act was amended to define the grade of nurse specialist in 2000. Currently, no specific mention is made in the international literature about NI in Taiwan; however, this is likely to change in the near future with the increasingly professional nature of the nursing workforce.[4]

Thailand is well along a pathway to developing a national health information system. In parallel, a nursing component to the system is also under development. The first step in the development of the nursing component is the identification of a nursing minimum data set (NMDS). This will involve comparing the Thai NMDS with other national nursing data sets, particularly those found in the U.S. The Thai NMDS translates the International Classification of Nursing Practice (ICNP®), with further work required to increase nurse's involvement in the process. Further iterative improvements are taking place. An article in the *Journal of Advanced Nursing* noted elements of the NMDS have been identified, but further work is required to improve buy-in from nurses, including increasing nurses' involvement with the process.[5]

Korea

Korea has a very active health informatics society with an NI special interest group and a regularly published journal. The next IMIA Nursing Informatics Conference will be held in Korea in 2006. Please refer to Case Study 29A for a description of EHR development in Korea.

Australia

Nurses in Australia enjoy some of the best working conditions in this region. For example, the state of Victoria requires that each nurse is only allocated four patients per shift. Considerable technological infrastructure is available to the nurse, depending on the location. Some areas already have local versions of an EHR, some of which include nursing information.

Health*Connect* is an extensive project being run by the Central Department of Health and Aging in Canberra. Health*Connect* is Australia's proposed national health information network to facilitate the safe collection, storage, and exchange of consumer health information between authorized health care providers. Under Health*Connect*, health-related information about a consumer would be collected, subject to the consumer's consent, in a standard electronic format at the point-of-care. This could include a hospital or general practitioner's (GP) surgery. Health providers, again with the consumer's consent, would be able to access information for subsequent episodes of care, regardless of their location. Consumers would also have access to this information.

The information collected under Health*Connect* would be in the form of standardized health event summaries. These summaries would include information such as basic details about the results of health treatments, a hospital discharge report, referral, the results of pathology tests, or medications prescribed. They would not contain all of the clinical notes made by the provider. Health event summaries, when stored, form the basis of the Health*Connect* EHR. In the longer term, event summaries for the GP consultation, pathology, community health care, hospital, etc., must be defined and agreed upon nationally.

Local EHR systems have existed for some time now, and the Health*Connect* project aims to ensure interoperability across the various states of Australia. Several of the Health*Connect* projects have evolved from pilot studies to full implementation in the pilot sites.

Following a Health Ministers' Conference in 2003, the Nursing Informatics Special Interest Group of the Health Informatics Society of Australia received funding to develop a strategic plan for NI capacity building, including a plan for the nursing profession's engagement with the Australian government and its informatics agenda.[2] The provision of funding for such developments is likely to assist NI progress in Australia and internationally.

A recent review undertaken on behalf of the newly established National Health Information Group (NHIG) and the Australian Health Information Council (AHIC) identified lack of nursing involvement as a significant impediment to the provision of better health care outcomes, safety, quality, and cost efficiencies. The adoption of health informatics principles is seen as an enabler of coordination between the many stakeholders. The review, undertaken in early 2004, was a first step in the development of a revised national health information management and communications technology strategy. The trend is toward greater coordination between providers with a strong emphasis on improving health outcomes.[2]

Many nurses in Australia are actively involved in various aspects of health informatics that may indirectly assist in the development of the Health*Connect* EHR model. In particular, nurses are involved in committees developing standards in health information. Nurses are working at all levels within Health*Connect* projects, although they may not be specifically working on EHR nursing developments. There are also many nurses who have been involved in health informatics organizations across Australia for several years. Case Study 29B from Cook and Conrick that follows this chapter outlines the considerable nursing involvement in the development of Health*Connect*.

New Zealand

New Zealand is ranked high in the development and application of patient management systems (PMS), second only to the United Kingdom in terms of PMS use within general practice (52 percent of GPs versus 59 percent), double that achieved to date in Australia (25 percent), and triple that of the U.S. (17 percent). Work is currently under way to develop systems that will allow sharing of this electronic information between clinicians.

As shown in Figure 29-1, New Zealand's health system is largely public and financed through taxes. Access to public health services is based on need. In 2000–2001, $9.884 billion was spent in New Zealand on health and disability support services (NZ$2601 per capita). The New Zealand government has moved away from market-based structures by combining the health care purchaser and provider functions to community-focused District Health Boards (DHBs).

Historically, there has been no sector-wide approach to developing information systems in New Zealand. Over the past five years, however, the DHBs have been replacing isolated departmental and clinical systems with more integrated and dynamic network-based technologies that support a more connected delivery network.

New Zealand has had a National Health Index (NHI) unique patient identifier since 1977, and there is strong political commitment to develop a comprehensive EHR, enabling health provider's access to electronic records. Several components required to develop an EHR are already being tackled, through the National Health Information Strategy in response to strategic recommendations to local initiatives aiming to fill gaps.[6] The existing health intranet will provide an EHR that is available to all via a secure network.

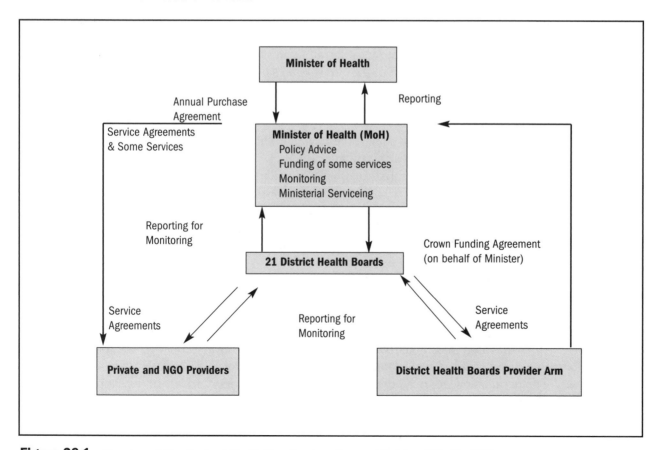

Figure 29-1. *Structure of New Zealand Health Care Services. Source: Ministry of Health, 2003.*

The ever-increasing workload of nurses in New Zealand means nurses themselves are searching for more efficient ways to deliver and record the care they give in an effort to reduce the amount of paper work. While this is certainly not new or specific to New Zealand nurses, the added requirements of delivering care in sometimes isolated areas with few medical specialists available has meant New Zealand nurses have become extremely innovative. Particular attention has been paid to inputting data electronically at the point of care to reduce the work of transposing data from paper forms to electronic forms.[7] Data is required in primary care delivery to make claims against contracts for care delivery. Without careful recording of this data, funding for services and nurses is at risk.

There is considerable development toward a more collaborative approach to care delivery, with integrated patient notes found in many areas, particularly intensive care and critical care units. With staff shortages and the changing roles of both nursing and medicine, the overlap of information requirements is now considerable, making the shared record the most sensible approach.

At present, the standards required to share information across disciplines do not exist in New Zealand, particularly a nursing language that is an accepted standard. This, as in most countries, is probably the single biggest hurdle to the implementation of an EHR in New Zealand. Standards development in health is well supported through the ministerial committee, and the Health Information Standards Organization (HISO), which endorses proposed standards following extensive stakeholder consultation and agreement. Currently, no nursing-specific standards are under consultation, development, or in HISO's prioritized work plan. Their most recent work is to develop the standards to support electronic referrals to other care providers, as well as electronic laboratory orders and results.

Nursing in New Zealand has long used electronic information for the assessment of patient acuity, linked with the staff roster system to ensure the appropriate skill mix is available for patients, but no other discipline has used this information. Patient acuity information has also been used as a handover tool—outlining the requirements for the patient for the next eight hours of care. This information is standardized as a tool set but allows for little individualization of the patient care information, and therefore may be limited in its contribution to the multidisciplinary EHR.

The considerable expansion of the nurse role in New Zealand has been highlighted by recent legislation allowing nurse practitioners, i.e., nurses with a master's degree qualification in a particular area of nursing (e.g., rural nurses and those with further education in pharmacology) to prescribe medications on a limited basis. Few nurses have thus far taken up the challenge. Those who have are mostly practicing in isolated locations where they are the only health care provider. The EHR and, in particular, access to effective electronic decision support would provide these isolated nurses with information at the time of prescribing. Other members of the care team at disparate locations would also have access to notes on the patient's progress and latest care plan.

Electronic prescribing is being implemented in many DHBs, at least at the hospital level, to improve the safety of drug administration by nurses, particularly to lower the rate of errors that can be attributed to illegible handwriting on prescriptions.[8] Electronic discharge summaries from hospitals to GPs are also common. Although these do not yet include a nursing discharge summary, there would be little work required to make this standard practice.

In primary care, considerable use is made of Practice Management Systems (PMS). These systems have clinical components for prescribing and taking clinical notes, and some are now providing interactive disease management through decision support. At this stage, these systems are not used extensively by practice nurses to assist in care delivery. A 2001 study found that:

> "nurses often lack buy-in toward information systems. They use them in a task-orientated way and have not really invested in them due to lack of computer literacy and education on how to use systems extensively."[9]

The Health Information Strategy for New Zealand outlines the proposed development of a component-based EHR, whereby components are developed in isolation as stand-alone applications, but would be compatible and interoperable, capable of delivering data to the centrally and regionally held systems.[10] At this stage, there is no plan to include nursing information at the central and regional level, and indeed, this may not prove useful. However, it may be advantageous for nurses to investigate where their information needs overlap with the proposed EHR components and ensure these needs are considered at the development phases. Locally held data on nursing care will provide extensive decision support to department managers and funders of care delivery. Further, the ability to "speak" to nursing colleagues and other disciplines through the locally held EHR will assist in the delivery of seamless care. It appears that now is the time for nursing in New Zealand to develop clear thinking about information requirements.

South Pacific

Health care in the South Pacific is public and free or at least is heavily subsidized. There are also a number of private hospitals and clinics, offering more services than available publicly for those who are able to pay or have insurance. A reduction in population affects most of the smaller island countries because many of the young people are leaving for Australia or New Zealand where they have automatic rights to live and work. Life expectancy is considerably lower than most Organization for Economic Co-operation and Development (OECD) country members, and diseases such as diabetes are prevalent. Local knowledge of prevalent disease is high and preventive care is encouraged through World Health Organization (WHO) programs and support.

The isolation encountered by doctors, nurses, and allied health workers working in remote South Pacific Island countries is considerable. For example, the northern group of the Cook Islands is a four-hour plane ride from the main island of Rarotonga. There is often only one health worker on each island. Low pay rates and political instability have increased the severe problem with recruitment and retention of qualified, experienced staff throughout the South Pacific.[8] Medical equipment and medications are in limited supply on the smaller islands; many patients need to be moved to the local hospital for complex problems. Paper-based summaries of care provided prior to transfer are sent with the patient, and the nurse receives similar information back following discharge.

It may be that nurses are the ones most isolated and in need of better information. Nurses are situated on the most remote outposts, often covering scattered villages and a population of around 300 people, on an entirely different island from any other medical assistance. Nurses are provided with radio or telephone contact with other nurses and medical staff at the local hospital (local may mean a journey of several hours by small fishing boat). Many nurses note how difficult it is to adequately care for patients.[8] Many health care professionals in the South Pacific note the urgent need for distance-consultation services that would enable the delivery of applicable health care advice between distant islands and other communities, including larger health care centers or even other countries with better specialization.

Many nurses in the Pacific Islands undertake their nursing training locally. The training is based on the three-year New Zealand or Australian nursing curriculum, with increased emphasis on public health. Ongoing education is also limited. Libraries, when available, are limited to a few mostly out-of-date books and journals. Nurses rarely have access to any journals, apart from in the main hospitals. Most health professionals find it difficult to gain access to up-to-date medical information. Further, there is little opportunity for postgraduate education due to geography, cost, and low staffing levels.[8]

The development of the EHR in Australia and New Zealand may at some point affect the Pacific Islands, particularly if Telehealth is included in the components. This is currently proposed in New Zealand, where there has been an increased interest in developing national policies, standards, and guidelines around Telehealth, with emphasis on Pacific countries requirements. Also, HealthConnect in Australia specifically outlines Telehealth as a strategic initiative in their EHR strategy.

Improvements in technology, particularly more affordable infrastructure and operational costs for connectivity between the islands, as well as more affordable basic equipment, such as PCs and digital cameras, are required before it would be feasible to implement even the most basic components of an EHR for nurses. In the meantime, it may be possible to include Pacific Island requirements in New Zealand or Australian developments in nursing standards to ensure they do not fall further behind in health care delivery advances. This would require changes to the curriculum of nurses in the South Pacific to include an outline of the EHR and a general overview of health informatics.

Nursing institutions and representative organizations in Australia and New Zealand have close links throughout the South Pacific, with educational visits made possible through international aid funding and private grants. This gives nurses in the Pacific Islands some exposure to health care technology. Although there are computers in the larger health care institutions in the South Pacific, many are not available to nurses, or nurses are not sufficiently trained to use them, as they are not seen as a nursing tool. Close links with ministries of health throughout the South Pacific and Australasia also provide educational training opportunities for better management of centrally held health care data.

Conclusion

New Zealand and Australia propose a component-based EHR. It is therefore possible, particularly with the NI expertise found in this region, to develop effective EHR components for nurses that comply with the overall requirements of the EHR and other health care providers. It is unlikely there could be an EHR that meets everyone's needs, but individual, interoperable components would provide the required flexibility for each discipline. Data would feed into a centrally managed health event summary system that would include multidisciplinary information for management and policy developers.

There is considerable potential for the EHR to capture nursing knowledge, and this is a great opportunity for nursing to be recognized for its contribution to health outcomes. Nursing education and research would also benefit through the clear documentation of decision making at the bedside, with subsequent discoveries leading to improved patient outcomes.

At present, much of the South Pacific makes use of the Telehealth services that provide connectivity between major hospitals. Could this connectivity be used for other types of health communication around the Pacific? A component-based EHR has the potential to link health services provided via Telehealth with the centrally held EHR to ensure all providers are aware of consultations. While at present it may not be feasible to implement a connected EHR in any country in the South Pacific, the opportunity to gain specific nursing knowledge of this population's needs may provide unforeseen benefits for all those caring for Pacific Islanders throughout Australasia.

In Asia, dramatic recent progress in all areas of e-health has taken place. The potential for understanding the nursing needs of the very mobile Asian populations may also provide Asian nurses with the impetus to continue to take part in new EHR developments.

It may not be feasible to expect the development of an EHR that meets everyone's requirements. Should nurses therefore work toward their own needs, taking into account the developments nationally and internationally? Nurses need not wait for central agencies to consider their needs, but should work on their own developments to ensure a nursing-led project that collaborates with central agencies when possible.

There is the danger of information technology (IT) specialists developing systems that do not meet nurses' needs—systems that are unable to respond to the complexity and subtlety of the world of nursing and midwifery. Therefore, it is in the best interests of nurses to remain involved at all levels of the development process. As migration and tourism grows dramatically around the region, and we are increasingly nursing a multicultural population, it is also important to be aware of the health needs of the whole of the Asia Pacific region in the development of the EHR.

References

1. Coenen A. The International Classification for Nursing Practice (ICNP) programme: advancing a unifying framework for nursing. *Online J Issues Nurs.* April 3, 2003. http://www.nursingworld.org/ojin/tpc7/tpc7_8.htm. Accessed 16.8.05.

2. Hovenga EJS, Carr R, Honey M, Westbrook L (2005): Pacific Rim In: Saba V, McCormick K. A 4th Ed 2005 *Essentials of Nursing Informatics,* McGraw-Hill, New York.

3. Singapore Nurses Association. Nursing informatics. Available at: http://www.sna.org.sg/cms/publish/article_62.shtml. Access date 16.8.05.

4. Taiwan Nurses Association. The nursing profession in Taiwan. Available at: http://www.twna.org.tw/eng-02-2.htm. 2004. Access date 13.12.04.

5. Volrathongchai K, Delaney C, Phuphaibul R. Nursing minimum data set development and implementation in Thailand. *J Adv Nurs.* 2003;43:588-594.

6. Wilson S, Roy D. KIWI nurse: an automated documentation solution for nursing education. In Marin H, Marques E, Hovenga E, & Goossen W. (Eds) *Proceedings of the 8th International Congress in nursing informatics-NI2003.* Rio de Janeiro: E-papers services Editorials Ltd.

7. New Zealand Ministry of Health. *Sharing Excellence in Health and Disability Information Management.* Wellington: New Zealand Ministry of Health; 2004.

8. Kerr K. *A Needs Assessment for Telehealth in the South Pacific* [master's thesis]. Wellington University of Otago; 2002.

9. Gibben B, Boustead C. *A Report for Investment Workstream, Health Information Management and Technology Plan.* Ministry of Health. Wellington 2001.

10. *Health Information Strategy Steering Committee.* New Zealand Health Information Strategy. Ministry of Health. Wellington; 2005.

Case Study 29A

Current Status and Evolution of Nursing Informatics in Korea

Myun-Sook Jung, PhD; Hyeoun-Ae Park, PhD; and
Jeongeun Kim, PhD, RN, Informatics Nurse Specialist

The evolution of Korean nursing informatics (NI), a field that has grown rapidly in this rapidly changing information society, has helped upgrade the position of nursing science in this country. Because nursing science supports nursing practice, active research, and academic activities, these areas also have been advanced.

As of 2004, there were 45,772 hospitals (including general hospitals, long-term-care facilities, and clinics), with a total of 340,988 beds in the Republic of Korea.[1] These data indicate an exploded health care system in immediate need of enhanced productivity through the computerization of work activities and that the role of nurses and informaticians will continue to grow.

The Nursing Special Interest Group of the Korean Society of Medical Informatics was established in 1993. Currently, it has about 600 members. In the past ten years, Korean NI has made dramatic progress in nursing practice, research, and education. This progress has been crucial to the development of the electronic health record (EHR). This case study discusses the state of the art in Korean NI, with a special focus on the EHR. It addresses a terminology-based electronic nursing record, describes the status of research trends to support the EHR, and delineates NI education and e-learning initiatives aimed at creating an information-literate nursing workforce.

A Terminology-based Electronic Nursing Record Component of the EHR

The use of computers in the South Korean health care system began in the late 1970s as part of an effort by hospital finance and administration departments to expedite insurance reimbursements. The focus of hospital computerization then shifted from finance to patient care, and clinics also began to use computers to support practice. More recently, hospitals have started implementing paperless EHR systems. Two tertiary-care hospitals now have completely paperless enterprise-wide EHR systems, and many more hospitals are expected to adopt them soon.

This section of the case study will focus on the implementation of a terminology-based electronic nursing record system as a component of the EHR in two Korean hospitals.[2-4] The Bundang Seoul National University Hospital, a tertiary-care facility with 563 beds, implemented an electronic nursing record system as part of a hospital-wide EHR system when it opened in May 2002. The electronic nursing record system supports documentation in eleven nursing units, e.g., the operating room, the post anesthesia care unit, three intensive care units, the dialysis room, and the emergency department. The system was subsequently upgraded to include decision support systems for nursing diagnosis and intervention. In October 2004, Seoul National University Hospital—one of Korea's largest facilities, with more than 1,200 beds—also implemented an electronic nursing record system.

Analysis of Nursing Notes

Development of the electronic nursing record system at Bundang Hospital began with an analysis of nursing documentation, including both structured and narrative nursing notes. The narrative nursing notes pertaining to patients were separated into phrases and coded by meaning. Analysis of nursing notes was halted when no new phrases were found. The phrases were further parsed into nursing concepts and cross-mapped with use of terms from the International Classification for Nursing Practice (ICNP®) beta version.[3,5] In this process, more than 400 new terms that did not map with the ICNP® were identified.

Development of a Terminology Server and a User Application System

A Web-based ICNP terminology server was developed at Bundang, the functions of which were ICNP navigation, concept management, and precoordinated-phrase management. Precoordinated-phrase management allows users to create, update, or delete a library of precoordinated phrases for describing nursing signs and symptoms, diagnoses, goals, interventions, and evaluations. Each precoordinated phrase may have attributes for detailed expression. For the development of the user application system, phrases from the narrative nursing notes were structured according to the nursing process. The design of this system took into consideration the cyclical process of ongoing nursing assessment, diagnosis, intervention, and evaluation. The terminology server and user application system share the same database; thus, the precoordinated phrases created by the ICNP terminology server are employed in the user application system.

Evaluation of the System

The Bundang electronic nursing record system was evaluated by surveying user satisfaction and time required to document nursing notes. The mean user-satisfaction score was 4.56 (of a possible 5.0 points); the mean time for data input was 2.3 minutes and the mean number of 3.7 precoordinated phrases used in nursing notes.

The domain completeness and expressiveness issues of the ICNP® were evaluated through the analysis of nursing notes from the electronic nursing record system. Of the total data input, 75.6 percent were entered using the dictionary of precoordinated phrases, 3.3 percent were free-text input, and 21.1 percent were a combination of precoordinated phrases and free text. Content analysis of the free-text input showed that 63 percent could be found in the dictionary of precoordinated phrases; 29.9 percent were used to describe non-nursing-care variables, such as patient complaints, references to the care plan, and physicians' orders; and 7.1 percent were used for supplementary purposes, e.g., adding a conjunction or a verb to make an expression grammatically correct. Only 0.1 percent of free-text items were not found in the dictionary of precoordinated phrases. This evaluation demonstrated that the ICNP® has enough compositional power to cover expressions typically used in a hospital clinical nursing setting.

Discussion

An ICNP-based system has been in use since May 2002 in Korea. It was not easy to develop a terminology-based electronic nursing record; there were no guidelines in place or mentors to consult. It was especially difficult to decide what to include in the dictionary of precoordinated nursing phrases, as well as which concepts best fit the vocabulary used in our local clinical system. Although an ad hoc committee within the nursing department was actively involved in development of the electronic nursing record system throughout all phases, from analysis to evaluation, committee members did not know which data are required by nurses and other health care providers to care for patients. If they had known this, it would have been much easier to standardize nursing phrases and nursing concepts. Committee members also came to realize how important it is to have a standard terminology that allows the exchange and sharing of information between departments and systems. They also came to appreciate the value of documenting nursing notes to determine the effectiveness of nursing interventions on patient outcomes.

Nursing Informatics Research Trends and the EHR in Korea

The growing interest in NI has been reflected in nursing research in the Republic of Korea. The number of studies related to NI has increased exponentially in the past ten years. A synthesis of these studies and their contributions to the EHR is both useful and necessary. The authors examined the research trends of Korean NI from 1995 to 2004. The *Journal of Korean Society of Medical Informatics,* launched in 1995, provided an excellent dissemination mechanism for NI research to support the EHR. The authors also searched for NI-related studies on numerous literature-based Web sites, including those of the National Digital Library, the Korean Nurses Association, the Korean Society of Medical Informatics, KoreaMed, and MedRIC. As a result of this search, analysis, and synthesis, specific research trends in Korean NI and its contribution to the EHR were identified. Because concepts addressed in NI are varied, they were classified into groups for the purpose of the literature search (see Table 29A-1).

Initially, the authors retrieved and reviewed the abstracts of research papers, excluding studies that were not directly related to NI research. Standardized nursing terminologies and studies utilizing a classification system were included, as were studies up to the stage of system (database) development. Studies that simply applied nursing classification systems [e.g., North American Nursing Diagnosis Association (NANDA), Nursing Interventions Classification (NIC), Nursing Outcomes Classification (NOC), the Omaha System, Home Health Care Classification (HHCC), and International Classification of Nursing Practice (ICNP)] to nursing records were grouped in the standardized language/classification category.

Table 29A-1. Numbers and Percentages of Research Papers According to Subject, 1995–2004

Subject	Journal of Korean Society of Medical Informatics	Master's Degree Theses/Doctoral Dissertations	Journal of Korean Academy of Nursing	Total for All Sources
System development & database Percentage of total Percentage of category	23 (53.5%) (29.1%)	13 (30.2%) (20.0%)	7 (16.3%) (50.0%)	43 (27.2%)
Electronic patient record Percentage of total Percentage of category	15 (51.7%) (19.0%)	9 (31.0%) (13.8%)	5 (17.2%) (35.7%)	29 (18.4%)
Standardized language/classification Percentage of total Percentage of category	12 (26.7%) (15.2%)	32 (71.1%) (49.2%)	1 (2.2%) (7.1%)	45 (28.5%)
Internet/Web/Education Percentage of total Percentage of category	22 (64.7%) (27.8%)	11 (32.4%) (16.9%)	1 (2.9%) (7.1%)	34 (21.5%)
Other Percentage of total Percentage of category	7 (100.0%) (8.9%)			7 (4.4%)
Total	79 (50.0%)	65 (41.1%)	14 (8.9%)	158

Number of Research Papers

Papers from the *Journal of Korean Society of Medical Informatics*, the *Journal of Korean Academy of Nursing*, master's degree theses, and doctoral dissertations—all published between 1995 and 2004 and focusing on NI—were retrieved and reviewed. There were seventy-nine papers in the *Journal of Korean Society of Medical Informatics*, fourteen papers in the *Journal of Korean Academy of Nursing*, and sixty-five master's degree theses and doctoral dissertations—for a total of 158 papers.

Nursing Informatics Research Subjects

The 158 papers were analyzed and grouped into five areas according to research subject: system development, database, EHRs, standardized language/classification, Internet/Web education, and other (Table 29A-1). A summary of each area follows.

System Development/Database. Studies focused on protocol development or early system consideration phases were excluded from this synthesis; those focused on system development and database were included. This subject category had the next-to-highest frequency of studies (forty-three papers, 27.2 percent), second only to the standardized language/classification subject.

Electronic Health Record. Some may believe this subject should be incorporated into the system development and database category. This review found that more than 45.5 percent of NI studies focused primarily on the EHR or system development.

Standardized Language/Classification. This subject category had the most NI studies (forty-five papers, 28.5 percent), and accounted for almost half of all NI-related dissertations (thirty-two papers, 49.2 percent). This indicates responsiveness to the scholarship demands of nursing practice. Moreover, there is a high commitment that clinical applications should be made after systematic studies on standardized language or classification. Although most dissertations written two to three years ago use terminologies related to NANDA or NIC, more recent dissertations reflect increasing interest in the clinical applications of ICNP, HHCC, and Omaha. NANDA-NIC nursing terminologies have been actively studied; however, their use and application in clinical practice are limited. Some studies have focused on development of the ICNP-based system. (As mentioned earlier, Seoul National University Hospital recently introduced and implemented an ICNP-based electronic nursing record in its hospital information system.)

Internet/Web Education. Including Jung's research,[6] there are many program developments and evaluations in this subject category. It comprises thirty-four papers, accounting for 21.5 percent of all NI studies. Most of these papers have appeared in the *Journal of Korean Society of Medical Informatics.*

Other. Seven papers (4.4 percent) did not match the criteria of the other categories. All were published in the *Journal of Korean Society of Medical Informatics.*

Findings

Based on the findings previously discussed, it is evident that the number of studies on NI is increasing, especially on the subject of standardized language/classification. Although there is great interest in the clinical applications of standardized nursing languages and classification systems, few Korean hospitals use computerized nursing records with standardized nursing language. The digitalization of nursing information should be strengthened in order to make the clinical utilization of information easier and smoother.

Nursing research, especially that pertaining to NI, can empower evidence-based practice. Knowledge-building creates the expertise to conduct comparative studies of nursing care, e.g., the study by Delaney et al.[7] This nursing research empowers Korea to be a leader in the International Nursing Minimum Data Set (iNMDS) project. Myun-Sook Jung leads the Korean participation in the iNMDS project. Hyeoun-Ae Park serves on the Steering Committee of the iNMDS Project as well as an International Medical Informatics Association (IMIA) NI representative for the Republic of Korea.

Nursing Informatics Education and e-Learning for Next-generation Korean Nurses and IT Competencies

Preparing nurses for the challenges in the rapidly evolving world of health care delivery and the EHR imperative is a daunting task. Korea has one of the highest levels of Internet penetration in the world, making it well-positioned to provide global leadership in nursing education by using e-learning technologies.

Brief History of Nursing Informatics Education in Korea

In 1992, the Department of Nursing Information Education established the first undergraduate informatics course in Korea. The course became available at the graduate level in 1996.[8] In the wake of the rapid changes in health care information technology (HCIT) that began in the early 1990s, some academicians took the initiative to offer medical and NI programs in an attempt to improve health care. In 1996, the Korean Nurses Association developed a self-study program in nursing, which it distributed through use of diskettes.

Several nursing academicians tried to enhance nursing education through informatics, leading to the establishment of nursing information programs in many universities. Seoul National University College of Nursing offered the first degree-earning NI program in Korea, establishing the Department of Nursing Information at the undergraduate level in 1997 and at the graduate level in 2000.

National Studies Measuring Nursing Informatics Education in Korean Nursing Education Institutions

The Korean Society of Medical Informatics Working Group on Medical Informatics Education conducted two surveys: one on the present state of education and training in NI at nursing colleges and the other on the professional consensus about the learning outcomes of NI education in Korea.[9] In the first survey, Kim et al[9] examined the curricula of nursing colleges in Korea, using the Internet and other published data. Of 115 nursing colleges studied, thirty-three (28.7 percent) had incorporated at least one nursing informatics subject into the regular undergraduate education program and six offered graduate-level courses. Most of the courses carried two or three academic credits and were offered to second- and third-year students in undergraduate programs.

This survey study was followed up with an in-depth look at the content and effectiveness of the NI curriculum in these nursing colleges. Using a Delphi method, the authors selected the panelists (experts) from a list of nursing informaticians who had at least one year of nursing college teaching experience. The questionnaire comprised items about the experts' perceptions of the curriculum and of the learning outcomes in terms of NI education at colleges. The experts categorized NI into four fields: general informatics, basics of NI, clinical/applied NI, and public/social aspects of NI. The three case studies presented below represent a sampling of the Delphi findings and serve to demonstrate the current status of NI curriculum offerings.

Case Studies of e-Learning Programs in the Korean Nursing Association

Case 1: Seoul National University College of Nursing

Seoul National University College of Nursing created its Web site in 1999, providing an e-learning platform for undergraduate courses. In 2004, the college decided to increase its online offerings in nursing and developed e-learning applications for the e-learning platform, which are accessible to undergraduate and graduate students and to those in special education programs. The e-learning solution is divided into three sections: nursing education, nursing intervention, and nursing research. The nursing education section can be used for sharing information and training students to function in a computerized world. The nursing intervention section provides information on nursing care for patients and the public. The nursing research section addresses the research process and building nursing knowledge. These content areas were essential to the successful implementation of the University hospital's EHR.

Case 2: e-Learning for Continuing Education at the Asan Medical Center

The Asan Medical Center ranks among the best teaching hospitals in Korea and maintains a cutting-edge information system. The Center took the lead in providing online continuing education. Newly recruited nurses are provided with access to e-learning programs for hospital orientation and with basic knowledge about their assignments before starting their work. The Center also offers a course to help nurses strengthen the English-language skills required for their work. The extensive course content is delivered in streaming video format using Flash software.

Case 3: Cyber Education Center of the Korean Nurses Association

The Korean Nurses Association (KNA) established a cyber continuing education center in 2004 in an effort to develop structured, effective educational programs committed to producing world-class nurses. This online continuing education initiative focuses on increasing learning opportunities for nurses free of the constraints of time and space. The KNA demonstrated a profound commitment to expeditiously addressing this initiative. The KNA issued a bidding announcement for the system developer in January 2003, signed an agreement with the system developer in May 2003, established a cyber education committee in June 2003, finalized the evaluation and grading system for students in January 2004, and launched the center in February 2004. Currently, a two-part course in geriatric nursing and a course on nurses and the law are offered through the e-learning center. The promise of this center for addressing state-of-the-art nursing and the demands of the electronic health care world is pervasive.

References

1. Korean Ministry of Health and Welfare. Health Resource Division. Available at: http://www.mohw.go.kr. Accessed July 15, 2005.

2. Cho IS, Park HA. Development and evaluation of a terminology-based electronic nursing record system. *J Biomed Inform.* 2003;36:304-312.

3. Cho IS, Park HA, Chung EJ, Lee HS. Formative evaluation of standard terminology-based electronic nursing record system in clinical setting. *J Korean Soc Med Infom.* 2003; 9(4):413-421.

4. Cho IS, Park HA. Evaluation of the expressiveness of ICNP terminology in a computerized nursing record system. In: Lorenz P and Dini P, eds. *Proceedings of the 4th International Conference on Networking (ICN '05), Reunion Island, France, April 17–21, 2005.* New York: Springer.

5. International Council of Nurses. International Classification for Nursing Practice Beta International Council of Nurses, Geneva: 1999.

6. Jung MS. Development of Web-based education program in nursing informatics. *J Korean Nurs Admin Acad Soc.* 2000.

7. Delaney C, Ruiz M, Clarke M, Srinivasan P, Knowledge Discovery in Databases: Data Mining the NMDS. [Paper] In Saba V, Carr R, Sermeus W, Rocha P (eds.). One Step Beyond: The Evolution of Technology & Nursing, Proceedings of the 7th International Congress on Nursing Informatics (pp.61-65). 2000.

8. Park HA, Kim JE, Yang YH, Hyun SK. A survey study of nursing informatics education in Korea. *J Korean Soc Inform.* 1999;5:1:11-25.

9. Kim JE, Chun BC, Choi SW, Hwang DH, Yum YH, Moon YJ. What should be educated to the nursing students in nursing informatics? In: Proceedings of the Asian-Pacific Association for Medical Informatics (APAMI) 2003 Congress, DaeKu, Korea. 2003;576.

Case Study 29B

Australia's Health*Connect:*
Delivering Value for Nurses and their Patients

Robyn Cook, BBus, MBA, RN, and Moya Conrick, PhD, RN

Australia's Health System

Australia's health system's structure reflects the country's model of governance, a complex combination of public and private service delivery models. The Commonwealth and state/territorial governments have overlapping responsibilities in providing health services. The Commonwealth Government's leadership role is in policy making, in particular, in national issues, e.g., public health, research, and national information management. The Commonwealth also funds most out-of-hospital medical services and health research.[1] In turn, the states are primarily responsible for service provision, although the Commonwealth influences this. The six Australian states and two territories cover the delivery and management of public health services, as well as relationships with health professionals.

Health services in Australia are a mix of Commonwealth and state-funded public hospitals, community aged care, and disability services. Universal access is provided through Medicare, a general taxation system. The Commonwealth exerts some control over the health agenda by directing state and territory funding of services through the Medicare Funding Agreement and by offering incentive payments to them. However, this funding agreement is often criticized by the states because the agreements are renegotiated every five years, and, according to the Commonwealth, meeting the financial pressure from the rising costs of and increasing demands for health care is always the responsibility of the states and territories. In 2004, the Commonwealth provided 47 percent of national health funding, the states provided 23 percent, and 30 percent came from nongovernment sources.[2] However, in some quarters, the current funding model is thought inadequate because of the cost of new drugs, technology, and rising wages.[3] This complex funding model leads to an equally complex arrangement for service provision.

Three key areas of service provision exist: community and private services, hospital and nursing home services, and public health services. They are provided by individual health professionals, the Commonwealth, or state government health care organizations. Public hospitals are the shared responsibility of the Commonwealth and state governments, as are some nursing home services. However, private sector and not-for-profit organizations are the major supplier of nursing home beds, and the Commonwealth provides payments to cover a percentage of the costs for residents, who often have to supplement the cost of their care. The private sector also offers a range of services and hospital beds. Although the system of joint governance over health care has been in place for some time, changes in demographics, escalating costs, a lack of clinical staff, and changes to the health care delivered have led to the need for a more cohesive and integrated health service, delivered much more efficiently. Central to this goal is the use of information technology (IT).

Nursing and Primary, Secondary, and Tertiary Services

Nurses deliver care across all health sectors, often in very isolated settings throughout Australia. Nursing is dominant in the primary health care setting, but as in many other countries, general practitioners regard themselves as the gatekeepers of the system and claim to be primary health caregivers, albeit it in a very narrow sense. Nursing is the largest group of health professionals in Australia with 290,000 registered personnel. Approximately 230,000 of those are actively working. The nursing workforce is growing older; the average age is around 42.2 years. The number of nurses has dropped to 1,024 full-time employed (FTE) nurses per 100,000 residents because fewer are entering the field. Across geographic regions, the level of supply ranges from 886 full-time employed nurses per 100,000 in remote areas to 954 per 100,000 in inner regional areas.[2]

In the primary setting, nursing responsibilities range from early childhood monitoring and supporting child and family development to coordinating all aspects of individual health care and broader population health programs in a rural or remote setting. Some nurse-led clinics are more than 600 kilometers from the nearest hospital or medical officer. At a secondary level, nurses are key to twenty-four hour, seven-day-a-week care and coordination in a range of settings. Nurse practitioners are gaining a greater role in health care, and nursing services that span hospital and community are becoming more common. Nurse practitioners prescribe medications, order diagnostic tests, and make referrals within approved guidelines. At a tertiary level, nurses provide extensive specialized nursing care.

Information Flow Challenges

As health care becomes more complex and the boundaries between the professions and health sectors (primary, secondary, and tertiary) become increasingly blurred, the ability to communicate effectively about patient care is essential. Information flow across all sectors of the health care system is less than satisfactory and does not support effective, efficient health care delivery.[4] The complex structure of the health system creates organizational boundaries that reduce information flows. This is significantly exacerbated by the lack of electronic clinical systems.[4]

The existing privacy policy frameworks in both Commonwealth and state jurisdictions have also impeded information flow. Significant discussion and review of privacy policies are in process; changes will be needed to support improved information flows within a consumer-agreed, consent model. Until recently, privacy was also problematic as the technologies did not provide a secure platform for the exchange of information. Significant research and development in this area has led to the availability of more cost-effective technologies to accomplish implementation of such a platform.

One of the greatest impediments to information flow in nursing is the lack of any standardization of data, leaving nurses unable to communicate efficiently across locations and geographical settings.[5,6] Changing community and clinical expectations about the management of data, and a growing expectation that health information should be available when it is needed, have also created an environment to support change. Whereas clinicians expect timely transfer of information to support care delivery, consumers are demanding it.

Health*Connect* Aims, Objectives, Initiatives, and Evaluation

In 1999, a task force, under the auspices of Commonwealth and state health ministers, was established to provide a coordinated approach to the development of a national Australian electronic health record (EHR). The task force recommended the establishment of a health information network for Australia, which was endorsed by the health ministers in 2000, to create Health*Connect* and a medications record (Medi*Connect*).[7] Health*Connect* is designed to provide an environment in which access to information can be exploited to support care delivery, improve health outcomes, support care planning, and foster further research. According to the Commonwealth, Health*Connect* will "improve the delivery of health care and provide better quality of care, consumer safety, and health outcomes for all Australians while enhancing the privacy and respecting the dignity of the health consumer."[8]

The governance arrangements for Health*Connect* involve an integrated approach to planning, resourcing and managing projects that involve sharing of costs and risks across jurisdictions and the private sector.[8] Governance arrangements are under review since a consulting report about the structure of Health*Connect;* the Stakeholder Reference Group was disbanded and a National Electronic Health Transition Authority (NeHTA) was set up by the Commonwealth. NeHTA's focus is e-health informatics standards and integrating infrastructure. This includes developing standards for the exchange of clinical information. The Health*Connect* project office is overseeing the operational component of implementing pilot EHR projects. Neither group has nursing representation at advisory levels.[9]

The Health*Connect* Model

Health*Connect* is underpinned by a draft systems architecture that describes in detail the building blocks for the EHR and what Health*Connect* should look like while providing the technical blueprint for how the system should be implemented. The blueprint includes plans for MediConnect, which began its life as a separate project, to be integrated into the Health*Connect* program. The Health*Connect* model is based on a series of health-related "event summaries," collected with the consumer's consent at the point of care. Within the consent framework, health care providers will have secure access to the summary information on subsequent occasions of service and consumers will also have some access to their records. It also provides for the creation and storage of other types of health information (X-rays and so forth).[10] Having more complete and up-to-date information available also means that consumers and their providers are better prepared to make decisions in partnership. Privacy and confidentiality have been pivotal issues in the development of Health*Connect.*

A three-stage development program was proposed to test, scope, and focus the Health*Connect* project. In the initial testing phase, seven questions were used to focus on the broad value of Health*Connect.* These concerned the technical feasibility, implementation models, private sector role, privacy management, governance, cost, and sustainability. These concepts defined key areas of work and have supported and informed the Health*Connect* trials. An incremental development model, building on state-based trials and integrating lessons learned, is ongoing. The private sector, involved since the program's inception, is an important part of the long-term provision of Health*Connect.* Private health providers, e.g., general practitioners and pharmacies, have been integral to both the Medi*Connect* and the Health*Connect* trials.

Health*Connect* has established an evaluation framework using a benefits realization approach. Through defining the benefits, the key processes impacted by Health*Connect* have been identified and an estimation of the change in health outcomes identified. The evaluation framework outlines key population groups, disease groups, and health care settings in which significant opportunities for cost and quality improvements could be realized in the initial phases. The framework also includes an economic evaluation tied to clear management accountabilities to ensure the continued delivery of benefits in later phases.[11]

Health*Connect* State-based Trials and Nursing Involvement

States and territories were invited to submit research proposals for trials. The first trials began in Tasmania and the Northern Territory for Health*Connect*, and in Launceston and Ballarat for MediConnect. Stage two Health*Connect* trials are now underway in the North Queensland, South Brisbane, and in the Western Australian Eastern Goldfields broadband trial. Several of the original trials have proceeded to implementation. Table 29B-1 below gives a succinct overview of the projects underway and nursing's involvement in them.

Nursing Involvement in Health*Connect*

Although nursing has fought for many years to be involved at the higher, decision-making levels of government, this has been refused repeatedly. Nursing involvement in the Health*Connect* trials has been serendip-

Table 29B-1. Health*Connect* Trials and Status

	Tasmania— Hobart & Launceston	Northern Territory— Katherine	North Queensland— Townsville	Brisbane— South Brisbane	New South Wales	South Australia	Western Australia
Population	Over 18 years with diabetes	Remote Aboriginal	Elective surgery	Adults with diabetes	Chronic Disease (1) and 0–15 age (2)	All patients	All patients
Scope	Test prototype of Health*Connect*	Indigenous mobile group and test concept	Test concept including privacy, consent, consumer participation and data storage	*open*EHR trial and test concept of value to people with specific disease	Test and evaluate core components, including opt out model of consent	OACIS—key source system for Health*Connect*	Provide Broadband access in rural and remote areas. Will test VOIP and VPN's.
Key Outcomes	Trial successful. Project now extended to whole of state.	Trial successful. Also acceptance by indigenous community.	Yet to report— anecdotal evidence points to success	Yet to report	Yet to report	Ongoing project	Secure e-mail communication between health care providers.
Nursing Involvement	Serendipitous— no specific Nursing	Serendipitous— no specific Nursing	Serendipitous— no specific Nursing	Serendipitous— no specific Nursing	Community Nursing active involvement	Not known	Serendipitous— no specific Nursing

itous rather than deliberate. Many nurses are involved because of their organizational skills and are managing trials or patient enrollments. Nurses have been involved on IT committees representing Australia's major nursing groups, e.g., the Royal College of Nursing Australia (professional issues) and the Australian Nursing Federation (industrial issues). These groups were represented by one individual on the Health*Connect* Stakeholder Reference Group, the open EHR Steering Committee, and the Clinical Information Project (CIP) working group. Nursing was granted observer status to the Health*Connect* Board for the last two meetings before it was recessed. The CIP has no nursing representative on its advisory committee, but it has actively engaged with nursing in developing clinical event summaries. Standards Australia has had a representative from the Royal College of Nursing Australia on its Health Informatics Committee (IT14) for many years; however, at a government advisory level and national standards level, no nursing representative has been sought nor nominated candidates accepted.

Initiatives to Support Health*Connect*

To ensure the viability of Health*Connect*, a number of key building blocks, e.g., standards, event summaries, health identifiers, connectivity, and privacy policies (regarding consent and access control) were earmarked for development. These, of course, are also essential to all other e-health initiatives.

Standards. Standards underpin the effective operation of EHRs, and it is acknowledged that the implementation of standards is essential to ensure the seamless movement of information across networks. The development of standards has accelerated since the inception of the Health*Connect* project and involves mainly the NeHTA, the Commonwealth government, and Standards Australia, with significant sharing of developments with the International Standards Organization (ISO), European Committee for Standardization (CEN), and Health Level 7 (HL7). These groups are developing standards for data security and authentication, messaging and communications, terminologies, coding, and classification systems.[12] The Commonwealth produced a substantial discussion paper to inform these developments. Archetype development that underpins the open EHR architecture in Health*Connect* is also being tested in demonstration pilots.

The Australian Catalogue of Medicines (ACOM), another type of standardization being undertaken will be a vital source of information on all prescription and nonprescription medicines, including complementary health care products, available within Australia. Each product will have a globally unique identification code or Global Trade Item Number (GTIN), and the catalogue will enable the reliable transmission of product details between health care providers. The ACOM will ensure that doctors, pharmacists, and hospitals refer to the same medicine and that information is consistent across all IT systems. This is another essential building block for Health*Connect* and should reduce the adverse events associated with medicine use, improve the accuracy of medicine information communicated between systems, and achieve quality use of medicine for all consumers.

Event Summaries and Other Content. Also vital to the development of Health*Connect* is the *Clinical Information Project* (CIP), which focuses on the content requirements for the health record. The CIP project involves development of the following: a framework and data model for determining clinical information capture and representation; a prototype that prioritizes health event summaries and EHR list views.[13] The overall objective of the CIP is to underpin electronic health information interchange and to facilitate semantic interoperability of clinical information across Australia.[13] CIP is also defining the concept of event summaries, which will provide an overview of a patient's health care event. An event summary will contain only the information that is relevant to the future health and care of the consumer, rather than the comprehensive notes that a doctor may keep as a record of a consultation. An event summary may be retrieved and shared in a timely fashion via a secure network between authorized health care providers, with the consumer's consent. Research and development work is ongoing around defining a framework that specifies what information should be included in an event summary and how the data will be recorded.

Security and Confidentiality. The need for a secure system of identification is a significant issue for Health*Connect*, as Australia does not have a unique identification number for users of health care services or for providers. Consumer identification in a national record, however, is essential to ensure that a consumer's medical information is unambiguously linked to that person and that there is no uncertainty about the transfer of clinical information. State and Commonwealth patient identifiers are currently being investigated via the ProviderConnect project and this will enable the unique identification of all health care providers—including nurses. NeHTA has assumed responsibility for nursing identification.

Providers and consumers will need to be assured that personal health information is adequately protected within Health*Connect* and that stringent access controls are enforced. Consent will involve seeking the agreement of consumers to record information in Health*Connect* and to access that information in the future.

Consent must be informed and voluntary with an opt-in system for both consumers and providers.[14] Consumers, however, will have the right to opt out of providing information overall or for a single visit. Many clinicians are concerned this policy will leave gaps in health care records, but consumers regard the choice as their right. Because of these concerns and the likelihood of higher costs to support an opt-in model, New South Wales is testing an opt-out model. According to Conrick and Newell,[15] on balance, this arrangement seems no different from the current disconnected method of collecting data in which patients can have many records spread across many organizations and private providers. They also feel that the EHR can be secured more easily than paper and should enhance privacy.

Models for secure access and consent have been tested as a priority throughout the Health*Connect* project. Consumers have control over the content of their record and determine which health care providers may access it, while passwords, audits, review processes, and other security mechanisms will prevent unauthorized access. However, providers and consumers must be confident in these measures or the record will languish.

Health*Connect* participants will register for a Medicare "smartcard," which will provide a unique identification number for each person. Kiosks equipped with smartcard readers will be available, and eventually, patients will be able to access their health records from home via a secure Internet link. Initially, the smartcard will store emergency information including allergies and adverse drug reactions. An option for the storage of a digital photo will also ensure patient identification in an emergency situation. Over time, other health data, e.g., child immunization records and donor status will be added.

However, a fundamental problem in Australia is the vast distances over which information needs to travel and the inadequacy of current mainly copper wire telecommunication systems. To achieve these levels of functionality, Health*Connect* will require broadband access.

State-based Implementations as Feeders to Health*Connect*

A number of states are working toward the implementation of core clinical systems that will be used at the point-of-care. These systems will form the basis of the electronic clinical (patient) record (in contrast to the EHR). Nursing will be a major contributor to the electronic clinical record as it will be the repository for all nursing documentation. Because these systems will feed summary data to Health*Connect*, it is important that they are implemented in the short to medium term (three-to-five years). This will reduce the need to document in different systems and ensure automated information flows. Such systems will increase NI skills and knowledge. Nurses are involved in many of the point-of-care clinical solution developments and implementations, particularly in the realm of clinical documentation.

Challenges for Nursing

IT supports clinicians by enabling much greater interaction and improvement in communication. If nurses in Australia are unable to engage because of incompatible work processes, lack of common language, person and facility identification, education, or interoperable systems, a large section of the nursing community will remain isolated and nursing's communication within the health system will be inconsistent.[16] Australian nurses must also decide on a governance framework through which a group with delegated decision-making authority will direct nursing's collective efforts. Further insight into these and many others issues affecting the ability of nurses to embrace IT are contained in a report to the Commonwealth Government by Conrick et al.[16] Some of the major issues from that report are discussed below.

The capacity of nursing to exploit IT is unknown, but anecdotal reports and generalized studies point to problems in this area. Few education and training programs are available at either the undergraduate or postgraduate level, and indeed there are very few informatics educators.[16] Nonetheless, it is essential that beginning practitioners have basic competencies in NI; in particular, they should understand the importance and use of clinical information systems. A national approach to the development of competencies and integration of these into curricula must be undertaken and academic incentives provided if governments are to demonstrate their commitment to informatics scholarship.[16]

The standardization of nursing language presents quite a challenge and, according to Conrick et al,[16] Australian nurses will probably not agree on or find a single classification that covers a whole nursing solution. A major problem is the lack of funding to initiate research into appropriate terminology that represents the spectrum of nursing practice. A comprehensive report of nursing data sets and terminologies currently in use needs to be compiled, as does an evaluation of available data sets and terminologies to assess their ability to adequately represent nursing concepts and meet nurses' information needs at all levels in the health industry.[16]

A record architecture that is independent of particular language, e.g., an open EHR, may provide an answer. However, if Health*Connect* were to adopt an open EHR approach, Australian nurses would need to develop archetypes that describe the concepts of their practice. As archetypes are not language-specific, agreement on particular data sets would not be crucial. The Commonwealth government's adoption of SNOMED-CT and SNOMED'S new international governance will help to alleviate these problems, but much work is still required. A study by Scott et al[17] demonstrates the difficulties of content coverage when mapping three different classifications to raw patient data. The highest hit rate was 68 percent returned by SNOMED-CT. Nursing has set up an archetype portal to support this work, but a governance framework for its management is also required.

As new technology is developed and implemented, personnel and organizations have to adjust; sometimes the adjustment is major. Nursing, as key participants and the largest stakeholder group in health care, will be most affected by the introduction of technology, and change management will be crucial to its uptake. Nurse leaders and managers will play vital roles to ensure the successful implementation of IT. If nurses are not involved and do not feel ownership in the early development of IT in Australia, future change management strategies may be at risk. Senior nursing personnel are aware and agree that information systems and technology are critical to improving clinical care. Consequently, nurse informaticians must take immediate action to raise the profile of NI and clinical information systems and to extol the benefits that technology can provide in supporting nursing practice.

Summary

In Australia, IT will significantly redefine the professional boundaries in health care and support health care workers across vast geographical distances by providing access to quality, timely data and information. IT opens up new possibilities for the dissemination and use of information that enable government initiatives, e.g., Health*Connect,* to demonstrate improved performance and outcomes across the health sector. The explosion of IT uses' and the Commonwealth's vision for the future of health care has made it urgent for nurses to engage and become partners in these developments.

Acknowledgements
Thank you to the following people for their contribution to this chapter:
- John Fletcher, Trial/Implementation Manager, Health*Connect* NT
- Sue Ashlin, Trial Manager, Tasmanian Health*Connect* Trial

References

1. Commonwealth of Australia. *The Australian Health Care System: An Outline.* Canberra: Commonwealth Department of Health and Aged Care Financing and Analysis Branch; 2000.

2. Commonwealth of Australia. *National Review of Nursing Education 2002.* Canberra: Department of Education, Science and Training; 2002.

3. Menadue J. *Breaking the Commonwealth/State Impasse in Health.* Sydney: Whitlam Institute, University of Western Sydney; 2004.

4. Commonwealth of Australia. Health*Connect Interim Research Report: Overview and Findings.* Vol 1. Canberra: Department of Health and Ageing; 2003.

5. Conrick M. *Introduction to information technology and information management.* In: M Conrick ed. Health Informatics: Transforming Health Care with Technology. Melbourne: Thompson Publishing. 2006 in press.

6. Conrick M. Nursing and the electronic health record. In: Barnard A, ed. *Nursing in a Technological World.* July 2003. Brisbane: Queensland University of Technology; 2003.

7. Commonwealth of Australia. Health*Connect.* Canberra: Department of Health and Ageing; 1999.

8. Commonwealth of Australia. *Report of the National Electronic Records Taskforce.* Canberra: Department of Health and Ageing; 2000.

9. Conrick M. Informatics professional roles and governance. In: Conrick M, ed. *Health Informatics: Transforming Health Care with Technology*. Melbourne: Thompson International (in press).

10. Commonwealth of Australia. Health*Connect Trials*. Department of Health and Ageing. Canberra: 2004.

11. DMR Consulting (2004). *Benefits Realisation Framework*. Canberra, Department of Health and Ageing. Canberra: 2004.

12. Walker S, Frean I, Scott P, Conrick M. *Classifications and Terminologies in Residential Aged Care: An Information Paper*. Canberra: The Ageing and Aged Care Division of the Commonwealth Department of Health and Ageing; 2004. Available at: http://www.NIAonline.org.au.

13. Commonwealth of Australia. *Clinical information project*. Available at: http://www.HealthConnect.gov.au/building/Building.htm#CIP. Accessed January 12, 2005.

14. Commonwealth of Australia. *National health privacy code*. Available at: http://www.health.gov.au/pubs/nhpcode.htm. Accessed March 2003.

15. Conrick M, Newell C. Issues of ethics and law. In: Conrick M, ed. *Health Informatics: Transforming Health Care with Technology*. Melbourne: Thompson Publishing (in press).

16. Conrick M, Hovenga E, Cook R, Laracuente T, Morgan T. *A Framework for Nursing Informatics in Australia: A Strategic Paper*. Health Informatics Society of Australia– Nursing Informatics Australia, Melbourne: Department of Health and Ageing; 2004.

17. Scott P, Jones L, Saad P, Conrick M, Foster J, Campbell M. Matching residential aged care terms to SNOMED CT, ICNP2Beta, and CATCH. In: Conrick M, Soar J, eds. *Proceedings from ACCIC04*. Brisbane: Health Informatics Society of Australia; 2004.

Case Study 29C

The New Zealand Approach to the Electronic Health Record

Lucy Westbrooke, DipNurs, GradDipBus, Health Informatics and Annie Fogarty, MA, BHS

New Zealand, with its population of just over four million, has traditionally embraced technology and often is at the forefront of electronic system use, e.g., in the banking sector. The use of technology has extended into the primary, secondary, and tertiary sectors of health. In line with many countries, New Zealand recognizes that to improve efficiency, safety, and quality of care, information exchange between health service providers must be improved. Electronic health records (EHRs) are recognized as a way to achieve this transfer of information and to promote improved health care outcomes for all. New Zealand is in a good position to embrace this, as much of the infrastructure needed to support the development and implementation of EHRs is already in place.

New Zealand Health Sector

The New Zealand health system is 77.5 percent publicly funded, with the remaining 22.5 percent privately funded.[1] Within the public sector, the health care purchaser and provider functions are combined and delivered by twenty-one individual district health boards (DHBs). These DHBs are responsible for primary, secondary, and community care, with some DHBs also providing tertiary and quaternary services. This model has highlighted the needs for information exchange and for a change to a sector-wide approach to the development and implementation of information systems.

Health Sector Strategies

Over the past few years, there have been a number of national health-related strategies developed by the New Zealand Ministry of Health, e.g., The New Zealand Health Strategy;[2] The Primary Health Care Strategy;[3] New Zealand Disability Strategy;[4] and From Strategy to Reality: The WAVE Project.[5] These strategies promote the collection and sharing of information and support the development of comprehensive EHRs. Development of EHRs is outlined as a goal in *From Strategy to Reality: the WAVE Project*.[5] This strategy came from the collaboration of a range of health sector players including government representatives, clinicians, health care managers, information technology (IT) managers, and system vendors. It describes an EHR as:

> An electronic longitudinal collection of health information, based on the individual patient, entered and accepted by health care professionals, which can be distributed over a number of sites and in a number of settings. The information is organized primarily in support of continuing, efficient, and quality health care. The record (or records) is under the control of an agreed access policy. Information does not form part of the health record until a health care professional has taken responsibility for it and entered it into the record. The data is typically stored in a single clinical data repository at each site. An EHR exists when a health care provider accesses health information from a clinical data repository(s) or a single national server, or multiple distributed servers, where the health information is stored, for information on their patient's health history. A longitudinal history is incrementally created for the patient as more health information is provided to these servers.

The strategy summarized the EHR recommendations as:

- Implement electronic exchange of information, e.g., referral letters and discharge summaries, between hospitals and health care providers.
- Develop standards for transmission of health event summaries between providers based on existing referral and discharge standards.
- Implement disease management programs, encouraging general practitioners (GPs) to use electronic clinical record software and hospitals to use clinical data repositories.

Components and Infrastructure Supporting EHRs

EHRs, by allowing providers access to clinical data about patients, can contribute to improved health care outcomes as well as efficiencies in health care delivery. New Zealand is fortunate that some of the core components to achieving this are already in place. Standards for messaging and coding, e.g., Health Level-7 (HL7) and International Classification of Diseases-10 (ICD-10), are accepted and utilized. Legislation, e.g., the Privacy Act 1993,[6] governs the collection, storage, access, and use of personal information; the Health Information Privacy Code 1994,[7] applies the Privacy Act to the health sector; and the Official Information Act 1982[8] provides controls on information. Some of the infrastructure, e.g., the National Health Index, which provides a unique patient identifier, and the Health Intranet and Healthlink,[9] which provide a secure network for transfer of information, are already in place. Other components, such as the Health Provider Index which supplies a unique identifier for all health care providers, are under development and due for release shortly.

Stakeholders in EHRs

Over the past three years, there has been a dramatic change in the way the health sector approaches development of information systems. Many legacy systems have either been replaced or have been integrated with other systems, often using dynamic Web-based technologies to provide seamless information delivery.

There are a number of parties participating in EHR initiatives in New Zealand: the IT Health Cluster,[10] which consists of health IT vendors and health informatics organizations, e.g., Health Informatics New Zealand (HINZ)[11] and Health Information Association of New Zealand (HIANZ);[12] standards organizations, e.g., the Health Information Standards Organization (HISO);[13] a range of professional organizations; and individual health care providers. The New Zealand government is taking a more active role in setting strategies for health information and is funding some initiatives that will support it. The approach focuses more on infrastructure and standards, leaving system implementations and change management to the local or regional levels.

One of the major stakeholders in EHRs is the patient or consumer. There are few published New Zealand studies on this, but one by Ryan and Boustead[14] concludes that "there is a low level of awareness and many misconceptions amongst the lay public about e-health information and patient rights. National awareness campaigns, as recommended by the WAVE project, could go some way to reversing this situation."[14]

Nurse involvement in EHR development is from a health informatics perspective rather than solely focused on nursing. Because nurses are traditionally patient-focused, they see the benefits of developing multidisciplinary EHRs.

Initiatives with EHRs in New Zealand

The EHR is still seen as the "Holy Grail," but by using the philosophy of "not letting the perfect get in the way of the good," New Zealand has decided that having some of the components of an EHR is better than waiting for the ultimate solution, which may be financially out of reach.

New Zealand is fortunate to have a number of health IT vendors who have worked with the health sector to provide an integrated view of information. Patient information is often held in a number of disparate systems, including patient management systems (for registration; admission, discharge, and transfer (ADT); and outpatient scheduling), laboratory and radiology systems and clinical systems. For health professionals, there is a need to see a patient-centric view of this information.

In the secondary sector, companies, e.g., Orion Systems International[15] and i-Health (now part of iSoft16), have products that allow a Web-based view of information from different systems, providing seamless access to patient-related information. Orion's Concerto product is a "Medical Applications Portal that is placed over multiple information systems to provide a single, seamless view of a patient's data," e.g., admissions, discharge, and transfer; laboratory; and radiology information. The Soprano product provides "solutions for clinical notes, discharge summaries, disease management, and an electronic provider index."[15]

i-Health's Clinician View™ "allows clinicians in hospital environments to create, view, and search an electronic patient record, check laboratory and radiology results, view clinical documents and images, check on medical warnings, create orders for tests and investigations, create referrals, view medication profiles, create prescriptions, communicate directly with other health care providers, and access many more clinical functions, e.g., clinical pathways and knowledge bases."[16]

Creation of template-based clinical documents to record a range of things, e.g., discharge summaries and referral letters, are used by a number of secondary providers. These documents often are prepopulated with selected information from other systems, such as visit details, diagnosis, laboratory, and radiology results. On completion, they can then be forwarded to other providers, e.g., general practitioners, using secure networks—Healthlink[9] and the Health Intranet, for example. There also are initiatives under way in the areas of e-referrals, order entry, and e-prescribing. Information from these will then form part of the EHR of the future.

Community-based caregivers are also using computerized systems that integrate patient administration and clinical data to provide an EHR. Because nurses deliver much of the community care, they have significant input into information held in the EHR. Most urgent is the need for a standardized terminology—the lack of which is a critical limitation on achieving an electronic record that allows for information sharing across providers and care venues.

The primary care sector has had a high uptake of electronic systems with an estimated 80 percent of clinic practices using practice management systems. Many of these systems also have clinical components. More than 50 percent of general practitioners use them for clinical note taking during patient encounters, as well as for electronic generation of prescriptions. Nurses working as practitioners in these areas are also contributing to the patient record.

Also, within the primary care sector, development of standards is badly needed to allow national coding of patient encounter information and data exchange between providers. Although there is a high uptake of electronic systems and use of clinical components, there is little information exchanged with other providers, as these systems only operate in the provider's environment. The electronic discharge summaries, laboratory, and radiology results—sent by specialists and private providers—are received by some of the systems and then added to the electronic record.

Decision support system initiatives are also under way. One of these projects assists primary care practitioners with care planning and referral for specific gynecological conditions by utilizing the Predict product from Enigma.[17] Chronic disease management initiatives are also being explored in the areas of cardiovascular diseases and diabetes. These decision support systems are integrated into some of the tertiary acute care centers, secondary community/home based care, and primary care health systems.

There is still a big gap in electronic systems designed to address the specific nursing requirements to aid assessment, planning, implementation, and evaluation of care. The Clinically Integrated System (CIS) model is one of the few systems in use in the secondary community care sector that takes an interdisciplinary approach to patient care.[18]

The CIS Model

The CIS model is an electronic interdisciplinary system that links evidence-based practice, clinical redesign, outcome management, and participatory action research into a single framework of patient care delivery and management. The model can be applied to any patient group regardless of condition or diagnosis. As a patient-focused system, an important component of the model is to capture and track individual patient and family perspectives of care delivery. The model also provides an opportunity to gauge the patients' reaction to using a computerized system to record their care, with preliminary feedback showing a positive response. This has been reflected in an increased number of patients requesting copies of information that is available on the CIS model, e.g., evidence-based guidelines. The concurrent collection and analysis of outcome data from a variety of perspectives, such as clinicians, patients, and relatives, has provided incentives for interdisciplinary teams to work more closely to resolve potential or actual adverse trends.

Issues with EHRs

EHRs carry legal, privacy, and other risks, but also have the potential for major benefits. For EHRs to work, there must be a balance between the benefits and risks. Electronic solutions are not perfect, but probably less risky than the current combination of paper and electronic systems. To reach a high level of EHR compliance, the system must have well-structured authentication, confidentiality, integrity, with anywhere accessibility and remain user friendly.

The New Zealand Privacy Act 1993 and the Health Information Privacy Code 1994 decreed that patients have the right to their stored information. This, however, does not extend to ownership of the electronic documents. In the move toward EHRs, technology and health policy need to consider how to provide access to this electronic information as per the law when a request is made. We are fortunate in that the New Zealand privacy legislation also considers criteria "reasonable in the circumstances."[19] Unfortunately, however, under current New Zealand law, there are components that should form part of the EHR but still require paper—prescriptions are one example. Until this type of legislation changes, these requirements need to be accommodated. Electronic recording of prescribed medication in a patient's record is allowed, but not the electronic transmission to authorize dispensing.

With the large number of health IT projects going on in New Zealand, there is concern that patients are not well-informed and are putting their trust in health care and IT professionals to "get it right."[20] Some health professionals believe there is some information that should not be stored in an individual's EHR. These areas need further debate before the country proceeds much further.

EHR's Future in the New Zealand Health Sector

Many of the components required for an EHR are available, but New Zealand has yet to achieve a totally patient-centric EHR that is available to patients and a range of providers.[21] New Zealand favors incremental steps toward EHRs, rather than the "big bang" approach. For New Zealand, the incremental approach is viewed as helping to minimize disruption, help gain stakeholder acceptance, track accountability for future proofing, and control costs.[22] The content of an EHR has yet to be fully debated in the New Zealand context, between health professionals and consumers.[23-25] The size of New Zealand and the work being done on health IT infrastructure, including the EHR component, does mean that we may one day be able to realize the dream of a national EHR for New Zealanders, but we still have a long way to go.[26] The technology may be ready, but there is still work to be done in the readiness of people, processes, and change management.

Summary

New Zealand is poised to capitalize on its unique EHR initiatives. Although information technologies play a significant factor in the country's future success, the focus on building collaborative partnerships between government, clinicians, and patients is seen as the ultimate key to ensuring that the EHR becomes an integral part of improving patient care.

References

1. Ministry of Health. Future funding of health and disability services in New Zealand. 2002. Available at: http://www.moh.govt.nz/moh.nsf/0/8C766E4FF69F86ADCC256F2B007F14A3/$File/futurefundingofhealthanddisabilityservicesinnewzealand.pdf. Accessed on July 30, 2005.

2. Ministry of Health. The New Zealand health care strategy. 2000. Available at: http://www.moh.govt.nz/moh.nsf/f872666357c511eb4c25666d000c8888/fb62475d5d911e88cc256d42007bd67e/$FILE/NZHthStrat.pdf. Accessed on July 30, 2005.

3. Ministry of Health. The primary health care strategy. 2001. Available at: http://www.moh.govt.nz/moh.nsf/0/7BAFAD2531E04D92CC2569E600013D04/$File/PHCStrat.pdf. Accessed on July 30, 2005.

4. Ministry of Health. The New Zealand disability strategy. 2001. Available at: http://www.odi.govt.nz/documents/publications/nz-disability-strategy.pdf. Accessed on July 30, 2005.

5. Ministry of Health. From Strategy to Reality: the WAVE Project. 2001. Available at: http://www.moh.govt.nz/moh.nsf/0/F34F8959738E992CCC256AF400177998/$File/TheWAVEreport.pdf. Accessed on August 8, 2005.

6. New Zealand Government. Privacy Act 1993. Available at: http://www.legislation.govt.nz/browse_vw.asp?content-set=pal_statutes. Accessed on August 8, 2005.

7. New Zealand Government. Health Information Privacy Code 1994. Available at: http://www.privacy.org.nz/comply/HIPCWWW.pdf. Accessed on July 30, 2005.

8. New Zealand Government. Official Information Act 1982. Available at: http://www.legislation.govt.nz/browse_vw.asp?content-set=pal_statutes. Accessed on July 29, 2005.

9. Healthlink. *Integration Suite*. Available at: http://www.healthlink.net/index2.htm. Accessed on August 25, 2005.

10. Health IT Cluster. Available at: http://www.healthit.org.nz/ Accessed on July 29, 2005.

11. Health Informatics New Zealand. Available at: http://www.hinz.org.nz. Accessed on July 29, 2005.

12. Health Information Association of New Zealand. Available at: http://www.hianz.org.nz/. Accessed on July 30, 2005.

13. Health Information Standards Organisation. Available at: http://www.moh.govt.nz/hiso. Accessed on July 30, 2005.

14. Ryan KM, Boustead AJ. Universal electronic health records: a qualitative study of lay perspectives. *New Zealand Fam Prac.* 2004;31:149–154. Also available at: http://www.rnzcgp.org.nz/NZFP/Issues/June2004/Ryan June04.pdf. Accessed July 29, 2005.

15. Orion Systems International. Available at: http://www.orionhealth.com/. Accessed July 28, 2005.

16. i-Soft PLC. *Clinical Solution Suite.* Available at: http://www.isoftplc.com/. Accessed August 8, 2005.

17. Enigma. *About Enigma.* Available at: http://www.enigma.co.nz/. Accessed August 8, 2005.

18. Ministry of Health. Sharing Excellence—Clinically Integrated System (CIS). Available at: http://www.moh.govt.nz/moh.nsf/f872666357c511eb4c25666d000c8888/b724d17ae05fa9f0cc256d7b00104014?OpenDocument. Accessed on August 8, 2005.

19. Wigley & Company. Electronic health records: legal issues. Presentation at: NZ Electronic Health Records Summit; 4, August 2004; Auckland. Also available at: http://www.wigleylaw.com/assets/_Attachments/ElectronicHealthRecords.pdf.

20. Hunter I. Patient attitudes to electronic medical records. Presentation to: The Privacy Forum; March 10, 2003; Auckland. Also available at: http://www.privacy.org.nz/media/Hunter.pdf. Accessed August 8, 2005.

21. Delany R. Creating quality in primary health care using electronic health records. *Health Care and Informatics Review Online™.* 2004;7(1). Also available at: http://www.enigma.co.nz/hcro/website/index.cfm?fuseaction=editorialdisplay&issueID=51. Accessed July 30, 2005.

22. Didham R, Martin I. A review of computerised information technology systems in general practice medicine. *Health Care and Informatics Review Online™.* 2004;8(1). Also available at: http://www.enigma.co.nz/hcro/website/index.cfm?fuseaction=articledisplay&featureid=040302. Accessed July 30, 2005.

23. Gillies J, Holt A. Anxious about electronic health records? No need to be. *New Zealand Med J.* 2003; 116(1182). Also available at: http://www.nzma.org.nz/journal/abstract.php?id=604. Accessed July 30, 2005.

24. Kerr K. The electronic health record in New Zealand. *Health Care and Informatics Review Online™.* 2004;8(1). Also available at: http://www.enigma.co.nz/ hcro/website/index.cfm?fuseaction=articledisplay&featureid=040304. Accessed July 30, 2005.

25. Leech K. The virtual patient record. *Health Care and Informatics Review Online™.* 2004;8(1). Available at: http://www.enigma.co.nz/hcro/website/index.cfm?fuseaction=articledisplay&featureid=040303. Accessed July 30, 2005.

26. Statistics New Zealand (2002). Information Technology Use in New Zealand 2001. Available at: http://www2.stats.govt.nz/domino/external/web/prod_serv.nsf/874ea91c142289384c2567a80081308e/c57aa3d688daaa80cc256bc7000ea3a5/%24FILE/ITUNZ01.pdf. Accessed July 30, 2005.

SECTION VI

The Near Future and Nursing

Section VI

Introduction

Neal Patterson, MBA

Medicine has always been about knowledge—information skillfully applied. Information technology (IT) is about effectively managing data, information, and knowledge. *Health care informatics,* the combination of medicine and IT, promises to transform our current health care delivery system. Nursing is and must be at the center of this transformation. The discipline of *nursing informatics* (NI) extends back merely a few decades, but the ideas behind it date back to Florence Nightingale. As long as there has been nursing, there has been nursing information—ranging from patient data to quantitative and qualitative information about nursing practice and theory. To get an idea of what the future holds, it is necessary only to reflect on the past and the present, and then observe the trends. Previous chapters have addressed the past and present. The chapters in this section touch on some of the topics that will have relevance to nurses in the next decade and beyond—the groundbreaking science of genomics and its impact on condition diagnosis, treatment, and education; the inclusion of nursing research as a significant part of a broad National Institutes of Health research strategy; the rise of e-consumerism around the globe; the continued shift to patient-centered models of care delivery; and the search for a professional home for NI. These are diverse topics, but highly reflective of the complexity of modern care and the breadth and depth of the scientific and specialized knowledge required of a twenty-first century nurse.

Much has been written about the impact of this century's convergence of science, demographics, IT, and consumerism on our system of health care. This convergence creates both the strong fundamental pressure and the environment for significant, even seismic, change. As health care consumers, there is no doubt that we will play an expanded role in directing our care, armed with our versions of the best science and research about our conditions and the next generation of treatment. The demographic and financial pressures will force society to develop new economic models, empowering us as individuals with the "accountable" knowledge of the financial consequences of our every health care decision. The successful sequencing of the human genome has launched a new era of personalized medicine, and it will evolve from the conceptual stage into mainstream practice over the next few decades. Organizations' current investments in clinically-based systems that automate the core clinical processes of nurses and physicians will result in structured electronic health records (EHRs) that will, in turn, unleash a series of second-order benefits, including providing a rich research medium for discovering new knowledge to fuel the evolution of evidence-based practice. NI will gain the most in this new transparent world, which will expose current nursing practices to scientific inquiry, investigation, and discovery of best practice.

Considered together, this convergence leads to information overload for almost every caregiver and practitioner in the system. Some of the chapters in this section address ways in which the glut of information can be thoughtfully harvested and applied in ways that make a difference in people's lives. It is clear that it will be impossible to survive and thrive in the near future without artificial aid to augment our memories and personal knowledge. In his 2005 address, "Personalized Medicine in the Postgenome Era," Dr. William Neaves, president and chief executive officer of the Stowers Institute for Medical Research suggests that computers and computing power be rightly viewed as a "mental prosthesis," eyeglasses to amplify our seeing; hearing aids to amplify our hearing; and a smart, networked computing device to amplify our thinking.[1]

Despite an increasing reliance on computers, the trained and experienced human mind is and will remain the most amazing "computing device." Hands-on clinical experience will remain the foundation of NI for its ability to inform and guide the process of discovery and care innovation. People, both patients and clinicians, are at once the drivers, the consumers, and the beneficiaries of

472

the revolution in health care informatics. The following chapters inform and support the view that the biggest breakthroughs will come when the finesse of the human mind is combined with the computational power of IT.

Reference

1. Neaves W. *Leaping beyond the genome—what lies ahead?* Association for Pathology Informatics' Clinical Information System/Life Science Roundtable, College of American Pathologists, Chicago, July 2002. Available at: http://www.cap.org/apps/docs/cap_today/feature_stories/genome_roundtable_feature.html. Accessed September 12, 2005.

CHAPTER 30

The Influence of Biomedical Informatics on Clinical Information Systems

By Kathleen A. McCormick, PhD, RN, FAAN, FACMI, and Mark Hoffman, PhD

In 2001, a map of the entire human genome was released to the public.[1,2] It has been said that this discovery will change the face of human health care in the twenty-first century. "By 2010 it is expected that validated, predictive genetic tests will be available for as many as a dozen common conditions."[3] But how can genomic information change the face of nursing unless its entry into clinical information systems and electronic health records (EHRs) has been planned in advance? Given that capturing the nursing process electronically took as long as the last twenty-five years, plans must be laid now to incorporate the genetic, genomic, proteomic, metabolic, and small molecule chemical pathway information into the EHR in readiness for the changes occurring in health care.[4]

The genome era will change the scope of nursing care in this century. Nurses will begin to determine the genetic causes of a nursing diagnosis and use genomic information in planning to prevent symptoms. For example, the genetic factors involved in wound healing are becoming better understood, and nurses can identify postoperative patients who might have compromised wound healing. The new genomic information will also have an effect on how the professional nurse needs to develop and redesign clinical trial systems, hospital information systems, EHR systems, and personal health records.

Because nurses are frequently the genetic counselors in health care environments, the development of new tools to incorporate genetic maps and pedigrees might be necessary. The structured capture of family health history and environmental data will become critical in nursing assessments. Nurses will require new tool-kits to determine the environmental causes of diseases and symptoms in persons who have a susceptibility to the disease, e.g., those suffering from asthma associated with environmental pollutants.

Single Nucleotide Polymorphisms (SNPs) and Haplotype Maps (HapMaps)

The analysis of the human genome showed that, between any two individuals, only about one in 300 nucleotide positions differ. We are all 99.9 percent alike at the genetic level, with about three billion base pairs of adenine, cytosine, thymine, and guanine nucleotides. The 0.1 percent difference accounts for individual physical differences and varying susceptibilities to disease. An international coalition has begun work to identify haplotype mapping (HapMap Project) of the human genome; the purpose is to construct a catalog describing the patterns of human genetic variations and how they are organized on chromosomes.[5] The map will serve as the tool to discover the common genetic variations in complex multifactorial diseases, rather than just the relatively simple single-gene diseases. It is also expected to help identify common variations responsible for differences in drug response. An early part of this endeavor was the Single Nucleotide Polymorphism Consortium that has already identified millions of genetic variants.

Genes to Genomes to Proteomes

What effect does this have on how nurses focus their clinical observations and care to help prevent, diagnose, and appropriately manage the patient? With genetic information about an increasing number of clinical conditions available, nursing health care practitioners are challenged to integrate genomic, biological, clinical, and behavioral tools into the current EHR and data capture tools. How can information-based tools help the nurse focus clinical observations and delivery of care to help prevent, diagnose, and appropriately manage the patient? To explore this topic, a summary of the current state-of-the-art in genomic health care is useful.

Although the pace of adoption of genomic technologies has been slower than expected, the genetic codes provide researchers with valuable tools that ultimately will lead to new drugs, new diagnostic tests, and a more complete understanding of human biology. These advances have a fairly lengthy development horizon, requiring between seven to twelve years before a new drug candidate can reach the marketplace.

Despite the slow pace of new drug releases, genomic medicine is becoming a reality. Recently, the U.S. Food and Drug Administration approved diagnostic devices based on microarray technology in which dozens, hundreds, or even thousands of genetic traits can be tested in a single run. Genetic traits that influence how well a patient responds to a clinical treatment are better understood and utilized to stratify patients by risk. The management of many infectious diseases relies heavily on molecular diagnostic technologies, speeding the time it takes to diagnose an infection accurately and to manage it. The incorporation of molecular diagnostic results into the EHR will dramatically affect the practice of nursing and thus the related information tools.

Bioinformatics

Bioinformatics is the application of information-intensive technologies, e.g., genome analysis algorithms, to the solution of biological challenges. *Biomedical informatics* is a subdiscipline focused primarily on the use of bioinformatics to support the development of new diagnostic tests and pharmaceuticals that are likely to offer new alternatives in patient care, although typically with a fairly long development cycle. *Clinical informatics,* of which nursing informatics (NI) is a subdiscipline, on the other hand, focuses on the exploration and development of information-based technologies that can improve the quality of patient care. The increasing adoption of genomics-based technologies to support the delivery of patient care requires us to recognize areas in which biomedical informatics and NI overlap. This chapter summarizes topics that illustrate the overlap between the two fields.

Family Health Histories

Capturing a clinical family history is often a responsibility of the nurse. In general, the information provided by patients about the medical histories of their family members is not currently structured in a way that can be leveraged by automated clinical decision support systems. The design of documentation dialogues that optimize family history information for integration with the molecular diagnostic and genetic findings is an area of active investigation. One topic of exploration is the pedigree map, currently utilized only by specialists in genetic counseling and clinical genetics. Map applications use symbols that are not generally a part of a nursing history unless the nurse is a genetic counselor.

The formalized capture of family history became a priority to the U.S. Department of Health and Human Services on November 8, 2004, when Surgeon General Richard H. Carmona declared Thanksgiving Day as National Family History Day. On that day, Americans are encouraged to ask family members about relevant family health history information that could benefit all members. To keep their record, family members can download a tool from www.hhs.gov/familyhistory.[6] Included in this tool are questions about the risks of heart disease, cancer, and diabetes. Links to the Agency for Healthcare Research and Quality can lead individuals to practice guidelines that help individuals and their health care professionals customize their prevention programs when they have known genetic diseases. The guidelines can be found at the National Guideline Clearinghouse at www.guideline.gov.

Recording family health histories has increasingly become more important with the new genetic information. A family history and its inherent risk factors can be the determining factors in deciding whether costly genetic tests are performed or treatments initiated. Francis Collins, Director of the National Human Genome Research Institute, acknowledges that family history is like a window into a person's genome.[7]

If nurses enable patients to keep track of their family history, personalized disease prevention plans can be developed for individuals. The family genetic history when embraced by the nursing profession as an assessment tool for genetic health entails the use of terms that might require evaluation by the American Nurses Association for inclusion in its recognized nursing vocabularies.

A Model for Studying Genetics in Health Care

One of the most impressive models describing the vision of where the Human Genome Project is going is shown in Figure 30-1.[7] Francis Collins et al[7] described a blueprint for the genome era. The figure defines six crosscutting elements needed to advance this science: (1) Constant resources for many years to come; (2) Expanded technology; (3) Better tools to analyze genetic data computationally; (4) Nurses trained as genetic scientists and social, legal, and ethical scientists and scholars to develop integrations between clinical care and genomic applications; (5) Examination of many ethical, legal, and social issues, e.g., race, in the context of genetics; and (6) Requisite genetics education for health care professionals and consumers.

How will these new developments converge with the EHR? The primary changes required to the current architecture of the EHR relate to the appropriate structuring of molecular diagnostic findings. Needed are clear differentiations between somatic and inherited mutations and between the results describing pathogens and those describing patients. Results describing inherited conditions should be structured to reflect their lifelong nature, an approach that is not always clearly managed in encounter-based systems. Other EHR extensions that support genomic medicine include the ability to link personal records in a manner that appropriately protects the privacy of the linked persons.

Representing the information known about a patient's genome poses challenges in terms of information density, data clarity, and appropriate representation and visualization. Two primary display options are available: physical representation and functional organization. *Physical representation* relies on biological accuracy, for example, indicating where amino acid substitutions are found in the three-dimensional structure of a protein or where a gene is located in the genome. *Functional organization* of genomic findings is more likely to be useful for the care provider—for example, a summary of patient-specific genetic findings grouped by the physiological function of a gene. One method of providing functionally grouped genetic test results is to use the Gene Ontology

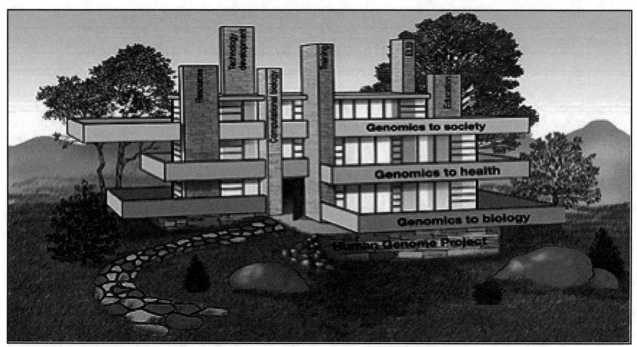

Figure 30-1. *The Future of Genomics Rests on the Foundation of the Human Genome Project*

(GO) to group genes by their cellular function or anatomic locations.[8] The GO is widely utilized by the biomedical informatics community to support the comparison of genes between species, but it has not yet been widely examined for its utility in supporting the care provider community. As experts in health care informatics explore the usefulness of the GO, they are likely to find gaps in its adaptability to the clinical setting.

New Controlled Vocabulary—The Clinical Bioinformatics Ontology™

The vocabularies that are familiar to the clinical informatics community, especially the Systematized Nomenclature of Medicine (SNOMED), Logical Observation Identifiers Names and Codes (LOINC®), and the International Classification of Diseases Version 9, Clinical Medicine (ICD-9CM) have not been expanded to support the precision needed to describe genomic observations. A new controlled vocabulary, the Clinical Bioinformatics Ontology™ (CBO)[9] has been developed to support standardization of genetic test findings generated by the molecular diagnostics and cytogenetics laboratory. The CBO includes concepts that represent discrete observations; for example, there is a concept representing the Philadelphia chromosome translocation associated with chronic myelogenous leukemia. This concept is, in turn, associated with concepts representing chromosome 9 and chromosome 22. Through this network of machine-readable relationships, systems that utilize the CBO can provide a much deeper context for genetic observations.

The benefits of the CBO include its utility as a controlled vocabulary and its usefulness in providing contextual information. As a controlled vocabulary, the CBO simplifies the process of designing systems that rely on standardization. Multifacility organizations can use the underlying controlled vocabulary to standardize information while preserving the freedom of each facility to display the most comfortable on-screen conventions. For example, the mutation associated with the most common form of cystic fibrosis has the CBO-coded value CBO AEO/PQD7LLZ5XY9cn4waeg. One site can display "CFTR.del508" while another might use "del508 of CFTR." The underlying association of either form to the CBO-coded value preserves the consistency of meaning between sites. By delivering machine-readable, context-defining information, such as the Online Mendelian Inheritance in Man (OMIM™)[10] value for a gene, the CBO also allows systems to deliver greater context to the users. The CBO allows users to associate findings, e.g., the observation of a specific gene mutation, with a coded value. These coded values can then be used as the basis for data exchange, standardization of documentation, and the design of decision support rules.

New Laboratory Information System and PathNet Helix™

The PathNet Helix™ laboratory information system module, developed by Cerner Corporation, Kansas City, Missouri, is an example for how genomic information and work flow can be incorporated into a clinical information system (CIS). For example, in the PathNet Helix™ laboratory system, users can view a cell in which a mutation result is displayed as well as detailed information about the mutation, including the intron or exon in which the site of the mutation is found. This new solution was developed specifically for the work flow and content needs of the molecular diagnostic and cytogenetics laboratory. PathNet Helix™ uses the CBO as a source of reference information that influences its behavior. For example, users entering results for a genetic test can right-click on the result accept cell and access context-defining information. Right-clicking on the representation of an orderable procedure branches the user to the OMIM Web site appropriate for the gene that is the target of testing. As NI solutions evolve to incorporate genomic information, similar access to context-appropriate resources should be provided in the clinical system.

Decision Support Rules

As genomic health care becomes a greater part of general clinical practice, many topics relevant to clinical informatics areas will require the ability to integrate genomics information and logic. Representative topics include EHR systems, nursing documentation, clinical decision support applications, and computerized provider order entry (CPOE). With genomic information becoming a significant part of the EHR, discrete information can be used as the basis for decision support rules. These rules can influence the design of patient care plans and can be instrumental in evaluating and influencing medication ordering decisions and other clinical activities that can be automated. Specifically, nursing research in knowledge management may have to expand to this area of decision logic to aid nurse clinicians in genetic implications for prevention, diagnosis, treatment, and cure.

To illustrate how these topics intersect with current and future clinical practice, examples from six clinical areas are discussed below.

1. Inherited Diseases

Genomic medicine is most readily appreciated in terms of inherited disorders. Indeed, a deep understanding of many genetic disorders was available prior to the dissemination of the genome map. The genes associated with cystic fibrosis, Huntington's disease, and other genetic conditions were mapped and their DNA sequences determined before the Human Genome Project was completed. Although this information made precise diagnostic tests possible, none of these conditions can be treated. Thus the recognition of a gene-disease association can provide information that is useful for family planning but that often does not immediately support the development of new treatments.

Often the genetic counselor, who works closely with patients managing an inherited condition, has a background in nursing. Information systems capable of integrating the results of molecular diagnostic tests with the information captured by a nurse can provide a more complete clinical picture than either resource could on its own. The EHR that is capable of this type of integration will thus enhance the capabilities of the primary care provider. Easy access to context-defining information, such as OMIM Web sites, is useful to the care provider, especially when managing a rare, less familiar condition.

Managing information related to inherited conditions requires the implementation of security policies and technologies. For example, the inadvertent disclosure of a positive test for Huntington's disease can have major consequences not only for the person who was tested but for family members as well. Likewise, documenting family histories can lead to delicate situations related to the paternity of a patient. Testing for genetic conditions consistently reveals that the person presented as the father and included in the testing regimen is actually not the biological father 5–10 percent of the time.[11] Clearly it is important to control whether and when these peripheral observations are revealed.

Related to inherited conditions are inherited risk factors. The associations between certain gene variants and the risk of adverse responses to medications or of developing a complication during a surgery are active areas of research. For example, persons with a mutation in the ryanodine receptor gene are at significant risk of developing malignant hyperthermia when exposed to halothane during surgery. Recognition of the demographic factors associated with this and other risks can be facilitated by clinical decision support systems, which can be used to support improvements in patient safety. Tools that aid the surgical nurse in recognizing how to integrate this information into a patient's care plan will become necessary.

In the first case of newborn screening, most nurses understand that testing for phenylketonuria (PKU) is a standard newborn screening procedure; in fact, it is the most widely utilized genetic screen. The nurse seeking information to share with the family of a child found to be affected by PKU could refer to HugeNet (www.HugeNet.gov).[12] There the nurse learns that PKU is a phenylalanine hydroxylase (PAH) deficiency that is "inherited in an autosomal recessive manner. At conception, the sibs of an affected individual have a 25 percent chance of being affected, a 50 percent chance of being asymptomatic carriers, and a 25 percent chance of being unaffected and not carriers. Prenatal diagnosis of PAH deficiency is possible in pregnancies at 25 percent risk either when direct DNA testing has revealed the disease-causing mutations in the PAH gene in an affected family member or when linkage analysis has identified informative markers. PAH deficiency is most commonly diagnosed upon routine screening of newborns. PAH deficiency can be detected in virtually 100 percent of cases by newborn screening utilizing the Guthrie card bloodspot obtained from a heelprick. The ability to translate this type of information into an explanation that any patient can understand will be a fundamental skill for current and future nurses.

2. Infectious Diseases

Many infectious diseases are increasingly managed with the help of information gathered using molecular diagnostic testing. For example, the management of a patient with the human immunodeficiency virus (HIV) routinely involves the use of a reverse transcriptase polymerase chain reaction (RT-PCR) to assess viral load. The viral load results are generally complemented by flow cytometric analysis of circulating CD4 positive T cells, an indicator of a patient's overall immune status. Because these tests are generally repeated periodically, clinical documentation tools and the EHR must be able to support the clear longitudinal representation of the findings, regardless of encounter. A relatively new aspect of HIV management is the use of viral genotyping. A patient who fails to respond to a therapy (as indicated by increased viral load and/or lowered CD4 counts) might have a viral strain resistant to the antiretroviral medication(s) utilized. To identify the optimal therapy, it has become standard practice to determine the nucleic acid sequence of the genes in the virus that encode the viral proteins (reverse transcriptase and protease) that are the targets of these drugs. Through applying algorithms that correlate mutations in the genes to drug resistance, the laboratory is able to infer which medications are most likely to be successful. One of the best characterized examples of pharmacogenomics in clinical practice, HIV viral genotyping has been shown to improve the management of acquired immunodeficiency syndrome (AIDS) by enhancing survival, lowering the cost of management by an average of $2,000 per year, and improving Quality-Adjusted Life Years (QALY).[13-15] Although the clinician does not generally need to see the original results that lead to the recommendation, a greater awareness of the methodology and its limitations can be provided by content integrated into the EHR.

Public health bioinformatics has also benefited from the use of molecular diagnostic technologies. For example, through the use of pulsed-field gel electrophoresis (PFGE) to analyze the bacterial genomes from multiple patients involved in a suspected disease outbreak, it can readily be determined whether the cases are of a common source (i.e., they share a genomic pattern) or of disparate origins. Likewise, the use of such technologies will increasingly be utilized in support of hospital infection control practices, another venue in which nurses are often the primary practitioners.

3. Cancer

Gathering information that can assist in the determination of whether a woman should be screened for the risk of hereditary breast cancer is a task often performed by a nurse. Accomplishing this goal will be enhanced by documentation tools that remind nurses of the questions to ask a woman who is a candidate for genetic screening: "Do you have a sister, mother, or grandmother who was diagnosed with breast cancer before the age of fifty years?" Through the use of structured documentation, a nurse interviewing a patient can ask a standard set of questions and contribute to a more consistent standard of care. Significantly, responses captured through the nursing documentation dialogue can be associated with clinical vocabularies or with genomics vocabularies, e.g., the clinical bioinformatics ontology.

The following scenario illustrates how family, genomic, and environmental factors come into play in the management of a complex condition: breast cancer. This is a possible scenario that a nurse practitioner will see on a recurring basis. A thirty-seven-year-old Ashkenazi Jewish woman comes to see a nurse practitioner for a routine pelvic examination and Pap (Papanicolau) test. Because the nurse practitioner has followed the patient's mother's history of breast cancer, the nurse is vigilant during routine breast examinations. The patient informs the nurse practitioner that her forty-three-year-old sister has just been diagnosed with breast cancer. Recognizing that risk-associated mutations in the BRCA1 and BRCA2 genes are most common in women of Eastern European heredity, should the nurse practitioner gather more information on family history and/or consider the possibility of genetic testing? To make the decision, the nurse practitioner might go to http://www.cancer.gov or www.HugeNet.gov. Race, ethnicity, gender, family history, and diagnostic results are all important factors in this scenario. The choice made by the nurse practitioner can make a difference in the diagnosis and potential cure of the disease.

Another example of nurse involvement in genetic screening is in the diagnosis and treatment of leukemia in children. One learns from genetic databases that acute myeloid leukemia in children is affected by a glutathione-S-transferase gene deletion. A search of the sites for the National Center for Biotechnology Information and the National Library of Medicine, linked to the Web site HugeNet, discloses that leukemia can arise from DNA translocations, inversions, or deletions of genes in regulating blood cell development and/or homeostatis. Folate deficiency has been associated with these aberrations.

4. Hypertension

The genes associated with pre-eclampsia in pregnancy and chronic essential hypertension have been analyzed. In persons with pre-eclampsia and hypertension, there was an increase in the AGT haplotype in genetic susceptibility to pre-eclampsia and chronic essential hypertension.

5. Obesity

In population studies of obesity, research has shown that genetics plays a role. Genes can directly cause obesity in disorders such as Bardet-Biedl syndrome and Prader-Willi syndrome.[16-18] However, genes do not always predict future health. Specific genetic variations combined with behavioral characteristics are additional assessment tools required for evaluating genetic health. Furthermore, in some cases, multiple genes may increase the susceptibility for obesity and require additional research before the complex matrix of their interactions can be used to predict or manage a patient at risk.

A relatively small proportion of obesity in the population can be explained by mutations in single genes. Despite the low percentage, researchers have gained a significant understanding of how fat stores are regulated from studying the biology and clinical presentations of the rare individuals and families, as well as the animal models of these conditions. These conditions exhibit autosomal recessive, autosomal dominant, or X-linked patterns of inheritance. Information about the genes, the clinical findings, and, when available, the treatment interventions is provided by means of links to the OMIM database. Although the conditions rarely occur in human populations, they are important in helping to understand the complex systems that regulate energy intake and expenditure in humans.

6. Pharmacogenomics

In the area of pharmacogenomics, advanced nurse practitioners will be able to examine an individual's genomic information to predict which drug will be most effective and produce the fewest side effects for the individual. Variability in drug responses is often caused by genetic differences in individuals that affect their ability to metabolize a drug or to activate the drug enzymatically.

In the future, the combined genetic and molecular information about disease pathways will likely lead to the development of rational drug treatments specifically for a given condition. Such drug development is occurring in cancer today; *imatinib* and *gefitinib* are examples of drugs developed for specific targets. In the future, drugs for specific types of diabetes and autoimmune conditions also are likely to be developed. Equally important will be the information about a drug, a dose, or a response to toxicity. The level at which some patients are likely to develop complications or side effects will be more specifically predictable than ever.

Nursing research will need to focus on the pharmacogenomic consequences of dosage and the metabolism of drugs that cause common side effects like nausea, vomiting, fatigue, and mucositis. The future goal for the pharmaceutical industry will be to develop medications with the greatest effect on the biological pathway and metabolism while being less toxic to the person. Pharmacogenomics may create another patient advocate area for nurses as they inform patients about genomic information, including such areas as prevention, screening, diagnostics, prognostics,

Table 30-1. Knowledge Needed by Health Care Professionals for Applying Genetics in Health Care

1.1	Basic human genetics terminology
1.2	The basic patterns of biological inheritance and variation both within families and within populations
1.3	How identification of disease-associated genetic variations facilitates development of prevention, diagnosis, and treatment options
1.4	The importance of family history (minimum three generations) in assessing predisposition to disease
1.5	The role of genetic factors in maintaining health and preventing disease
1.6	The differences between clinical diagnosis of disease and identification of genetic predisposition to disease (genetic variation is not strictly correlated with disease manifestation)
1.7	The role of behavioral, social, and environmental factors (lifestyle, socioeconomic factors, pollutants, etc.) to modify or influence genetics in the manifestation of disease
1.8	The influence of ethnoculture and economics in the prevalence and diagnosis of genetic disease
1.9	The influence of ethnicity, culture, related health beliefs, and economics in the client's ability to use genetic information and services
1.10	The potential physical and/or psychosocial benefits, limitations, and risks of genetic information for individuals, family members, and communities
1.11	The range of genetic approaches to treatment of disease (prevention, pharmacogenomics/prescription of drugs to match individual genetic profiles, gene-based drugs, and gene therapy)
1.12	The resources available to assist clients seeking genetic information or services, including the types of genetics professionals available and their diverse responsibilities
1.13	The components of the genetic-counseling process and the indications for referral to genetic specialists
1.14	The indications for genetic testing and/or gene-based interventions
1.15	The ethical, legal, and social issues related to genetic testing and recording of genetic information (e.g., privacy, the potential for genetic discrimination in health insurance and employment)
1.16	The history of misuse of human genetic information (eugenics)
1.17	One's own professional role in the referral to genetics services, or provision, follow-up, and quality review of genetic services

selection of treatment, and monitoring of treatment outcomes. Patient education related to these new options is likely to become a responsibility of the nurse.

Nursing Competency and Skills Needed

The National Coalition for Health Professional Education in Genetics[19] is a national organization that develops core competencies in genetics for health professionals. The impetus for developing the core competencies was to help health care providers integrate genetic knowledge into routine health care for individuals and families. The core competencies that are recommended for all health professionals are listed in Table 30-1.

Knowledge of genetics is a basic requirement for persons who are going to design information systems that integrate genetic information. Some of the skills required of persons involved in genetic-based information system implementations are shown in Table 30-2. These skills include the ability to gather genetic information from patients and families that is credible and that can help health care providers identify the required resources. Additional skills are required for genetic health professionals, and genetic education programs are recommended for all health professionals (see http://www.nchpeg.org).

Putting It All Together

Figure 30-2[3] is a diagram from the National Human Genome Research Institute[20] that maps the relationships among basic biology, genetics, and practical applications in diagnosis and treatment. From

Table 30-2. Skills of Health Professionals Related to Genetics

2.1	Gather genetic family history information including an appropriate multigenerational family history
2.2	Identify clients who would benefit from genetic services
2.3	Explain basic concepts of probability and disease susceptibility, and the influence of genetic factors in maintenance of health and development of disease
2.4	Seek assistance from and refer to appropriate genetics experts and peer support resources
2.5	Obtain credible, current information about genetics for self, clients, and colleagues
2.6	Use new information technologies effectively to obtain current information about genetics
2.7	Educate others about client-focused policy issues
2.8	Participate in professional and public education about genetics

the timetable shown, it is clear that the nurse practitioners will need guidance in ordering tests, clear and concise genomic information, clinical genomics documentation capabilities, decision support embedded in order entry, and a family medical and nursing record. Particularly, the questions are when is it appropriate to order a genetic test and where are the tests sent for analysis? (see http://www.genetests.org.)

Summary

One of the best ways that nurses can prepare for the genome era is to explore some of the resources mentioned in this chapter. Already EHRs provide linkages to these resources. However, further integration of clinical data with geneticgenomic data is currently a necessity in diagnosis and treatment only in research environments.

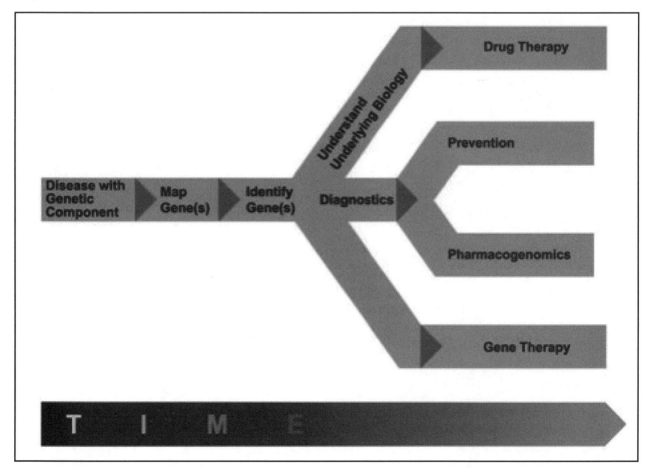

Figure 30-2. *Genome Timetable.*

This chapter described models for the integration of clinical and genomic data with social and ethical dimensions. It also provided sample nursing knowledge and skills, developed by those in professional organizations who have been involved in genetic counseling for many years. The future of genetics is being described as the next revolution in health care. As the largest number of health care practitioners in the U.S., nurses should become familiar with the body of knowledge related to clinically applied genomics and utilize the available information resources to assist them in gaining and managing this knowledge.

References

1. Lander ES, et al. Initial sequencing and analysis of the human genome. *Nature.* 2001;409(6822):860-921.
2. Venter JC, et al. The sequence of the human genome. *Science.* 2001;1; 291(5507):1304-1351.
3. Collins F. Genomics: the coming revolution in medicine. *Global Agenda.* 2003;152-154. Available at: http://www.nhgri.nih.gov. Accessed August 18, 2005.
4. McCormick KA. Future directions. In: Saba VK, McCormick KA. *Essentials of Nursing Informatics.* 4th ed. New York: McGraw-Hill; 2005.
5. Collins FS. An interview with Francis S. Collins, MD, PhD, Director, National Human Genome Research Institute. *Assay and Drug Development Technologies.* 2003;1:1-2.
6. Department of Health and Human Services. HHS launches new family history initiative. Available at: http:www.hhs.gov/familyhistory. Accessed August 18, 2005.
7. Collins FS, Green ED, Guttmacher AE, Guyer AS. A vision for the future of genomics research. Available at: http://www.genome.gov/11007524. Accessed August 18, 2005.
8. Harris MA, Clark J, Ireland A, et al. The gene ontology (GO) database and informatics resource. *Nucleic Acids Res.* 2004;32; (database issue):D258-D261.
9. Hoffman M, Arnoldi C, Chuang I. The clinical bioinformatics ontology: a curated semantic network utilizing refseq information. *Pac Symp Biocomput.* 2005;139-150.
10. McKusick-Nathans Institute for Genetic Medicine, Johns Hopkins University (Baltimore, MD) and National Center for Biotechnology Information, National Library of Medicine (Bethesda, MD). Online Mendelian inheritance in man, OMIM™. Available at: http://www.ncbi.nlm.nih.gov/omim/. Accessed August 18, 2005.
11. Neale M, Neale B, Sullivan P. Nonpaternity in linkage studies of extremely discordant sib pairs. *Am J Hum Genet.* 2002;70:526-529.
12. Centers for Disease Control and Prevention. HugeNet. Available at: http://www.cdc.gov/genomics/hugenet/default.htm. Accessed August 18, 2005.
13. Chaix C, Grenier-Sennelier C, Clevenbergh P, et al. Economic evaluation of drug resistance genotyping for the adaptation of treatment in HIV-infected patients in the VIRADAPT study. *J Acquir Immune Defic Syndr.* 2000;24(3):227-231.
14. Durant J, Clevenbergh P, Halfon P, et al. Drug-resistance genotyping in HIV-1 therapy: the VIRADAPT randomised controlled trial. *Lancet.* 1999;353(9171):2195-2199.
15. Saag MS. HIV resistance testing in clinical practice: a Qaly-fied success. *Ann Intern Med.* 2001:134(6):475-477.
16. Hirsch J, Leibel RL. The genetics of obesity. *Hosp Pract.* 1998;33(3):55-59,62-65,69-70.
17. Perusse L, Bouchard C. Gene-diet interactions in obesity. *Am J Clin Nutr.* 2000;72(supplement):1285S-1290S.
18. Perusse L, Chagnon YC, Weisnagel SJ, et al. The human obesity gene map: the 2000 update. *Obesity Res.* 2001;9(2):135-169.
19. National Coalition for Health Professional Education in Genetics. Available at: http://www.nchpeg.org. Accessed August 18, 2005.
20. Collins FS. Genomics: the coming revolution in medicine. *Global Agenda.* Available at: http://www.nhgri.nih.gov. Accessed August 18, 2005.

CHAPTER 31

Nursing Informatics and the NIH Roadmap

By Patricia Flatley Brennan, PhD, RN, FAAN, FACMI

Nursing informatics (NI) holds the key to the success of the National Institutes of Health (NIH) Roadmap Initiatives, a multiyear commitment to accelerate scientific discoveries that will improve health on a global scale. By stimulating new pathways to such discovery, encouraging the creation of new types of research teams, and facilitating re-engineering of the clinical research enterprise, the NIH Roadmap Initiatives strive to capitalize on biological knowledge emerging from the Human Genome Project.[1] Accomplishing these goals requires the active participation of all nurses, particularly those who specialize in NI.

Nursing informatics is a combination of computer science, information science, and nursing science, designed to assist in the processing of nursing data, information, and knowledge, with the goals of supporting the practice of nursing and the delivery of nursing care.[2] Recognized as a specialization within nursing and as a key discipline within biomedical informatics,[3] NI addresses the formalization and manipulation of a phenomenon of concern to nursing: the diagnosis and treatment of human responses.[4] Nurses who specialize in NI will play a major role in delivering on the promise of genomic discoveries by:

1. Helping to make available terminologies used to describe people and their problems along dimensions uniquely known by nursing, which involve how individuals and families respond to health, illness, and physical insult
2. Designing and facilitating computerized information systems (IS) that will support nurses in clinical practice everywhere
3. Developing knowledge resources and devising pathways to the most relevant set of electronic resources, ensuring that knowledge will be available at the point of care
4. Creating patient educational resources and consumer health informatics innovations that will promote an understanding of health and disease in a molecular world
5. Ensuring patients' rights to autonomy, privacy, and control over access to and release of their personal, life state, and family systems information

The full range of NI specialists—investigators, clinical systems designers, developers, analysts, system implementation specialists, chief nursing informatics officers—have important contributions to make to the achievement of the NIH Roadmap. The purpose of this chapter is to review the vision and major directions of the NIH Roadmap and to describe where it intersects with nursing and which contributions of NI are most essential.

NIH and the NIH Roadmap

In its mission statement, the National Institutes of Health, a division of the U.S. Department of Health and Human Services describes itself as "the steward of medical and behavioral research for the Nation."[5] Comprising twenty-seven institutes and centers, the NIH hosts a wide variety of intramural laboratories and disperses approximately $25 billion annually for research and research training directed toward the development of health-related knowledge. Some NIH institutes, such as the National Institute on Aging and the National Cancer Institute, focus on specific body systems, conditions, or diseases, whereas others, e.g., the National Institute of Biomedical Imaging and Bioengineering, target emerging technologies. The National Institute of Nursing (NINR), established in 1993, is one of the few institutes with a mission that is defined by the nature of a

Table 31-1. Themes of the NIH Roadmap

Theme	Title
1	New Pathways To Discovery
2	Research Teams of the Future
3	Reengineering the Clinical Research Enterprise

profession's knowledge base. In fiscal year 2004, the NINR expended $134 million to support clinical and basic research aimed at establishing the scientific basis of care for individuals across their lifespan.

NI researchers receive support from many NIH agencies, including NINR and the National Library of Medicine. Other federal institutes and agencies, including the Agency for Health Care Quality and Research (AHRQ) and the Health Resources and Services Administration (NRSA), also support research and research training in NI. For the purposes of this chapter, however, we will confine our discussion to the NIH and the NIH Roadmap initiatives.

The NIH Roadmap, which was promulgated in 2003, arose from the concerted efforts of the NIH and national biomedical leaders.[6] Although NIH investment has led to significant improvements in health and well-being, scientific leaders recognized that accelerating the pace of discovery would require complex, interdisciplinary efforts that were not feasible within any single institute or center. Thus, the Roadmap provides a blueprint for cross-institutional research investment. The goal of the Roadmap Initiatives is to define a "compelling, limited set of priorities that can be acted upon and are essential to accelerate progress across the spectrum of the institute missions."[1] The Roadmap represents both a strategic vision and a framework for setting priorities, dispersing funds, and organizing intramural and extramural research and research training initiatives.

The Roadmap was developed on the basis of three key themes: the provision of opportunities for new approaches to scientific discovery, the establishment of interdisciplinary approaches to research, and expansion of the capacity for clinical research (see Table 31-1).

The Roadmap is not simply a new type of strategic plan; it is a commitment to concerted action that demands the full participation of all clinical and basic science disciplines. Under the theme "New Pathways to Discovery," shared resources will be developed that will relieve individual research enterprises of the burden to create and recreate methods needed to enhance scientific discovery (see Table 31-2).

These shared resources represent a change in philosophy, from the creation of large isolated centers to the development of a network-accessible infrastructure that will leverage investments for multiple uses. Because NI specialists frequently find themselves to be the only investigators in their specialty at a given institution, this emphasis on cross-institutional resource sharing will better unify their solitary efforts into a coordinated contribution. The patient care interventions that arise from these discoveries will in turn necessitate the development and deployment of NI tools for patient education and self-monitoring.

NI specialists will also create needed terminologies to ensure that human health and disease processes are delineated broadly enough to extend beyond the arbitrary boundaries of their current characterization. Nursing language systems describe disease not only from the biological perspective but also from human experience. Hope, fear, support, and perseverance all contribute to the experience of disease and its management and mitigation.

Under the second theme, the "Research Teams of the Future" are envisioned as interdisciplinary groups capable of taking on high-stakes projects (see Table 31-3).

This dimension of the Roadmap (Table 31-3) focuses on increasing the pipeline of researchers skilled in interdisciplinary investigation as well as on creating institutional and organizational environments that will better support interdisciplinary scholarship. Interdisciplinary research is a natural extension of the long-standing interdisciplinary nature of nursing and NI. Nursing informatics researchers and practitioners have central roles to play as members of the "research teams of the future." These initiatives mandate interdisciplinary training and research and require the participa-

Table 31-2. Theme 1: New Pathways to Discovery—Groups and Initiatives

Group	Initiative	Outputs
Building Blocks, Pathways, and Networks Implementation Group	National Technology Centers for Networks and Pathways	• New tools to describe the dynamics of protein interactions • Instruments, methods, and reagents for quantitative measurements at sub-cellular resolution and very short timescales
	Metabolomics Technology Development	• Novel technologies to study cellular metabolites
	Standards for Proteomics and Metabolomics/Assessment of Critical Reagents for Proteomics	• Quality and data standards for proteomics and metabolomics • Advice regarding critical reagents required to enhance future research in proteomics
Molecular Libraries and Imaging Implementation Group	Molecular Libraries Screening Center Network (MLSCN)	• Public collection of chemically diverse small molecules • High-throughput screening to identify compounds active in target- and phenotype-based assays • Public database of screening data
	Cheminformatics	• Database of chemical structures and their biological activities • PubChem
	Technology Development	• Improvement of chemical diversity • Assay flexibility • Screening instrumentation/robotics prospective characterization of chemical compounds' metabolism and toxicology properties
	Development of High Specificity/High Sensitivity Probes to Improve Detection	• Probe detection sensitivity 10- to 100-fold within 5 years
	Comprehensive Trans-NIH Imaging Probe Database	• Specialized portion of the PubChem database • Catalog imaging probe information, describing the specificities, activities, and applications of imaging probes
	Core Synthesis Facility to Produce Imaging Probes	• Known imaging probes for the research community • Novel imaging probes for biomedical research and clinical applications
Structural Biology Implementation Group	Protein Production Facilities	• Development of rapid, efficient and dependable methods to produce protein samples that scientists can use to determine the three-dimensional structure, or shape, of a protein
Bioinformatics and Computational Biology Implementation Group	National Centers for Biomedical Computing	• National software engineering system • Supercomputing network to share and analyze data, using a common set of software tools
Nanomedicine Implementation Group	Planning for Nanomedicine Centers	• New funding opportunity (RFA) for planning the Centers • Quantitative measurement of biological processes at the nanoscale • Engineering of new tools to intervene at the nanoscale or molecular level synthetic biological devices

tion of nurses. NI researchers can avail themselves of the training opportunities that will arise under these efforts.

Parallel to the basic science aspect of the "New Pathways to Discovery" theme, the "Re-engineering of the Clinical Research Enterprise" theme targets accelerating the processes and practices of clinical research (see Table 31-4).

Relying on a network model, efforts connected to this theme will lead to more sophisticated clinical trials that in turn will stimulate translational research activity. The primary point of

Table 31-3. Theme 2: Research Teams of the Future—Groups and Initiatives

Group	Initiative	Activities
High-Risk Research Implementation Group	NIH Director's Pioneer Awards	
Interdisciplinary Research Implementation Group	Interdisciplinary Research Centers	• Interdisciplinary research programs that will address significant and complex biomedical problems • Interdisciplinary research consortium
	Interdisciplinary Research Training Initiative	• New model of funding
	Innovations in Interdisciplinary Technology and Methods (Meetings)	
	Removing Structural Barriers to Interdisciplinary Research	
	NIH Intramural Program as a Model for Interdisciplinary Research	
	Interagency Conference on the Interface of Life Sciences and Physical Sciences (See NIH House Appropriations Report 108-188, p. 94)	
Public Private Partnerships Implementation Group	Designation of a Public-Private Sector Liaison	
	High-level Science-driven Partnership Meetings	

contribution for NI will be to apply language systems and innovations in both clinical and personal health records to enhance the dynamic assessment of patient-reported chronic disease outcomes.

Nursing Informatics and the NIH Roadmap

It is fortunate that thirty years of efforts in NI have resulted in terminology systems, technology-mediated patient care innovations, and robust tools for knowledge development and dissemination. Although much work remains to be done, the accomplishments to date articulate well with the data needs, IS architectures, and interdisciplinary research efforts proposed by the NIH Roadmap. Nursing is essential to the NIH Roadmap Initiatives because of its expertise in characterizing the experiences of patients, reaching them where they receive care, live, and work and producing well-trained scholars.

Table 31-4. Theme 3: Re-engineering the Clinical Research Enterprise—Groups and Initiatives

Group	Initiative	Activities
Clinical Research Implementation Group	Clinical Research Networks/NECTAR	• National Electronic Clinical Trials and Research (NECTAR) Network
	Clinical Research Policy Analysis and Coordination	
	Clinical Research Workforce Training	• Development of clinical researchers • Multidisciplinary Research Career Development Program • National Clinical Research Associates (NCRAs) initiative
	Dynamic Assessment of Patient-Reported Chronic Disease Outcomes	• Measurements of self-reported health states and outcomes across a wide range of illnesses and disease severities
	Translational Research	• Regional Translational Research Centers • Translational Research Core Services

NI research, both that is supported by NINR and that is funded through other agencies such as the National Library of Medicine and Agency for Health Care Quality and Research has developed mechanisms for achieving two major goals: (1) characterizing patients' experiences with regard to health, recovery, pain and coping, and family and community environments, which are not encompassed in languages developed by other disciplines, in a computerizable way that can allow them to be linked conceptually to genetic structures and formalizations of biological pathways; and (2) effectively using IT to reach all individuals, sick and well, empowered and underserved, with information and skill-building strategies that can help them to participate actively in their own health care.

Because it is replete with unfamiliar terminology, e.g., *metabolomics* and *membrane protein production facilities,* the Roadmap may at first not seem to have direct relevance to NI. However, there are several points of articulation between the accomplishments of NI and the themes of the Roadmap. Specific to NI is its emphasis on the acceleration of biomolecular discovery linked to human function. NI oversees the development of computerizable terminologies that describe human function; these language systems provide unique characterizations of human phenomena, in a manner that can be integrated with the basic scientific discoveries.

As nursing IS designers and implementers facilitate large-scale implementations of computerized patient record systems that encompass automated descriptions of patient phenomena, they ensure that clinical care data are more easily captured for use in research studies.

Stimulation of Interdisciplinary Research Teams

NI specialists are uniquely equipped to capture and manage clinical information and to make it accessible to the research enterprise. The inclusion of NI specialists on research teams will ensure sufficient opportunities for identifying points of articulation where better specification of nursing phenomena may enhance biological discovery and its clinical consequences. These points of articulation may, in turn, require new NI tools and language systems.

Reliance on Public-Private Partnerships

NI specialists, particularly those who work at the intersection of vendor-developed IS and clinical care facilities, have broad-ranging experience in creating and maintaining relationships between the private sector and the not-for-profit environment of health care. Thus, they can offer expertise and strategies for creating successful public-private partnerships.

Nurses in practice have developed efficient ways to deploy evidence-based approaches to patient care, and these pathways can serve in the rapid translation of biological and nanotechnological innovations into people's everyday lives. Nursing research already encompasses a plethora of problem-solving strategies to assist patients in managing illness and responding to health threats. NI has the terminologies and proven technology-mediated care models to extend benefits from the biomolecular laboratory to the households and hospital bedrooms of all patients.

Nursing and the NIH Roadmap

Nursing also stands to gain from the achievements of the Roadmap Initiatives. The creation of large-scale computer tools will support not only biological discovery but also the analysis of large data sets, from which we may devise new ways to develop nursing knowledge. Rationalization of the clinical research enterprise and achievement of interoperable health information will increase the integration of our research findings, yielding greater benefits. The creation of new informatics technologies for capturing data at the point of care and of new methodologies for deploying enriched information resources throughout the care trajectory hold great potential for helping NINR to achieve its goal of reducing health care disparities.

Over the last twenty years, we have developed systematic, computerizable languages to describe human experiences. Using these languages, scientists can link the genetic structure of an individual and that person's pedigree to the health behaviors, home environments, and community influences that mediate the relationship between genes and destiny. Additionally, nurses who work in communities have developed strategies for linking universities with the communities they serve and for characterizing the health of those communities.

Basic nursing languages that provide terms to characterize human phenomena include the Nursing Diagnoses, the Nursing Interventions Classification, and the Nursing Outcomes Classification. NI researchers have built on these semantics-based systems to make them more valuable to nursing and to patient care.

The Nursing Minimum Data Set (NMDS) and the International Nursing Minimum Data Set (i-NMDS) provide an organizing structure for disparate vocabularies to ensure an integrated view of patient experiences. Parallel work has been done to ensure the robustness of clinical terminologies and to make them amenable to computerization.[7,8] Nurses already understand the interconnections among individuals, families, and communities. This knowledge, linked seamlessly with the outputs of biomolecular discoveries, portends an even greater understanding: that of how human pathways interact with and extend biological pathways.

Nursing might be the discipline that is best equipped to help fill in the blanks between biology and destiny. Nursing research that sheds light on human behavior—its antecedents, motivations, consequences, and reinforcements—can help to make the link between biological susceptibility to physical insult and the realization of the ultimate experience of the individual, the family, and the community.

References

1. Zerhouni E. The NIH roadmap. *Science*. 2003; 302: 63-65.
2. Graves JR, Corcoran S. The study of nursing informatics. *Image: J Nurs Scholarship*. 1989;21:227-231.
3. American Nurses Association. Task Force on the Scope of Practice for Nursing Informatics. *Scope of practice for nursing informatics*. Washington, DC: American Nurses Publishing, 1994.
4. American Nurses Association. *Nursing: A Social Policy Statement*. Washington, DC: American Nurses Association, 1995.
5. National Institutes of Health (NIH). NIH mission. Available at: www.nih.gov. Accessed March 20, 2005.
6. National Institutes of Health (NIH). NIH Roadmap Initiatives. Available at: http://nihroadmap.nih.gov/index.asp. Accessed March 20, 2005.
7. Goossen WT, Ozbolt JG, Coenen A, et al. Development of a provisional domain model for the nursing process within the Health Level 7 reference information model. *J Am Med Inform Assoc*. 2004;11:186-194.
8. Bakken S, Cashen MS, Mendonca EA, O'Brien A, Zieniewicz J. Representing nursing activities within a concept-oriented terminological system: evaluation of a type definition. *J Am Med Inform Assoc*. 2000;7:81-90.

CHAPTER 32

Citizen Empowerment: eHealth Consumerism in Europe

By Kaija Saranto, PhD; Patrick Weber, MA, RN; Kristiina Häyrinen, MSc; Pirkko Kouri, MNSc, PHN; Jari Porrasmaa, MSc; Jorma Komulainen, MD; Martti Kansanen, PhD, MD; Esa Kemppainen, MSc (Eng)/Information Technology; Kaija Hämäläinen, PHN; and Annikki Jauhiainen, PhD, RN

This chapter explores the growing consumer activism happening in health care across Europe as more individuals use the Internet to access expert medical information and as countries extend their national electronic health record (EHR) initiatives to include access by the individual at home. Practice-based, Internet communication also offers consumers a secure method to make queries to their health care providers, obtain health information, and access personal clinical information.[1] The rapid growth of the Internet has been one of the most remarkable developments in the telecommunications sector in recent years. The number of personal computers used in homes with Internet connectivity has doubled annually throughout the 1990s and such connectivity has been the constant, lifetime companion of an entire generation of young adults. This informal "network of networks" that started as a creation of the United States' military, was initially used exclusively by by universities. Its explosive worldwide growth is reflected in an ever-increasing range of enticing communication services. As a case example, we describe Finland's current efforts to leverage its national EHR infrastructure to support numerous eHealth initiatives. These projects aim to make health information and Internet access available to targeted populations in schools, community centers, in the home and health facilities.

Health Care in Transition

Consumerism is driving profound changes in the culture and social organization of health care that will significantly impact clinicians and care delivery processes. As consumer empowerment becomes increasingly expressed in the health care arena, it will push transition from old to new. In this transition state, health care will bridge from the traditional, authoritarian state, in which physicians were the undisputed experts and sole owners of an individual's medical data, to a care team model in which the individual patient is at the center of decision making.

Consumers are increasingly using the Internet to access the latest science in the management and treatment of a given medical condition; the literature is full of stories of patients coming in to see a specialist armed with the latest results from clinical trials.[2-5] In addition, Web sites for particular medical conditions exist in which patients and patients' family members share their knowledge and experiences, complete with recommendations regarding the various treatments.[2-5] Studies that measure use of the Internet to access medical information show a logarithmic rate of adoption around the world.[2-5] Truly, citizens are becoming avid consumers of health information to the extent that in 2005, it is unlikely that health care professionals will encounter a patient who has not used information technology (IT) to influence his/her knowledge of health behavior. The availability of health information on the Internet makes it possible for patients to gain sufficient information to engage as full-fledged participants in their own care and decision making; thus, the patients' role is rapidly changing from passive recipients to active participants in their own care.

It is evident that relationships between patients and health care professionals will change as a result of Internet use.[2-5] As patients become better informed, participative discussions between patient and physician about the alternatives in care will become more common. The role of professionals will change from one of authority to that of processor of information. Patient-physician encounters will change from health care professional-centered to patient-controlled events. Numerous benefits resulting from patients' Internet use have been reported.[5] Physicians have identified the information, advice, and social support derived from patients' Internet use as benefits, although improved coping and self-care were identified as the main benefits from the health service's perspective due to decease in utilization and costs.[5-7]

It is to be expected that some clinicians will experience consumerism behavior in health care as disruptive and confusing, but it is a trend that will only continue to grow. Technology, personal computers, and ubiquitous Internet access make this an irreversible change that is happening simultaneously on a global scale. Health professionals will need to shift their thinking to focus on supporting and empowering patients to realize their potential for managing their own health and for controlling the decisions made in their health care.

As health care systems move toward the concept of a single EHR, ownership of an individual's medical record will become an outdated concept. The very reason for the EHR is to make the person's medical data accessible to all who have a need to know at any time and from any location, including the individual patient. Increasingly, each person will be responsible for his/her health data and the role of health care providers will be to add their updates to an individual's EHR. This phenomenon also is driving the need for a growing focus on the new discipline of consumer health informatics, as described by Eysenbach:[6]

> "Consumer health informatics is the branch of medical informatics that analyses consumers' needs for information; studies and implements methods of making information accessible to consumers; and models and integrates consumers' preferences into medical information systems."[6]

In many countries, consumer informatics has a growing importance.[7] Goldsmith and Safran[7] (2003) urge policy makers and clinicians to support consumerism because of its great potential to improve patient care and care management. According to Goldsmith and Safran,[7] EHR applications are designed to enhance communication and decision making between providers, patients and their families. Fuller participation in decision making and care by the patient and family members has been shown to result in improved outcomes.[6] Also, it is widely held that the safest and most effective care happens when individuals control his/her medical data and actively participate in disease management and care decision making.[7] In spring 2000, the American Medical Informatics Association (AMIA) published a position paper recommending that the patient-provider partnership be supported to provide more patient-centered health care.[8] Supportive activities are called for in five main areas: research, provider support, information access, new patient record system, and evaluation and policy and regulation.[8]

Health-related Information Consumption Through the Internet

Use of the Internet to search for health care related topics is becoming a common and expected practice. According to a 2001 Pew survey in the U.S., more than 52 million Americans used the Internet to search on health-related topics.[9] These usage numbers increased to 70 million in 2002,[10] 93 million in 2003,[11] and 95 million in 2004.[12] It was estimated in 2003 that half of all Internet queries are searches for health related information.[11] Although this data is not available for European population's Internet usage, it is known that approximately 260 million, or 35.5 percent of the population use the Internet, compared with 200 million, or 67.8 percent in the U.S. This would suggest that Internet adoption is more pervasive in the U.S. than in Europe, which has significance for consumerism in health care also.[13]

Using the U.S. experience as an example for what may be in store for Europe's future, the Pew 2005 survey found that 80 percent of American Internet users have searched for information on at least one major health topic online and also found that many users searched for several kinds of information related to that topic. The types of health topics requested in these searches are shown in Table 32-1.

Table 32-1. Major Domains for Internet Queries

Health Topics	%	Health Topics	%
Specific disease or medical problem	66	Depression, anxiety, stress, or mental health issues	23
Certain medical treatment or procedure	51	Experimental treatments or medicines	23
Diet, nutrition, vitamins, or nutritional supplements	51	Environmental health hazards	18
Exercise or fitness	42	Immunizations or vaccinations	16
Prescription or over-the-counter drugs	40	Sexual health information	11
Health insurance	31	Medicare or Medicaid	11
Alternative treatments or medicines	30	Problems with drugs or alcohol	8
A particular doctor or hospital	28	How to quit smoking	7

Interestingly, more than half of the Internet users in the U.S. who had recently conducted searches did so on behalf of someone else—a spouse, child, friend, or other loved one—and not for themselves.[11] This finding demonstrates the degree to which relatives are involved in investigating health-related information research. This practice of a family member accessing health information on behalf of the patient should be taken into account in the patient encounter. Nurses will want to include this family broker in health care decisions as well as patient education and planning of care to ensure effective communication and engagement.

Vast amounts of health information for health professionals are also available on the Internet, with most professional journals now accessible in electronic format at the journal's Web sites and through various sources, e.g., PubMed. While health professionals may be the targeted audience for these sites, the general public may also access these sites and read published papers and postings. The ready availability of online published journals, government funded research results, and professional organizations' information postings further acts to lessen the distance between the provider specialist and the patient (or patient's advocate).

Governmental Actions and Consumerism

The World Health Organization (WHO) is actively working on the use of information and communication technologies (ICT) because of their potential for both high- and low-income countries. The secretariat of the WHO executive board describes this potential: "Today, eHealth—understood in this context to mean use of information and communication technologies locally and at a distance—presents a unique opportunity for the development of public health. The strengthening of health systems through eHealth reinforces fundamental human rights by improving equity, solidarity, quality of life and quality of care."[14] The eHealth resolution was accepted May 25, 2005 at the 58th World Health Assembly.[15] The WHO eHealth resolution charges health care leaders with facilitating the development of model solutions, which could be established in national centers and would serve as a health network.[16]

In 2002, the European Union (EU) Commission adopted a five-year, community action program to improve public health and wellness. The recommendations call for creating and coordinating an advisory structure to guide the overall planning process for implementing systems in the following fields:

1. Lifestyle and other health determinants (including sexual and reproductive health aspects)
2. Mortality and morbidity (including cancer and rare diseases)
3. Health systems (including prevention and promotion aspects)
4. Health and environment (including specific settings, e.g., workplace, school, and hospital settings)
5. Mental health
6. Accidents and injuries (including self-inflicted injuries, suicide, and violence aspects)
7. Community health indicators / network of working party leaders[17]

The community action plan, eEurope 2005, accepted by the EU Commission on April 30, 2004, describes in just 26 pages what needs to be done through 2010 to empower citizens across the EU countries in the use of eHealth. The broader goal of the plan is to promote general awareness of electronic services in the different fields to make them more accessible and user-friendly for the general public. These initiatives are to be carried out in collaboration with businesses and local authorities.[18] Access is planned by gradual equipping of regional service points with customer terminals at locations such as, schools, libraries, public service points, and municipal offices. These access points would be open to the general public and would provide Internet connections, as well as advisory services, including health information and services as a key component.[18] Specifically targeted are uses of e-Health to improve access to health care and to boost the quality and effectiveness of ICT across the whole range of functions that affect the health sector.[15]

The EU Commission also encourages joint work between biology, medical, and behavioral social sciences for a more integrated and holistic team approach to the research dimensions brought to a given endeavor. This field is called *bioinformatics* (conjunction of medical informatics, bioinformatics, and neuroinformatics). Over the last 10 years, the EU has awarded approximately 460 million Euros across 476 European research projects. For the next 10 years (2003–2014), the EU is prioritizing funding support for initiatives that support well-being, health knowledge information structure, and biomedical informatics for individualized health care.[15,19] Similar to the U.S., in Europe, the new devices using Internet are under studies with a focus on the convergence of research efforts in bioinformatics.

Developments in biomedical informatics have contributed to the emergence of a new e-Health industry that has the potential to become the third largest industry in the health sector with a turnover of 11 billion. By 2010, the e-Health industry could potentially account for 5 percent of the total health budget. At present, the e-Health industry in Europe—mainly comprised of small- and medium-sized enterprises—has a competitive advantage, but it still needs to enjoy a more favorable position in the business environment. EU member states have shown that they are keen to take an e-Health agenda forward, drawing on best practices and experience from across the EU. The EU support should enable a move toward a "European e-Health Area," that is, an emerging framework built on a wide range of European policies and initiatives for concerted actions and synergies in e-Health that will provide a favorable environment for the integration of related policies at a community level.[15]

The EU commission encourages nursing projects to integrate into the European e-Health action plan because it is realized that it primarily will be nurses at the front line when a citizen needs health-related information. A 2000 survey of more than one thousand U.S. health care consumers found that 89 percent of respondents would use a nurse triage service to help them manage a chronic medical condition when available and that they would like this service to be available via the telephone and the Internet. Consumers would also like to have available a nurse triage service to answer questions after regular office hours.[20]

In 2002, Cambridge University held an invitational conference to develop a consensus statement on patient involvement and consumerism. Five expert panels from across the EU countries participated in this review and development of recommendations. In a report entitled, "The Informed Patient," which refers to a research initiative aimed at guiding future policy on the provision of information to patients in Europe, the major conclusion is that the future of health care in Europe will demand that far greater health-related information be made available for patients and citizens if the goal of fully informed patients is to be achieved. The report further recommends that information and knowledge support be available at both the level of the EU/member states and at the regional/local level to assure sufficient access, educational resources, and appropriateness to local context. "The Doctor-Patient Partnership" (DPP) project in the United Kingdom is an example of an initiative that aims to provide health information at a local level with access support. A project of the United Kingdom's National Health Service, the DPP demonstrates that it is possible for a government to make relevant patient information easily available through the Internet. The DDP (www.dpp.org.uk) is free to the public and aims to encourage better communication between patients and health care professionals, promote responsible use of NHS services, and offer practical advice on self-medication.[21]

Studies show that systems in which patients and doctors could access the medical record through the World Wide Web improved the patients' understanding of their health and created better communication with health care providers.[22] Findings also show, however, that some patients have difficulty understanding their medical record, and others became more worried and pessimistic after reading their psychiatric record.[23] Physicians and nurses will therefore need to acquire new skills that focus on teaching patients how to read their medical record with interpretation of meaning that can be positively channeled into their health behavior and care decisions. This new dimension to the patient-provider role will most likely fall to nurses as an education and case management function, especially if the time is provided for patients to ask help in reviewing their medical record.

Trustworthiness of Health Information on the Internet

The quality of the information available on the Internet is crucial to its serving as an expert source for health information. The most common problem reported with the use of the Internet for health information was receiving misinformation. Nonreliable information could have a tremendous effect in the health care field; therefore, efforts are underway to help the voluntary-based effort to reach a sufficient level of quality. Health On the Net Foundation (HON) took the first initiative to define a code of conduct (HONCode) and to provide a credentialing label for a Web site that follows the HONCode. The HONCode addresses three main domains: identification of the site editors and their competencies; citation of references to external sources; and a clear distinction between advertising and scientific editorials.[24] Another creditable source is the Internet Healthcare Coalition and its edited eHealth Code of Ethics which is used internationally and is translated into many languages.[25] It is exceedingly important that Internet editors of health-related information follow one of these two code of ethics and apply the credentialing label to give the reader better confidence regarding the content. The last available study conducted by HON shows a positive attitude toward the certified sites. Approximately 66 percent of persons who answered the patient section only (N = 1,318) think that certification and/or accreditation of medical Web sites may help resolve the issues previously discussed, whereas 71 percent of professionals (N = 1,294) expressed a similar opinion. Among all respondents, 59 percent favor certified Web sites, with the rest stating that they did not favor them (25.3 percent) or did not answer the question (15.6 percent).[26]

Technology Brings Life-Long Learning to All

The Nursing Perspective
Working as a nurse in the information society requires wide and versatile know-how. Nursing informatics (NI) is one of the core issues for future nurses.[27,28] NI consists of basic skills related to information and communication, e.g., skills related to word processing and the use of graphics and spreadsheet applications; skills related to electronic data transfer and messaging; skills for data processing, e.g., retrieving, storing, and utilizing the collected data; skills related to acting on the basis of data security; and skills for using versatile EHRs. The positive attitude toward information and computer technology (ICT) and a motivation toward using ICT solutions and different applications as daily tools are essential for advanced nurses.[28-30] Furthermore, NI competencies include recognition of the ergonomic aspects related to the use of ICT[29] and the applied use of telecommunications techonology for health services, care delivery, and education.[28] Information literacy and the use of versatile databases are a fundamental part of evidence-based nursing.[27,31,32]

In the recent study by Jauhiainen,[28] NI competencies were strongly integrated in nursing care. Ideally, the nurse should have the capabilities necessary for assessing and using ICT, based on the needs of the customer or patient. The best customer service emphasizes that the nurse should assess the patient's computer literacy and his/her willingness to use e-services as a part of the care service, the ICT tools used by the patient, and the functioning network infrastructure. A newly added aspect of the nurse's role will be to guide and to encourage the use of qualified reference databases. Skills that future nurses will need include the ability to search for versatile data from different databases; the ability to assess the quality and accuracy of information searched; and the ability to apply different educational methods to e-service interactions when teaching the customer. The nurse should maintain her/his teaching strategies and compare his/her ICT literacy skills to those with the client's. In the virtual environment to which much interaction will be referred, the lack of facial expressions and gestures and all other lack of sense perceptions or other matters related to the e-situation may hamper the nurse/patient interaction. The ethical considerations and responsibilities of patient care involve quality communication between the nurse and the customer/patient. To close the gap that may initially appear that may hamper such communication, nurses will be called on to work in both worlds for a while and it will be important to respect the patient's decisions irrespective of whether the customer/patient chooses the traditional way of service/care or the "e-facilitated" way in order to enhance his/her health and well being/welfare.[28]

As has been noted by earlier chapters in this book, in order to provide future nurses with the NI expertise that will be needed for the new era, NI should now be integrated into the entire nursing curriculum—both in theory and in clinical practice.[28,32] Education should include information retrieval, data storage, and the adaptation of data in versatile care situations, both in theoretical studies and in patient care. Moreover, the teaching of knowledge use, e.g., terminology and classification, electronic documentation, and the use of electronic records, should also be added to the curriculum. Web-based/virtual education is a teaching method that allows a virtual training model to demonstrate how to carry out nursing care and how to counsel patients on the Internet. Nursing faculty need supplementary education and training in NI in clinical settings in order to implement informatics as part of their teaching and to enhance knowledge and skills in NI among graduating nurse students.[28]

Today, many nurses lack NI competencies. The developed and new ICT applications and programs require constant education, training, and familiarizing in practice. Realizing that NI competencies accumulate with working experience and lifelong learning, nurse education reform extends into the work setting and calls for continuing education that can provide the informatics skills needed by today's nursing workforce.[28,33] There is need for learning in the fields of information retrieval, electronic documentation, nursing terminology and classifications, and in the use of evidence-based nursing literature. Further and supplementary education must be planned with the objective of meeting the needs and competence of the nurses.[28] Staggers et al[34] (2001) have drafted descriptions of the competence level for the different levels of nurses from novice to expert, extending to nurse specialist and to innovator in NI. The descriptions of competences needed in the literature[27-30,34] and the scenarios outlining the future use of NI all speak to the urgent need to develop educational strategies for NI competencies needed broadly across the nursing workforce.[28] Ehnfors and Grobe[33] (2004) recommend a global education strategy for versatility and standardization in NI. In Chapter 5, Skiba and colleagues[35] (2006) outline the shift needed to bring informatics competencies as core components into the nursing curriculum and practice skills in the nursing workforce.

Information Literacy Among Consumers

According to the American Libraries Association,[36] an information-literate consumer is able to determine the extent of information needed, access the needed information effectively and efficiently, evaluate information and its sources critically, incorporate selected information into his/her knowledge base, use information effectively to accomplish a specific purpose, understand the economic, legal, and social issues surrounding the use of information, and access and use information ethically and legally. IT skills enable a consumer to use computers, software applications, databases, and other technologies to achieve a wide variety of work-related, educational, and personal goals. Jääskeläinen's[37] 2000 findings suggest that in order to prevent a "digital divide," information literacy should be included as an obligatory part of compulsory education. The digital divide refers to the gap that exists between those who have and those who do not have access to technology, e.g., computers and Internet access. The divide is applicable to all population sectors, encompassing different ages with particular focus on the underserved segments of the population: low-income, rural, and multicultural areas; disabled or elderly individuals; and women.[37,38] Health care information is often provided in a written form, which combined with the complexity of the health care system, may be overwhelming for individuals with limited literacy skills. These limited skills often translate into problems understanding even the simplest written instructions, accurately completing intake forms, or appropriately prescribing medication for consumers/patients. Clearly, the goal is to provide consumers with health information that is understandable and easy to access.[37,39]

Finland Case Example: Bringing IT to Consumers

The Finns have been among the most enthusiastic users of the Internet. The Finnish University and Research Network (FUNET), founded in 1984, committed itself early on to the TCP/IP protocol, which is the foundation of the Internet. The choice was an auspicious one, as Finland today has more computers per capita connected to the Internet than any other country in the world. According to the host count carried out by Network Wizards, there were approximately half a million Internet nodes registered in Finland, although now only one quarter of those are in the network of organizations belonging to the FUNET.[40]

Currently, the big question for Finnish health professionals is not where to find information but rather how to interpret this information to accommodate their patients' needs. The national evidence-based medicine (EBM) guidelines have been developed in various countries; in Finland, the Finnish Medical Society Duodecim organizes this process. The work started in 1994, and currently there are 54 EBM guidelines published on the Internet.[41] In addition to the Internet, these guidelines are also available for downloading to mobile devices. The rationale behind electronically published, evidence-based guidelines is to ensure that doctors and nurses have the best and the most reliable information for their treatment decisions. An optimal response to this professional concern would be that these guidelines are directly integrated into an EHR. To enable the inclusion of medical guidelines into the EHR, the data elements should be structured and coded for at least diagnoses, medications, laboratory and other examinations, as well as for surgery and other treatments and procedures. This integration requires standardization of physicians' documentation and their medical record systems. Therefore, the Finnish Medical Society Duodecim is currently developing automatic decision support tools based on the EBM guidelines that in the future will be implemented into the EHR systems.[42]

In Finland, the infrastructure of the EHR illustrates the possibilities of ICT to empower the consumer and the possibilities of the consumers to use or be involved in the eHealth service and the decision-making process. Finland's national EHR project is described in Case Study 27B in this book.[43] In the following Finnish case examples, we present four consumer informatics initiatives that illustrate the ways Internet-based health information applications support the special needs of consumers from early childhood to elderly individuals. The information literacy skills of both health care professionals and consumers must be taken into account and the essential education must be planned accordingly. As patients increasingly use the Internet and online consumer services, a huge concern is the risk of misinformation. On the other hand, online messaging with health care practices provides opportunities to educate consumers/patients to improve health.[44,45] Consumers who currently communicate online with health care providers report high levels of satisfaction with these services and find them easy to use.[46] However, computer literacy skills are still a challenge for segments of patient population, as well as for some professionals.[7,47] Deficient literacy skills that are the most troublesome relate to consumer's ability to investigate health information on the Web and to evaluate the quality and validity of that information.[2] While the Internet constitutes an easy way to obtain information, it also requires a critical attitude toward the quality of information.

Eysenbach and Köhler[48] (2002) report that consumers tend to trust Web sites of what are perceived as official authorities, and this is increased when the site uses a professional layout, understandable and professional writing, and scientific reference citations. Furthermore, greater trust toward online health information was observed when the same information was repeated on multiple Web sites. In general, consumers tend to judge commercial sites as untrustworthy.[4]

The trustworthiness of health care Web sites could be guaranteed by requiring validation of a code of ethics conducted by an impartial international organization. If such validation were required, in conjunction with the use of Web site guidelines, regulation of health information on the Internet would be possible.[49] Given the difficulty in accomplishing regulation, the safest approach for controlling the quality of health information is to educate consumers and to post third party evaluations of the information.[50] Health portals also play an important role in health consumerism. Sites that are updated by a trusted organization offer the possibility of maintaining quality. Health portals complement public health services, and the trend in Finland is for health-related associations to update them. Planning for a health portal for consumers is being developed by a trusted organization as part of the Finnish EHR project.[47]

New record systems are needed to integrate care with use of informatics tools rather than through either the patient or the provider. A new model of care should be developed to transcend the brief patient-clinician encounter, and records should encompass the entire process of care. Based on our experiences in Finland, informaticians need to design new clinical record systems that will:

1. Be longitudinal, organized around the person, in addition to institutions or providers, and relevant to individual patients in managing their own care.
2. Situate care in the context of a patient's life, and not only in the business of the institution, with records that extend across a lifetime and across institutions.
3. Allow pathways to and through information services across a number of institutions, including the records a patient keeps at home.
4. Link to knowledge resources that may be dynamic.
5. Integrate knowledge that patients and providers each need.
6. Integrate information and care across institutions, requiring a balance between information integrity and care needs.
7. Support epidemiological, public health, and statistical analysis in order that the information can be useful to clinicians.
8. Give attention to identity, security, privacy, and trust issues.[8]

Having a well-defined plan for the development of an EHR system should allow including new technologies as they emerge. These technologies will be those that help the patient to gain access to data and to send data to the health care center. Self-monitoring systems using the Internet are becoming available for tracking patients who have chronic diseases, e.g., diabetes, hypertension, arrhythmia, and others. Investments toward these are currently being made in the U.S., as in the European Union. Millions of dollars will be available for such developments, with a high emphasis on the empowerment of the citizen and a decrease of total costs.[51,19] As new devices are put into use, biomedical informatics will play an increasingly central role because of new areas of data generated. The enormous volume of data generated from these biomedical devices will require processing with high capacity for analysis, grid computing, security considerations, and three dimensional image analysis.[52]

In Finland, ongoing projects are continuously seeking new technologies to be used in health care. The *All-wireless Hospital Project* (2004–2006) focuses on the development of the wireless local area networks and the ultra wideband technologies in health care and piloting them in real life in a hospital environment at the Oulu University Hospital. The research serving as the basis for the project has two main objectives: to develop technologies for wireless monitoring of patients; and to create wireless interfaces between medical patient-monitoring devices and hospital data systems.[53]

Using eHealth to Meet Consumer Needs: Children to Elderly Individuals

Over the years, various patient groups have used technology for counseling and support. For instance there are online support groups for those addicted to alcohol, drugs and the Internet, as well as groups for patients who have diabetes and their caregivers, which are moderated by a nurse or doctor who provides health information, such as the Finnish Diabetes Association.[54,55] The following four projects represent targeted community populations in which health information is specifically designed and forwarded to designated portals.

Kidmednet Finland Project

One example of a project aiming toward producing trusted health information with the intention of its being passed from child to child is the *Kidmednet Finland Project.* The other goals of the project are to introduce children to World Wide Web programming and to inspire them with further knowledge of the human body. The topics for the pilot projects in 2003 were selected with two purposes in mind: the topics had to be interesting and also had to be as simple as possible. Thus, children in one school were asked to produce information about human development, whereas those in another school were asked to familiarize themselves with the functioning of the human heart. The next step was to teach the children about their topics. For that, a consultant pediatrician gave two lectures, one in each school. After the lectures, the children were asked to produce text and pictures about what they had just learned. Afterwards, these primary products were used as basis for further workup. Subsequently, children studied more of their topics under the direction of their teachers. They utilized both literature as well as various electronic databases, with some help from the project personnel. During their learning process, they produced text, pictures, and animations about what they were studying. Before closing this project, the consultant pediatrician checked the material, and the products were thoroughly discussed in groups including the children, their teacher, the project personnel, and the pediatrician. As the result, the works of the children were published on the Internet six months after the start of the project.[56]

Net Clinic for Pregnant Families

The *Maternity and Infant Clinic* (Net Clinic) is an example of a solution designed to facilitate communication between health care professionals and to ease consumers' access to information. In order to use the Maternity and Infant Clinic, both parents receive personal passwords and user instructions at their first contact with maternity care professionals. The pregnant families can send questions or comments to the maternity care professionals in both primary care and specialized care. There is also a discussion group for families that allows anonymous participation. Professionals monitor the conversation and, as necessary, make comments—always using their own name. Professionals' answers to frequently asked questions and information about topical issues are available on a bulletin board that is updated regularly. In addition, all users can provide feedback. The team responsible for the service goes through the feedback and, when necessary, forwards relevant issues to the health care professionals for follow-up or further processing. The Net Clinic offers an extensive information retrieval system through which clients and maternity care professionals can obtain information on maternity and baby care as well as on services and issues related to the health and well-being of families, e.g., maternity care guidelines, such as good clinical practice, daily instructions for both professionals and families as well as scientific publications and reports for professional use. Furthermore, the site promotes communication and thus develops a model for joint e-Work and education for professionals.[45]

Virtual Childbirth Tour

The ongoing project called *Tutuks* (familiarizing birth environment via virtual tour) is a new health and welfare service available on the Internet. The virtual tour through the maternity ward is especially helpful to families expecting a baby. The *Tutuks* service provides information on childbirth and nursing on the maternity ward. A demonstration version of the virtual tour has been produced as preparation for the project in 2005. Although during development of the project the target group was inhabitants of the North Savo province in Finland, the service will be available to everyone on the Internet in 2006.[57]

Extending Technology to the Elderly

ICT-based services for elderly care are developing in a service home called *Levänen*, which is a part of the *Health Kuopio Programme*. The main focus of the program is on wellness expertise in the areas of health, environment, and social welfare, with a particular focus on health technology. The Levänen service home plays a key role as a test bed for solutions when developing new health and welfare/well-being innovations in order to enhance the functional capacity and the quality of life for both elderly and disabled individuals. Furthermore, the development program seeks to use current working solutions for the health care professionals. The service home Levänen has 67 round-the-clock beds, and the home offers daytime activities for both the residents and the elderly individuals living nearby. The building has a special infrastructure, which gives possibilities to test, and even adapt, new health and welfare technology, and the environment aims toward user-friendly solutions. To enhance the user-friendliness, the Levänen service home chose a special decoration/furnishing plan called the "stress-free area." This new Finnish solution eliminates or minimizes the sources of negative stress. The new stress-free environment encompasses choices in furniture, cutlery, design, acoustics, lightning, colors, and working clothes. Both the customers and health care professionals evaluate and give feedback on the functioning of both the test environment and the modern tools.

As part of the project, the Levänen service home personnel are writing a test manual that describes the rules for living in the home as well as the mutual development approach used to create this stress-free environment. The manual will also contain ethical considerations and instructions on how to evaluate the efficacy of the technology solutions implemented in the health care processes. The manual will be completed by 2006, when the first pilot phase will be initiated. Finally, the most important goal is to provide good care for the elderly citizens of Kuopio with the help of skilled and innovative health care professionals and modern technology.[58]

In Finland, consumers have been able to get a Computer License degree for more than ten years. At the beginning of 2002, the 100,000th computer license was awarded.[59] Internationally, the European computer driving license (ECDL) is the world's largest vendor-neutral, end-user, computer skills certification awarded. The ECDL is internationally recognized as the global benchmark in this area. In 2005, the ECDL has over 4 million participants. The ECDL is currently available in 138 countries around the world, and the license has been translated into thirty-two languages, making it the world's leading certification program. The license shows that the consumer has certain ICT skills, e.g., basic IT skills for information management, media literacy, and the use of electronic services. This kind of education well aligns Finland with the eEurope2005 Action Plan and will enable Finns to have the basic computer literacy skills to take full advantage of all the eEurope2005 initiatives, including health care.

Summary

Consumer health informatics, with its focus on health information systems specifically designed for use by the public, is an evolving branch in informatics. Until now, EHR projects mostly have focused on issues concerning health care professionals and organizations. The benefit for consumers is to obtain better health care services. The health portals for consumers are important and must help them to get the right information in the right time. This trend and the impact of consumer health behavior will increase as the public sector's use of Internet online services increases. From the consumer's point-of-view, the online services enable them to use services irrespective of the time or the place. Those people who do not have access to computers nor the skills for using online services also have the greatest health care needs, e.g., elderly individuals or people suffering from chronic illnesses. Special services targeting these vulnerable populations will need to be included in any nation's strategy for consumerism in health care.

In the future, the role of citizens as active consumers of health care information will increase. We can fully expect that consumers with information literacy skills will assume and demand more responsibility for their own health and health care. This consumer behavior in turn will increase the demand for health care information comprehensible for a lay person[1,36,50] and health personnel with informatics skills to support patients' use of and access to IT to manage their own health.

References

1. Eysenbach G, Jadad A. (2001). Evidence-based Patient Choice and Consumer health informatics in the Internet age. Journal of Medical Internet Research 3(2):e19. Retrieved March 11, 2005, from http://www.jmir.org/2001/2/e19/>3:2:e19.

2. Hart A, Henwood F, Wyatt S. (2004). *The Role of the Internet in Patient-Practitioner Relationships: Findings from a Qualitative Research Study.* Journal of Medical Internet Research 6(3):e36. Retrieved March 11, 2005, from http://www.jmir.org/2004/3/e36/.

3. VanBiervliet A, Edwards-Schafer P. (2004). *Consumer Health Information on the Web: Trends, Issues, and Strategies.* Dermatology Nursing 16 (6), 519-523.

4. Bernhardt JM, Felter EM. (2004). *Online Pediatric Information Seeking Among Mothers of Young Children: Results From a Qualitative Study Using Focus Groups.* Journal of Medical Internet Research 6(1):e7. Retrieved March 11, 2005, from http://www.jmir.org/2004/1/e7/.

5. Potts HW, Wyatt JC. (2002). *Survey of Doctors' Experience of Patients Using the Internet.* Journal of Medical Internet Research 4(1):e5. Retrieved March 11, 2005, from http://www.jmir.org/2002/1/e5/.

6. Eysenbach G. *Recent Advances: Consumer Health Informatics.* BMJ 2000; 320: 1713-16.

7. Goldsmith D, Safran C. Collaborative Healthcare. In Nelson R, Ball M. Consumer Informatics. New York: Springer-Verlag 2003 pp 9-19.

8. Kaplan B, Brennan PF. Consumer Informatics Supporting Patients as Co-Producers of Quality, JAMIA Vol 8 Nr 4 Jul/Aug 2001 pp 309-316.

9. Gerber BS, Eiser AR. *The Patient-Physician Relationship in the Internet Age: Future Prospects and the Research Agenda* J Med Internet Res 2001;3(2):e15 http://www.jmir.org/2001/2/e15/. Accessed May 2005.

10. Nelson R. Preface in Nelson R, Ball MJ. Consumer Informatics Springer 2004.

11. Fox S, Fallows D. Internet Health Resources. PewInternet & American life, July 2003.

12. Fox S. Health Information Online. PewInternet & American life, May 2005.

13. Internet usage statistics. http://www.internetworld-stats.com/stats.htm. Accessed May 2005.

14. Secretariat. eHealth. WHO executive board Dec 16th 2004.

15. Commission of the European Communities, e-Health - making healthcare better for European citizens: An action plan for a European e-Health Area, SEC (2004) 539.

16. Agenda item 13.17. eHealth. WHA 58.28. 25 May 2005.

17. EU. Operating the health information and knowledge advisory system in the Programme of Community action in the field of public health 2003-2008. EU commission. Luxembourg 21.11.2003.

18. eEurope 2005. Retrieved March 11, 2005, from http://www.eeurope2005.org/intro.html.

19. Iakovidis I. Biomedical informatics in support of genomic medicine. Workshop on Biomedical Informatics Brussels 18 March 2004.

20. Wong N. *Consumers Demand Combination of "High Tech" and "High Touch" Personalized Services to Manage Healthcare Needs.* Harris Interactive 17 October 2000 http://www.harrisinteractive.com/news/allnewsbydate.asp?NewsID=166. Accessed June 2005.

21. Detmer DE, Singelton p.PD., MacLeaod A, Wait S, Taylor M, Rdjwel J. The Informed Patient, Study Report, March 2003. Cambridge University Health.

22. Cimino J-J, Patel VL, Kushnirk AW, *What Do Patient Do with Access to Their Medical Records.* In Patel V. L. & al MEDINFO 2001 IOS press pp 1440-1444.

23. Ross SE, Lin C-T, The Effect of Promoting Patient Access to Medical Records: A Review JAMIA Vol 10 Nr 2 Mar/Apr 2003 pp 129-138.

24. Apple R. Boyer C. *Steps Towards Reliable Online Consumer Health Information.* In Nelson R, Ball M.J. Consumer Informatics. Springer 2004 pp 80-89.

25. Internet Healthcare Coalition. EHealth Code of Ethics. http://www.ihealthcoalition.org/ethics/ethics.html. Accessed 06/05.

26. Boyer C, Provost M, Baujard V. Highlights of the 8th HON Survey of Health and Medical Internet Users. Health On the Net Foundation, 2002. URL: http://www.hon.ch/Survey/8th_HON_results.html. Accessed 06/05.

27. Greiner AC, Knebel E. (eds.) (2003). *Health Professions Education: A Bridge to Quality.* Board on Health care Services, Institute of Medicine, The National Academic Press, Washington. Retrieved March 11, 2005, from http://nap.edu/catalog/10681.html.

28. Jauhiainen A. (2004). Information and communication technology in future nursing. Views of an expert panel on scenarios and qualifications of nursing in the year 2010. Doctoral dissertation Abstract in english. Kuopio University Publications E. Social Sciences 113. Kopijyvä, Kuopio.

29. Saranto K, Leino-Kilpi H. (1997). Computer literacy in nursing: developing the information technology syllabus in nursing education. Journal of Advanced Nursing 25, 377-385.

30. Hobbs SD. (2002). *Measuring Nurses' Computer Competency: An Analysis of Published Instruments.* CIN: Computers, Informatics, Nursing 20 (2), 63-73.

31. Stevens KR, Weiner EE. (2001). Informatics for Nursing Practice. In: Chaska, NL. (ed.) *The Nursing Profession. Tomorrow and Beyond.* Sage Publications, Thousand Oaks, California, 461-476.

32. Saranto K, Hovenga EJ. (2004). Information literacy-what it is about? Literature review of the concept and the context. International Journal of Medical Informatics, 73(6), 503-513.

33. Ehnfors M, Grobe, SJ. (2004). Nursing curriculum and continuing education: future directions. International Journal of Medical Informatics 73, 591-598.

34. Staggers N, Gassert CA, Curran C. (2001). *Informatics Competencies for Nurses at Four Levels of Practice.* Journal of Nursing Education 40 (7), 303-316.

35. Skiba DJ, Carty B, Nelson R. Growth in nursing informatics education programs: Skills and competencies. In, CA Weaver, CW Delaney, P Weber, RL Carr (eds), Nursing and Informatics for the 21st Century: International look at Practice, Trends and the Future. Chicago: HIMSS Publishing 2006, Chapter 5, in press.

36. ALA (2001). *Information Literacy Competency Standards for Higher Education.* Retrieved March 11, 2005, from http://www.ala.org/acrl/ilcomstan.html.

37. Jääskeläinen P. (2000). Through knowledge and skills towards a citizens' information society. Studies in knowledge and skills as resources for participatory and autonomous citizenship - pension knowledge and information technology skills as examples. Doctoral dissertation. Abstract in English. The Central Pension Security Institute. Studies 2000:1. Helsinki.

38. Rogos A, Latta J. Digital Divide. Retrieved March 11, 2005, from http://www.fourthwave.com/DigitalDivide.htm.

39. Davis T, Wolf M. (2004). *Health Literacy: Implications for Family Medicine.* Family medicine 36:8, 595-598.

40. Communications Superpower (2003). Retrieved March 11, 2005 from http://virtual.finland.fi/netcomm/news/showarticle.asp?intNWSAID=25850.

41. Current Care guidelines. Ministry of Social Affairs and Health http://www.kaypahoito.fi/ Accessed June 2005.

42. Häyrinen K, Porrasmaa J, Komulainen J, Hartikainen, K. (2004). *The Core Data Elements of EHR.* Final report. Publications and publisher the Network of Excellence Centers 5/2004. In Finnish http://www.oskenet.fi/asp/system/empty.asp?P=1&VID=default&SID=384957562278141&S=1&C=27600, Accessed October 6, 2005.

43. Kouri P, Saranto K, Hayrinen K, Porrasmaa J, Komulainen J, Kansanen M. Finland's National Health Project and the EHR. In, CA Weaver, CW Delaney, P Weber, RL Carr (eds), Nursing and Informatics for the 21st Century. An International Look at Practice, Trends and the Future. Chicago, HIMSS Publishing, 2006 in press, Ch 27b.

44. Patt MR, Houston TK, Jenckes MW, Sands DZ, Ford DE. (2003). Doctors who are using e-mail with their patients: a qualitative exploration. Journal of Medical Internet Research 5(2):e9. Retrieved March 11, 2005, from http://www.jmir.org/2003/2/e9/.

45. Kouri P, Antikainen I, Saarikoski S, Wuorisalo J. (2001). Beginning Life project aimed at developing and producing social innovations. Abstract in English. Helsinki 2001. Publications of the Ministry of Social Affairs and Health.

46. Liederman E, Morefield C. (2003). Web messaging: a new tool for patient-physician communication. Journal of the American Medical Informatics Association: JAMIA, 10(3), 260-270.

47. Working Group Steering the Implementation of EHR Systems. (2005). *Final Report of the Working Group Steering the Implementation of EHR Systems.* Working Group Memorandum 2004:18. Abstract in English. Ministry of Social Affairs and Health, Finland.

48. Eysenbach G, Köhler C. (2002). *How Do Consumers Search for and Appraise Health Information in The World Wide Web?* Qualitative Study Using Focus Groups, Usability Tests, and In-depth Interviews. British Medical Journal 324, 573-577.

49. Dyer KA. (2001). Ethical Challenges of Medicine and Health on the Internet: A Review. Journal of Medical Internet Research 3(2):e23. Retrieved March 11, 2005, from http://www.jmir.org/2001/2/e23/.

50. Eysenbach G. (2000). Consumer health informatics. British Medical Journal, 320, 1713-1716.

51. Forkner-Dunn J. *Internet-based Patient Self-care: The Next Generation of Health Care Delivery* J Med Internet Res 2003;5(2):e8 http://www.jmir.org/2003/2/e8/ Accessed May 2005.

52. Martin-Sanchez F, Iakovidis I, Norager S, Maojo V, De Groen P, Van Der Lei J. et al. *White Paper: Synergy Between Medical Informatics bioinformatics: Facilitating Genomic Medicine for Future Healthcare.* EC-IST 2001 35024.

53. Health Informatics Europe. (2004). Finns plan all-wireless hospital. Retrieved March 11, 2005 from: http://www.hi-europe.info/files/2004/9960.htm.

54. Communications Superpower (2003). Retrieved March 11, 2005 from http://virtual.finland.fi/netcomm/news/showarticle.asp?intNWSAID=25850.

55. Finnish Diabetes Association, http://www.diabetes.fi/english/index.htm.

56. Kidmednet Finland. Retrieved March 11, 2005, from http://www.kidmednet.fi/main.asp?sid=3.

57. Tutuks. Retrieved March 11, 2005, from http://hermes.savonia-amk.fi/tutuks/Tutuks_englanniksi.pdf.

58. Health Kuopio, http://www.tervekuopio.fi/freimstart.htm.

59. Tietokone.fi. Retrieved March 11, 2005, from http://www.tietokone.fi/pda/uutinen.asp?news_id=16521#.

CHAPTER 33

Patient and Family Centered Care in an Academic Medical Center: Informatics, Partnerships and Future Vision

By Patricia Sodomka, MS, FACHE; Harold H. Scott, BS Computer Sciences (Hons), MA Management and Supervision; Angela M. Lambert, MBA, RN; and Barbara D. Meeks, MBA, RN

Patient- and family-centered care (PFCC) has been embraced as an important aim of the health care system of the twenty-first century.[1] Patient- and family-centered care is defined as:

> *"...an approach to planning, delivery, and evaluation of health care that is grounded in mutually beneficial partnerships among patients, families, and health care providers."[2]*

In 1993, the Medical College of Georgia (MCG) took the first small steps toward what would later become a significant shift in its patient care culture. MCG, which is the health sciences university of the university system of Georgia, located in Augusta, began its cultural transformation journey in the planning of a new, 150-bed children's hospital. The change process started when we involved a group of approximately twenty parents in the formal planning process for the new facility. These were parents of children who had been patients in the existing children's units located within the adult hospital. In addition to the parents, a group of children (former and existing patients) acted as an advisory council. During the facility planning project, these two groups taught us to see care delivery through the eyes of patients and their families, an experience that revolutionized the thinking of MCG's organizational leaders. Indeed, the project launched a twelve-year journey of learning how to move an entire health care system toward a patient- and family-centered approach to care.

This chapter will describe MCG's approach to driving major cultural transformation, including the role nursing played, the enabling of information technology (IT), the settings implemented, the results achieved, and our vision for the future.

The Early Years: Development of a New Children's Hospital

MCG, one of the oldest and largest medical education institutions in the U.S., comprises five schools—medicine, allied health, nursing, dentistry, and graduate studies. The clinical system includes a 482-bed adult medical center, a 150-bed children's medical center, an organized multi-specialty physician practice with approximately 350 physicians, a large ambulatory care center in Augusta, and 110 specialty clinics located throughout Georgia and South Carolina. In 2004, there were more than 22,000 admissions and 455,000 ambulatory care visits. Total employment for the campus exceeds 6,000 full-time equivalents.

The Children's Medical Center (CMC) is a tertiary pediatric facility with a full spectrum of medical and surgical subspecialties, including a Level III neonatal intensive care unit, pediatric critical care, a trauma center, and cardiovascular and oncology services. Plans for building a free-standing children's hospital took shape in the early 1990s. The group of parents served as influential members of the planning team in the development of the 212,000-square-foot, five-story facility. The process began with the development of a core values statement, a foundational document that drove the planning process. We developed the core values statement to uphold CMC's belief in honoring each child and family as unique and recognizing their values, needs, environments, cultures, resources, and strengths. CMC sees parents and their children as integral members of the health care team.

Parents participated on every design team for the new hospital and then came together as a group to review plans for the overall facility. In the discussions that followed, nursing and other staff came to understand that the existing care culture was rigid and inflexible regarding access to information, family participation, and physical layout. For example, a pediatric intensive care unit policy allowed parents to see their children only at specified times of day, treating parents as visitors to their hospitalized children. Through the exchange of perspectives among parents, nurses, and faculty, we came to understand that the visitation rules actually interfered with the ideals for patient care. If parents were the experts in their children's lives, then they were valuable partners in the care process itself, not just distant observers of a technical care system. The process of parents sharing personal stories directly with health care professionals shaped the new vision for care and for the new facility. Because of this initiative, caregivers have developed a much greater understanding of parents' value in helping children achieve the best health outcomes in terms of quality and safety.

As explained by the parent group, the key elements of family-centered care are access to information and participation in actual hands-on care or care-making decisions. IT provides a vital tool for both. Kiosks offer parents and children access to reference information on the CMC intranet as well as links to key health information sites on the Internet. An IT initiative currently in process will allow MCG to share the patient's electronic health record (EHR) among care providers and support information exchange between parents and clinicians. A family resource center, located centrally within the facility and staffed by volunteers, provides families with access to printed and electronic materials. Patient rooms are single bedrooms configured with accommodations for at least two adults to allow the consistent presence of family to support care delivery.

With the opening of the new $53 million CMC in December 1998, we completed our first patient- and family-centered care undertaking. The cultural shift extended even into the architecture of the units, e.g., layout of the lobbies, the materials and colors used, and the inclusion of services and gardens—all of which reflected input from the family and former patient groups. Today, family-centered care is a hallmark of the architectural design and operation of the CMC, which has twice been recognized by *Modern Healthcare,* a benchmark in the industry.[3,4] Patient satisfaction has consistently ranked in the ninety-fifth to ninety-ninth percentile of Press Ganey since this measurement was first used in 2000. Market share has grown 40 percent from 1996 through 2003, and discharges have increased 83 percent during the same period.

Leadership for Change

CMC's adoption of a family-centered care philosophy and the facility design process were led by the chief operating officer, senior nurse executives, and key physician leaders. Vital to the success of the initiative was this sustained collaboration of nursing, physician, and patient leaders over several years. Nursing leadership provided crucial support by driving the vision and commitment across all disciplines within the care team. Nurse managers served as drivers of cultural change at the front line, consistently asking of every potential decision, "Is this family-centered or not?" Executive team leaders collaborated with patients and families to promote positive change.

Middle Years: Experimentation and Diffusion

From the time the CMC opened in 1998, hospital leadership recognized that PFCC principles applied to all patients, yet a clear path to progress in adult care was elusive. At the same time, a major reorganization of the clinical system was under way, moving the hospital from state operation under the Board of Regents to a separate 501c3 corporation. Leaders created a strategic plan for the advancement of PFCC.

Two Levels of Work

Work in the health system took shape at two levels. First, where opportunities existed to work in clinical microsystems within the medical center, leaders supported efforts to undertake change. Second, team members addressed the health system infrastructure, developing enabling policies and structures. These included human resources policies and programs, facilities development, strategic planning, designation of a dedicated role to support PFCC, creation of patient advisory councils, and involvement of patients in a variety of ways in the educational program of the university. Patient participation was highly desirable. For example, the steering committee for the clinical information system (CIS) selection included a patient who had experienced a delay in diagnosis of a significant condition resulting from lack of communication of an important test result.

Clinical Microsystems in Adult Care: Two Successful Experiments

A *clinical microsystem* is a group of health care professionals working together with a group of patients who share a common set of health care experiences. Two clinical microsystems at the MCG Medical Center (MCGMC) provided interesting insights.

Breast Health Center: Mammography

The first area in which MCGMC leaders expressed an interest in bringing PFCC to adult care was in breast health. Reinventing the mammography services in the radiology department occurred between 2001 and 2002. A breast cancer survivor partnered with clinical and administrative staff in this effort. This initiative yielded another significant victory—major gains in quality and patient satisfaction indicators and, of equal importance, added to our organization's knowledge of how to drive a cultural shift to PFCC beyond the pediatric setting. An important discovery in this project was the need to rethink the concept of mammography from a "diagnostic test" to "a woman doing something good for herself." This drove change in every aspect of breast care, including the physical environment and staff attitudes.

Neurosciences Center of Excellence—Cross-care Continuum

The second microsystem MCGMC transformed was the neuroscience service. In late 2002, the administrative director of the Neuroscience Center of Excellence—a strategic business unit of the health system structured to organize and align the academic departments of neurology and neurosurgery along with all related clinical, academic, and research efforts—began to create a PFCC agenda. Work began in one organized program of the center, the multiple sclerosis (MS) clinic. The physician director and administrative director convened a meeting with a group of patients. Here again, as with the Breast Health Center, profound discoveries occurred. The leadership of the neuroscience center envisioned a significant research agenda for MS as a high-priority undertaking. Patients, however, expressed more fundamental needs:

1. "We want help with independence."
2. "We cannot use the bathroom in the clinic."
3. "No one calls us back."
4. "We need support."

With the patient advisors' input, the efforts of everyone involved came into closer alignment. Addressing the patients' issues became the primary concern. To this end, the clinic has been moved and is co-located with Rehabilitation Services to streamline the care and treatment process for patients with MS.

Based on the experience with the MS clinic, it became possible to discuss redesigning the entire inpatient Neuroscience Center of Excellence. The staff now had a sense of what it meant to truly partner with a group of patients to improve care. The medical center had a need to expand access to intensive care unit (ICU) beds. This led to the opportunity to create a twenty-bed neurological unit with ten universal ICU rooms and ten regular medical surgical rooms in the adult medical center. Experienced patient advisors from the MS clinic and other staff were part of the redesign team. The unit underwent a partial renovation. Physical barriers that impeded collaboration and communica-

Table 33-1. Changes in Press Ganey Patient Satisfaction Scores for Children's Medical Center (CMC), Medical College of Georgia

	Before		After	
	Score	Percentile	Score	Percentile
CMC Since 1998			88.0	96th
Breast Health	88.9	40th	91.4	93rd
Neurosciences	79.7	10th	86.4	95th
Source: MCG Health Inc. Strategic Support Department, Press Ganey Results, 2005.				

tion between patients, families, and caregivers were torn down. Designers ensured space for families at the end of patients' beds in the universal ICU. They created a small nursing substation with visibility into two patient rooms.

The chief nursing officer and nurse manager were vital to the success of this transformation. They enabled staff and patient advisors to work together. They also responded to patient suggestions and ideas. The neurosciences leadership team developed a small information resource center for patients and families offering written materials and computer links to important Web sites. Patient suggestions for pet therapy and a healing arts program were adopted. Staff also created "doc/talk" cards for inpatient and outpatient services. These paper-based cards are offered to patients prior to office visits to help them express concerns, questions, and other pertinent information to facilitate communication and information sharing with care providers.

The neurosciences leadership team also invited patient advisors to interview all neuro unit staff individually and to interview the faculty as a group prior to opening the new unit. The results achieved in the neurosciences unit, significant in promoting PFCC, include:

1. Patient satisfaction with neurosciences improved from the tenth percentile to the ninety-fifth percentile (see Table 33-1 for more Press Ganey results).
2. The RN vacancy rate dropped from 7.5 percent to 0 percent on the neurosciences unit, which had a waiting list of five RNs as of March 1, 2005.
3. Neurosurgery length of stays decreased 50 percent.
4. Discharges from the service line increased 15.5 percent.
5. Reported perceptions (morale) of staff and physicians are highly positive.
6. Medication errors dropped by 62 percent.

Role of Informatics

MCG views a full EHR as a key component to its strategic IT plan and commitment to achieving PFCC delivery. Full participation in care decisions and delivery means that information must be shared with the patient and family members as it is generated during episodes of care. This need for exchange of information is not limited to acute care. Capturing health care delivery information that occurs across the care continuum is essential for continuity, timeliness, basic safety, appropriateness of interventions, higher quality of care delivered, and best practice hand-off across different sectors (home, ambulatory/community, and acute care). Enabling the patient and family to have access to the full, cross-continuum record with the ability to actively exchange information with the primary care providers is the enabling IT infrastructure needed to achieve full transformation to best practice within PFCC. MCG has implemented the basic infrastructure for an EHR and is currently engaged in delivering a portal capability for accessing personal health records, where patients can record information related to their personal health practices (e.g., use of over-the-counter and herbal medications, exercise frequency, adherence to a specific care plan) useful to the clinician providing their care. The portal will also facilitate communication with clinicians and scheduling of appointments. These initiatives are basic to MCG's organizational commitment to PFCC.

Information Sharing and Patient Involvement

It is apparent that informatics has taken center stage on the national agenda. On April 27, 2004, President George W. Bush called for the majority of Americans to have interoperable EHRs within ten years. The first National Coordinator for Health Information Technology, David J. Brailer, MD, PhD, was charged with developing a strategic plan to guide the nation toward accomplishment of this goal. The framework for this strategy includes significant involvement of the consumer/patient in the delivery of their care.

Engaging the Patients

Individuals are acutely sensitive to their physical environments. Malcolm Gladwell observes about such environments, "relatively small elements can serve as Tipping Points"[3] in the environment, influencing behavior to change. Small changes, such as lowering a reception desk or eliminating a high wall around a nursing station, can change the way the space supports the patient-caregiver partnership. Likewise, it is believed the structure and processes used in producing and managing clinical information have the potential to tip the environment toward a PFCC when designed appropriately. Donnelly[4] advocates reform of the medical record:

> "...the conventional, problem-oriented medical record (POMR) is a pathology-oriented record that helps perpetuate a disease focused, biomedical model of practice."[4]

Donnelly goes on to say, "the medical record can become an effective way of teaching both physicians-to-be and their mentors to practice patient-centered medicine." Our view at MCG that the patient's and family's story must be a central part of the team's plan of care is directing every design decision as we build and continue to roll-out components of our EHR system."

The opportunity for the design of a CIS to significantly support patient partnering in all health care settings cannot be overstated. Consumers report that they often do not feel that they are the principal decision maker for their health care and may feel instead that their clinician or their health plan is making the critical choices. Dr. Brailer's framework includes encouraging the use of personal health records as a means of engaging the patient in his or her own health care process.[5]

Presently, e-health applications are being developed that permit secure e-mail communication between provider and patient, along with the ability to monitor certain conditions on a real-time basis. In addition, the design of a CIS should be flexible enough to allow for a future world where hospitalized patients and families can, in real time, document their experiences (what is going right and what is not), access test results, link to robust sites for information about their condition and health concerns, ask questions, and express concerns, all from the bedside. A rounds report, a report that is generated by the CIS to list all activity, including clinical test results and medications administered for each patient and is currently available in our facility, can be a means to share information among all doctors, nurses, and patients each day. If there were explicit options for patient and family participation in record creation, this could have a transforming effect and enable PFCC ideals of patient-caregiver partnerships to be achieved more easily.

Lessons Learned and a Vision for the Future

The Medical College of Georgia has learned many lessons from implementing these PFCC care delivery models. Real cultural change occurs in clinical microsystems in which everyone can understand and appreciate each other's perspective, especially that of the patient and family, and receive encouragement and support throughout the change. The power of patients' personal stories that describe what care "feels" like is essential to creating the desire in providers to change how they deliver care. Even small changes in the environmental context, i.e., health care setting, can help support desired behavior changes. The patient's need for access to information about diagnosis, treatment, and care is an essential element of a PFCC environment. The ultimate vision for the caring experience is created through the partnership of patients, their families, and caregivers.

Based on the successes described in this case study, in summer 2004, MCG determined that the PFCC model of care and the underlying principles would become a strategic goal for the entire university. The creation of a center for Patient- and Family-Centered Care facilitated the transformation of care toward a PFCC model for the health system as a whole. In addition, the core principles of PFCC were added to the curricula of all the schools. A new research agenda to demonstrate the linkage of PFCC to outcomes, including quality and safety measures, cost effectiveness, patient satisfaction, and staff satisfaction and engagement was developed. University leadership believes that a key part of the solution to today's expensive, unsafe, poor quality, and dissatisfying health care experience lies in a model that embraces those cared for as true partners.

These efforts, along with others directed at gaining and maintaining the participation of the patient and family in the care delivery model, have produced outstanding measurable results. They are consistent with the national vision of delivering high-quality care in a manner that will result in fewer medical errors, fewer unnecessary treatments, and fewer variations in care, which should be helpful to all.[5] And they are meaningful to those we serve.

MCG believes that moving to a PFCC culture is a critical change for any organization or individual health care professional to make. To those already embarked on this journey, a partial vision of what is possible emerges early in the process. Through collaboration with patients and caregivers, new ideas and ideals for patient care take shape. Satisfaction improves for both patients and caregivers. Participants discover alignment of interests and common ground for improvement. As an organization that has now experienced twelve years of sustained success in PFCC, we suggest the rewards of this journey far outweigh the effort.

References

1. Institute of Medicine. *Crossing the Quality Chasm.* Washington, DC: National Academy Press; 2001.
2. Institute for Family Centered Care. Available at: www.familycenteredcare.org. Accessed August 22, 2005.
3. Gladwell M. *The Tipping Point.* New York: Little, Brown and Company; 2002.
4. Donnelly WJ. Viewpoint: patient-centered medical care requires a patient-centered medical record. *Acad Med.* 2005;80(1):33-38.
5. Thompson TG, Brailer DJ. *The Decade of Health Information Technology: Delivering Consumer-centric and Information-rich Health Care, Framework for Strategic Action.* Washington, DC: Department of Health and Human Services; 2004.

CHAPTER 34

Looking to the Future: Informatics and Nursing's Opportunities

By Heather Strachan, MSc, Dip.N, RGN, MBCS; Connie W. Delaney, PhD, RN, FAAN, FACMI; and Joyce Sensmeier, MS, RN, BC, CPHIMS, FHIMSS

Nursing informatics (NI) has developed in tandem with the science and practice of nursing. NI's focus is on the collection, analysis, and use of nursing information to improve health outcomes. This encompasses the use of information to support nurses' clinical decision making and to show the value of nursing to improve outcomes within clinical information systems. Nurse informaticians defined the concept of nursing information *as that of information that is specific and necessary for nursing practice and research on nursing practice. Harriet Werley (1982)[1] first presented this nursing information concept as the nursing minimum data set (NMDS). Dr. Werley defined a set of 16 data elements that cover who the patient is as a sociocultural person, problems assessed, interventions used, and goals/outcomes and the care context.[2,3] This informatics approach to defining nursing practice put quantifiable form and structure to the evolving yet sometimes invisible science of nursing.*

Werley's NMDS defined the data elements needed to capture the essence of nursing in a care delivery context. Importantly, it gave nursing the data and information to leverage the qualitative and quantitative scientific methods and technology tools to examine itself in an increasingly sophisticated scientific manner. Not only did the NMDS allow nursing to discover what it is that nursing does, these same informatics tools provided the means to begin to demonstrate to other health professionals and to society nursing's contribution to patient outcomes, costs, and satisfaction measures.

Efforts to operationalize the NMDS immediately called into question the need for nursing to have a standardized language. In contrast to medicine, nursing evolved without a language and lacked a coded standardized terminology system to enable naming what it is that nurses do that is unique to nursing. Over the past two decades, numerous nursing research teams and professional organizations have worked to build this reference terminology that could serve as an international standard.[4-14] In 2005, we are finally able to name what it is that nursing does, link these interventions for patient health to nurse-sensitive outcomes, and to analyze these data on large, aggregated, population-based clinical databases generated from electronic health record (EHR) systems.

Before we peer through this looking glass to examine what this alignment of information technology (IT) infrastructure, NMDS, and standardized nursing terminology holds for the science, profession, and practice of nursing, it is appropriate that we pause and review the current state. Just as McBride's and Skiba et al's earlier chapters in this book point out, NI will continue to propel nursing forward—beyond a specialty—to become an integral component in research, practice, and education. Therefore, it is important to take a critical look at the international similarities and variations that exist on the status of NI, its affiliation within professional nursing, and the external world of health care.

Nurses and Informatics

NI has only recently begun to find its professional home even though nursing information and knowledge discovery, building, and representation have always existed. There are numerous definitions of NI, but an agreed international definition states: "Nursing informatics is the integration of nursing, its information, and information management with information processing and communication technology, to support the health of people worldwide."[15] NI's growth and development are closely linked to nursing's evolution to professional status. For many years, nursing was identified as a semi-profession because it lacked autonomy, a university-based education, and a theoretical and research basis for its independent knowledge domain. From Florence Nightingale's 1850s to the 1960s, however, nursing advanced from a capacity as assistant to the physician, a scenario in which the physician diagnosed and prescribed and the nurse performed prescribed tasks, to an independent role with autonomous practice and as a full member of the health care team. The introduction of the nursing process model and practice framework in the 1970s positioned nurses to be able to describe the elements of nursing, not only in terms of what they did but also in terms of their decision-making process, the evidence on which care was based, and the outcomes of that care.[16]

In the U.S., United Kingdom (U.K.), and most Commonwealth countries, once nursing education began moving from hospital-based training programs to university-degree tracked programs in the 1960s, nursing's professional status changed quickly. Beginning in the late 1960s, nursing gained wide professional status and recognition by demonstrating the required attributes which include: a code of conduct; theory development; community services orientation; continuing education; research, development and use of evaluation; self-regulated autonomy; professional organization participation; publication; and communication.[17] Development of nursing higher-level degree programs at the master's and doctoral level were in place by the 1970s. These graduates further extended nursing research and served as faculty who came to academic appointments with more clearly defined professional research paths. Over the last 40 or more years, this shift to university-based nursing education has been adopted gradually throughout the world, with Ireland graduating its first baccalaureate nursing class in spring 2006. Internationally, this higher education has resulted in nurses being broadly educated with a knowledge base that has allowed these generations to ascend to the highest leadership positions in government, organizations, and businesses. NI's growth parallels this same 40-year time frame as nursing's move to university-based education. There can be no doubt that NI occurred in direct response to the rapid growth of IT's use in health care. However, the sheer numbers of nurse informaticians in key leadership positions were enabled by their university-based education.

In the early 1960s, nurses recognized the potential value of information and communications technologies and their ability to provide nurses with powerful tools to support the management of nursing information in everyday practice.[3,5,18,19] These early pioneers promoted the practice, science, and profession of nursing by raising the profile of nursing information and supporting the development of nursing knowledge. As technology evolved, so did nurses' use of these tools. Early computers required batched processing but later moved to online data communication and real-time processing, making information more accessible than previously and therefore useful for clinical decision making, as well as for management decision making.

Today, around the globe, the most profound changes occurring in our health care systems are being driven from extensive adoption and use of the Internet and the World Wide Web as a source of expert knowledge and the latest science. For the first time in history, the health care expert is not the sole holder of knowledge and scientific facts that have served to differentiate the health professional from a lay person. In today's world, from Africa to Newfoundland, the patient or family member can access this same body of knowledge over the Internet. In many instances, the patient and/or family may even be better informed of the latest clinical trial and treatment results than the generalists, and sometimes even the specialists caring for them. The Internet-empowered informed patient has created the movement of consumerism and has led to redefining the power relationship between patient and clinician to that of equal partner in decision making and care management. This shift highlights a pivotal role for the nurse, as the only member of the interdisciplinary team that is in constant contact with the patient in acute care and who coordinates care across all venues from hospital to home. Nurses are required to act as knowledge facilitators, translators, and interpreters of scientific information to support patient preference and the development of individualized care pathways to support improved health outcomes. IT serves as a tool to support nurses in managing information and knowledge, educating the consumer/patient, and care delivery in new "telehealth" modes.

Nursing's Professional Evolution and the Need to Manage Information

Environmental, political, economical, and professional forces influence nursing's domain. Nursing's practice and science are shaped by health care needs and nurses' ability to influence them. Changes in health care needs have been influenced by emerging concepts of health and illness, technology and science advancements, disease patterns, population structures, and the increasing ability to meet those needs through new health care technologies and knowledge. The demand for health care has increased exponentially although the economic and political status of each country has determined the extent and degree of health services offered. In countries with government purchased health care, for example, escalating costs resulted in a need to scrutinize how taxpayer's money was being used. As a trend that crossed many industrialized countries in the 1990s, health care organizations became accountable to the tax-paying public and consumers for efficient and effective services and for ensuring value for cost.

In the United Kingdom specifically, political recognition of consumer demands for account-ability led to a number of government inquiries and initiatives which in turn recognized the impor-tance of having thorough and accurate information to manage health care resources. As the biggest cost component of health care, nursing has always been a target when efficiencies are examined. These wide-ranging accountability and quality issues influenced not only NI but also the entire nursing profession. Reporting demands required nurse managers and informaticians to focus on nursing-specific information and to define what data should and could be collected, how to analyze the data, and how the data should be used to promote greater efficiency and effectiveness of health care to improve the populations' health.

Nursing Informatics and Organizational Structures

A United Kingdom and United States Comparison

The international context in which nursing, nursing education and NI have developed varies consid-erably across the globe. As we look at the future for the nursing profession, it is clear that informat-ics holds a central and foundational position with a role that ranges from ensuring basic competencies needed for direct patient care, to applying sophisticated research methodologies and to using state of the art teaching strategies. Thus, it is important to recognize the diversity that presents in the current state and the cultural and structural reasons for this variation. The following two examples compare the United Kingdom and the U.S. to illustrate this variability, as well as to show core similarities and significance for going forward in mapping the preferred future with greater uniformity across countries.

U.K. Exemplar

Within the U.K., nursing regulation is structured in a way that has not lent itself to incorporating NI as a specialty. The Nursing and Midwifery Council, which is the statutory regulatory body respon-sible for overseeing standards for nursing in the U.K., has initial registration at the diploma level for four branches of nursing; these include adult, children's, mental health, and learning disability nursing. Two other areas, midwifery and health visiting (public health nursing), are regarded as sep-arate professions although still within the nursing family. Specialist Practitioner status, at the degree level, exists in the areas of adult, children, mental health, and learning disabilities, with either an inpatient or community focus. Additional specialities are general practice nursing (primary care), school nursing, and occupational health nursing. Specialist practitioner status tends therefore to be either client/environment or practice focused rather than theme focused, as NI could be considered. However, non-client-related, theme-focused recordable qualifications are emerging, including lecturer/practice educator and three "nurse prescribing" levels. These recordable qualifications could provide a regulatory place to NI as a nursing specialty qualification. Without specialty recognition for NI, formal education and qualification programs in the United Kingdom have tended to fall under health informatics programs in universities. Advanced nursing practice status still is being debated and as yet is not formalized within the Nursing and Midwifery Council. Current thinking is that advanced nursing practice will require master's level qualifications. This would be congruent with the emerging role of "consultant nurses" who are prepared at the master's or doctorate level and who perform at an advanced practice level. Another possibility for NI to emerge as a distinct speciality would most probably be at the nurse consultant level.

Despite the U.K. context for the evolution of nursing specialities, NI emerged early on as a significant voice for both nursing and other health informatics disciplines. The Computer Projects Nursing Group, formed in 1974, was involved in organizing an international conference, The Impact of Computers on Nursing—An International Overview in 1982. As mentioned later in this chapter, from this conference emerged the formation of an international NI group under the auspices of the International Medical Informatics Association.

Within this mid-1970s time frame, the British Computer Society (BCS) had a Medical Specialist Group, and the CNPG felt it made sense to affiliate with the BCS alongside the Medical Group for their national professional organization presence. This affiliation provided nursing informaticians an instant structure and platform for participation within the United Kingdom and internationally in the emerging field of health informatics. It was also a professional society giving NI added professional credibility. The BCS, formed to promote standards in computing, was incorporated in 1984 by Royal Charter, by order of the Privy Council, as a chartered body and has since become a Chartered Engineering Institution and awarded Chartered Scientist Status. It has its own standards, code of ethics, level of entry according to educational status, and knowledge base, and university-based degrees.[20]

The BCS Nursing Specialist Group (NSG) had its first Annual General Meeting in May 1983 and over the intervening two decades, the medical group affiliation has been replaced by the Health Informatics Forum within the BCS. Health informatics has emerged, as one of the strongest and most active of the BCS specialties. The recently formed BCS Health Informatics Forum is comprised of six health-related specialist groups, four regional health informatics specialist groups, which are multidisciplinary, and a primary care and nursing group. Today, the NSG continues to play a leading role within this interdisciplinary group as the voice for NI. The NSG has developed links with Government Health Departments across the four countries in the United Kingdom, as well as with professional nursing, midwifery, and home health visiting Royal Colleges. The NSG has become one of the most influential constituencies in the BCS' Health Informatics Forum. This parallels the development of nursing as a profession: no longer content with being a component of medicine but establishing itself as a distinct discipline, in its own right, working equally alongside other health professionals.

For the historical reasons previously described, the professional home of NI within the United Kingdom has emerged as a hybrid of the nursing profession and the computing profession. Its educational background was acquired from nursing and the broader field of health informatics, because NI courses currently do not exist. This partnership with other health informaticians is deepening with the establishment of the U.K. Council for Health Informatics Professions.[21] Formed in 2002 to promote professionalism in health informatics, the Council operates a voluntary registration scheme for all health informatics professionals who agree to work in accordance with clearly defined standards. The Council's formation stemmed from a desire to improve the safety of health information systems by ensuring that those designing, implementing, and managing them were appropriately qualified. Secondly, this Council also aims to improve the credibility and status of those working in health informatics in the United Kingdom. The BCS and other health informatics organizations are major sponsors of this initiative.[21] In the near future, the Health Service will expect anyone working in health informatics to be registered, and eventually it is envisioned that statutory registration will be introduced in order to protect the interests of the public. NI leaders in the United Kingdom anticipate that the U.K. Council for Health Informatics Professions will support the emergence and recognition of NI as a specialty/profession—equal collaborators, yet distinct from other health informatics specialities.

U.S. Exemplar

In contrast to the development of NI in the United Kingdom, NI did evolve into a specialty in the U.S. This evolution is, however, a reflection of the context of nursing in general in the U.S., just as was the situation in the United Kingdom. As described in Bickford's case study 25B, nursing in the U.S. has a long history of establishing, recognizing, and regulating nursing specialty practice.[22] In general, this practice builds upon a foundation of nursing generalists who have acquired license through a national examination, controlled within each state. Predominately, generalists pursuing the specialty practice preparation build on the bachelor's degree and most acquire master's and/or doctoral degrees. Certification examinations are controlled by the American Nurses Association (ANA) or specialty organizations themselves.

NI in the U.S. emerged within this traditional framework and is consequently supported by educational programs within the higher education model, both in terms of master's and doctoral level study within other specialties, e.g., nursing administration, gerontological nursing. Additionally, NI as a specialty itself now has master's and doctoral degrees in nursing or health informatics.[23,24] Moreover, the NI specialty has also emerged within both the professional organizations, e.g., the ANA, nursing accreditation organizations in the form of the Commission on Collegiate Nursing Education and the National League for Nursing, and research organizations, e.g., the Midwest Nursing Research Society. In fact, as described earlier by Dreher et al in Chapter 4, calls for educational reform were replete with the demand for the integration of nursing and health informatics into all nursing curricula. Simultaneously, the demand for master's level prepared clinical specialists and doctorally prepared academicians, researchers, and industry leaders has been profound (see Section II and Section III).

For more than three decades, the American Medical Informatics Association (AMIA) has been the primary professional organization for the academics, researchers, government, and applied information services leaders who worked in the field of applying IT in health care. AMIA members have worked to strengthen the nation's ability to create and manage the science and knowledge base of health care. Through its International Medical Informatics Association (IMIA) membership, AMIA has been an active participant in informatics at a global level. NI has maintained a key positioning within AMIA as one of its largest working groups. The Nursing Informatics Working Group (NI-WG) promotes the advancement of NI within the larger multidisciplinary context of health informatics. The organization and its members pursue this goal in many arenas: education, research, industry, professional practice, governmental and other services, and professional organizations. NI-WG represents the interests of NI for its members within AMIA and provides member services and outreach functions. Thus since the 1970s, AMIA NI-WG has been the key home base for NI.

Increasingly, organizations that are implementing health care information systems and technology are recognizing the importance of addressing the needs of nursing work flow and practice. As a result, health care organizations are creating new roles for nurse informaticians related to guidance for purchasing and implementing clinical information systems.[25] Health care IT vendors and suppliers are also recognizing the role of nursing by seeking their involvement with the design and implementation of systems. In order to provide content expertise for solution development, resources, and educational programs needed by nurse informaticians, the Healthcare Information and Management Systems Society (HIMSS) convened the Nursing Informatics Task Force in 2004. This group provides strategic guidance for the programs and activities of the Nursing Informatics Community within HIMSS. In the past year, there has been a 100 percent increase in HIMSS members with a nursing background, further reflecting the rapid growth of this specialty.[25]

The growth in HIMSS NI membership in just two years reflects the intensity of health care's adoption of IT in the U.S. The immense and extensive developments of NI within nursing and the interdisciplinary context in the U.S. set the stage for dramatic and revolutionary changes in nursing and health care—a twenty-first century synergy. However, to capitalize on these opportunities, nursing leadership needed to organize in order to gain a unified voice in health policy and to be included in the national research agendas. Key health policy areas in which this unified NI voice was needed include: IT standards development; shared communication and networking opportunities; development of a consistent core curricula and certification process; and promotion of collaborative research initiatives. Importantly for the advancement of NI, there is a need to establish a NI research agenda in collaboration with multidisciplinary research initiatives and governmental and non-governmental funding sources.

Finding a Professional Home

NI as a professional body is dispersed across numerous generalist organizations, smaller local or regional voluntary organizations, and informatics and information systems health care organizations. The discipline faces the current challenge of organizing at a national and international level to give nursing a unified voice that can be market-facing and to gain representation in health policy making. In the U.S. context, there are two primary professional organizations for nursing informatics—AMIA and HIMSS. At an international level, NI organizes under the IMIA as a special interest working group

By 2003, there were more than twenty NI organizations in the U.S. These local, regional, and national, volunteer-based NI groups represent a wealth of energy, expertise, and experience. They also provide a valuable and accessible support system for education and networking opportunities for practicing nurse informaticians. Given the national emphasis on IT health policy that started under the presidental administration in 2004, an opportunity for nurse informaticians to participate in health IT policy presented. The NI community recognized that to capitalize on these developments, they needed to have a forum that would provide them a single, unified voice. This unified voice would allow for consistent representation and participation in the public health care policy process and most importantly, would allow nursing to represent itself and be visible as a large and significant stakeholder.

The opportunity to coalesce this talent, energy, and membership into a single alliance was spearheaded by nurse leaders in the AMIA and HIMSS organizations in early 2004. The advantage that the AMIA and HIMSS organizations have over the other voluntary NI organizations is that they have paid staff and established programs, publications, meetings, and the organizational resources to maintain and support their own NI activities. Importantly, this infrastructure provided the support needed to establish a collaborative entity for all U.S. NI. These formalized efforts to coordinate NI groups resulted in the forming of the Alliance for Nursing Informatics (ANI) in October 2004.[26] The ANI represents more than 3,000 nurses with informatics expertise and brings together more than 20 NI groups in the U.S. The ANI Steering Team consists of representatives from member organizations and acts to define and operationalize the strategic goals and activities of the Alliance. The ANA assisted in developing the Alliance and is an ad hoc member of all ANI activities.

The importance of the ANI for U.S. NI is that it allows nursing to speak with a single, unified voice on health policy, standards, and relevant professional issues. The ANI also provides the structure and synergy needed to support the NI professionals' efforts to improve delivery of health care by sharing knowledge and best practice across its members. The ANI represents an unprecedented commitment to the power of collaboration within the NI community. National health information technology strategic initiatives will benefit from the ability of the ANI to act as a whole, responding to and participating in informatics-related issues and opportunities. The contribution that nursing plays in the consumer-centric, information-rich EHR initiative will benefit from the plethora of nursing education, research, and practice knowledge, given a voice through the Alliance.[26]

IMIA: Nursing Informatics at the International Level

IMIA has provided a key focus for health informatics activities over the past twenty-five years,[27] and nursing, in particular, has been active as a Special Interest Group within IMIA. Tallberg, Saba and Carr's Chapter 6 in Section I describes in rich detail the formulative history of IMIA and nursing's participative role in the organization. This review focuses on NI growth under the IMIA structure.

Nursing falls under the IMIA umbrella as a Special Interest Group on Nursing Informatics (IMIA-NI SIG). As mentioned by Tallberg, Saba and Carr earlier, the idea for creating the IMIA-NI SIG group followed from a group of international nurses that attended an International Conference, The Impact of Computers on Nursing: an International Overview, held in London in 1982.[28] The proposed purpose of the IMIA-NI SIG group was to promote NI in practice, education, and research, and to support its development in countries broadly across the world. Maureen Scholes, then Director of Nursing at the London Hospital, U.K., proposed the formation of the working group, which had its first meeting in August 1983 in Amsterdam, Holland.

IMIA-NI SIG was formed as a result of this 1983 British-led proposal, and it has been in existence now for more than twenty-one years. The aims of the group have remained constant. The activities it undertakes to achieve these aims, however, have considerably broadened over the past two decades, aided greatly by the Internet and through the hard work and collaboration of its officers, national and honorary members, and working group's members. IMIA-NI SIG's current vision is to provide leadership in the development, implementation, and evaluation of NI worldwide, as an inter-related component of health informatics, to ensure that NI supports the nursing profession, organizations, communities, and patients in pursuing and achieving health for all.

The achievements of IMIA-NI SIG have been significant in relation to establishing NI as a significant component within the broader health informatics disciplines at an international level. Within IMIA, the NI group is the most active and wide-reaching of all the special interest groups. These achievements have been met in a number of ways, including through eight active working groups that include: Education, Evidence Based Practice, Consumer Health Informatics, IMIA-NI History, Nursing Informatics Management, Concept Representation, Standards, and Open Source Software. Many of IMIA-NI achievements are orchestrated through its national members' expertise and networks. To date, the group has three officers, twenty-eight national representatives, fourteen honorary members, and two institutional members from a total of thirty-three countries.[15] In terms of output, it has held eight international congresses on NI from 1982 to 2005. Each conference has published proceedings and a working conference report. Its members' representatives have authored numerous publications, and special editions of health informatics journals. Through assigned mentors, IMIA-NI SIG members have engaged with nurses and nursing organizations across the world, particularly in developing countries, to support informatics development.

Some of IMIA-NI's most notable accomplishments include producing an international standard for a reference terminology and NMDS in collaboration with the International Council of Nurses[29-31] and developing competency certification in NI. Member participation within IMIA has insured that nursing content and perspectives are included in the IMIA conferences, working groups, and strategic direction. The strong nursing leaders that make up the country representatives have engaged their extensive networks, professional organizations, and policy bodies to move nursing leadership forward. IMIA-NI SIG works closely with organizations, e.g., the World Health Organization and the International Council for Nursing in project and standards initiatives. IMIA-NI SIG has ensured a professional focus of NI through developing and sharing of a body of know-ledge and by contributing to the development of educational competencies and informatics standards. As a component of IMIA, it has an ethical framework within which to work.[32] Through its members' expertise and commitment to NI at a national and international level, IMIA-NI SIG has served as the sole international body to provide direction, leadership, and support to nursing informaticians worldwide.

Nursing's place within IMIA was initially viewed as a beginning strategy to get NI organized. The British proposal under Maureen Scholes' leadership in 1983 that launched the NI special interest group within IMIA makes this clear. In a letter seeking membership, it was stated that "the group should develop within the IMIA framework and it might eventually lead to a sister organization—The International Nursing Informatics Association."[28] This suggestion was perceived as a challenge to the evolving discipline of health, biological and medical informatics, which had been thought to encompass all health care disciplines. However, it should be noted that recommendations to broaden the name from *medical* to *health informatics* have been resisted at the international level in IMIA. This same question needs to be posed to the national informatics organizations comprising IMIA's national members, e.g., AMIA.

Over the intervening two plus decades, nursing has not acted to establish an independent entity from IMIA but has stayed within the broader context of medical informatics professional organizations. In 2005, the medical informatics label is again being challenged with nurses actively participating in this challenge. It is evident that as IMIA now is comprised of a range of distinct professional disciplines, all of whom sit alongside the discipline of medicine, not under it, the broader term of *health informatics* represents an equality between the participating disciplines. Some nations started their informatics organizations under the name of *health informatics*. Australia, New Zealand and the United Kingdom have recognized the issue and use the umbrella term *health informatics* rather than *medical informatics*. NI as a key component of health informatics has grown in acceptance internationally, particularly because the nursing profession has demonstrated such a significant contribution to the field.

Looking to the Future: Nursing and Informatics

Nurses are at the leading edge of the transformation of our health care systems worldwide. This is demonstrated by the wide range of new and extended roles that have been adopted and continue to be developed by nurses in recent years in order to meet the huge challenges facing the need to deliver safe, sustainable, effective and efficient health care. Nursing is in a state of rapid change and now, as never before, the possibilities exist for nurses to develop their careers in response to service demands, professional aspirations, policy drivers, and most importantly, patient need. To ensure that nursing develops to benefit patients and clients, nursing must be able to name its unique knowledge base in order to measure and evaluate its impact. At present, universally agreed terminology to describe nursing is just becoming available. Nurse informaticians have been working on the challenging task of developing a standardized nursing terminology for more than two decades. They have contributed to international standards in the form of ICNP® (International Classification for Nursing Practice), and SNOMED CT®, which are emerging for use in clinical systems to support nursing documentation.[28,33]

The significance of this development—that of international standardized nursing terminologies that are available for use within clinical information systems—has profound importance for nursing practice and science. At the most basic level, nursing will be in a position for the first time in its modern history to capture, in a quantitative way through codified data, what nursing does that is uniquely nursing and what impact nursing has to patient outcomes. Given the large population-based databases that are generated with EHR systems, nurse researchers will have a natural laboratory to support the most rigorous of quantitative research methodologies to generate new nursing knowledge and to evaluate effectiveness of current best practices. Nursing has never before had these research tools available to support its science and practice. We stand on this threshold. The advances will happen quickly once a critical mass in EHR adoption occurs across nations, and these systems include standardized nursing terminology for nursing documentation.

Nurse informaticians have been leaders among nurses, adopting many of the attributes of an advanced practitioner.[4] Nurses come into the informatician role already experts in nursing. These nurses have taken theories, models, and principles from information and computer science and applied them to nursing theory and practice. In doing so, these nurse leaders have recognized the complexities of the nature of nursing knowledge and its use in decision making. Nurse informaticians have embraced both the art and science of nursing by using technology with a human interface. Their informatics focus extends to examining what nurses do, how they make decisions and have applied the findings to support the further development of nursing practice and educational strategies. Nurse informaticians recognize their accountability to the patient and the need to ensure efficient use of limited resources. Collaboration and working as part of multidisciplinary teams has been a consistent theme in professional organization participations, as well as the work setting. And finally, in their leadership roles within the informatics teams, they have supported the management of change and have promoted evaluation of the impact of technology on health care and patients.

Dedicated nursing informaticians across the globe have recognized the importance of informatics for enabling the nursing profession in defining, developing, and delivering nursing knowledge, in recognizing nursing's unique value base to transform healthcare and its contribution to support the health of people worldwide. NI pioneers include June Clark, Margareta Ehnfors, Kathryn Hannah, Evelyn Hovenga, Norma Lang, Elly Pluyter-Wenting, Virginia Saba, Maureen Scholes, Marianne Tallberg, Harriet Werley, and many others who have held on to this vision and have worked tirelessly over these past two decades to make these developments a reality. Informatics holds the future of nursing, and it is important that we capture this moment prior to stepping across this threshold and honor these leaders among nurses who have made it possible.

And finally, the question of finding a professional home still looms by virtue of the international and many national informatics organizations that are under the "medical" umbrella both in name and structure. Nurse informaticians are increasingly questioning whether this professional affiliation serves nursing well, as the name does not convey an equitable or collaborative working relationship or recognition of nursing contributions to health informatics. Since its inception, NI has emphasized the importance and significance of naming—naming patient problems within the domain of nursing, naming nursing interventions, and naming outcomes specific to nursing care. Should not the name of our professional NI home reflect back to nursing's focus, significance, and advocacy?

References

1. Werley HH. "Nursing Research". HCA TV Network Productions, WQED Pittsburgh PBS, Computers in Nursing Series,© RL Simpson, 1983.
2. Werley HH, Lang NM. (eds) Identification of the Nursing Minimum Data Set. New York: Springer, 1988.
3. Werley HH, Devine EC, Zorn, CR. Nursing Minimum Data Set. Collection Manual, Milwaukee, WI: University of Wisconsin, Milwaukee, School of Nursing, 1990.
4. Clark J, Lang N. Nursing's next advance: an international classification for nursing practice. International Nursing Review 39 (4):109-112, 1992.
5. Saba VK. The classification of home health care nursing diagnoses and interventions. Caring 11 (3): 50-57, 1992.
6. Saba VK. Home Health Care Classification (HHCC) System two terminologies: HHCC of nursing diagnoses and HHCC of nursing interventions with 20 care components. Appendix A, in, VK Saba, KA McCormick (eds), Essentials of Computers for Nurses, New York: McGraw-Hill, 1999 3rd edition, pp 529-533 and available at http://www.dml.georgetown.edu/research/hhcc.
7. Martin KS, Scheet NJ. The Omaha System: Applications for Community Health Nursing. Philadelphia PA: WB Saunder, 1992.
8. McCloskey JC, Bulechek GM. Nursing Interventions Classification St Louis, MO: Mosby, 1996 2nd edition.
9. Johnson M, Maas M. Nursing Outcome Classification. St Louis, MO: Mosby, 1997.
10. Ozbolt JG. From minimum data to maximum impact. Using clinical data to strengthen patient care. Advanced Practice Nursing Quarterly 1: 62-69, 1997.
11. International Council of Nurses. Nursing's Next Advance: Development of an International Classification for Nursing Practice: A Working Paper. Geneva, ICN: 1993.
12. International Council of Nurses. The International classification for Nursing Practice: A Unifying Framework: The Alpha Version. Geneva, ICN: 1996.
13. Casey A. Standard terminology for nursing: results of the nursing, midwifery and health visiting terms project. Health Informatics 1 (2): 41-43, 1995.
14. Gliddon T, Weaver C. The community nursing minimum data set Australia: from definition to the real world. In, SJ Grobe, ESP Pluyter-Wenting (eds), Nursing Informatics: An International Overview for Nursing in a Technological Era. Amsterdam: Elsevier, 1994.
15. International Medical Informatics Association, Nursing Informatics-Special Interest Group, http://www.imia.org/ni/index.html, definition adopted, August 1998, Seoul, Korea.
16. Roper N, Local W, Tierney A., The Elements of Nursing. Churchill Livingston, Edinburgh 1980.
17. Adams D, Miller B. Professionalism in nursing behaviours of nurse practitioners. *J Prof Nurs.* July 2001;17:203-210.
18. Scholes M, Bryant Y, Barber B, eds. *The impact of computers in nursing: an international review.* North Holland: Elsevier Science Publishers BV; 1983.
19. Knight JE, Streeter J. the computer as an Aid to Nursing Records, Nursing Times, February 19 1970.
20. British Computer Society. About the BCS. Available at: http://www.bcs.org/BCS/AboutBCS. Accessed July 15, 2005.
21. UK Council for Health Informatics Professions. Available at: http://www.ukchip.org. Accessed July 15, 2005.
22. American Nurses Association at: http://www.nursingworld.org and Nursing Alliance

Organization at http://www.nursing-alliance.org accessed September 23, 2005.

23. AMIA (2005) Nursing Informatics-Working Group, Nursing Informatics programs available in the United States, accessed Sept 23, 2005 available at: http://www.amia.org/mbrcenter/wg/ni/education.asp.

24. Skiba DJ, Carty B, Nelson R. Growth in nursing informatics education programs: Skills and competencies. In, CA Weaver, CW Delaney, P Weber, R Carr (eds), Nursing and Informatics for the 21st Century: International look at Practice, Trends and the Future. Chicago: HIMSS Publishing 2006, Chapter 5 in press.

25. HIMSS (2005). 2005 Leadership Survey: Trends in Healthcare Information Technology. Available at: http:www.himss.org/2005survey/healthcareCIO_final.asp. Accessed July 15, 2005.

26. Alliance for Nursing Informatics, available at: http://www.allianceni.org Accessed September 23, 2005.

27. International Medical Informatics Association, available at: http://www.imia.org Accessed September 30, 2005.

28. Scholes M. The use of computers in nursing-Historical Perspective. In: Fokkens O, (ed) MED-INFO 83 Seminars, North Holland, Amsterdam 1983 p 310-311.

29. International Council of Nurses. *International Classification for Nursing Practice (ICNP®) Version 1.0.* Geneva, Switzerland, 2005.

30. Goossen W, Delaney C, Semeus W, Junger A, Saba V, Oyri K, Coenen A. (2004). Preliminary Results of a Pilot of the International Nursing Minimum Data Set (i-NMDS) [Abstract] In *Proceedings of MedInfo 11th World Congress on Medical Informatics of the International Medical Informatics* Association.S103.

31. Goossen W, Delaney C, Coenen A, Saba V, Sermeus W, Warren J, Marin H, Park HA, Junger A, Hovenga A, Oyri K, Casey A. The International Nursing Minimum Data Set: iNMDS. In, CA Weaver, CW Delaney, P Weber, R Carr (eds), Nursing and Informatics for the 21st Century: International look at Practice, Trends and the Future. Chicago: HIMSS Publishing 2006, Chapter 24, in press.

32. Kluge EH. A Handbook of Ethics for Health Informatics Professional. Swindon, UK: The British Computer Society, 2003.

33. SNOMED International. SNOMED CT®Mappings to NANDA, NIC, and NOC now licensed for free access through National Library of Medicine. News Release, January 25, 2005, available at: http://www.snomed.com/news/documents/012505_E_NursingMapsLicenseToNLM-Final._001.pdf, Accessed September 30, 2005.

Index

t = table entry
f = figure entry